STRESS-INDUCED ANALGESIA

ANNALS OF THE NEW YORK ACADEMY OF SCIENCES
Volume 467

STRESS-INDUCED ANALGESIA

Edited by Dennis D. Kelly

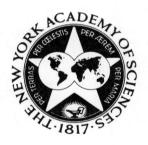

The New York Academy of Sciences
New York, New York
1986

Library of Congress Cataloging-in-Publication Data

Stress-induced analgesia.

(Annals of the New York Academy of Sciences, ISSN 0077-8923 ; v. 467)
Papers presented at a conference held by the New York Academy of Science on May 1-3, 1985 in New York City.
Includes bibliographies and index.
1. Analgesia—Congresses. 2. Stress (Physiology)—Congresses. I. Kelly, Dennis D. II. New York Academy of Sciences. III. Series. [DNLM 1. Analgesia—congresses. 2. Pain—physiopathology—congresses. 3. Stress—physiopathology—congresses. W1 AN626YL v. 467 / WL 704 S9151 1985]
Q11.N5 vol. 467   500 s   86-12727
[QP451.4]   [152.1'824]
ISBN 0-89766-329-2
ISBN 0-89766-330-6 (pbk.)

A / PCP
Printed in the United States of America
ISBN 0-89766-329-2 (cloth)
ISBN 0-89766-330-6 (paper)
ISSN 0077-8923

ANNALS OF THE NEW YORK ACADEMY OF SCIENCES

Volume 467
June 5, 1986

STRESS-INDUCED ANALGESIA [a]

Editor
DENNIS D. KELLY

CONTENTS

[a] The papers in this volume were presented at a conference entitled Stress-Induced Analgesia, which was held by the New York Academy of Sciences on May 1-3, 1985.

Financial assistance received from:

- AIR FORCE OFFICE OF SCIENTIFIC RESEARCH
- AMERICAN CYANAMID COMPANY (LEDERLE LABORATORIES)
- LILLY RESEARCH LABORATORIES/DIVISION OF ELI LILLY AND COMPANY
- McNEIL PHARMACEUTICAL
- MERCK, SHARP & DOHME/RESEARCH LABORATORIES
- NATIONAL SCIENCE FOUNDATION
- NORWICH EATON PHARMACEUTICALS, INC.
- OFFICE OF NAVAL RESEARCH
- AH ROBINS COMPANY
- SCHERING CORPORATION
- SQUIBB CORPORATION
- STUART PHARMACEUTICALS/DIVISION OF ICI AMERICAS INC.

Range of Environmental Stimuli Producing Nociceptive Suppression: Implications for Neural Mechanisms

RONALD L. HAYES

Division of Neurosurgery
Medical College of Virginia
Virginia Commonwealth University
Richmond, Virginia 23298

and

YOICHI KATAYAMA

Department of Neurosurgery
Nihon University School of Medicine
Tokyo, Japan

IMPORTANT CHARACTERISTICS OF NOCICEPTIVE MODULATION IN THE RAT PRODUCED BY ENVIRONMENTAL STIMULI: FUNCTIONAL IMPLICATIONS

More than ten years ago, as a graduate student in David Mayer's laboratory, I initiated the first studies of the range of environmental stimuli that could modulate the behavioral responses of rats to noxious stimuli.[1,2] We established several important characteristics of this nociceptive modulation that have important implications for the possible functional roles of the neural systems mediating this modulation: (1) Exposure of rats to a variety of environmental stimuli results in modulation of nociceptive responses. (2) Environmentally induced nociceptive modulation is mediated by supraspinal systems regulating nociceptive input at the level of the spinal cord. (3) Regulation of nociceptive input within the spinal cord can be learned by exposure to classical conditioning procedures. (4) Noxious stimuli are sufficient but not necessary to produce nociceptive suppression. (5) Stress is not sufficient to produce nociceptive suppression. (6) Multiple modulatory systems, both non-narcotic as well as narcotic, could mediate environmentally induced analgesia. (7) Environmentally induced nociceptive modulation includes both suppression and facilitation of nociceptive responses.

These early observations had several important implications for understanding the functional features of environmentally induced nociceptive suppression. First, while previous studies had established that the nervous system contains supraspinal mechanisms capable of selectively modulating nociceptive input at the level of the spinal cord,[3-8] such studies had emphasized the roles of exogenous agents (such as narcotic analgesics) or invasive procedures (such as brain stimulation). No studies had systematically explored the possibility that certain environmental stimuli could initiate activity within endogenous neural

1

systems capable of ongoing regulation of pain perception. The observation that suppression of a spinally integrated flexion reflex could be classically conditioned further supported the hypothesis that the perceived intensity of painful stimuli can be dynamically regulated at the level of the spinal cord by normally occurring neural processes.

We also demonstrated that stressful environmental stimuli were not always sufficient to produce nociceptive suppression. It is clear that certain types of environmentally induced analgesia (EIA), especially those mediated by humoral mechanisms, may require the presentation of stressful stimuli (see L. Watkins and P. Mayer, this volume). However, excessive emphasis on stress-related analgesia by many researchers has limited studies of the range of environmental contexts producing nociceptive suppression and handicapped efforts to describe neural mechanisms mediating EIA. It is important to remember that many neuro-physiological, humoral, and psychological changes accompany exposure to stressful situations, one or more of which could contribute to the resultant analgesia. Studies to date have not carefully examined these factors and their possible contributions to analgesia in non-stressful contexts.

Another feature of EIA was the observation that the nervous system might contain multiple systems capable of modulating nociceptive responses. Previous research had largely ignored the possibility of endogenous non-narcotic analgesic systems.[3-12] Since it seems unlikely that these physiologically different systems would serve purely redundant roles, it seemed reasonable to speculate that these systems might mediate modulatory functions in addition to regulating sensory information on noxious stimuli. The observation that some environmental conditions could increase nociceptive responses certainly indicated that environmentally induced nociceptive modulation might produce hyperalgesia as well as hypoalgesia. These and other observations lead us to suspect that neural mechanisms mediating at least some forms of EIA could be related to mechanisms mediating more general modulating processes associated with selective attention, orienting, or arousal.

The possibility that the brain contains multiple systems capable of bi-directionally modulating nociception in a variety of non-stressful and stressful situations posed important questions about relationships between specific features of environments producing nociceptive modulation, the nature of the resultant modulation, and the neural systems mediating this modulation. However, the environmental stimuli examined in these first papers (i.e., electric grid shock, centrifugal rotation, intraperitoneal injections of hypertonic saline, ether anesthesia, and horizontal oscillation; FIGURE 1) provided little insight into the nature of nociceptive modulation associated with environmental contexts more typically encountered during animals' normal activities. These studies also provided no details on the nature of cognitive, attentional, and/or motivational processes contributing to environmentally related nociceptive modulation. For example, could distraction or changes in attentional demands influence nociceptive modulation? In addition, these studies provided no electrophysiological data on environmentally induced changes in response properties of dorsal horn neurons implicated in the encoding of sensory-discriminative nociceptive. Such data would lend further, more direct support to the hypothesis that certain environmental contingencies can alter the perceived intensity of pain by regulating nociceptive input at the level of the spinal cord.

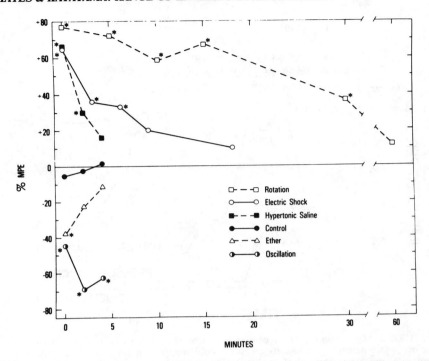

FIGURE 1. The effects of various environmental manipulations on nociceptive suppression as assessed by increased latencies of rats to withdraw their tails from a radiant heat source. Changes in latencies are expressed as a percentage of the maximum possible effect (% MPE: + % MPE = increased latencies; − % MPE = decreased latencies). Centrifugal rotation, a stressful but non-noxious manipulation, increased tail-flick latencies as compared to control rats that were simply repeatedly tested. Electric grid shock and intraperitoneal injections of hypertonic saline, noxious manipulations, also increased tail-flick latencies. Brief ether anesthesia (not producing ataxia) and horizontal oscillation, stressful but non-noxious manipulations, decreased tail flick latencies. These data indicate that stressful situations are not always sufficient to produce nociceptive suppression. Moreover, some environmental manipulations may facilitate nociceptive responses. (From Hayes *et al.*[1] With permission from *Brain Research*.)

MODULATION OF MEDULLARY DORSAL HORN NEURONS IN THE PRIMATE BY STIMULUS RELEVANCE, STIMULUS PREDICTABILITY, AND VIGILANCE DEMANDS

In collaboration with Ronald Dubner and Donna Hoffman, I studied the influence of different behavioral situations on the responses of nociceptive neurons.[13-15] The purpose of these studies was to evaluate in a reasonably natural

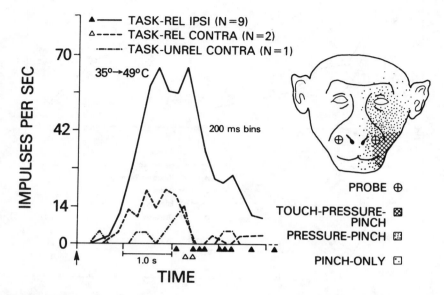

FIGURE 2. Modulation of the receptive-field size of a wide dynamic range nociceptive neuron. The neuron first had its receptive field mapped in response to experimenter-presented mechanical stimuli (face sketch). The neuron had a sensitive central focus (cross-hatched area). Within this zone, increasing intensities of mechanical stimuli from light touch to pressure and finally noxious pinch result in corresponding increases in the frequency of neuronal discharge. Outside this focus, a less sensitive zone responded differentially only to pressure and pinch (densely stippled area). Finally, there was a fringe of the receptive field, which responded only to noxious pinch (lightly stippled area). The circled cross shows the two probe loci, one (ipsi) within the receptive field zone and the other (contra) on the opposite side of the monkey's face. The post-stimulus histogram on the left plots the neuronal response of the same nociceptive neuron to 49°C heat stimuli presented during three different experimental situations. The 49°C stimulus was presented on monkey-initiated trials with the probe inside (task-rel ipsi, nine trials averaged) or outside (task-rel contra, two trials averaged) the experimenter-determined receptive field. Triangles show the discrimination or escape latencies with the probe inside (filled) and outside (open) of the receptive field. The monkey also was presented 4.0 sec, 49°C stimuli during the inter-trial interval with the probe outside of the experimenter-determined receptive field (task-unrel contra, one trial). Note that when the probe was placed outside the receptive field and presented within the inter-trial interval, a time during which the monkey could not terminate the brief noxious stimulus, the neuron responded minimally to a 49°C stimulus (task-unrel contra). However, with the probe in the same spot, the neuronal response was enhanced during trials on which the monkey could terminate the 49°C stimulus (task-rel contra). Thus, receptive field properties of nociceptive neurons can be influenced by the relevance of stimuli to certain tasks. (From Hayes et al.[13] With permission from *Journal of Neurophysiology*.)

context the modulatory effects of environmental manipulations on responses of dorsal horn nociceptors coding sensory-discriminative information such as the locus and intensity of noxious thermal stimuli.[14] Activity was recorded from cells in the medullary dorsal horn (trigeminal nucleus caudalis) of awake monkeys trained in a thermal task to respond differentially to noxious and innocuous stimuli applied to the face. The same monkeys also were trained in a visual task to detect the onset of a variable intensity light. In the visual task, behaviorally irrelevant thermal stimuli of a fixed duration were applied to the face on some trials.

Behaviorally relevant thermal stimuli presented during performance of the thermal task produced a greater neuronal response than equivalent irrelevant thermal stimuli presented either during the intertrial interval in the thermal task or during performance of the visual task. Behaviorally relevant noxious thermal stimuli also produced a neuronal response when applied outside of receptive fields that had been determined with irrelevant stimuli (FIGURE 2). Neuronal responses to mechanical stimulation produced by lip movements under the thermal probe were less during performance of the visual task than during the thermal task.

The effects of changes in attentional demands were studied in the visual task by systematically reducing the intensity of the light cue. A reduction in light intensity required monkeys to attend more rigorously to the light cue and was associated with a reduction in neuronal responses to noxious and innocuous thermal stimuli. When the light intensity was further reduced to levels resulting in behavioral disruption, the magnitude of neuronal responses to thermal stimuli returned to levels observed with maximum light intensity. In the thermal task, attentional demands also were reduced by having the experimenter rather than the monkey initiate the trials and reward the monkey independent of his behavior of innocuous thermal trials. Reduced neuronal responses to thermal stimuli were observed on experimenter-initiated trials.

A warning signal preceding noxious heat simuli presented during the thermal task produced systematic differences in response to those stimuli. The warning signal reduced the latency and maximum neuronal discharge frequency in the first monkey and increased the maximum discharge frequency in the second monkey, as compared to unsignaled noxious heat stimuli. These differences between the two monkeys may be related to the fact that the warning signal did not reliably predict the onset of noxious heat stimuli in the second monkey.

These results indicate that behavioral variables influence the responses of medullary dorsal horn and nociceptive neurons coding sensory-discriminative information about thermal and mechanical stimuli applied to the face. The tasks confronting the monkeys in these experiments required them actively to seek and evaluate stimulus information relevant to their goal of securing a reward, thereby maximizing the opportunities for behavioral variables to influence sensory processing. We assumed that the performance of such tasks approximated the demands placed on monkeys in a natural environment in which the extraction of significant stimulus information is necessary for survival. The study of central nervous system activity during such behaviors strongly suggests that higher order neural processes invoked by changes in stimulus relevance, stimulus predictability, and vigilance demands are involved in the altering of sensory input at the first central synapse. This filtering can result in increased as well as decreased responses of nociceptors. In this same series of experiments, we also observed task-related responses of dorsal horn mechanoreceptors and thermal nociceptors that were independent of stimulus parameters and appeared to result from the integration of sensory input and the central neural evaluation of its behavioral relevance or significance.[15] Such data further emphasize the complexity of modulating influences on spinal integration of sensory transmission.

However, this research provided no information on specific neural mechanisms, either opiate[16-18] or non-opiate,[1,2,19] mediating the observed behavioral modulation. Indeed, there is no reason to suspect that any one modulatory system underlies every behavioral effect reported here. Descending midbrain and medullary pathways have been described[20,21] and appear to modify the responses of medullary and spinal dorsal horn neurons to noxious stimuli.[22-24] Descending projections from the locus coeruleus to the spinal cord also have been implicated in the modulation of nociceptive input.[25,26] There also are multiple descending cortical projections to the dorsal horn.[27]

An additional possible neural substrate mediating modulation observed in these primate studies was described in a series of experiments outlined below. In contrast to the primate studies, which did not address mechanisms mediating behavioral modulation, these experiments examined the role of a physiologically characterized neural system in nociceptive modulation associated with environmental events animals may expect to encounter in their normal environment.

STUDIES OF THE CHOLINOCEPTIVE PONTINE INHIBITORY AREA IN THE CAT: FUNCTIONAL ROLE IN ENVIRONMENTALLY INDUCED NOCICEPTIVE SUPPRESSION

In a recent series of experiments, conducted in collaboration with Yoichi Katayama and Linda Watkins,[28-32] we characterized anatomical and pharmacological properties of a muscarinic cholinoceptive pontine inhibitory area (CPIA) as well as the differential behavioral consequences of activation of various sites within CPIA. These studies indicated that an endogenous, nonnarcotic analgesic system represented a subcomponent of a larger cholinergic system principally involved in regulating animals' responsiveness to external stimuli, in part by influencing segmentally organized behaviors. Moreover, we provided evidence that this same subcomponent of CPIA functions physiologically to modulate nociceptive responsiveness to certain normally occurring environmental stimuli but not to others.

In these studies we examined the effects of bilateral injections of the cholinergic agonist carbamylcholine (carbachol) into the rostral pontine tegmentum of the cat.[28] We observed a variety of functions supporting animals' responsiveness to external stimuli including postural somatomotor; sympathetic visceromotor and nociceptive somatosensory functions were differentially affected depending upon the injection sites (FIGURE 3). Sites associated with maximal effects on each of these functions were clustered in the dorsal pontine tegmentum, i.e., cholinoceptive pontine inhibitory area (CPIA). In a medial area of CPIA, which corresponds to an area caudal to the ventral tegmental nucleus of Gudden and ventromedial to the principal nucleus of locus coeruleus, postural somatomotor and sympathetic visceromotor functions were maximally suppressed. In a laterally adjacent area ventral to the principal nucleus of locus coeruleus, somatomotor function was predominantly suppressed. Nociceptive somatosensory function was primarily suppressed following microinjections into a more lateral area surrounding the lateral half of the brachium conjunctivum.

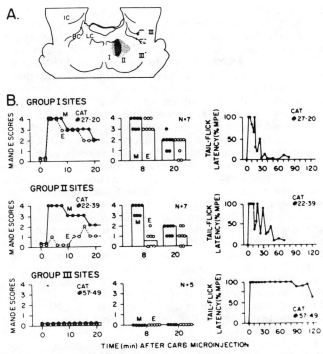

FIGURE 3. (A) Schematic representation of regional extent of sites associated with differential effects of carbachol microinjections into cholinoceptive pontine inhibitory area (CPIA) of the cat. (B) Time courses for behavioral effects associated with carbachol microinjections in each of these regions. M scores reflected the responsiveness of postural muscles and were scored by assessing the animal's best momentary response to maximal external stimuli (e.g., M0 = normal locomotor and running abilities, M4 = complete absence of responsiveness). E scores reflected eye-opening responses to external stimuli and evaluated the responsiveness of non-postural muscles and sympathetic visceromotor function by grading the lowest intensities of stimuli necessary to produce the responses of palpebral widening and retraction of nictitating membranes (e.g., E0 = eyes open in absence of stimulation, E4 = unresponsiveness even to maximal external stimuli). Nociceptive suppression was inferred by evaluating the latency to withdrawal of the tail from a noxious radiant heat source. Increased latencies were expressed as a percentage of the maximum possible effect (% MPE). Group I sites were associated with maximal suppression of postural and non-postural and sympathetic visceromotor functions. Group II sites were associated with maximal effects on postural somatomotor function but effects on non-postural and sympathetic visceromotor functions were much less than seen in Group I sites. Group III sites were associated with suppression of nociceptive responses in the absence of effects on M or E score functions. Group III' sites were associated with significant nociceptive suppression (>80% MPE) accompanied by evidence of some modest suppression of postural and non-postural somatomotor function and reduced sympathetic visceromotor tone. These observations, together with other data, suggested that CPIA is a system that primarily regulates animals' responsiveness to external stimuli, in part by influencing segmentally organized behaviors. The exclusive suppression of nociceptive responses seen in Group III sites is only one of several functional capacities of CPIA. (From Katayama *et al.*[28] With permission from *Brain Research.*)

Subsequent research[29] showed that in the dorsal aspect of this lateral region, carbachol microinjection produced no generalized sensory, emotional, or motor deficits, indicating that nociceptive transmission was primarily affected. Carbachol microinjection into the ventral part of this lateral region resulted in slight suppression of motor responses in addition to profound nociceptive suppression (FIGURE 3). Carbachol-produced analgesia (CPA) blocked supraspinally as well as spinally integrated responses normally elicited by either phasic or tonic noxious stimuli. Atropine sulfate, but not mecamylamine hydrochloride, significantly antagonized CPA, indicating that muscarinic receptors mediate this phenomenon. The opiate antagonist naloxone, systemically administered either prior to or after carbachol microinjection, did not reliably attentuate CPA. Microinjection of morphine into the sites from which CPA had previously been obtained did not produce significant effects on nociceptive responses. Thus, opiate mechanisms appear not to be necessary either for the activation of this system or for the production of the resultant analgesia. These findings indicate that the neural population examined in these studies is anatomically and pharmacologically distinct from previously identified opiate-mediated pain inhibitory systems.

We further noted a number of anatomical and pharmacological similarities between CPA and non-opiate analgesia induced by brief hind-paw shock. Both CPA and analgesia produced by hind-paw shock are mediated by supraspinal structures that (1) originate caudal to the intercollicular level;[28,29,33] (2) contain muscarinic cholinoceptive neurons;[29,31] and (3) require the integrity of pathways descending in the dorsolateral funiculus of the spinal cord.[19,30] These similarities suggested that pathways arising in the lateral aspect of CPIA could compose at least one non-opiate pain-mediating analgesia resulting from exposure to certain environmental stimuli.

Thus, we studied the effects of bilateral microinjections of the muscarinic antagonist atropine into lateral aspects of CPIA on nociceptive suppression produced by exposure of food-deprived cats to novel environmental changes or the opportunity to eat. Atropine microinjections reliably decreased nociceptive suppression produced by placing animals in a novel testing environment or by presenting them with novel stimuli in a familiar environment (FIGURE 4). Atropine failed to reduce nociceptive suppression when microinjected outside of regions in CPIA-mediating analgesia. Atropine also failed to attenuate nociceptive suppression produced by presumably non-novel but highly relevant stimuli associated with food consumption (FIGURE 4).

These data indicate that muscarinic cholinoceptive cells in the parabrachial region could function physiologically to modulate nociceptive responsiveness in the presence of certain environmental stimuli. It may be that pain inhibitory systems arising in the lateral aspect of CPIA are preferentially involved in nociceptive suppression associated with certain categories of environmental events (e.g., novel stimuli) more than others. Future studies employing more sophisticated behavioral paradigms may provide additional insights into the contribution of this cell group to neural processes supporting other behaviors possibly related to attentional mechanisms including responses associated with habituation and dishabituation to environmental stimuli.

CONCLUSIONS

The possibility that the brain contains at least two endogenous, physiologically distinct systems capable of regulating spinal integration of nociceptive responses

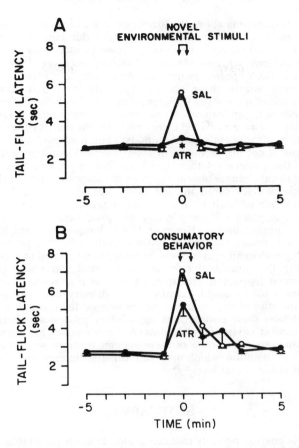

FIGURE 4. (A) The effect of atropine microinjection into the parabrachial region on tail-flick suppression accompanying presentation (10 sec) of a novel object emitting irregular clicks. Closed dots, trials ($N = 6$) 15–35 min after saline microinjection (SAL) into the parabrachial region open circles, trials ($N = 6$) 15–35 minutes after saline microinjection into the parabrachial region. Note that atropine (ATR) microinjection significantly attenuated tail-flick suppression observed during presentation of novel environmental stimuli (*) as compared to saline microinjection, ($p < 0.0005$, paired t-test). (B) The effect of atropine microinjection into the parabrachial region on tail-flick suppression during consummatory behaviors (30 sec) in cats food-deprived for 24 hours. Closed dots, trials ($N = 6$) 15–35 min after atropine microinjections into the parabrachial region; open circles, trials ($N = 6$) 15–35 min after saline microinjection into the parabrachial region. Tail-flick suppression observed during consummatory behavior was not significantly attenuated by atropine as compared to saline microinjection ($p < 0.05$, paired t-test). The magnitude of reduction is significantly smaller than that observed in A ($p < 0.05$, paired t-test). These data indicate that a function of one region of CPIA is to modulate nociceptive responses in the presence of novel non-relevant stimuli but not in the presence of relevant but non-novel stimuli. (From Katayama et al.[32] With permission from *Brain Research*.)

poses significant questions about the functional roles of these systems. It seems unlikely that such systems evolved as purely redundant pain modulatory mechanisms. In addition, nociceptive suppression produced by various experimental manipulations, whether electrical brain stimulation, drug administrations, or electric shock applied to the extremities, may not produce changes in functional activity within these systems approximating that seen in more physiologically relevant contexts. While these approaches have proven extremely useful in describing many features of nociceptive modulation, it is doubtful that these manipulations have provided direct evidence for the physiological role of these modulatory processes in normal animals. Thus, it is possible that regulation of noxious input is not the exclusive, or even principal, consequence of normal activity within these systems. Other significant, but as yet undetected or poorly described behavioral changes may accompany the responses used to characterize analgesia. Such changes could include subtle alterations related to affect or attention, which are difficult to assess. Most researchers recognize that such changes may take place following many analgesic manipulations, including systemic opiate administration. However, these changes have not been widely studied, and few researchers have systematically related changes in other behavioral categories to analgesia. Thus, important and related questions remain concerning both the functional roles and behavioral features of endogenous systems implicated in pain modulation, as well as interactions between such systems. Future studies should examine more directly not only whether the modulatory capacities of such systems extend beyond the regulation of noxious input but also how these endogenous modulatory processes operate in more functionally relevant environmental contexts. Such studies, for example, could include examinations of the roles of these systems in more general modulating processes, such as attention, which may well influence integration of nociceptive responses even at the spinal level.[13,34]

SUMMARY

Initial studies of environmentally induced analgesia in the rat established several important characteristics of this phenomenon. We demonstrated that stressful environmental stimuli were not sufficient to produce nociceptive suppression. However, emphasis by many researchers on stress-related analgesia has limited studies of the range of environmental contexts producing nociceptive suppression and handicapped efforts to describe neural mechanisms mediating EIA.

Another feature of EIA was the observation that the nervous system might contain multiple opiate and non-opiate systems capable of modulating nociceptive responses. Although previous research had recognized the possibility of endogenous opiate analgesic systems,[3-12] little attention had been given to non-opiate analgesic mechanisms. Since it seems unlikely that multiple systems would serve purely redundant roles, it seemed reasonable to speculate that at least some of these systems may mediate other modulatory functions in addition to regulating sensory information on noxious stimuli. The observation that some environmental conditions could increase nociceptive responses certainly indicated that environmentally induced nociceptive modulation was not restricted to analgesia. These and other observations lead us to suspect that neural mechanisms mediating at least some forms of EIA could be related to mechanisms mediating more general modulating processes associated with selective attention, orienting, or arousal.

Subsequent studies in the primate established that changes in vigilance demands, stimulus relevance, and stimulus predictability could modulate responses of medullary dorsal horn nociceptors coding sensory-discriminative information on noxious thermal stimuli. However, these studies provided no information on the neural mechanisms mediating this modulation.

Later studies in cats described an endogenous, non-narcotic analgesic system representing a subcomponent of a larger cholinergic system principally involved in regulating animals' responsiveness to external stimuli. Research also indicated that this cholinergic analgesic system could function physiologically to modulate nociceptive responsiveness in the presence of certain environmental stimuli but not others.

Considered together, data from these studies indicate that, while stress is not sufficient to produce analgesia, a variety of environmental conditions can modulate nociceptive input. A number of different neural systems could contribute EIA associated with various stimuli. It is possible that the regulation of nociceptive input is not the exclusive, or even principal, consequence of normal activity within certain of these systems.

REFERENCES

1. HAYES, R. L., G. J. BENNETT, P. G. NEWLON & D. J. MAYER. 1978. Behavioral and physiological studies on non-narcotic analgesia in the rat elicited by certain environmental stimuli. Brain Res. 155:69–90.
2. HAYES, R. L., D. D. PRICE, G. J. BENNETT, G. J. WILCOX & D. J. MAYER. 1978. Differential effects of spinal cord lesions on narcotic and non-narcotic suppression of nociceptive reflexes: Further evidence for the physiologic multiplicity of pain modulation. Brain Res. 155:91–101.
3. REYNOLDS, D. V. 1969. Surgery in the rat during electrical analgesia induced by focal brain stimulation. Science 164:444–445.
4. MAYER, D. J. & J. C. LIEBESKIND. 1974. Pain reduction by focal electrical stimulation of the brain: an anatomical and behavioral analysis. Brain Res. 68:73–93.
5. SOPER, W. Y. 1976. Effects of analgesic midbrain stimulation on reflex withdrawal and thermal escape in the rat. J. Comp. Physiol. Psychol. 90:91–101.
6. ADAMS, J. E. 1976. Naloxone reversal of analgesia produced by brain stimulation in the human. Pain 2:161–166.
7. RICHARDSON, D. E. & H. AKIL. 1977. Pain reduction by electrical brain stimulation in man. Part 2: Chronic self-administration in the periventricular gray matter. J. Neurosurg. 47:184–194.
8. HOSOBUCHI, Y., J. E. ADAMS & R. LINCHITZ. 1977. Pain relief by electrical stimulation of the central gray matter in humans and its reversal by naloxone. Science 197:183–186.
9. HUGHES, J. 1975. Isolation of an endogenous compound from the brain with pharmacological properties similar to morphine. Brain Res. 88:295–308.
10. PASTERNAK, G. W., R. GOODMAN & S. H. SNYDER. 1975. An endogenous morphine-like factor in mammalian brain. Life Sci. 16:1765–1769.
11. CHANG, J.-K., B. T. W. FONG, A. PERT & C. B. PERT. 1976. Opiate receptor affinities and behavioral effects of enkephalin: structure-activity relationship of ten synthetic peptide analogues. Life Sci. 18:1473–1482.
12. PERT, C. B., A. PERT & J.-F. TALLMAN. 1976. Isolation of a novel endogenous opiate analgesic from human blood. Proc. Natl. Acad. Sci. USA 73:2226–2230.

13. HAYES, R. L., D. S. HOFFMAN & R. DUBNER. 1981. Neuronal activity in medullary dorsal horn of awake monkeys trained in a thermal discrimination task. II. Behavioral modulation of responses to thermal and mechanical stimuli. J. Neurophysiol. 46(3):428–443.
14. HOFFMAN, D. S., R. L. HAYES & R. DUBNER. 1981. Neuronal activity in medullary dorsal horn of awake monkeys trained in a thermal discrimination task. I. Responses to innocuous and noxious thermal stimuli. J. Neurophysiol. 46(3):409–427.
15. DUBNER, R., R. L. HAYES & D. S. HOFFMAN. 1981. Neuronal activity in medullary dorsal horn of awake monkeys trained in a thermal discrimination task. III. Task-related responses and their functional role. J. Neurophysiol. 46(3):444–463.
16. MAYER, D. J. 1979. Endogenous analgesia systems: neural and behavioral mechanisms. In Advances in Pain Research and Therapy. J. C. Liebeskind & D. Albe-Fessard, Eds. 3:385–410. Raven Press. New York.
17. SHERMAN, J. E. & J. C. LIEBESKIND. 1980. An endorphinergic, centrifugal substrate of pain modulation: recent findings, current concepts, and complexities. In Pain. J. J. Bonica, Ed. 58:191–204. Raven Press. New York.
18. MAYER, D. J. & D. D. PRICE. 1976. Central nervous system mechanisms of analgesia. Pain 2:379–404.
19. WATKINS, L. R. & D. J. MAYER. 1982. Organization of endogenous opiate and non-opiate pain control systems. Science 216:1185–1192.
20. BASBAUM, A. I., C. H. CLANTON & H. L. FIELDS. 1978. Three bulbospinal pathways from the rostral medulla of the cat: an autoradiographic study of pain modulating systems. J. Comp. Neurol. 178:209–224.
21. CASTIGLIONI, A. J., M. C. GALLAWAY & J. D. COULTER. 1978. Spinal projections from the midbrain in monkey. J. Comp. Neurol. 178:329–337.
22. BASBAUM, A. I. & H. L. FIELDS. 1978. Endogenous pain control mechanisms: review and hypothesis. Ann. Neurol. 4:451–462.
23. HABER, L. H., R. F. MARTIN, J. M. CHUNG & W. D. WILLIS. 1980. Inhibition and excitation of primate spinothalamic tract neurons by stimulation in region of nucleus reticularis gigantocellularis. J. Neurophysiol. 43:1578–1593.
24. WILLIS, W. D., L. H. HABER & R. F. MARTIN. 1977. Inhibition of spinothalamic tract cells and interneurons by brain stem stimulation in the monkey. J. Neurophysiol. 40:968–981.
25. NYGREN, L. G. & L. OLSON. 1977. A new major projection from locus coeruleus: the main source of noradrenergic nerve terminals in the ventral and dorsal columns of the spinal cord. Brain Res. 132:85–93.
26. COMMISSIONG, J. W., S. O. HELLSTROM & N. H. NEFF. 1978. A new projection from locus coeruleus to the spinal ventral columns: histochemical and biochemical evidence. Brain Res. 148:207–213.
27. COULTER, J. D. & E. G. JONES. 1977. Differential distribution of corticospinal projections from individual cytoarchitectonic fields in the monkey. Brain Res. 129:335–340.
28. KATAYAMA, Y., D. S. DEWITT, D. P. BECKER & R. L. HAYES. 1984. Behavioral evidence for a cholinoceptive pontine inhibitory area: Descending control of spinal motor output and sensory input. Brain Res. 296:241–262.
29. KATAYAMA, Y., L. R. WATKINS, D. P. BECKER & R. L. HAYES. 1984. Non-opiate analgesia induced by carbachol microinjection into the pontine parabrachial region of the cat. Brain Res. 296:263–283.
30. HAYES, R. L., Y. KATAYAMA, L. R. WATKINS & D. P. BECKER. 1984. Bilateral lesions of the dorsolateral funiculus of the cat spinal cord: Effects on basal nociceptive reflexes and nociceptive suppression produced by cholinergic activation of the pontine parabrachial region. Brain Res. 311:267–280.
31. WATKINS, L. R., Y. KATAYAMA, I. B. KINSCHECK, D. J. MAYER & R. L. HAYES. 1984. Muscarinic cholinergic mediation of opiate and non-opiate environmentally induced analgesia. Brain Res. 300:231–242.
32. KATAYAMA, Y., L. R. WATKINS, D. P. BECKER & R. L. HAYES. 1984. Evidence for

involvement of cholinoceptive cells of the parabrachial region in environmentally induced nociceptive suppression in the cat. Brain Res. **299**:348–353.

33. WATKINS, L. R., I. B. KINSCHECK & D. J. MAYER. 1983. Failure of decerebration or periaqueductal gray lesions to abolish opiate or non-opiate foot shock analgesia. Brain Res. **276**:317–324.
34. HAYES, R. L. 1980. The multiplicity of physiological and behavioral variables modulating pain responses. Behav. Brain Sci. **3**:311.

Analgesia Following Defeat in an Aggressive Encounter: Development of Tolerance and Changes in Opioid Receptors[a]

KLAUS A. MICZEK[b]

Department of Psychology
Tufts University
Medford, Massachusetts 02155

and

MICHAEL L. THOMPSON AND LOUIS SHUSTER

Department of Biochemistry and Pharmacology
Tufts University
Boston, Massachusetts 02111

INTRODUCTION

Stress-induced analgesia may actually by a misnomer for an array of phenomena that are relevant to the perception of and the response to pain. Neither the physical properties of a stressor nor the acute response of the pituitary-adrenal axis to this stimulus predict clearly whether or not the organism is rendered analgesic. Instead, the biological significance of the stimulus situation and the adaptive reaction to it appear to be of paramount importance for endogenous pain modulation. One such situation is that of an aggressive confrontation between a resident animal and an intruder. Both opponents display an intricate sequence of behavioral and physiological adaptations to the conflict; the intruder ultimately is defeated and fails to respond to painful stimuli. We have studied analgesia in mice that have been defeated by an opponent, and have explored several behavioral and physiological processes that characterize this phenomenon. Our evidence suggests that the analgesia in defeated mice is mediated by brain opioid peptides. Of particular interest are the observations suggesting long-term adaptations to the analgesia-causing events, a process that is closely similar to opiate tolerance.

Stress-induced analgesia or the antinociceptive effects of stress may be produced by exposure to various physical and chemical stimuli, conditioned or

[a]Supported in part by U.S. Public Health Service research grants DA02632 and AA05122 (K.A.M.), DA01626 (L.S.), and DA 03797 (M.L.T.).

[b]Address correspondence to: K.A. Miczek, Research Building, Tufts University, 490 Boston Ave., Medford, MA 02155.

14

unconditioned, under controlled experimental conditions. A complex, often inconsistent set of findings has emerged on which forms of stress-induced analgesia are (1) reversed, at least in part by opiate antagonist drugs, (2) show some degree of cross-tolerance to opiate agonist drugs, (3) are correlated with changes in the release of opioid peptides or activation of opioid receptors. Which types of opioid peptides and which pools of these peptides are critically important for analgesia to occur also remain matters of conflicting evidence.[1,15,18,22] Also, the nature of the stress, i.e. its severity and its physical and temporal parameters, and its behavioral significance have been shown to be important determinants for opioid mediation of analgesia.[13,19]

So far, studies with defeated mice and rats have provided surprisingly consistent and clear evidence for a significant role of brain opioid peptides in the mediation of analgesia.[18,19,25,26] After summarizing our initial behavioral, pharmacological, endocrinological, and genetic observations on analgesia following defeat, we will address two issues in particular: (1) The non-essential contribution of pituitary-adrenal "stress" responses to the development of analgesia in defeated mice and (2) the development of tolerance and its potential mediation by changes in opioid receptors in brainstem processes for analgesia, even after a single defeat experience.

CHARACTERISTICS OF ANALGESIA IN DEFEATED MICE

Aggressive behavior during confrontations between a territorial resident male mouse (*M. musculus*) and an intruder male is a significant and necessary part of the behavioral repertoire, serving to disperse reproductively active male members of the species.[5,8] The pattern of attack, threat, and pursuit behavior is vigorous, robust, and in most instances non-injurious; it is readily studied under controlled laboratory conditions.[17] Most research has focused on the behavioral and neurobiological processes of the attacking animal; yet, recently behavioral and hormonal aspects of the recipient of the attack behavior, the intruder animal, have begun to be studied.[12] Behaviorally, the intruder initially retaliates, then engages in defensive reactions such as the defensive upright posture and escape attempts; eventually, the intruder displays a submissive response pattern or "defeat" behavior. This defeat behavior includes several characteristic features: upright body posture, limp forepaws, upwardly angled head, and retracted ears (FIGURE 1). As a matter of fact, once defeated, mice show these behavioral features even before being attacked, squeal before being bitten, and most distinctly, fail to orient toward the approaching opponent.

In initial experiments, we found that intruder mice of the B6AF$_1$/J strain did not react to a heat stimulus that was focused on their tails (i.e. tail-flick assay[9]) after they were defeated by resident animals. This analgesic response was large and long-lasting. FIGURE 2 portrays the magnitude of the analgesia as function of the "stress" stimulus. Expressed in this traditional fashion, it appears that the intruder mice respond with increasingly longer latencies to the heat stimulus when they are exposed to an increasing number of bites. In fact, these group averages obscure the all-or-none mode of analgesia in individual subjects. Actually, it is the proportion of animals showing significant analgesia (i.e. three to four times longer latencies than baseline) that increases when individuals are attacked more often.

Another potentially misleading feature of this form of data portrayal is the

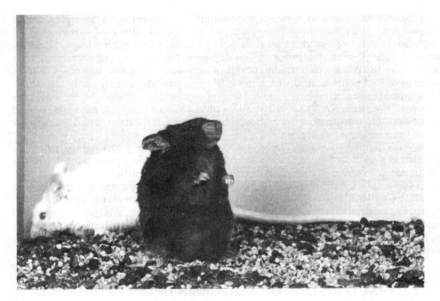

FIGURE 1. Intruder mouse in characteristic "defeat" posture. (From Miczek et al.[19] With permission from *Science*.)

implication that the magnitude of the analgesic response is related to the number of bites, which presumably are painful; that is, exposure to pain produces pain blockade. However, it is not the number of bites, but whether or not the bites caused the defeat response that predicts the emergence of analgesia. Individual mice showed full analgesia after receiving as few as 20 bites, others again failed to show any evidence of analgesia when we terminated the experiment after 100 attack bites. Moreover, an equivalent number of pinches with forceps in the back and tail region by the experimenter failed to produce any analgesia.

The tail-flick assay, relying on a relatively simple spinally mediated reflexive response, reveals unambiguously the magnitude and time course of the analgesia in defeated mice. In additional sets of mice, we measured the latency to react to a hot plate or, alternatively, to exhibit a writhing response in reaction to injection with 0.6% acetic acid. In both the hot-plate as well as the acid-writhing assays, defeated mice showed significant analgesia.

Mice of the $B6AF_1/J$ strain were selected for our initial experiments, because of their substantial and uniform response to morphine.[28] Analgesia following defeat is also apparent in strains of mice other than the $B6AF_1/J$ mice, albeit to varying degrees.[18] Significantly longer tail-flick latencies were recorded after exposure to 70 attack bites from resident stimulus animals in mice of the BALB/cBy, C57B1/6J, C57B1/6By, and DBA/2J strains and in Swiss-Webster–derived mice (CFW). Of particular interest are CXBK mice; these mice show a very small analgesic response to morphine and a very low number of [³H]naloxone binding sites in brain.[2] When challenged with attack bites from a resident animal, they increase their tail-flick latency to a very small degree.[19] In general, the magnitude of the analgesia following defeat correlates well with the degree of morphine analgesia in the various strains of mice.

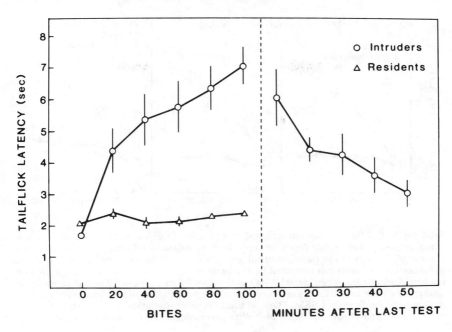

FIGURE 2. Tail-flick latencies in intruder mice ($N = 9$) as a function of being bitten, or in resident mice ($N = 5$) as a function of attacking an intruder. Values are means ± standard errors. Latencies were determined before any fighting experience and after 20 bites. The heat stimulus was automatically terminated at 8 sec if no flick occurred. (From Miczek and Thompson.[18] With permission from Alan R. Liss.)

The first critical evidence for a significant role of opioid peptides in the analgesic response of defeated mice came from studies with naloxone and naltrexone. Both opiate receptor blockers effectively antagonized the analgesia following defeat at doses of less than 1 mg/kg.[19] However, quaternary naltrexone, which does not cross the blood-brain barrier, failed to antagonize the analgesia in defeated mice. Recently, we prepared mice with permanently implanted intracranial cannulae and injected naloxone into the periaqueductal grey area and into the region of the arcuate nucleus. Doses as low as 1 microgram completely blocked analgesia in mice subjected to as many as 100 bites from a stimulus animal (FIGURE 3).[20] It appears that even smaller doses may be effective in attenuating analgesia in defeated mice, if it would be technically feasible to verifiably administer nanoliter amounts to freely moving mice.

DEFEAT PRODUCES ANALGESIA AND PITUITARY-ADRENAL ACTIVATION: HOW ARE THEY RELATED?

Being attacked, threatened, and pursued in a confrontation with an opponent results in pituitary-adrenal activation. This form of social stress causes the release of ACTH and, consequently, corticosterone.[4] We have confirmed these observa-

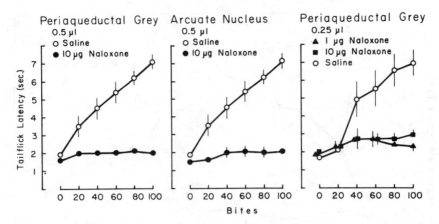

FIGURE 3. Tail-flick latency (in seconds) as a function of exposure to attack bites from a stimulus animal. *Left*: Saline (open circle) or 10 μg naloxone (solid circle) were injected in a volume of 0.5 μl into the periaqueductal grey area. *Center*: Saline (open circle) or 10 μg naloxone (solid circle) were injected in a volume of 0.5 μl into the region of the arcuate nucleus. *Right*: Saline (open circle), 1 μg naloxone (solid triangle), or 10 μg naloxone (solid square) in a volume of 0.25 μl were injected into the periaqueductal grey area. Vertical lines in data points indicate ± 1 SEM. The heat stimulus was automatically terminated at 8 sec if no flick occurred. (From Miczek *et al.*[20] With permission from *Psychopharmacology*.)

tions and asked whether or not the level of corticosterone in plasma is related to the degree of analgesia as mice are exposed to an increased number of bites from an opponent. Specifically, male CFW mice, housed in groups of 10, were individually exposed to either 0, 30, 60, or 90 bites by resident stimulus mice. Before and after the introduction into the cage of the stimulus animal their response to pain was determined with the tail-flick assay. The intensity of the heat stimulus was adjusted so that baseline reaction times were 5–6 sec in duration. Thereafter, the animals were killed by decapitation and trunk blood was collected for determination of corticosterone levels via radioimmunoassays.

Significantly elevated plasma corticosterone was found in mice that were exposed to 60 and 90 attack bites (FIGURE 4A); this change was paralleled by significant increases in tail-flick latencies in the same groups (FIGURE 4B). When these effects are expressed as a function of the number of bites, i.e. amount of stress stimulation, the data suggest a correlation between pituitary-adrenal activation and analgesia. However, inspection of each individual's values for corticosterone and analgesia reveals large variations. When each mouse's value for corticosterone is plotted as a function of its tail-flick latency, the wide scatter of the points demonstrates the absence of a clear systematic relationship (FIGURE 4C). Corticosterone values of less than 5 μg/100 ml plasma to up to more than 23 μg/100 ml plasma are associated with similar tail-flick latencies. At the highest possible tail-flick latencies, 18 sec being the cut-off at the currently used low-intensity stimulus, many corticosterone values are higher than 30 μg/100 ml plasma. It is possible that a threshold level of corticosterone has to be exceeded in order for a large analgesia to develop. However, this issue remains unresolved, because the animals that showed these high corticosterone values were also exposed to the greatest number of bites. It would be informative to measure corticosterone in animals that fail to show analgesia after being exposed to a large number of bites.

The poor correlation between an individual's elevation in plasma corticosterone and reduced responsiveness to pain brings into question the existence of an essential functional relationship between these two responses and their mediating processes.

Direct manipulations of pituitary and adrenal activity should provide more compelling evidence concerning the contributions of these two glands to the development of analgesia in defeated mice than correlational data. In order to assess whether or not the pituitary and adrenal glands are necessary for the development of analgesia, several treatments were selected for blocking the output from either gland.[29,30]

Separate groups of mice were either injected with dexamethasone (1 mg/kg 30 min prior to defeat) or presented with hypertonic saline solution (2%) as drinking fluid for 3 days. Thereafter, these mice and their respective controls were subjected to attacks by stimulus resident mice, and their response to pain was determined with the tail-flick assay. Analgesia developed at the same rate and to the same extent in mice whose pituitary endorphin activity was suppressed by dexamethasone or hypertonic saline as it did in control animals; after exposure to 60–80 attack bites from an opponent, animals in all groups showed tail-flick latencies up to the 8-sec cut-off limit.

In a further series of experiments, mice were either injected with corticosterone (1 mg/kg) or, alternatively, had their adrenal glands surgically removed. In confrontations with resident animals the treated mice were attacked and their response to pain subsequently assessed. Again, no evidence for an essential contribution of adrenal secretions to the analgesia in defeated mice was found. Adrenalectomized mice as well as corticosterone-treated mice actually showed a large analgesic response (i.e. up to the 8 sec cut-off limit) in reaction to a smaller number of bites than their respective controls. Instead of blocking or attenuating the analgesia in defeated mice, these treatments enhanced this response.

These results add to others that show little or no effect of compromising pituitary-adrenal activation on other forms of stress-induced analgesia.[3,6,14,31] Our observations are also consistent with the demonstration that corticosterone injections increase the submissive behavior of mice that are attacked by an opponent.[12]

The secretion of endogenous opioid peptides in response to stress from cells of the anterior and intermediate lobes of the pituitary gland, and from chromaffin cells in the adrenal medulla, as well as the existence of a common precursor molecule for ACTH and endogenous opioid peptides, suggested a possible role for these substances in stress-induced analgesia. Yet, in defeated mice the analgesic response and the activation of the pituitary-adrenal axis appear to be independent processes.

TOLERANCE

In our initial experiments on analgesia in defeated mice we were quite confused and dismayed by our inability to replicate the large analgesic response within the same subject on subsequent occasions. This disappointment turned into a

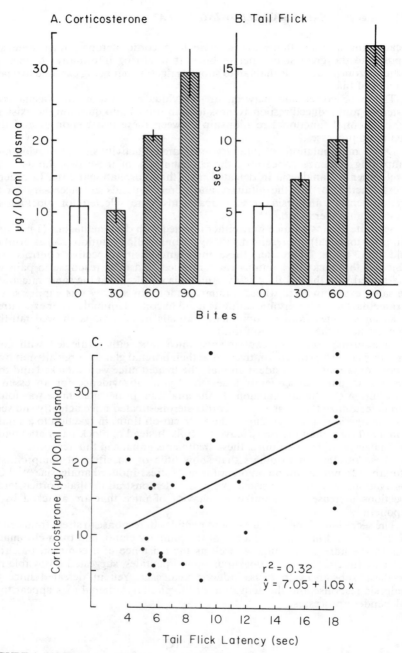

FIGURE 4. (A) Plasma corticosterone (μg/100 ml) in mice that were exposed to either 0, 30, 60, or 90 bites from resident mice. (B) Tail-flick latencies (seconds) in mice that were exposed to either 0, 30, 60, or 90 bites from resident mice. Vertical lines in each bar represent ± 1 SEM. (C) Corticosterone values (μg/100 ml plasma) as a function of latencies to flick the tail in reaction to a heat stimulus. Each point represents data from a single mouse.

fascination with one of the most significant features of this analgesic response, namely the development of tolerance. Apparently, mice exposed to a brief defeat experience every day for a number of days would show less and less analgesia, resembling in many aspects the tolerance that develops to repeated morphine injections.

Initial reports of tolerance development to stress-induced analgesia involved prolonged exposure to the stressor for as much as two weeks. Thus, in designing our initial experiment we assumed that a relatively long period with repeated defeats would be necessary for the development of tolerance to the analgesic response. FIGURE 5A portrays the time course of tolerance development to the analgesic effects of defeat in a group of mice that was exposed to 100 bites by stimulus resident mice. Twenty-four hours after the last defeat experience, the mice were challenged with an injection of morphine (5 mg/kg). In contrast to the

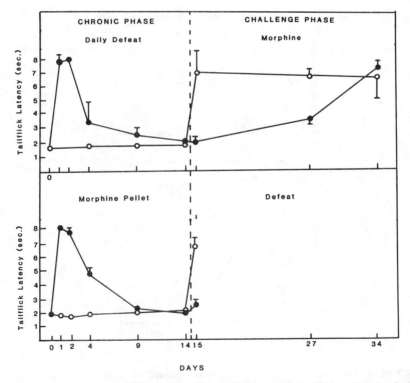

FIGURE 5. Cross-tolerance between morphine analgesia and defeat-induced analgesia. (A) Tail-flick latencies in intruder mice ($N = 6$) subjected to 100 bites by resident mice every day for 14 days (solid circle) and in control mice ($N = 6$) not subjected to attack (open circle). On days 15, 27, and 34 the defeated mice and the controls were administered 5 mg/kg morphine sulfate and tested 30 min later. (B) Tail-flick latencies in mice implanted with a 75 mg morphine pellet ($N = 10$; solid circle) or with a placebo pellet ($N = 5$; open circle). On day 15, mice with morphine or placebo pellets were exposed to 100 bites and tested for tailflick latency. (From Miczek *et al.*[19] With permission from *Science*.)

concurrently treated non-defeated control animals, chronically defeated mice failed to show morphine analgesia. A comparable time course of tolerance and cross-tolerance was evident in mice that were chronically exposed to morphine (FIGURE 5B).[19]

In a subsequent series of experiments we pursued the question of whether tolerance in defeated mice extends to morphine-sensitive functions other than responsiveness to pain.[21] In a conditioning test situation, food-deprived mice performed an operant response that was reinforced by milk after every 30th response (Fixed Ratio schedule 30). The dose-dependent effects of morphine on schedule-controlled response rates and on the response to pain were investigated over a period of about 6 weeks. The mice were then exposed to attack bites by resident animals once every day for 5 days before their tail-flick response was measured, and before they were placed into the conditioning chamber. FIGURE 6 (top) portrays the decrease in rate of operant performance as a result of the

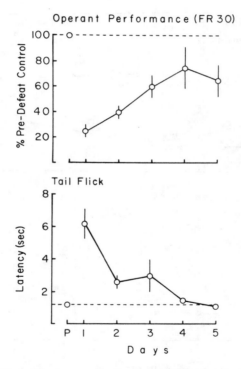

FIGURE 6. *Top*: The response rate of mice maintained on a fixed-ratio 30 schedule of reinforcement over consecutive daily defeat experiences. The mice were exposed to bites from resident mice before being placed in the conditioning chamber. The data are expressed as percent of pre-defeat control level. *Bottom*: The tail-flick latencies (in seconds) of mice after they were attacked by resident mice but before they were placed in the conditioning chamber. Dotted lines represent pre-defeat control levels; vertical lines in each data point indicate $\pm$ 1 SEM.

preceding defeat experience on the first day of exposure to an attack opponent. At the same time, these mice showed a pronounced analgesic response in the tail-flick assay (FIGURE 6, bottom). Over the course of the 5 days of defeat experiences, the baseline rate of operant responding was nearly recovered, and the tail-flick latencies returned to baseline level. During the subsequent 5–6 weeks the dose-effect determinations for morphine on operant behavior and response to pain were repeated.

FIGURE 7 depicts the morphine dose-effect functions for operant performance (top) and tail flick (bottom) before and after the 5-day defeat experience. It is evident that defeat produced a four-fold shift to the right of the dose-effect function for morphine analgesia, whereas no change in dose-effect curve for morphine effects on operant performance was seen. These results provide evidence for tolerance to the analgesic effects of defeat and for cross-tolerance to morphine's analgesic effects that are large and long-lasting, even though the defeat experiences were substantially shorter than in our initial studies. Moreover, no comparable shift in dose-effect curve for morphine's effects on operant

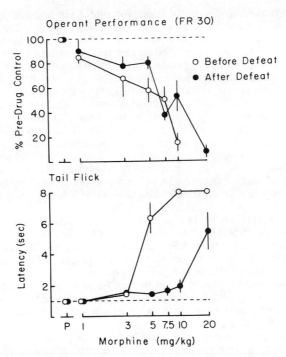

FIGURE 7. Effects of morphine on operant performance maintained by a fixed-ratio 30 schedule of reinforcement (*top*), and on tail-flick latencies (*bottom*) before (open circles) and after (solid circles) 5 days of defeat experience. Operant performance is expressed as percent of pre-drug control. Dotted lines represent control levels; vertical lines in each data point indicate ± 1 SEM.

performance was detectable in spite of the fact that a gradual waning of the disruptive effects of defeat was observed with repeated exposure. This selective tolerance development suggests that different opioid receptor subtypes mediate the two response systems.

Tolerance to the effects of defeat, and cross-tolerance to morphine, may result from chronically altered synthesis and release of endogenous opioid peptides and subsequent changes in opioid receptors.[11,16] We used the opiate antagonist diprenorphine to search for potential changes in *in vivo* opioid receptor binding in mice following acute or chronic exposure to defeat. Diprenorphine is a potent opiate antagonist that binds to opioid receptor subtypes nonselectively; therefore, the potential for observing effects of defeat on binding is enhanced. It has been assumed that decreases in diprenorphine binding following stress reflect the exclusion of the ligand from the receptors by stress-related release of endogenous opioid peptides, as shown recently after either acute footshock or cold-water swim stress.[27]

A rapid filtration method was employed to allow assessment of stereospecific *in vivo* binding.[24] Mice were injected subcutaneously with a tracer amount of [³H]diprenorphine (4 μCi in 0.05 ml NaCl, 2 μg/kg) immediately after a tail-flick assessment of the response to pain, which followed exposure to 100 bites. The brains were removed and rapidly dissected into four regions (FIGURE 8, top panel).[10] Binding in the defeated mice was compared to that in mice not subjected to defeat. Two additional groups of mice were also assessed for the effects of repeated exposure to defeat on [³H]diprenorphine binding. One group was subjected to defeat for 7 days to produce adaptation or tolerance to the effects of defeat, with binding being assessed immediately after the 7th test. Binding in these mice was contrasted to that of mice similarly treated but not exposed to defeat on the 7th day. This comparison allows an analysis of the effects of repeated defeat independently from the acute effects of defeat.

Diprenorphine binding was reduced by 11–25% in all three brain areas of defeated mice, but significantly so only in the brainstem (medulla-pons) region (FIGURE 8). In mice that were subjected to repeated defeat (i.e. defeat-adapted), this consistent reduction in binding in response to defeat was not observed. There was no significant increase or decrease in [³H]diprenorphine binding in response to defeat on the 7th day. Interestingly, however, mice adapted or tolerant to the effects of defeat showed significantly elevated (25–35%) [³H]diprenorphine binding in the brainstem when compared to naive mice. These results suggest that repeated exposure to defeat leads to an increase in the number of opioid receptors in the brain, or alternatively that repeated defeat leads to a depletion of opioid peptides below the levels present in naive mice, thus providing less competition for receptors following [³H]diprenorphine injection.

These results were supported by additional *in vitro* binding studies using the relatively μ selective agonist dihydromorphine. Mice exposed to 5 days of defeat showed an apparent increase in the number of μ receptor sites without apparent change in affinity (TABLE 1).

If in fact tolerance to analgesia in defeated mice is based on changes in brain opioid receptors, it may be possible to precipitate withdrawal responses akin to those seen after chronic morphine exposure. We investigated this possibility in mice subjected to 100 bites per day for 7 days. FIGURE 9 shows the large analgesic response in these mice after the first exposure to attack bites and the return to baseline latencies in response to pain over the course of the 7-day behavioral treatment. The magnitude and time course of analgesia in these mice matched those of a further group of mice that were injected daily with morphine (5 mg/kg).

Brain dissection scheme:

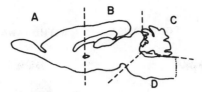

^{3}H − Diprenorphine binding (in vivo)

D. Medulla − Pons

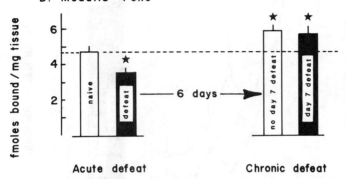

FIGURE 8. *In vivo* [^{3}H]diprenorphine binding in B6AF$_1$/J mice following a single or repeated defeats. *Upper panel*: Brains were rapidly removed after defeat and divided into four regions as shown.[10] *Lower panel (left)*: Binding in medulla and pons (region D) in mice after being bitten 100 times (dark bar) compared to that observed in naive mice not subjected to attack (open bar). [^{3}H]Diprenorphine (4 µCi, 2 µg/kg s.c.) was injected immediately after defeat, and mice were sacrificed 20 min after injection. *Lower panel (right)*: Binding in mice exposed to chronic defeat. The dark bar depicts binding in mice injected with [^{3}H]diprenorphine immediately after defeat on day 7, while the open bar shows [^{3}H]diprenorphine binding in chronically defeated mice not exposed to defeat on day 7. Values are means ± SEM: $N = 6$ for each group. Star indicates a significant ($p < 0.05$) difference from the naive group on day 1.

TABLE 1. [^{3}H]Dihydromorphine Binding in Defeat-Tolerant Mice

Group	N	K_D (nanomoles)	B_{max} (fmoles/mg protein)
Naive	6	3.11 + 0.34	13.03 + 0.84
Tolerant	12	4.48 + 0.38	17.02 + 0.61[a]

Scatchard analysis of *in vitro* [^{3}H]dihydromorphine binding in mice subjected to 5 days of repeated defeat. Binding was assayed according to the procedure of Cremins and Shuster.[32] Whole brains (minus cerebellum) were rapidly removed and homogenized in ice-cold Tris buffer with a Brinkman polytron. Aliquots were incubated with [^{3}H]dihydromorphine at 25°C for 45 min in the presence or absence of unlabeled levorphanol. Following incubation, receptor-bound ligand was collected on GF/B filters under vacuum, washed with ice-cold buffer, and counted in a scintillation counter. Stereospecific binding at ten different concentrations of [^{3}H]dihydromorphine (0.05–10 nM) was determined. Estimates of K_D and B_{max} were calculated by a least-squares curve-fitting analysis program (LIGAND[23]). [a]indicates significant difference, $p < 0.05$.

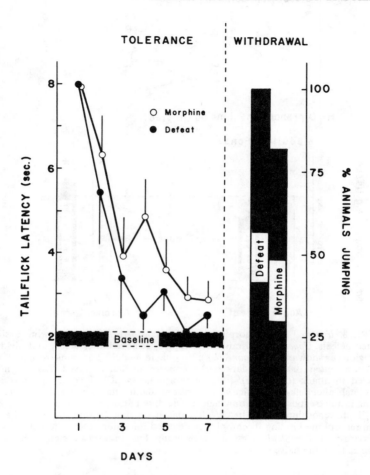

FIGURE 9. *Left*: Development of tolerance and withdrawal signs in mice subjected to repeated defeat. Intruder mice ($N = 6$; solid circles) were bitten 100 times daily by resident mice for 7 days. A second group was injected with morphine (5 mg/kg i.p.) every day for 7 days ($N = 6$; open circles). Tail-flick latency was assessed immediately after the 100th bite in the defeated animals and 30 min after injection in the morphine group; values are daily means ± SEM for each group. There were no significant differences between the two groups on any day. *Right*: The percentage of mice in each group showing naloxone-precipitated withdrawal jumping on day 7, when naloxone (10 mg/kg i.p.) was injected immediately after the daily defeat or 30 min after the daily injection of morphine.

On the seventh day immediately after the defeat test or the morphine injection, respectively, the mice were injected with naloxone (10 mg/kg).

Withdrawal jumping was observed in all mice that were exposed to attack bites for 7 days and in 5 out of 6 mice that received daily morphine injections (FIGURE 9). Under appropriate conditions, mice that are treated chronically with morphine as well as those that have been subjected to attacks by an opponent show a comparable initial analgesic response, and develop tolerance as well as naloxone-precipitated withdrawal responses. This pattern of effects suggests that chronically defeated mice show physical dependence to endogenously released opioid peptides.[7]

The striking long-term consequences of defeat can be observed after only a single brief behavioral experience. We have seen significant shifts to the right in dose-effect curves for morphine analgesia as measured over the course of 5–6 weeks in mice that were exposed to a single defeat experience.[21] FIGURE 10 illustrates the long-lasting reduction in analgesic response to a challenge with morphine (5 mg/kg) after a defeat. The magnitude of morphine analgesia was greatly reduced in those groups of mice that received morphine 3, 5, or 7 days after a single exposure to the attacks of stimulus animals.

CONCLUSION

The development of analgesia in defeated mice represents an important behavioral and physiological adaptation to a biologically significant "stressor."

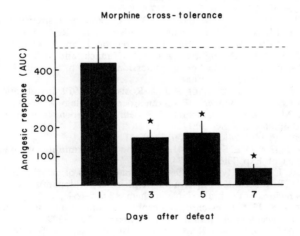

FIGURE 10. Time course of development of cross-tolerance to morphine following a single defeat. Analgesic response is portrayed as area under the response curve (AUC). Separate groups of $B6AF_1$ mice ($N = 6$ per group) were subjected to 100 bites on day 0 and subsequently tested for analgesic response to morphine (5 mg/kg i.p.) at 1, 3, 5, or 7 days after the defeat test. Values are means ± SEM; star indicates a significant ($p < 0.05$) difference from the morphine response of a control group of mice not exposed to attack (dotted line).

The analgesic response in defeated mice is large and long-lasting, and it is similar to that produced by morphine in many respects. Analgesia in defeated mice can be blocked by opiate receptor antagonists, whether injected systemically or intracerebrally. Tolerance develops to the analgesic response in mice that are exposed to attack bites by an opponent. When challenged with naloxone, tolerant mice show withdrawal signs comparable to those after repeated morphine exposure. Cross-tolerance to morphine can be detected after a single defeat. It appears that the cross-tolerance to morphine is selective for the analgesic effects of the drug. Binding assays with the non-selective opiate antagonist diprenorphine indicate increased receptor occupancy by endogenous opioid peptides after a single defeat, whereas changes in the opposite direction are seen after repeated defeats.

ACKNOWLEDGMENTS

We gratefully acknowledge assistance and comments by Drs. R. Kream and K. Noda, and J. T. Winslow.

REFERENCES

1. AMIR, S., Z. W. BROWN & Z. AMIT. 1980. The role of endorphins in stress: Evidence and speculations. Neurosci. Biobehav. Rev. 4:77–86.
2. BARAN, A., L. SHUSTER, B. E. ELEFTHERIOU & D. W. BAILY. 1975. Opiate receptors in mice: Genetic differences. Life Sci. 17:633–640.
3. BODNAR, R. J., D. D. KELLY, M. BRUTUS & M. GLUSMAN. 1979. Stress induced analgesia: Neural and hormonal determinants. Neurosci. Behav. Rev. 4:87–100.
4. BRAIN, P. F. 1979. Hormones, drugs and aggression. Eden Press. Montreal.
5. BRAIN, P. F. 1981. Differentiating types of attack and defense in rodents. In Multidisciplinary Approaches to Aggression Research. P. F. Brain & D. Benton, Eds.:53–78. Elsevier. Amsterdam.
6. CHANCE, W. T., G. M. KRYNOCK & J. A. ROSECRANS. 1979. Investigation of pituitary influences on autoanangesia. Psychoneuroendocrinology 4:199–205.
7. CHRISTIE, M. J. & G. B. CHESHER. 1982. Physical dependence on physiologically released opiates. Life Sci. 30:1173–1177.
8. CROWCROFT, P. 1966. Mice All Over. Foulis. London.
9. D'AMOUR, F. E. & D. L. SMITH. 1941. A method for determining loss of pain sensation. J. Pharmacol. Exp. Therap. 72:74–79.
10. GLOWINSKI, J. & L. L. IVERSEN. 1966. Regional studies of catecholamines in the rat brain. I. The disposition of [^{3}H]norepinepherine, [^{3}H]dopamine, and [^{3}H]DOPA in various regions of the brain. J. Neurochem. 13:665–664.
11. KUSCHINSKY, K. 1975. Does chronic morphine treatment induce a supersensitivity of dopamine receptors in rat brain? Psychopharm. 42:225–229.
12. LESHNER, A. I., S. J. KORN, J. R. MIXON, C. ROSENTHAL & A. K. BESSER. 1980. Effects of corticosterone on submissiveness in mice: Some temporal and theoretical considerations. Physiol. Behav. 24:283–288.
13. LEWIS, J. W., J. T. CANNON & J. C. LIEBESKIND. 1980. Opioid and nonopioid mechanisms of stress analgesia. Science 298:623–625.
14. MAREK, P., I. PANOCKA & G. HARTMANN. 1982. Enhancement of stress-induced analgesia in adrenalectomized mice: Its reversal by dexamethasone. Pharmacol. Biochem. Behav. 16:403–405.
15. MAYER, D. J. & L. R. WATKINS. 1981. Role of endorphins in endogenous pain control systems. In Modern Problems of Pharmacopsychiatry. T. A. Ban, Ed. 17:68–96. S. Karger. Basel.

16. McGIVERN, R. F., S. MOUSA, D. COURE & G. G. BERNSTON. 1983. Prolonged intermittent footshock stress decreases met and leu enkephalin levels in brain with concomitant decreases in pain threshold. Life Sci. **33**:47–54.

17. MICZEK, K. A. & J. M. O'DONNELL. 1978. Intruder-evoked aggression in isolated and nonisolated mice: Effects of psychomotor stimulants and l-dopa. Psychopharmacology **57**:47–55.

18. MICZEK, K. A. & M. L. THOMPSON. 1984. Analgesia resulting from defeat in a social confrontation: The role of endogenous opioids in brain. *In* Modulation of Sensorimotor Activity during Altered Behavioral States. R. Bandler, Ed.:431–456. Alan R. Liss. New York.

19. MICZEK, K. A., M. L. THOMPSON & L. SHUSTER. 1982. Opioid-like analgesia in defeated mice. Science **215**:1520–1522.

20. MICZEK, K. A., M. L. THOMPSON & L. SHUSTER. 1985. Naloxone injections into periaqueductal grey area and arcuate nucleus block analgesia in defeated mice. Psychopharmacology **87**:39–42.

21. MICZEK, K. A. & J. T. WINSLOW. 1985. Response to pain and operant performance in socially defeated mice: Selective cross-tolerance to morphine and antagonism by naltrexone. J. Pharmacol. Exp. Therapeutics (Submitted for publication.)

22. MILLAN, M. J. 1981. Stress and endogenous opioid peptides: a review. Modern Problems Pharmacopsych. **17**:49–67.

23. MUNSON, P. J. & D. RODBARD. 1980. LIGAND: A versatile computerized approach for characterization of ligand-binding systems. Anal. Biochem. **107**:220–239.

24. PERT, C. B. & S. H. SNYDER. 1975. Identification of opiate receptor binding in intact animals. Life Sci. **16**:1623–1634.

25. RODGERS, R. J. & C. A. HENDRIE. 1983. Social conflict activates status-dependent endogenous analgesic or hyperalgesic mechanisms in male mice: Effects of naloxone on nociception and behaviour. Physiol. Behav. **30**:775–780.

26. RODGERS, R. J., C. A. HENDRIE & A. J. WATERS. 1983. Naloxone partially antagonizes post-encounter analgesia and enhances defensive responding in male rats exposed to attack from lactating conspecifics. Physiol. Behav. **30**:781–786.

27. SEEGER, T. F., G. A. SFORZO & C. B. PERT. 1984. *In vivo* autoradiography: Visualization of stress-induced changes in opiate receptor occupancy in the rat brain. Brain Res. **305**:303–311.

28. SHUSTER, L. 1975. Genetic analysis of morphine effects: Activity, analgesia, tolerance and sensitization. *In* Psychopharmacogenetics. B. E. Eleftheriou, Ed.:73–98. Plenum Press. New York.

29. THOMPSON, M. L. & K. A. MICZEK. 1983. Analgesia in defeated mice: Evidence for mediation via central rather than pituitary or adrenal endogenous opioids. Neurosci. Abstr. **9**:134.

30. THOMPSON, M. L., K. A. MICZEK & L. SHUSTER. 1981. Changes in brain beta-endorphin and tolerance to morphine analgesia after a single defeat in mice. Neurosci. Abstr. **7**:881.

31. WATKINS, L. R., D. A. COBELLI, H. H. NEWSOME & D. J. MAYER. 1982. Footshock induced analgesia is dependent neither on pituitary nor sympathetic activation. Brain Res. **245**:81–96.

32. CREMINS, J. & L. SHUSTER. 1982. A genetically controlled difference in morphine analgesia and narcotic receptors in mice. Fed. Proc. **41**:13–14.

Vaginal Stimulation–Produced Analgesia in Rats and Women[a]

BARRY R. KOMISARUK AND BEVERLY WHIPPLE

Institute of Animal Behavior
Rutgers—The State University
Newark, New Jersey 07102

INTRODUCTION

A major contribution by many of the participants in this volume is the identification and characterization of a variety of sensory stimuli that produce analgesia and the neuropharmacological, neuroanatomical, and psychological bases of the analgesia. The unifying concept "stressor" has been applied to these analgesia-producing stimuli. They include foot shock, centrifugal rotation, and hypertonic saline injected intraperitoneally[1,2] cold water swim,[3-5] noxious mechanostimulation of the skin,[6,7] defeat,[8] trigeminal nerve stimulation,[9] immobilization,[6] and acupuncture and transcutaneous nerve stimulation.[10] Liebeskind and co-workers[11] and Akil and co-workers[12] have included the analgesia produced by vaginal stimulation as a member of this class of stress-induced analgesias.

We published the first evidence of vaginal stimulation (VS)–produced analgesia in our demonstration in 1971 that it blocks withdrawal responses to noxious cutaneous stimulation.[13] Subsequently, we presented evidence that VS is analgesic and not anesthetic or merely paralytic, based on our sensory studies in rats.[14] Conclusive evidence that VS produces analgesia requires a human verbal report. Our most recent publications present evidence that VS does indeed produce analgesia in humans.[15,16] What is particularly interesting and relevant to this volume is that the most effective analgesia occurs when the VS is perceived by the women as pleasurable, not stressful or painful. This leads us to examine more carefully the categorization of this analgesia as stress-induced. We shall address this question of whether or not VS-produced analgesia is stress-induced after reviewing the findings that led us to the conclusion that VS produces analgesia. We also review the neuropharmacological basis of the VS-produced analgesia.

VS-PRODUCED ANALGESIA IN LABORATORY RATS

Rats become unresponsive to intense noxious stimulation applied throughout the body surface immediately upon onset of VS.[13] VS totally blocks leg flexion to foot pinch[13] and strongly suppresses vibrissa retraction to ear pinch.[13] Some other characteristics of VS are that it blocks tail flick to radiant heat[17] and eye blink to

[a]The human studies were supported by funds from the Dean's Office, Institute of Animal Behavior, and Zoology Department, Newark Campus and the Research Council of Rutgers University. The animal studies were supported by National Science Foundation grant BNS-7824504 (B.R.K.). This is contribution No. 432 from the Institute of Animal Behavior.

corneal stimulation.[13] As VS intensity is increased, the vocalization threshold increases in a "dose-response" relationship.[18] The ability of VS to block the leg withdrawal response to compression of a foot far exceeds the effect of 2 mg/kg of morphine[19] and recently we have found that VS elevates tail-flick latency more than does 8 mg/kg of morphine. The VS effect has been replicated in other laboratories.[20-23]

There is evidence that VS specifically produces analgesia, rather than non-specific anesthesia or inability to show withdrawal response to noxious stimulation. The ventrobasal nuclear complex of the thalamus (VBT) was used to establish this. The VBT complex is a relay station for nociceptive input, where these neurons show increased firing rates in response to noxious stimulation (e.g. skin pinch) in rats[24,25] and monkeys.[26] We found that VS markedly attenuated responses of VBT neurons to noxious stimulation. Moreover, neuronal response to innocuous tactile stimulation remained unaffected by VS.[14] Suppression of behavioral and neuronal responses to noxious stimulation by VS has been replicated and extended in other laboratories with rats[20,21,27,28] and cats[29,30] in several brain sites and in spinal cord.

We believe that VS activates an intrinsic spinal gating mechanism that prevents the noxious but not innocuous input from reaching the thalamus. This is based on findings that after spinal transection, withdrawal responses to noxious stimulation below the level of the transection are blocked by VS.[13] In rats whose spinal cord is transected at T2, VS significantly elevates tail-flick latency, but to a significantly lesser degree than in intact or decerebrate rats.[31,32] In contrast, a cranial nerve-mediated withdrawal reflex (vibrissa withdrawal to ear pinch), which is attenuated by VS in intact rats, is no longer attenuated after spinal transection.[13]

This effect of VS is due to a spinal mechanism rather than to a blood-borne analgesic factor. If a blood-borne factor (e.g. endogenous opiates) of brain, pituitary, or adrenal origin[33] mediated the VS-produced attenuation of withdrawal reflexes, the responses rostral to, as well as caudal to, the level of transection would be affected by VS. However, only the responses caudal to the transection were found to be inhibited by VS.[13]

The VS-activated spinal mechanism apparently utilizes endogenous spinal opioids because naloxone administered either systemically or directly to the spinal cord significantly reduces the effect of VS on elevating the latency to flick the tail away from a radiant heat source.[34] There is apparently a test-specific naloxone antagonism of VS-produced analgesia. We first published a study showing no VS antagonism by naloxone or morphine tolerance on the vocalization threshold to tail shock.[35] Then Hill and Ayliffe[22] published a study showing a naloxone antagonism of the VS effect on tail-flick latency to heat. In replication experiments we have subsequently confirmed both these sets of findings. We have extended the study of Hill and Ayliffe[22] by finding that induction of morphine tolerance significantly attenuates VS-produced analgesia by 38%[34] on the tail flick test.

In further analysis of the role of neuropeptides in VS-produced analgesia (VSPA), we have recently found that intrathecal spinal administration of leupeptin, which inhibits the enzymatic breakdown of peptides, significantly prolongs the effect of VS after the VS is terminated. The leupeptin itself does not produce analgesia.[36] Evidence for a glycinergic component in VSPA is that strychnine, a specific glycine receptor antagonist, when administered intrathecally, significantly attenuates the vocalization threshold-elevating effect of VS.[37]

In addition to intrinsic spinal opioid and glycinergic mediators of VSPA, there is also good evidence of mediation by spinal alpha-adrenergic and serotoninergic mechanisms. VSPA was attenuated by injection of phentolamine intrathecally via chronically implanted catheters.[17] Consistent with this, microinjection of 6-hydroxydopamine at the level of the rostral spinal cord significantly reduced VSPA.[38] These data provide consistent evidence that VSPA is mediated in part by an alpha-adrenergic mechanism in the spinal cord.

As evidence of a serotoninergic component, VS has been shown to produce an increased uptake of 2-deoxy-D-glucose in midbrain dorsal raphe[39] which contains 5-hydroxytryptamine (5-HT) cell bodies with terminals in the spinal cord.[40,41] The descending 5-HT neurons with their cell bodies in the raphe nuclei course through the dorsolateral funiculus of the spinal cord.[42-45] When the dorsolateral funiculus is transected, analgesia produced by electrical stimulation of the raphe nuclei is attenuated.[46] We found that the VS-produced increase in tail-flick latency is attenuated by dorsolateral funiculus transection.[32]

In addition, we found that the VS produces a twofold increase in the levels of norepinephrine and serotonin released into spinal superfusates.[17] These findings provide evidence that VSPA is mediated in part by the descending noradrenergic and serotoninergic system.

Thus, VS apparently blocks transmission of nociceptive activity to the thalamus by two mechanisms: one an intrinsic spinal opioid and glycinergic component; the second, a descending alpha-adrenergic and serotoninergic component that is activated by vaginal afferents.

It is not at all surprising that multiple neurochemical systems are involved in the effects of VS since VS exerts multiple neuroendocrine and musculoskeletal actions. Release from the pituitary of LH, prolactin, and oxytocin[47] on the one hand, and immobilization plus facilitation of lordosis elicited by tactile stimulation on the other[48] are all produced by VS, in addition to pain threshold elevation. It is likely that these various physiological and behavioral responses utilize various and different neurotransmitters.

The studies reviewed above have presented behavioral and neurophysiological evidence that VS produces analgesia, and the pharmacological basis for the analgesia. However, conclusive evidence was lacking that VS suppresses pain. Consequently, we performed a series of studies using humans in which we used a verbal report to measure pain thresholds and tactile thresholds in relation to VS.

ELEVATION OF PAIN THRESHOLDS BY VAGINAL STIMULATION IN WOMEN

We have completed three studies using 10 women in each. Permission to perform the studies with women was obtained first from the Rutgers University Institutional Review Board for the protection of human subjects in research. Gynecological screening by the subject's own physician and psychological screening by a licensed psychologist were performed to eliminate any subject with a psychiatric illness or a gynecological condition that would contraindicate participation in the study. All of the subjects signed an informed consent form prior to participation and all were naive to the hypotheses of the studies.

The subject relaxed in a reclining chair in the human laboratory and was instructed in each step of the procedure by one of the investigators (B.W.). A specially designed cylinder with a force transducer (Precision Measurement, Inc., Ann Arbor, MI), attached to a digital strain gauge was used for the self-applied VS. The entire assembly was sterilized with Cidex (Surgikos, Inc., Arlington, TX) and then covered with a condom. All pressure and stimulation was self-applied by the subject and the subjects were their own controls.

A Ugo-Basile Analgesy Meter (Milan, Italy) was used to apply a compressive force to each finger of the left hand during control and experimental conditions. The subject places her finger on the point of the Analgesy Meter as the beam is lowered and a controlled amount of pressure is applied. A motorized drive moves the weight out along the calibrated beam, thereby increasing the pressure on the finger. The subject was instructed to say *pain* when pain was first detected on the finger and then to say *stop* when the pain on the finger became too uncomfortable to continue. The first statement, *pain*, is recorded as pain detection threshold, the second statement, *stop*, is recorded as pain tolerance threshold.

Tactile thresholds to innocuous stimulation of the dorsal surface of the left hand were obtained by using an aesthesiometer (Stoelting, Inc., Chicago, IL). This consists of a series of force-calibrated nylon monofilaments (von Frey fibers). The tactile threshold is defined as the force at which the subject identifies that she feels the fiber three out of three times using an ascending/descending method of limits. The tactile threshold was determined during each control and experimental condition.

Experiment 1. VS Produces Analgesia

In the first study, we found that pressure applied to the anterior vaginal wall produced an increase in pain detection threshold that was significantly greater by 41.7% than the pre-VS control. When the women applied VS in such a way that it felt pleasurable by their own description, rather than by simply maximizing the force, the pain detection threshold was somewhat higher (53.7%) and the increase was significantly higher over all the control stimuli, i.e. no-VS, pressure applied to knee, and voluntary contraction of pelvic muscles.[15,16] It is interesting to note that whereas anterior wall VS produced a significant elevation of pain detection threshold, posterior wall VS did not.

The pain tolerance threshold showed a similar trend but the magnitude of the effect was lower, reaching significance only when the VS was reported as pleasurable.

By contrast, no significant effects of any stimulation conditions were found for tactile threshold. Thus, there was a striking difference in the effect of VS between pain and touch thresholds. This is directly parallel to the effect that was observed in the behavioral and neurophysiological studies in rats. These data are supported by the verbal reports of the women who said that "I knew my finger was being squashed but it didn't hurt," "I was aware of the sensation but it didn't feel painful," "The sensation was there but it was distant."[16]

Experiment 2. Control for Distraction

A second experiment controlled for possible confounding factors. We determined the effect on pain thresholds of a distracting film segment shown on a

TV monitor (the train-chase scene from *The French Connection*) and a pleasurable distraction, i.e. a fur mitt brushed against the skin by the subject.

The elevation in pain tolerance thresholds in response to vaginal pressure at one minute was significantly greater than that in the pre- or post-VS controls or the TV or fur mitt conditions (showing a 40.3% increase over post-VS control levels). After one minute of VS self-applied in a way reported by the subjects to be pleasurable, and prior to orgasm, there was a significant increase (53.6%), which was greater than the controls. After 5 minutes of this stimulation, the tolerance threshold increase was 62.9%, which was significantly greater than VS at one minute. Four of the women reached orgasm from purely vaginal stimulation and during this condition showed the highest mean percent increase in tolerance threshold (74.7%) of all the conditions (FIGURE 1).[16]

The pain detection thresholds showed a similar but more exaggerated pattern. Vaginal pressure alone produced a significant (47.4%) increase whereas pleasurable vaginal stimulation at 5 minutes produced an 84% significant increase and the detection threshold at orgasm was significantly increased by 106.7% over a resting control of no stimulation (FIGURE 2).[16]

Again tactile thresholds showed no significant changes with any of the stimulation conditions (FIGURE 3).

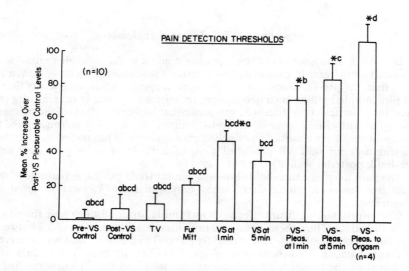

FIGURE 1. Pain detection thresholds during the various stimulus conditions of Experiment 2. Values shown are group mean (± S.E.M.) percent increases over control (post-VS pleasurable control) levels. Significant differences (based upon ANOVA and subsequent Student-Newman-Keuls tests, $p < .05$) between pairs of conditions are represented as follows: the value of any condition in which a letter is preceded by an asterisk is significantly greater than any other condition with the same letter that is not preceded by an asterisk. Example: the VS condition at 1 min is significantly greater than the Pre- or Post-VS control, TV or fur mitt conditions, but not the VS-at-5 min condition.

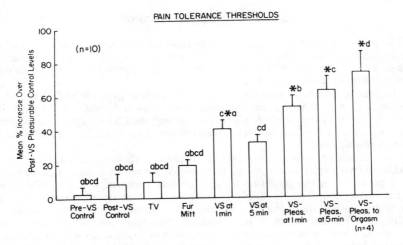

FIGURE 2. Pain tolerance thresholds during the various stimulus conditions in Experiment 2. The same conventions as in FIGURE 1 pertain.

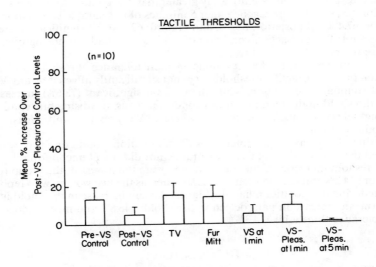

FIGURE 3. Tactile thresholds during the various conditions in Experiment 2. The same conventions as in FIGURE 1 pertain.

Experiment 3. Regional Specificity

The purpose of the third study was to replicate our previous studies and to systematize the areas of stimulation in order to determine the relative effectiveness of anterior or posterior vaginal wall or clitoral pressure and pleasurable stimulation in elevating pain thresholds.

The previous findings were replicated in that vaginal pressure and pleasurable self-stimulation increased pain thresholds over control conditions. As with the results in the previous studies, all values are reported as group mean percent increase over the non-stimulation reference threshold obtained at the end of each subject's testing session.

The increase in pain tolerance threshold during VS pressure on the anterior wall (26.8%) was significantly greater than that of the no-VS control, but the effect of VS pressure on the posterior wall or clitoral pressure was not. When the subjects were instructed to apply stimulation so that it was experienced as pleasurable rather than just as pressure, stimulation of each site showed a significantly greater increase in threshold than the control condition. As pleasurable stimulation continued to a maximum of 5 minutes, the pain tolerance threshold increased further to 55.7%, anterior wall, 43.5%, posterior wall, and 47.3%, clitoral, all of which were significantly greater than the control condition. A distraction control of reading a selected passage out loud did not elevate the pain tolerance threshold.

The results for the pain detection threshold were similar, the percent increases tending to be greater than for the pain tolerance threshold. This was the same as in our previous studies.

The pain detection threshold during VS anterior wall pressure (35.7%) was significantly greater than control, whereas during VS posterior wall pressure or clitoral pressure it was not significantly greater than the control. The highest pain detection thresholds were reached after 5 minutes of pleasurable stimulation (VS anterior: 67.4%, VS posterior: 62.8%, and clitoral: 62.5%), all significantly greater than control. The distraction condition of reading out loud did not significantly increase the pain detection threshold.

Again, in contrast to the elevations in pain tolerance threshold and pain detection threshold, tactile thresholds were not significantly affected by any VS or clitoral stimulation condition, while there was a significant (78.6%) increase in tactile threshold in the reading control condition. Thus, the distracting condition (reading) elevated tactile thresholds, whereas VS pressure and pleasurable conditions did not.

During the pleasurable anterior wall stimulation condition, two women reported that the VS did not feel pleasurable, nor did it feel uncomfortable. The pain threshold increases of these two women were the lowest in the group (pain detection: 14.2% and pain tolerance: 15.2%), whereas the two women who reported orgasm during this condition had the highest percent increase in threshold in the group (mean increase in pain detection threshold: 146.8% and mean increase in pain tolerance threshold: 114.3%).

DISCUSSION

In the context of this volume, the question is raised as to whether to consider the analgesia produced by VS as a form of stress-induced analgesia. The answer depends on whether one defines stress as necessarily aversive, or whether one includes in the category of stress the strong non-aversive arousal that occurs at orgasm. For example, both in response to noxious stimulation[49,50] and also during orgasm,[51] heart rate, blood pressure, respiration rate, and pupil diameter all increase markedly, indicative of the increased net sympathetic autonomic tone. Similar effects are also produced by exercise.[52] If both orgasm and exercise are defined as stressful, then "stress" need not be aversive. In that case, the analgesia that occurs during orgasm in our studies[15,16] or after exercise as in Janal et al.'s study,[53] are forms of stress-induced analgesia. Under this categorization, stress and pain are not synonymous and the concept of stress should be made sufficiently inclusive to incorporate exertion and strong pleasurable arousal. Under this definition, VS-produced analgesia could be considered to be one of the class of stress-induced analgesias. This follows Selye's concept that "stress" includes "distress" (from the Latin dis = bad) as well as "eustress" (from the Greek eu = good), during both of which conditions "... the body undergoes virtually the same nonspecific responses to the various positive or negative stimuli acting upon it."[54]

However, if stress is defined as requiring an aversive component, then the analgesia produced by VS is in a class apart from stress-induced analgesia, since our subjects described the vaginal self-stimulation as non-aversive. Indeed, a greater degree of analgesia was obtained during vaginal pleasurable stimulation than just vaginal pressure stimulation. Furthermore, the highest degree of analgesia was observed during orgasm and these were certainly pleasurable by the subjects' reports.

It is noteworthy that stimulation applied as pressure to the clitoris did not produce analgesia, but when the stimulation was self-applied in a pattern that was reported as pleasurable by the subjects, a significant elevation in pain threshold was observed. Thus, we have found that a sensory evoked sensation of pleasure elevates pain thresholds.

We are therefore presented with the choice that either pleasurable stimulation is one of the stressors that produces analgesia or pleasurable stimulation is a form of sensory stimulation that is different from stress but that also produces analgesia. We are led to conclude that whichever definition is chosen, it becomes necessary to conceptualize pleasurable sensations as an entity that antagonizes pain.

Pleasurable sensation can not readily be dismissed simply as one of a class of distractants because we have found it to differentially antagonize nociceptive but not tactile thresholds. Moreover, the tactile test we selected was not insensitive to distraction, since the distractant, reading a passage from a history text, did produce a marked elevation in tactile thresholds, and yet this distractant produced no significant elevation in pain thresholds. Thus, we found a dissociation of the effect of pleasurable stimulation on elevating pain thresholds but not tactile thresholds, in addition to a dissociation of the effects of distraction on elevating tactile thresholds but not pain thresholds. This leads us to conclude that pleasurable stimulation activates an analgesic process that is distinct from a distraction process.

Of course, these findings were obtained in a highly structured experimental paradigm and may be restricted to the paradigm. However, these findings provide the hypothesis that pleasure is an entity that antagonizes pain, a hypothesis comparable to that forming the theme of this volume, i.e. that stress is an entity that antagonizes pain.

ACKNOWLEDGMENTS

We gratefully acknowledge Dr. Susan Esquilin for performing the psychological screening tests, Dr. Judith Steinman for her help in developing the human studies, Leslie Hullett for technical assistance, and C. Banas for the graphics.

REFERENCES

1. HAYES, R. L., G. J. BENNETT, P. G. NEWLON & D. J. MAYER. 1978. Brain Res. **155**:69–90.
2. WATKINS, L. R., D. A. COBELLI & D. J. MAYER. 1982. Brain Res. **245**:97–106.
3. BODNAR, R. J., D. KELLY, S. STEINER & M. GLUSMAN. 1978. Pharmac. Biochem. Behav. **8**:661–668.
4. BODNAR, R. J., D. KELLY, A. SPIAGGIA, C. EHRENBERG & M. GLUSMAN. 1978. Pharmac. Biochem. Behav. **8**:667–672.
5. SPIAGGIA, A., R. J. BODNAR, D. D. KELLY & M. GLUSMAN. 1979. Pharmac. Biochem. Behav. **10**:761–765.
6. AMIR, S. & Z. AMIT. 1978. Life Sci. **23**:1143–1152.
7. LEBARS, D., A. H. DICKENSON & J. M. BESSON. 1982. *In* Brain Stem Control of Spinal Mechanisms. B. Sjolund & A. B. Bjorklund, Eds.: 381–410. Elsevier Biomedical Press. Holland.
8. MICZEK, K., M. L. THOMPSON & L. SHUSTER. 1982. Science **215**:1520–1522.
9. MCCREERY, D. B. & J. R. BLOEDEL. 1976. Brain Res. **117**:136–140.
10. WATKINS, L. R. & D. J. MAYER. 1982. Science **216**:1185–1192.
11. TERMAN, G. W., Y. SHAVIT, J. W. LEWIS, J. T. CANNON & J. C. LIEBESKIND. 1984. Science **226**:1270–1277.
12. AKIL, H., S. J. WATSON, E. YOUNG, M. E. LEWIS, H. KHACHATURIAN & J. M. WALKER. 1984. Ann. Rev. Neurosci. **7**:223–255.
13. KOMISARUK, B. R. & K. LARSSON. 1971. Brain Res. **35**:231–235.
14. KOMISARUK, B. R. & J. WALLMAN. 1977. Brain Res. **137**:85–107.
15. KOMISARUK, B. R. & B. WHIPPLE. 1984. Abst. Soc. Neurosci. **10**:675.
16. WHIPPLE, B. & B. R. KOMISARUK. 1985. Pain **21**:357–367.
17. STEINMAN, J. I., B. R. KOMISARUK, T. L. YAKSH & G. M. TYCE. 1983. Pain **16**:155–166.
18. CROWLEY, W. R., R. JACOBS, J. VOLPE, J. F. RODRIGUEZ-SIERRA & B. R. KOMISARUK. 1976. Physiol. Behav. **16**:483–488.
19. KOMISARUK B. R., V. CIOFALO & M. B. LATRANYI. 1976. *In* Advances in Pain Research and Therapy 1. J. J. Bonica & D. Albe-Fessard, Eds.: 439–443. Raven Press. New York.
20. PETTY, L. C. 1975. Unpublished doctoral dissertation. Virginia Commonwealth University. Richmond, VA.
21. CHIODO, L. A., A. R. CAGGIULA, S. M. ANTELMAN & C. G. LINEBERRY. 1979. Brain Res. **176**:385–390.
22. HILL, R. D. & S. J. AYLIFFE. 1981. Pharmac. Biochem. Behav. **14**:631–632.
23. CARGILL, C. L., J. L. STEINMAN & W. D. WILLIS. 1982. Soc. Neurosci. Abst. **9**:471.
24. MITCHELL, D. & R. F. HELLON. 1977. Proc. R. Soc. Lond. B. **197**:169–194.
25. OLESON, T. D. & J. C. LIEBESKIND. 1976. *In* Advances in Pain Research and Therapy 1. J. J. Bonica & D. Albe-Fessard, Eds.: 487–494. Raven Press. New York.
26. FOREMAN, R. D., R. F. SCHMIDT & W. D. WILLIS. 1977. Brain Res. **124**:555–560.
27. HORNBY, J. B. & J. D. ROSE. 1976. Exp. Neurol. **51**:363–376.
28. MAEDA, H. & G. J. MOGENSON. Unpublished manuscript.
29. PACHECO, P., C. BEYER, G. MEXICANO & K. LARSSON. 1976. Physiol. Behav. **17**:699–703.
30. HENRY, J. L. 1983. Neurosci. Lett. **38**:257–262.
31. WATKINS, L. R., P. L. FARIS, D. J. MAYER & B. R. KOMISARUK. 1982. Soc. Neurosci. Abst. **8**:771.

32. WATKINS, L. R., P. L. FARIS, B. R. KOMISARUK & D. J. MAYER. 1984. Brain Res. **294**:59–65.
33. FREDERICKSON, R. C. A. & L. E. GEARY. 1982. Prog. Neurobiol. **19**:19–69.
34. STEINMAN, J. L., L. A. ROBERTS & B. R. KOMISARUK. 1982. Soc. Neurosci. Abst. **8**:265.
35. CROWLEY, W. R., J. F. RODRIGUEZ-SIERRA & B. R. KOMISARUK. 1977. Psychopharmacology **54**:223–225.
36. HELLER, S., B. R. KOMISARUK, A. GINTZLER & A. STRACHER. 1986. Ann. N.Y. Acad. Sci. (This volume.)
37. ROBERTS, L., C. BEYER & B. R. KOMISARUK. 1985 Life Sci. **36**:2017–1023.
38. CROWLEY, W. R., J. F. RODRIGUEZ-SIERRA & B. R. KOMISARUK. 1977. Brain Res. **164**:317–322.
39. ALLEN, T. O., N. T. ADLER, J. H. GREENBERG & M. REIVICH. 1981. Science **211**:1070–1072.
40. OLIVERAS, J. L., F. REDJEMI, G. GUILBAUD & J. M. BESSON. 1975. Pain **1**:139–145.
41. OLIVERAS, J. L., G. GUILBAUD & J. M. BESSON. 1979. Brain Res. **181**:1–15.
42. DAHLSTROM, A. & K. FUXE. 1965. Acta Physiol. Scand. **232** (Suppl. 1–55).
43. BASBAUM, A. & H. L. FIELDS. 1978. Ann. Neurol. **4**:451–515.
44. WATKINS, L. R., G. GRIFFIN, G. R. LEICHNETZ & D. J. MAYER. 1980. Brain Res. **181**:1–15.
45. BJORKLUND, A. & G. SKAGERBERG. 1982. *In* Brain Stem Control of Spinal Mechanisms. B. Sjolund & A. Bjorklund, Eds.: 55–88. Elsevier Biomedical Press. Holland.
46. BASBAUM, A. I., N. MARLEY & J. O'KEEFE. 1976. *In* Advances in Pain Research and Therapy. J. J. Bonica & D. Albe-Fessard, Eds.: 439–443. Raven Press. New York.
47. KOMISARUK, B. R., E. TERASAWA & J. F. RODRIGUEZ-SIERRA. 1985. *In* Neuroendocrinology of Reproduction. N. T. Adler, Ed.: 349–376. Plenum Publ. Co. New York.
48. KOMISARUK, B. R. 1982. *In* Brain Stem Control of Spinal Mechanisms. B. Sjolund & A. B. Bjorklund, Eds.: 493–508. Elsevier Biomedical Press. New York.
49. MOUNTCASTLE, V. B. 1974. *In* Medical Physiology. V. B. Mountcastle, Ed.: 355. C.V. Mosby. St. Louis, MO.
50. LOWENSTEIN, O. & I. E. LOWENFELD. 1961. Trans. N.Y. Acad. Sci. **23**:579–586.
51. MASTERS, W. & V. JOHNSON. 1966. Human Sexual Response. Little Brown. Boston, MA.
52. MILNOR, W. R. 1974. *In* Medical Physiology. V. B. Mountcastle, Ed.: 977. C. V. Mosby. St. Louis, MO.
53. JANAL, M., E. W. D. COLT, W. C. CLARK & M. GLUSMAN. 1984. Pain **19**:13–25.
54. SELYE, H. 1976. The Stress of Life (revised edition). p. 74. McGraw Hill. New York.

Conditioned Fear-Induced Opiate Analgesia: A Competing Motivational State Theory of Stress Analgesia[a]

MICHAEL S. FANSELOW

Department of Psychology
Dartmouth College
Hanover, New Hampshire 03755

Endogenous analgesic systems may play a critical role in modulating the behavioral responses that evolved as antipredator defense. Animals can innately recognize certain environmental danger signals and can learn to recognize others. To such danger stimuli they react with complex and coordinated innate defensive behavioral patterns.[1] Bolles and I have pointed out that nociceptive stimulation delivered by the predator to the prey may disrupt these defensive behavioral patterns.[2] For example, limping on an injured leg would compromise flight; the movements involved in licking a wound could attract a predator's attention. If endogenous analgesic mechanisms were activated by the same stimuli that activate defensive behaviors, analgesia could function to prevent these disruptive influences of nociception on coordinated defensive activities. We incorporated such a role for endogenous analgesia into a more general model of aversively motivated behavior that we call the perceptual-defensive-recuperative model.[2,3]

THE PERCEPTUAL-DEFENSIVE-RECUPERATIVE MODEL

Components of the perceptual-defensive-recuperative (PDR) model are diagramed in FIGURE 1. Central to this model of defensive behavior is what I have labeled the defensive motivational system, a neurophysiological network that selects appropriate defensive responses to a variety of environmental danger signals (for reviews see[2,4–6]). Several stimuli have the ability to activate this system without prior experience. For the rat, examples of these innate danger stimuli include certain predators (e.g. cats and weasels[5,7]), tactile stimulation given to the dorsal area,[8] and pheromonal cues released by stressed conspecifics.[9] Neutral stimuli that do not innately activate the defensive system may acquire the ability to do so through the process of Pavlovian conditioning. It has been demonstrated that tones, lights, and even observation chambers can come to activate the defensive system, if they have a history of being associated with a nociceptive stimulus like electric shock.[10,11] Activation of this defensive system results in specific behavioral consequences, the animal's behavioral repertoire becomes

[a]Preparation of this paper was supported by National Institute of Mental Health grant #MH39786-01. Naloxone was a gift from Endo Laboratories. Naltrexone was provided by the National Institute of Drug Abuse. Portions of this research were supported by funds provided by the Faculty Research Committee of Dartmouth College.

40

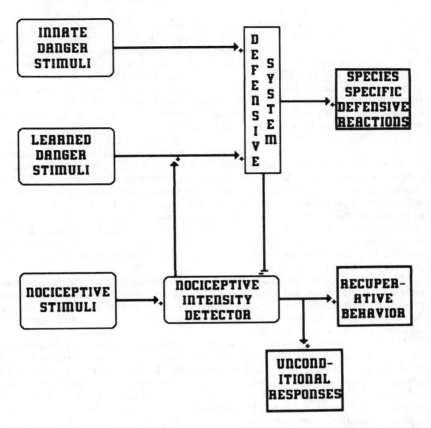

FIGURE 1. An illustration of the components of the perceptual-defensive-recuperative model. All links are excitatory (marked with a+) except for the link between the defensive system and the nociceptive intensity detector (marked with a−). This inhibitory link corresponds to an analgesic process.

dominated by species-specific defensive reactions (SSDRs). For the rat the dominant SSDR is the freezing response.[5] Freezing is an immobile crouching posture accompanied by shallow, rapid respiration. It is cryptic, in that it helps a prey avoid detection by the predator. Since prey movement is an important releasing stimulus for attack by many predators, freezing may also help prevent attack once the prey is detected.

Presentation of nociceptive stimuli often have very different consequences from presentation of innate and learned danger stimuli. Nociceptive stimuli may unconditionally elicit reflexive behaviors, many of which are withdrawal reflexes. However, if a nociceptive stimulus causes enduring tissue damage, more complex behaviors may be directed toward the locus of the injury. These behaviors can be termed recuperative behaviors because it is hypothesized that they can facilitate recovery and healing of the injury. Both these responses to nociceptive stimuli can be illustrated by a rat's reaction to a subcutaneous injection of a dilute formalin solution into a paw.[12] Upon contact with the subcutaneous tissue the formalin elicits a reflexive paw withdrawal. Twenty min later the animal's responses to the injury are quite different. The animal holds the injured paw close to the body. It will also spend considerable time licking the site of the injury. It seems probable that in the presence of a predator such reactions to a nociceptive stimulus could compromise the effectiveness of an animal's SSDRs.

The nociceptive system subserving recuperation, and the antipredator defensive system, can be viewed as independent systems that serve very different biological functions.[2,13,14] However, there are two important points of interaction between these systems. The first is that if a neutral stimulus comes to predict a nociceptive stimulus, the neutral stimulus will acquire the ability to activate the defensive system. That is, the neutral stimuli become Pavlovian conditional stimuli, the conditioned response being activation of the defensive system. Such stimuli are designated as learned danger stimuli in FIGURE 1. Notice that according to this model the conditioned responses (CRs) to stimuli that predict nociceptive events (SSDRs) differ from the unconditioned response (UR) to nociceptive events. This difference should not be considered idiosyncratic because modern Pavlovian theory recognizes many situations where the CR and the UR are different in form.[14-16]

The second point of interaction between the defensive and recuperative systems is the defensive system's ability to activate endogenous analgesic processes that reduce the impact that nociceptive stimuli have upon the defending organism. We have already discussed why this would confer an advantage to the defending animal.

While any one of the several endogenous analgesic mechanisms described in this volume could serve the antinociceptive function of the defensive system, available evidence suggests that the mechanism has three characteristics: (1) it appears to be readily antagonizable by opiate antagonists such as naloxone and naltrexone;[13,17,18] (2) it is not affected by hypophysectomy;[19,20] and (3) it is activated by comparatively mild stimulation—but it is the same stimulation that activates defensive behaviors.[21]

As can be seen in FIGURE 1, there is an inhibitory link between the defensive system and the nociceptive intensity detector. This link corresponds to the analgesic mechanism. The nociceptive intensity detector could be a cell assembly that responds selectively to nociceptive information, with a response that is directly proportional to the intensity of the nociceptive stimulus (for a review see[22]). Thus activation of the endogenous analgesic mechanism by the defensive system should reduce the perceived intensity of any nociceptive stimuli presented to the animal while the defensive system is activated. Since activity in the nociceptive intensity detector has three consequences (unconditional responses, conditioning of acquired danger stimuli, and recuperative behavior) endogenous analgesia should be able to suppress all three types of reactions. Therefore, the model predicts that danger stimuli that have the ability to activate the defensive system should result in a suppression of all three types of reactions. Since opioid antagonists should block this analgesia, a second prediction from the model is that opioid antagonists should be able to enhance all three types of reactions, provided that the test of nociceptive reactivity is conducted in the presence of danger stimuli.[23] The next section of this paper will describe research that supports these predictions as far as learned danger signals are concerned. The final section will present data indicating that similar effects are obtained with innate danger cues.

LEARNED DANGER STIMULI

Predictions from the PDR model have been primarily tested with learned danger stimuli as activators of the defensive system. Arbitrary stimuli associated with nociceptive electric shock rapidly acquire the ability to control defensive behavior. Such artificial stimuli offer a practical advantage over more ecologically valid stimuli because they are easier to control and therefore allow for a more rigorous analysis of the model's predictions. This section examines the effects of shock-associated stimuli and opioid antagonists on the three types of responses engendered by nociceptive stimuli that were outlined above.

As a measure of recuperative behavior I have used a modification of the formalin test developed in Melzack's laboratory.[12,24,25] A small amount of a dilute formalin solution is injected just beneath the dorsal surface of a rat's hind paw. Twenty to thirty min following injection the animal is observed for instances of recuperative behavior—stereotypical pawlicking and pawlifting responses. As is shown in FIGURE 2, reactivity to the injection increases with the concentration of formalin. The more intense the nociceptive stimulation, the greater is the reaction. Demonstration that the measure of reactivity to formalin varies with the physical intensity of the nociceptive stimulus is important, for it indicates that this measure should also reflect alterations in perceived intensity caused by activation of endogenous analgesic mechanisms. If stimuli that have acquired the ability to activate the defensive system also activate analgesia, then the analgesia should reduce the perceived intensity of the injury. This should be reflected in a reduction in formalin-induced recuperative behavior. To test this, Marlene Baackes and I first established one set of environmental stimuli as a conditioned danger cue by associating it with a mild (.5 mA, .5 sec) electric shock.[13] The cue was a distinctive observation chamber. A second distinctive chamber served as a control stimulus. Animals were exposed to each chamber for 8 min/day for 8

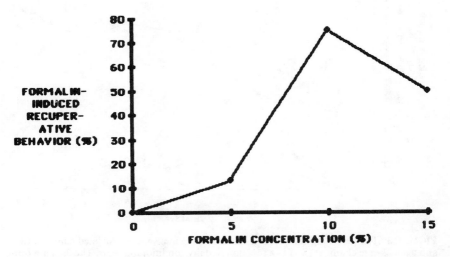

FIGURE 2. The percentage of formalin-injected rats showing recuperative behavior as a function of formalin concentration. (These data are based on Fanselow & Baackes.[13])

days. As can be seen in FIGURE 3, a conditional freezing response was acquired to the shock-associated chamber (designated S+) but not to the control chamber (designated S−). This indicates that the shock-associated chamber acquired the ability to activate the defensive system. On the ninth day of the experiment the animals were injected with formalin and later placed in either the shock-associated or control chamber. Some of these animals had been pretreated with the opioid antagonist naltrexone (7 mg/kg) and others were given a saline placebo. No shock was administered on this day. The levels of freezing on this test day were comparable to those on Day 8 of conditioning (FIGURE 3). As can be seen in FIGURE 4, there was considerable recuperative behavior in S−. However, recuperative behavior was abolished in S+. While naltrexone did not alter recuperative behavior in S−, it restored recuperative behavior in S+. These data are consistent with the model's prediction that stimuli that have acquired the ability to activate the defensive system (1) produce an analgesia that can suppress recuperative behavior elicited by injurious stimulation and (2) that that analgesia is susceptible to blockade by opiate antagonists.

We can now turn to a nociceptive stimulus' ability to act as a Pavlovian unconditional stimulus capable of bestowing a neutral stimulus with the ability to activate the defensive system. The previous experiment demonstrated that pairing a distinctive environment with a nociceptive shock conditions that environment so that it can produce a freezing response (FIGURE 3). There is considerable evidence that in such situations the freezing response is purely a conditional

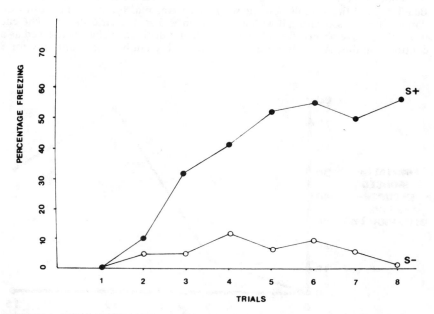

FIGURE 3. The percentage of time rats spent freezing in a shock-associated chamber (S+) and a shock-free chamber (S−) as a function of daily conditioning trials. The data are from a 5 min pre-shock period. (From Fanselow & Baackes.[13] With permission from Academic Press.)

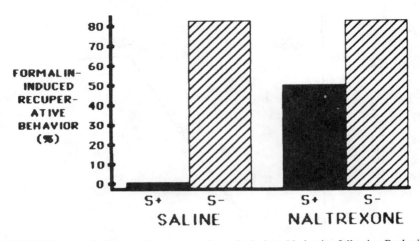

FIGURE 4. A shock-free test day to assess formalin-induced behavior following Pavlovian differential conditioning of S+ and S− (FIGURE 3). All animals were treated with formalin prior to testing. Naltrexone (7 mg/kg) or saline placebo treatments were also given prior to testing. (These data are based on Fanselow & Baackes.[13])

response to shock-associated stimuli.[11] FIGURE 5 shows that as the intensity of the shock is increased, a greater freezing response is conditioned. This indicates that the shock's ability to condition depends on its physical intensity and that the magnitude of the freezing response should reflect the perceived intensity of shock. According to the model, we would expect that the presence of a conditional stimulus that has already acquired the ability to activate the defensive system and its accompanying analgesia would reduce a subsequent shock's perceived intensity. A previously conditioned CS should therefore reduce a shock's ability to condition fear to a second stimulus. Students of Pavlovian conditioning should recognize this as the blocking effect.[26] The model also predicts that an opiate antagonist should eliminate this reduction in perceived intensity and restore the US's ability to condition.

We have obtained results consistent with this prediction.[3] One set of animals received 15 forward pairings of a 30 sec tone and shock, and a second set served as controls receiving backward pairings of the same stimuli. The next day these animals were given an intraperitoneal (i.p.) injection of either naloxone or a saline placebo. Then they were placed in a novel environment. Three min later all animals were presented with the tone followed by a shock. An 8 min post-shock observation period determined the amount of conditioning that accrued to this novel chamber.

FIGURE 6 shows the conditional freezing behavior that occurred during the tone. What the figure indicates is that the forward conditioning procedure enabled the tone to activate the defensive system but the backward conditioned stimulus did not. Naloxone did not affect this tone-evoked behavior. FIGURE 7 shows freezing in the presence of the apparatus cues that were conditioned by the signaled shock. Substantial conditioning occurred in backward controls; naloxone did not affect that behavior. In contrast, the forward conditioned stimulus

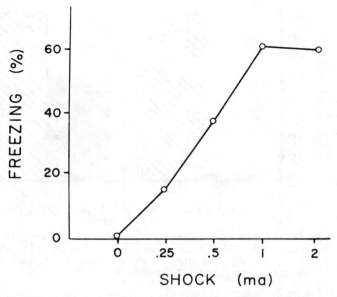

FIGURE 5. Percentage of time that rats spent freezing during an 8 min post-shock test period as a function of shock intensity. Each rat received two (.75 sec) shocks spaced twenty sec apart. (From Fanselow & Bolles.[18] With permission from the American Psychological Association.)

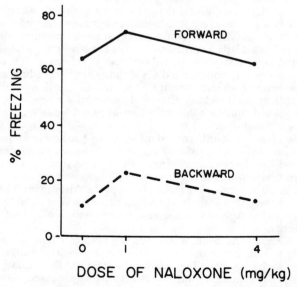

FIGURE 6. The percentage of time rats spent freezing during a 30 sec tone that had previously received forward or backward pairings with shock as a function of naloxone pretreatment. (From Fanselow & Bolles.[3] With permission from the Psychonomic Society.)

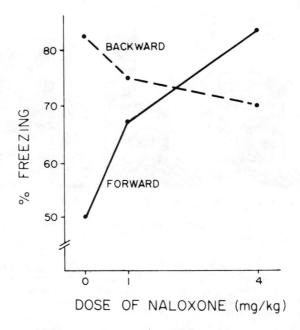

FIGURE 7. The percentage of an 8 min post-shock period that rats spent freezing as a function of naloxone pretreatment. Shock was signaled in a forward manner by a tone that had previously received either forward or backward Pavlovian conditioning. (From Fanselow & Bolles.[3] With permission from the Psychonomic Society.)

reduced conditioning to the chamber cues. Both doses of naloxone prevented this reduction in conditioning. These results can be explained by assuming that when the tone acquired the ability to activate the defensive system, as indicated by its ability to produce the freezing response, the tone also acquired the ability to activate a naloxone-reversible analgesia that reduced the perceived intensity of shock, and hence, the shock's ability to condition apparatus cues.

We can now turn to an unconditional reaction elicited by shock. When shock is administered to an animal, the shock elicits an immediate and unconditional burst of activity. Eventually, that activity burst gives way to the conditional freezing response, but a subsequent shock will again elicit an activity burst that disrupts freezing.[27] It is possible to measure the unconditional reaction to shock in the presence of activation of the defensive system by measuring the latency of the rat to resume freezing following shock. Again, if the activity burst is to be a measure of perceived shock intensity, we must first demonstrate that the duration of this response varies with the physical intensity of shock. FIGURE 8 shows this to be the case. The experiment depicted here consisted of a training day and a test day. On the training day all groups of animals were given the same treatment, 4 shocks (1 mA, .75 sec) in an observation chamber. The next day, the test day, the rats were placed in the same chamber and freezing was measured throughout an 11 min session. No stimuli were presented for the first 3 min to allow recording of the baseline level of freezing. Then each rat was subjected to a single, 0.75 sec

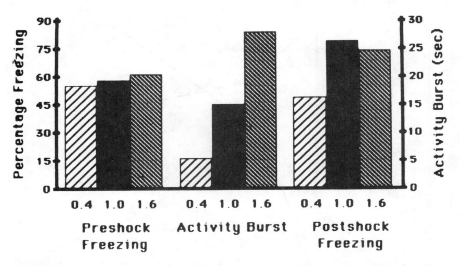

FIGURE 8. The percentage of time rats spent freezing during a 3 min pre-shock period (preshock freezing with axis to left), the latency for rats to resume freezing (activity burst with axis to the right) following a single .75 sec shock at the indicated intensity, and the percentage of the 8 min post-shock period spent freezing (postshock freezing with axis to the left). (After Fanselow.[27])

shock, at one of three intensities. Observations continued for the 8 min post-shock period. FIGURE 8 shows that for the three pre-shock min all animals froze at the same level reflecting the baseline training that occurred the day before. Latency to freeze following shock termination increased as a positive function of the testing shock intensity; that is, stronger shocks elicited a longer unconditional activity burst. You may also note that the stronger shocks resulted in more conditional freezing over the full course of the test session.

The freezing that occurred during the 3 min preshock period indicates that the baseline shocks conditioned the observation chamber so that it could activate the defensive motivational system. Therefore, we might expect that the perceived intensity of the shock that these animals experienced was reduced by the analgesia activated in conjunction with the defensive system. If naloxone pretreatment were substituted for the shock intensity manipulation it should enhance perceived shock intensity. In other words, the effects of naloxone administration should parallel those of increasing shock intensity. FIGURE 9 depicts the results of an experiment that showed just that. The design was the same as the above experiment except in two respects. All shocks were .8 mA and naloxone (4 mg/kg) or placebo pretreatments were administered just prior to the test session. Naloxone did not effect the pre-shock level of freezing. However, it increased the duration of the activity burst. The drug also increased the overall level of freezing during the 8 min post-shock test period. Note that very specific effects of naloxone rule out an account in terms of a drug influence on motor activity—naloxone's effects on freezing varied depending upon freezing's relationship to the test shock. Since the activity burst is an unconditional reaction, the

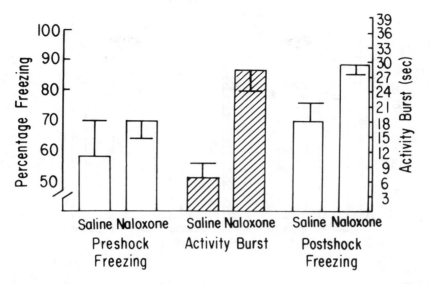

FIGURE 9. The percentage of time rats spent freezing during a 3 min pre-shock period (pre-shock freezing with axis to left), the latency for rats to resume freezing (activity burst with axis to the right) following a single shock, and the percentage of the 8 min postshock period spent freezing (post-shock freezing with axis to the left). Naloxone-pretreated groups received a 4 mg/kg dose. (From Fanselow.[20] With permission from the American Psychological Association.)

drug's influence on this measure can not be attributed to an influence on memory or associative processes. However, the drug's effects directly parallel the effects of increasing test shock intensity; the naloxone-treated rats behaved as if they had received a more intense shock than the control animals. Such results support the hypothesis that the baseline training shocks not only conditioned freezing to the environmental cues, but also conditioned activation of a naloxone-sensitive analgesic process that acted to reduce the perceived intensity of the test shock.

I will describe one more experiment utilizing the activity burst procedure that demonstrates that these effects of naloxone are specific to nociceptive stimuli. The procedure was the same as the last experiment except that a non-nociceptive startling stimulus was substituted for the test shock. Rats still received four .8 mA, 75 sec shocks during the baseline training period. However, instead of a test shock, the chamber's lights turned off, a loud tone was sounded, and a vibrator shook the floor. As can be seen in Figure 10, this non-nociceptive startling stimulus, which was .75 sec long, did cause an activity burst but naloxone did not increase this response. In fact, it caused a significant reduction in the duration of this response. Also note that when this stimulus was used in testing, naloxone had no effect upon post-stimulus freezing. This experiment suggests that naloxone's ability to enhance shock-related behaviors is specific to the nociceptive properties of shock. That is, naloxone, by antagonizing an endogenous analgesic response, acts to increase the perceived intensity of nociceptive, but not non-nociceptive stimuli.

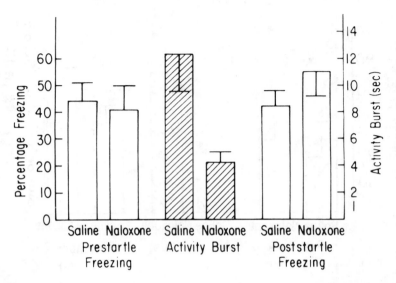

FIGURE 10. The percentage of time rats spent freezing during a 3 min pre-startle period (pre-startle freezing with axis to left), the latency for rats to resume freezing (activity burst with axis to the right) following a startle stimulus, and the percentage of the 8 min post-startle period spent freezing (post-startle freezing with axis to the left). Naloxone-pretreated groups received a 4 mg/kg dose. (From Fanselow.[20] With permission of the American Psychological Association.)

INNATE DANGER STIMULI

The research I have reviewed so far has concentrated on the ability of conditioned environmental cues to activate the defensive system. According to the PDR model innate danger stimuli should have effects similar to those of acquired danger stimuli. Therefore, my laboratory has recently begun investigating more natural-istic stimuli that innately, or unconditionally, activate the defensive system. The post-shock freezing paradigm offers a powerful way of determining if such stimuli cause a naloxone-reversible modulation in perceived intensity. TABLE 1 demonstrates that naloxone has no effect upon post-shock freezing if the freezing is precipitated by a single unsignaled shock. However, if the rat is examined following two shocks spaced 20 sec apart, naloxone does result in an increase in post-shock freezing. I have taken this as an indication that some priming stimulus must first activate the defensive system and its accompanying analgesia, before an effect of naloxone on perceived intensity can be observed. Any stimulus that is capable of activating the defensive system, if presented at the appropriate interval preceding shock, should be able to trigger a naloxone enhancement of the freezing that follows a single shock. However, naloxone never increases the freezing that follows a single brief shock unless that shock is primed by some stimulus that activates the defensive system. An example of such an outcome is provided by the Fanselow and Bolles experiment described earlier.[3] In that

TABLE 1. Comparison of Naloxone's Ability to Enhance Post-Shock Freezing

Number of Shocks	Shock Intensity (mA)	% Freezing in Saline Controls	% Change Caused by Naloxone	Difference Reliable at $p < .05$
1	0.5	10	−10	no
1	1.0	23	−8	no
1	1.3	22	5	no
1	1.6	11	−18	no
1	2.0	25	−12	no
2	0.4	9	267	yes
2	0.5	20	120	yes
2	1.0	54	30	yes
2	2.0	51	18	no

NOTE: Freezing is measured for 8 min following one versus two shocks. After Fanselow & Bolles.[18]

experiment (FIGURE 7), naloxone did not increase freezing following a single shock if that shock was preceded by a backwards conditioned control stimulus. However, if that shock was preceded by a Pavlovian forward conditioned stimulus, i.e. a stimulus that acquired the ability to trigger the defensive system, naloxone enhanced the freezing that followed a single shock. A stimulus that has the innate ability to activate the defensive system should function just like an acquired danger signal, producing a similar effect. In other words, freezing following a single shock should be enhanced by opioid antagonists when the shock is signaled by an innate danger cue whereas freezing following a single unsignaled shock should not.

In a series of as yet unpublished studies, R. A. Sigmundi and I used this single shock procedure and demonstrated that this is the case for at least two stimuli known to be unconditional activators of the defensive system: odors of a stressed conspecific and dorsal stimulation. Two experiments with 2 × 2 factorial designs were conducted. One factor in both experiments was i.p. administration of naltrexone (7 mg/kg) or a saline placebo; the other factor was the presence or absence of the innate danger signal. In the stress odor study, stress odors were produced by subjecting a conspecific donor to a series of brief electric shocks and then testing the experimental animal moments later in the uncleaned chamber. Aside from residual stress odors, the experimental animals had not been stressed. Control animals were tested in a cleaned chamber (such cleaning is standard procedure in my laboratory). In the dorsal stimulation study, the innate danger stimulus was the dorsal constraint administered by the experimenter's hand that is necessary to administer the i.p. injection. Since it was necessary to administer this stimulus to all animals, the control animals were simply adapted to handling for 10 days to familiarize them with this stimulus (this handling procedure is routinely used in all experiments in my laboratory). The experimental animals were given no such handling. It should be noted that in a separate series of studies, Dr. Sigmundi demonstrated that dorsal constraint functions as an unconditional stimulus capable of eliciting defensive struggling and of conditioning the freezing response to apparatus cues. He found that lifting a rat with a ventral approach, or by the tail, did not produce similar effects. We have also

noted that familiarizing the animal to handling eliminates the animal's unconditional reactions to dorsal constraint.

Immediately after the i.p. injection, the animals were placed in an observation
chamber (a clean chamber for all animals except those in the two stress-odor
tested groups). Six min after placement a single 1 mA, .75 sec shock was delivered.
The standard 8 min observation period followed. The data of the two experiments
are presented in FIGURE 11. Notice that naltrexone had no effect on post-shock
freezing in the control groups of either experiment. However, animals exposed to
either innate danger signal prior to shock evidenced a naltrexone enhancement
effect. Thus, just like an acquired danger signal, these innate danger signals
appear to produce activation of an opioid analgesic response.

In a third experiment, Sigmundi and I found that in response to dorsal
constraint, previously unhandled animals showed an elevated jump latency on
the hot plate test of pain sensitivity. This provides a converging line of evidence
that for animals not familiarized to handling, dorsal constraint activates an
analgesic response. Similarly, I have found that the odors of a stressed conspecific
increase the latency for a rat to show formalin-induced recuperative behavior.[28]
This increase in latency was reversed by naltrexone. I also found that a variety of
control odors produced no change in latency to recuperate. Thus, unstressed rats
react to the odor of stressed conspecifics with a naltrexone-reversible analgesia
that is capable of inhibiting recuperative behavior.

Rodents have a remarkable innate ability to recognize animals that prey upon
them.[29] This recognition is evidenced by the fact that animals with no prior
history of being preyed upon react to predators with defensive behaviors even
before any physical contact is made. For example, rats will show considerable
freezing in response to a cat.[7] Recently, Laurie Lester and I found that the mere
presence of a cat will cause an increase in the rat's latency to react with
recuperative behaviors to a formalin injection.[30] Naltrexone caused a complete
reversal of this analgesia. Thus we have evidence that rats react to three innate
danger stimuli (dorsal constraint, odors of stressed conspecifics, and cats) not
only with SSDRs but also with an opioid form of analgesia.

CONCLUSIONS

Taken as a whole, these data strongly support the hypothesis, derived from the
perceptual-defensive-recuperative model, that endogenous analgesia plays a role
in supporting a rat's antipredatory defensive behavior. The model points to the
biological utility that pain-inhibitory systems may serve in normal, (i.e. non-
pathological) functioning. Understanding the biological utility of pain-modu-
latory systems may improve our understanding of pathology in these systems.
Knowledge of the normal function of analgesia may further our ability to
influence these systems toward clinical ends.

The papers in this volume illustrate the difficulty in specifying the necessary
and sufficient antecedent conditions for activating endogenous analgesic processes. Nociceptive stimuli alone appear to be neither necessary nor sufficient.[19,31]
The same is true of stressful stimuli (defined by activation of the adrenocortical
system).[32] An important predictor of the ability of a stimulus to activate certain
forms of endogenous analgesia may be the role of that stimulus in controlling
species-specific defensive behavior.

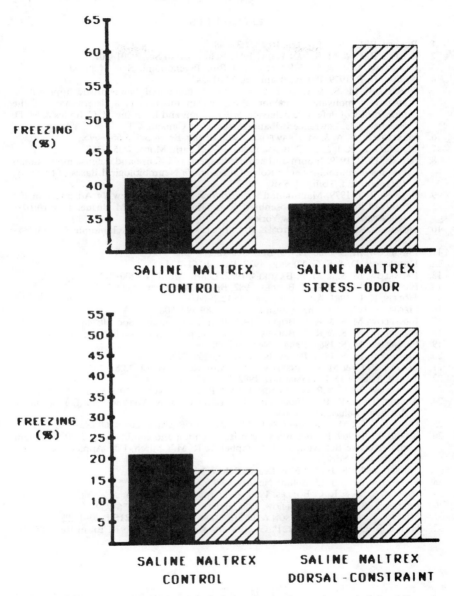

FIGURE 11. The percentage of freezing during an 8 min observation period that followed a single 1 mA, .75 sec shock as a function of naltrexone (7 mg/kg) or placebo pretreatment. The stress-odor test groups were tested in the presence of the odors of a stressed conspecific but were otherwise unstressed. All other animals were tested in deodorized chambers. The animals in the dorsal constraint group had not been previously adapted to the dorsal grab of an experimenter but all other groups had been adapted.

REFERENCES

1. BOLLES, R. C. 1970. Psychol. Rev. 71:32–48.
2. BOLLES, R. C. & M. S. FANSELOW. 1980. Behav. Brain Sci. 3:291–301.
3. FANSELOW, M. S. & R. C. BOLLES. 1979. Bull. Psychonomic Soc. 14:88–90.
4. ADAMS, D. B. 1979. Behav. Brain Sci. 2:201–241.
5. FANSELOW, M. S. & L. S. LESTER. 1986. A functional behavioristic approach to aversively motivated behavior: Predatory imminence as a determinant of the topography of defensive behavior. In Evolution and Learning. R. C. Bolles & M. D. Beecher, Eds. Lawrence Erlbaum Assoc. New Canaan, CT.
6. MASTERSON, F. A. & M. CRAWFORD. 1982. Behav. Brain Sci. 5:661–696.
7. BLANCHARD, R. J. & D. C. BLANCHARD. 1971. Learn. Motiv. 2:351–362.
8. ADAMS, D. B. 1979. Inborn and acquired aspects of offense and defense motivational systems in muroid rodents: Role of memory. In Neurobiological Bases of Memory. T. Oniani, Ed. Tbilisi, USSR.
9. BROWN, R. J. 1979. Mammalian social odors: A critical review. In Advances in the Study of Behavior. J. S. Rosenblatt, R. A. Hinde, L. Beer & M. Busnel, Eds. 10:103–160. Academic Press. New York.
10. SIGMUNDI, R. A., M. E. BOUTON & R. C. BOLLES. 1980. Bull. Psychonomic Soc. 15:254–256.
11. FANSELOW, M. S. 1980. Pav. J. Biol. Sci. 15:177–182.
12. DUBUISSON, D. & S. G. DENNIS. 1977. Pain 4:161–174.
13. FANSELOW, M. S. & M. P. BAACKES. 1982. Learn. Motiv. 13:200–221.
14. FANSELOW, M. S. & R. C. BOLLES. 1982. Behav. Brain Sci. 5:320–323.
15. HOLLIS, K. L. 1981. Adv. Study Behav. 12:1–64.
16. SIEGEL, S. 1975. J. Comp. Physiol. Psychol. 89:498–506.
17. FANSELOW, M. S. & R. C. BOLLES. 1977. Bull. Psychonomic Soc. 10:246.
18. FANSELOW, M. S. & R. C. BOLLES. 1979. J. Comp. Physiol. Psychol. 93:736–744.
19. FANSELOW, M. S. 1984. Behav. Neurosci. 98:79–95.
20. FANSELOW, M. S. 1984. Behav. Neurosci. 98:269–277.
21. BOLLES, R. C. & M. S. FANSELOW. 1982. Ann. Rev. Psychol. 33:87–101.
22. YAKSH, T. L. & D. L. HAMMOND. 1982. Pain 13:1–85.
23. FANSELOW, M. S. & R. A. SIGMUNDI. 1982. Physiol. Psychol. 10:313–316.
24. ABBOTT, F. V., K. B. J. FRANKLIN, R. J. LUDWICK & R. MELZACK. 1981. Pharmacol. Biochem. Behav. 15:637–640.
25. DENNIS, S. G., M. CHOINIERE & R. MELZACK. 1980. Exp. Neurol. 68:295–309.
26. KAMIN, L. J. 1969. Predictability, surprise, attention and conditioning. In Punishment and Aversive Behavior. B. A. Campbell & R. M. Church, Eds. Appleton-Century-Crofts. New York.
27. FANSELOW, M. S. 1982. Anim. Learn. Behav. 10:448–454.
28. FANSELOW, M. S. 1985. Behav. Neurosci. 99:589–592.
29. HIRSCH, S. M. & R. C. BOLLES. 1980. Z. Tierpsychol. 54:71–84.
30. LESTER, L. S. & M. S. FANSELOW. 1985. Behav. Neurosci. 99:756–759.
31. MICZEK, K. A., J. L. THOMPSON & L. SHUSTER. 1982. Science 215:1520–1522.
32. HAYES, R. L., G. R. BENNET, P. G. NEWLON & D. J. MAYER. 1978. Brain Res. 155:69–90.

Stressor Controllability and Stress-Induced Analgesia

STEVEN F. MAIER

Department of Psychology
University of Colorado
Boulder, Colorado 80309

The existence of multiple forms of stress-induced analgesia (SIA) focuses attention on factors that determine which form occurs. Experimental work has tended to focus on the physical characteristics of the putative stressor. Thus some investigators have compared the type of analgesia that follow exposure to different types of stressors (such as electric shock, cold water swim, rotation, etc.),[1] while others have studied the differential effects of the same type of stressor (e.g., electric shock) administered with different parameters,[2] or to different parts of the body.[3] Instead, we have explored the importance of a psychological dimension of the stress situation, the degree to which the organism can exert behavioral control over the stressor (alter by its behavior the onset, termination, intensity, or temporal pattern of the stressor), as a factor in determining the type of analgesia produced by the stressor.

In a typical study in our laboratory one group of rats is given a series of electric shocks each of which can be terminated by a behavioral response (turning a small wheel in the front of the chamber), while each member of a second group is yoked to a member of the first and is given the identical shocks as determined by the behavior of its partner. Thus both groups receive physically identical shocks, but one group has control over the termination of each shock (escapable shock) while the other does not (inescapable shock). A third group does not receive shock. Thus, the effects of exposure to shock per se and the impact of control versus lack of control can be isolated.

This experimental design has revealed that controllability exerts important modulatory effects on both behavioral and physiological changes produced by exposure to a stressor. Rats exposed to a series of 80 moderate intensity uncontrollable shocks later (1) fail to learn to escape or avoid shock or other stressors in different situations in which escape and avoidance is possible;[4] (2) are inactive in the presence of aversive events;[5] (3) show reduced aggression and social dominance;[6,7] and (4) show impairments in their ability to attend to relationships between their own behavior and shock termination.[8] None of these behavioral changes follow exposure to physically identical but escapable shock and so depend on the uncontrollability of the stressor rather than on mere exposure to the stressor. Behavioral outcomes such as these, which depend on the controllability/uncontrollability of the stressor, have been called "learned helplessness" effects.[9] Similarly, a variety of neurochemical changes produced by stressors depend on the controllability of the stressor.[10,11]

REINSTATED ANALGESIA AND STRESSOR CONTROLLABILITY

Our initial SIA experiments were initiated in the context of exploring mechanisms that might account for why inescapably but not escapably shocked subjects are later inactive in the presence of shock. An obvious possibility was that inescapable shock might elicit an analgesic reaction, possibly by altering an opiate system, thereby resulting in decreased movement. Indeed, the stressors used in all existing SIA studies had been nominally uncontrollable, thereby allowing this hypothesis. This sort of notion also had intuitive appeal. When an aversive situation is behaviorally uncontrollable it might be adaptive to withdraw from the situation and conserve energy resources until a time when behavioral coping becomes possible. It has been argued that the activation of opiate systems tends to function to conserve energy in a variety of emergency situations,[12] and decreased pain sensitivity/reactivity would make it easier to withdraw and conserve energy in a painful situation. If behavioral coping is possible it might be beneficial to act behaviorally rather than withdrawing and conserving energy. Thus we reasoned that learning that an aversive event is uncontrollable might be a critical determinant of analgesic processes.

An immediate difficulty was that SIA seemed to persist for at most an hour following stressor treatment, yet the reduced activity could be measured 24 hr following inescapable shock. However, activity measurement involved exposing the subjects to footshock. It seemed possible that even though SIA dissipates, the system(s) responsible might remain in a sensitized state for at least 24 hr so that the analgesia could be readily rearoused, thereby resulting in reduced activity.

We sought to determine whether a small amount of footshock administered 24 hr after inescapable shocks identical to those used in the behavioral controllability experiments referred to above might produce an analgesic reaction. Rats were given either 80 escapable 1.0 mA shocks, an identical series of yoked inescapable shocks, or were merely restrained in the apparatus. As in the controllability experiments the shocks were administered directly to the tail of the rat through attached electrodes. After 24 hr half of the animals in each group were placed in a shuttlebox and administered five 5 sec 0.6 mA gridshocks, while the other half were not shocked. In separate experiments either tail-flick or hot plate testing followed 3 min later in a different room. The results were that neither escapable nor inescapable shock were sufficient to produce changes in pain sensitivity/reactivity 24 hr later. Moreover, the five gridshocks did not by themselves lead to an analgesic reaction. However, animals previously exposed to inescapable shock and given the five reexposure shocks became analgesic, while animals initially given identical escapable shocks did not.[13]

The fact that this long-term reinstated analgesia depended on the escapability of the initial shocks did not insure that it was analogous to other learned helplessness effects. Learned helplessness effects are characterized by their extreme sensitivity to the control dimension. Thus exposure to escapable shock before inescapable shock is known to block the usual consequences of the inescapable shock. For example, escapable shock given before inescapable shock prevents the escape learning deficits that normally follow.[14] Similarly, exposure to shocks that can be controlled after inescapable shock counteracts the learning deficits that would be observed.[14] It has been argued[9] that a critical first step in the production of learned helplessness effects is the organism's learning that it has no control over the inescapable shock, and either prior or subsequent experience with escapable shock would be expected to counter such learning.

We thus sought to determine whether the analgesia that occurs upon reexposure to shock 24 hr after inescapable shock is similarly sensitive to experiences with control over shock both before and after the inescapable shock. The first experiment[15] involved three days of treatment. Three groups received 80 5 sec inescapable tail-shocks on Day 2 (designated by P in FIGURE 1), while the other two groups were merely restrained (R in FIGURE 1). All groups were given five brief footshocks on Day 3 followed by tail-flick testing. The critical differences between groups occurred on Day 1, the day before the usual inescapable shock procedure. One of the groups given inescapable shock on Day 2 received escapable shock in a totally different apparatus (E in FIGURE 1), another received yoked inescapable shock in that apparatus (designated by Y), while the third was merely restrained in the apparatus (R). One of the groups given restraint on Day 2 received the escapable shock on Day 1, while the other was restrained.

The results are shown in FIGURE 1. The first letter of each group designation indicates the Day 1 treatment, the second letter the Day 2 treatment. As can be seen, the data replicate the usual reinstated analgesia following inescapable shock (Group RP). The critical group is EP, which received escapable shock 24 hr before the inescapable shock. Escapable shock completely blocked the analgesic effect of the inescapable shock treatment! Moreover, this "immunization" effect depended on the controllability of the Day 1 shocks—yoked inescapable shock did not mitigate the analgesia produced by the Day 2 inescapable shocks.

We next employed a similar design to determine whether an experience with controlling shock after the inescapable shock would counteract the analgesia that would normally occur. Here[15] rats were given either escapable or yoked inescapable shock 4 hr after inescapable shock or restraint. Again, different

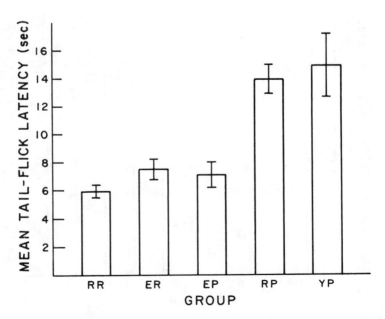

FIGURE 1. Mean tail-flick latencies for subjects given escape training (EP), yoked inescapable shock (YP), or restraint (RP) prior to a session of inescapable tail shock. The other groups received either escape training followed by restraint (ER) or were only restrained on both occasions (RR).

environments were used for the two treatments. The usual five footshocks and tail-flick testing occurred 24 hr after the initial shock treatment. The results can be seen in FIGURE 2. Inescapable shock produced a long-term reinstated analgesia (Group PR). The important group is PE, which received escapable shock between inescapable shock exposure and testing. Again, experience with escapable shock completely prevented the analgesia that is produced by inescapable shock. As before only escapable and not inescapable shock had this "therapy" effect.

These experiments suggest an extreme sensitivity of this reinstated SIA to the controllability dimension and support the notion that the analgesia does not result from exposure to shock per se but rather from what the organism learns about the shock. They also establish a parallel between the analgesia and learned helplessness effects. This potential parallel was further substantiated in a series of experiments comparing the analgesia to other aspects of learned helplessness. For example, learned helplessness effects such as shuttlebox escape learning and activity deficits following inescapable shock have a time course, with the effect dissipating by 48 hr following inescapable shocks with parameters as those used here. The analgesia reinstated by five footshocks had a similar time course—it too no longer occurs 48 hr after inescapable shock.[16]

The findings thus far presented raise a number of obvious questions. What is the relationship between the analgesic and other behavioral consequences of inescapable shock—does one cause the others? What is the relationship between

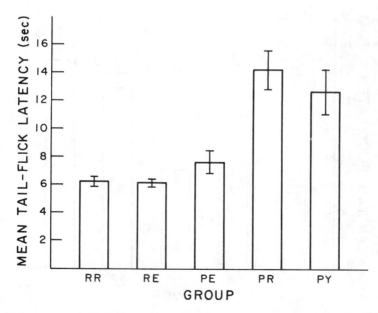

FIGURE 2. Mean tail-flick latencies for subjects given escape training (PE), yoked inescapable shock (PY), or restraint (PR) 4 hr after a session of inescapable tail shock. The other groups received either no inescapable tail shock followed by escape training 4 hr later (RE), or were not shocked at all (RR).

the long-term reinstated analgesia that depends on stressor controllability and the short-term analgesia that immediately follows exposure to the stressor that others study? What physiological mechanism(s) mediates the long-term reinstated analgesia? Only the last two of these questions can be discussed in the present chapter.

PHYSIOLOGICAL MECHANISMS

SIA exists in both opioid and nonopioid forms.[17] In practice, this means that SIA is sometimes reversed by opiate antagonists and cross tolerant with morphine and sometimes is not. FIGURE 3 shows the results of administering naltrexone before the inescapable shock session. Naltrexone completely and dose dependently blocked the long-term reinstated analgesia that occurs 24 hr later. Naltrexone administered before the reexposure shocks 24 hr later rather than before the inescapable shock treatment had the same effect.[18] Similarly, there was complete cross tolerance between morphine and the reinstated analgesia.[19] Rats were given 13 days of either morphine (12.5 mg/kg s.c.) or saline followed by inescapable shock or restraint on Day 14. All rats received five reexposure shocks 24 hr later followed by tail-flick testing. The results can be seen in FIGURE 4 and show that inescapable shock no longer produced analgesia in morphine-tolerant animals (a separate experiment established that the present regimen did produce morphine tolerance).

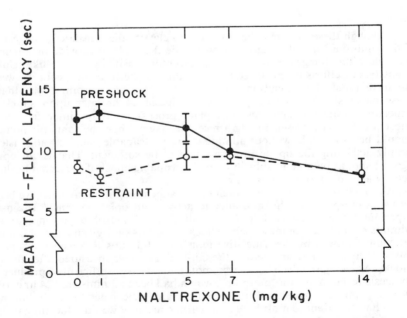

FIGURE 3. Mean tail-flick latencies for subjects given either saline or naltrexone before inescapable shock or restraint.

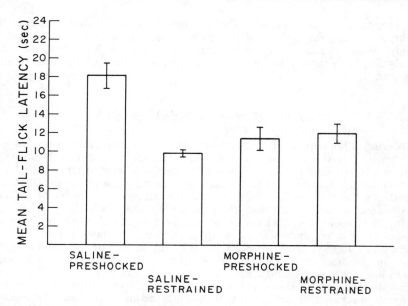

FIGURE 4. Mean tail-flick latencies for subjects given 13 days of saline or morphine, and then inescapable shock or restraint on Day 14.

Although these data may be sufficient to classify the reinstated analgesia as fitting into the "opioid category," it would be desirable to provide biochemical data showing changes in opiate levels, receptor sensitivity, or the like. Unfortunately, our efforts in this direction have thus far been unsuccessful. However, we have pursued a somewhat different strategy. Our reasoning was that if inescapable shock exposure produces analgesia 24 hr later upon shock re-exposure because it activates an opiate process, thereby either facilitating subsequent release or sensitizing a receptor system, then the same phenomena should be producible without administering inescapable shock at all. Instead, simply activating the opiate process ought to be sufficient. That is, an opiate agonist should be able to substitute for inescapable shock if inescapable shock acts by activating an opiate system.

Although we did not know which opiate system might be involved, we began by using morphine as the substance to activate an opiate system.[20] The usual experiment was conducted, but a small dose of morphine (4 mg/kg) was administered instead of inescapable shock. Thus rats were given either morphine or saline followed by the usual five footshocks (Groups R) or no (Groups N) shock 24 hr later. FIGURE 5 shows the tail-flick latencies measured after the five shocks. As usual, the five shocks were not in themselves sufficient to produce an analgesic reaction nor was morphine, which had been administered 24 hr earlier. However, the five footshocks produced an analgesic reaction in the animals which had experienced morphine 24 hr earlier, just as it would if the animals had received inescapable shock.

If morphine sensitized the analgesic reaction to footshock 24 later by the same

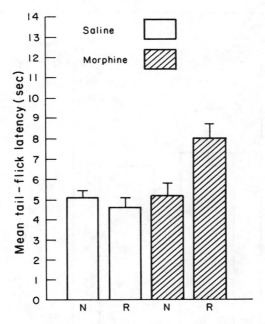

FIGURE 5. Mean tail-flick latency for subjects given saline or morphine followed by five footshocks (Groups R) or no shock (Groups N) 24 hr later.

mechanism as does inescapable shock, then it too should be sensitive to stressor controllability. Recall that a prior experience with controllable shock blocks the reinstated analgesia that follows inescapable shock. Thus we[21] sought to determine whether a prior exposure to escapable shock would block the effect of morphine! Animals were first given restraint, escapable shock, or yoked inescapable shock. After 4 hr, they received either morphine (4 mg/kg) or saline, followed by the five footshocks and tail-flick testing 24 hr later. As before, morphine led to an analgesic reaction upon exposure to five footshocks 24 hr later and exposure to inescapable shock 4 hr earlier did not disturb that effect. However, exposure to escapable shock completely blocked the effect of morphine!

The present logic suggests that we ought to be able to reverse these experiments and find that exposure to inescapable but not escapable shock would actually increase the organism's reactivity to morphine itself. This would follow if the two acted via the same mechanism. Thus we[22] gave rats either restraint, escapable shock, or yoked inescapable shock, followed by morphine (2 mg/kg) 24 hr later and simply measured the analgesia produced by the morphine. It should be noted that 2 mg/kg morphine produces only a marginal analgesic reaction with our testing conditions. The results can be seen in FIGURE 6. Prior exposure to inescapable but not physically identical escapable shocks exaggerated the organism's analgesic reactivity to morphine! Moreover, inescapable but not escapable shock enhances naloxone-precipitated withdrawal reactions from

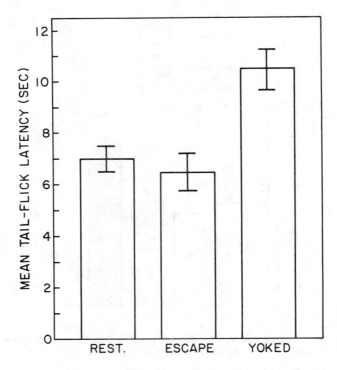

FIGURE 6. Mean tail-flick latency for subjects given morphine 24 hr after escapable shock, yoked inescapable shock, or restraint.

morphine as well as simple morphine reactivity. Williams and Maier[23] gave rats shocks of differing controllability followed by morphine 24 hr later. Naloxone was then administered and withdrawal reactions observed. The results can be seen in FIGURE 7. Clearly, prior inescapable but not escapable shock exaggerated the subject's withdrawal behavior. Finally, the morphine-sensitizing effect of inescapable shock can itself be blocked by prior exposure to escapable shock.[21] It would thus appear that morphine and inescapable shock can be substituted for each other in the production of these analgesic phenomena. Thus either inescapable shock or morphine leads to long-term reinstated analgesia, and prior exposure to escapable shock blocks either effect. Analogously, inescapable but not escapable shock sensitizes the analgesic reaction to later shock or morphine, and this too can be blocked by experiences with control. These data support the notion that inescapable but not escapable shock activates an opiate system involved in the production of SIA.

Opioid analgesia has a number of characteristics other than reversibility by opiate antagonists and cross tolerance with morphine. In particular, both morphine analgesia and opioid SIA act in part by inhibiting spinal cord transmission via descending messages conveyed through the dorsolateral funiculus.[24] Thus dorsolateral funiculus lesions can reduce both morphine analgesia

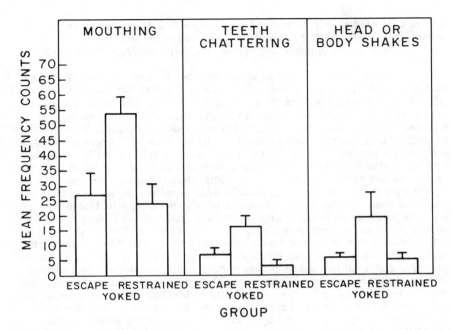

FIGURE 7. Mean frequency counts of three withdrawal measures for subjects given a naloxone challenge 30 min following morphine. The subjects had received escapable shock, yoked inescapable shock, or restraint, 24 hr earlier.

and SIA. In addition, the analgesic action of both morphine and opioid SIA is mediated, at least in part, by a spinal opiate synapse since the intrathecal administration of naloxone can block both kinds of analgesia.[25,26]

In collaboration with Linda R. Watkins and David J. Mayer we sought to determine whether the reinstated analgesia studied here also had these two characteristics. Both dorsolateral funiculus lesions[27] and intrathecal naloxone (2 μg) administered to lumbosacral cord completely blocked the reinstated analgesia produced by our usual inescapable shock procedure. Thus the long-term reinstated SIA produced by our 80 inescapable tail-shock procedure shares these characteristics of morphine analgesia. Again, these data support the notion that extended inescapable shocks activate an opiate system responsible for analgesia.

SHORT-TERM ANALGESIA AND STRESSOR CONTROLLABILITY

The data reported above raise an obvious difficulty. The SIA produced by our shock procedure appears opioid in nature, yet a large number of investigators have found the short-term SIA that immediately follows stressor administration to be insensitive to opiate antagonists and not cross tolerant with morphine. This state of affairs led us to inquire into the conditions that determine whether opioid or non-opioid SIA occurs. If learning that one has no control over the stressor is really a critical factor in producing opioid SIA, then learning variables ought to be crucial.

An obvious learning variable is the number of exposures to the shock, assuming that the shock is inescapable. Learning that the shock cannot be controlled is a complex form of learning and should take many trials. This argument suggests that the organism might sequentially exhibit non-opiate followed by opiate analgesia as it experiences a series of inescapable shocks and gradually learns that the shocks are inescapable. Thus we[20] exposed rats to a series of 80 inescapable tail-shocks in a restraining tube. Tail-flick tests were conducted after 0, 20, 40, 60, or 80 shocks without removing the subject from the apparatus, and naltrexone or saline was administered before the session. Control groups were merely restrained, given naltrexone or saline, and tested at the same points in time. The results of this experiment can be seen in FIGURE 8. First examine the group given saline followed by inescapable shock (Group SI). The 80 shocks produced a double peaked pattern of analgesia. Twenty shocks were sufficient to elicit an analgesic reaction, the analgesia dissipated by 40 shocks but again appeared after 60 and 80 shocks. Twenty shocks are not sufficient to produce behavioral learned helplessness effects such as poor escape learning.[28] We would thus expect the analgesia after 20 shocks to be naltrexone insensitive, whereas the analgesia after 80 shocks should be blocked. An examination of the naltrexone group (Group NI) reveals precisely this pattern—naltrexone had no effect on the analgesia produced by 20 shocks but completely eliminated the SIA after 80 shocks. This result holds regardless of the time of naltrexone administra-

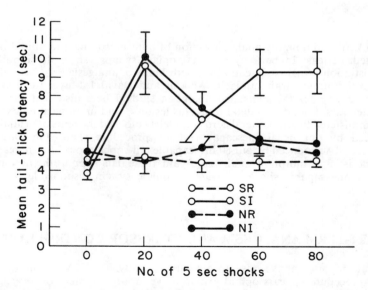

FIGURE 8. Mean tail-flick latency for subjects given either saline (S) or naltrexone (N) followed by 80 inescapable shocks (I) or an equivalent period of restraint (R).

tion or dose.[22] No dose in the range of 1.0 to 28.0 mg/kg naltrexone affected the first analgesic peak.

If this pattern occurs because the organism learns across trials that the shock is inescapable, then 80 escapable shocks should not produce the same pattern. In particular, the second opioid peak should not occur. We thus administered 80 escapable or yoked inescapable shocks and tested analgesia after 0, 20, 40, or 80 shocks. The shock session was preceded by either naltrexone or saline. FIGURE 9 shows the results. Escapable shock produced a double peaked pattern of analgesia just as did inescapable shock. Moreover, the first peak was insensitive to naltrexone for both types of shock. However, the second peak was insensitive to naltrexone when shock was escapable but was blocked when shock was inescapable. Finally, the SIA produced by 80 escapable and inescapable shocks proved to have quite different characteristics. For example, the analgesia after 80 escapable shocks dissipated quite rapidly, but was still present 2 hr after 80 inescapable shocks.[29]

If the second naltrexone-sensitive analgesic peak occurs because the organism learns that the shock is uncontrollable, then prior experience with escapable shock should block the peak just as it blocks reinstated SIA, and prior experience

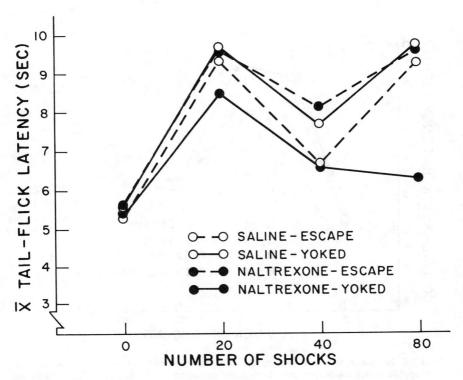

FIGURE 9. Mean tail-flick latency after either 0, 20, 40, or 80 escapable or yoked inescapable shocks for subjects injected with either saline or naltrexone.

with uncontrollable shock should lead to its earlier occurrence. We[29] thus exposed rats to escapable or yoked inescapable shock followed 24 hr later by 80 inescapable shocks. The inescapable shock session was preceded by either naltrexone or saline administration. Tail-flick testing occurred after 0, 5, 20, 40, or 80 shocks. The results of this experiment are shown in FIGURE 10. First examine the subjects given inescapable shock (in a different apparatus) before the 80 inescapable shock session. SIA no longer dissipated between 20 and 40 shocks and was now naltrexone reversible after 40 rather than 60–80 shocks. Now examine the data from the animals given escapable shock before the inescapable shock session. Escapable shock had no effect on the first analgesic peak but completely prevented the occurrence of the second analgesic peak. Indeed, escapable shock was as effective as naltrexone and duplicated its effects—it blocked the second but not the first analgesic peak.

The data presented in this section indicate that 60–80 inescapable shocks of the type used here are required to produce opioid SIA. Our interpretation is that it takes this many exposures for the organism to learn that the inescapable shocks are uncontrollable. The explanation given to the long-term reinstated analgesia and the morphine hyperreactivity produced by inescapable but not escapable shock was that the inescapable shock led the organism to learn that it had no control over shock and that it was this learning that activated an opiate system. If

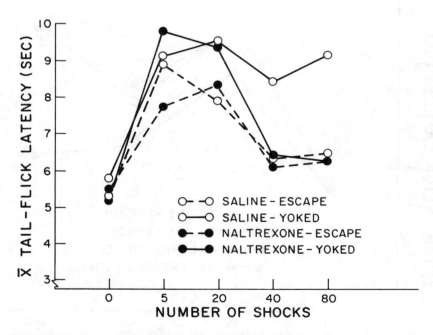

FIGURE 10. Mean tail-flick latency for subjects previously exposed to escapable or inescapable shock 24 before test. Tests were conducted following 0, 5, 20, 40, and 80 inescapable shocks with subjects receiving either naltrexone or saline 30 min prior to test.

the learning of uncontrollability requires 60–80 inescapable shocks, then the production of reinstated analgesia and morphine hyper-reactivity should also require 60–80 inescapable shocks.

To examine this possibility Grau *et al.*[20] gave rats either 0, 20, 40, 60, or 80 inescapable shocks followed by five reexposure shocks 24 hr later. The tail-flick latencies measured after the reinstating shocks are shown in FIGURE 11. Indeed, the reinstated analgesia only occurred following 60 or 80 inescapable Day 1 shocks. In a second experiment rats were given either 0, 40, or 80 inescapable tailshocks followed by either saline or morphine 24 hr later. FIGURE 12 shows tail-flick latencies taken after the morphine injection. Again, 80 inescapable shocks were required in order to obtain the usual effect. Thus both long-term reinstated analgesia and morphine hyperreactivity depend on using shock conditions necessary to produce a short-term opioid SIA. Neither escapable shock nor inescapable shocks fewer than 60–80 produce immediate opioid SIA, and neither produce these subsequent Day 2 effects. As noted previously, 60–80 inescapable shocks are required to produce behavioral learned helplessness effects such as poor shuttlebox escape learning. There is thus a correspondence between conditions required to produce opioid SIA and learned helplessness.

RELATIONSHIP TO RESULTS OF OTHER INVESTIGATORS

A number of investigators have explored conditions that act to determine whether SIA is opioid or non-opioid, and a consideration of stressor controllability may help to understand their results. For example, Lewis, Cannon, and Liebeskind[2] found 3 min of continuous 2.5 mA footshock to produce non-opioid SIA, whereas 20 min of intermittent 2.5 mA footshock led to opioid SIA. Obviously, a 3 min

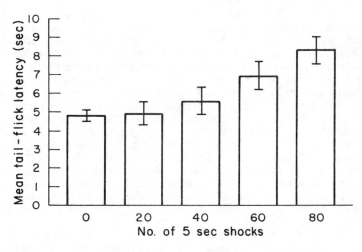

FIGURE 11. Mean tail-flick latency for subjects given five footshocks 24 hr after 0, 20, 40, 60, or 80 inescapable shocks.

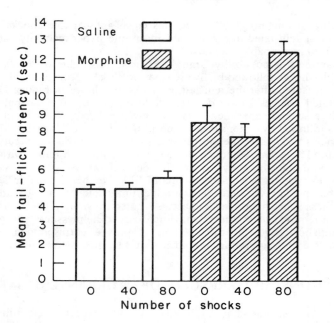

FIGURE 12. Mean tail-flick latency for subjects given saline or morphine 24 hr following 0, 40, or 80 inescapable shocks.

exposure to shock might be insufficient to allow for the learning of uncontrollability. In collaboration with Sherman, Lewis, Terman, and Liebeskind, we sought to examine this possibility. The shocker and gridbox used by Lewis et al.[2] was brought to our laboratory and we explored whether the Lewis et al.[2] shock procedures would produce a behavioral learned helplessness effect. We[28] administered either our usual 80 tailshock procedure, 3 min of continuous footshock using the Lewis et al. procedure, 20 min of intermittent footshock as in Lewis et al., restraint, or no treatment. All subjects were tested for shuttlebox escape learning 24 hr later using standard procedures. FIGURE 13 shows that 80 tailshocks produced their usual interference with escape learning. Trials terminated automatically after 35 sec of no response. Thus the 30 sec latencies observed indicate complete failure to learn in most subjects. Importantly, the Lewis et al. 20 min intermittent footshock procedure produced an equally severe impairment in escape learning, while the brief continuous footshock procedure failed to lead to interference with subsequent escape learning. Moreover, the 20 min procedure led to reinstated analgesia upon shock reexposure 24 hr later, but the 3 min procedure did not, further supporting the parallel being drawn. Thus there would appear to be a strong relationship between conditions that produce learned helplessness and opioid SIA.

Unfortunately, the present argument encounters obvious difficulty because not all procedures reported to produce opioid SIA are ones likely to lead to the learning of uncontrollability. There are a variety of conditions under which shock

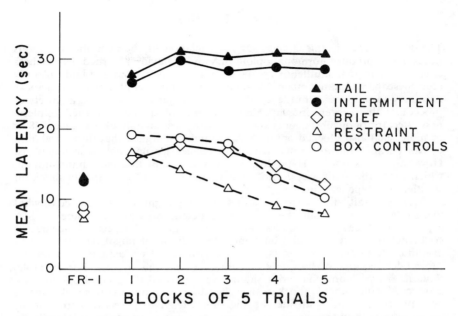

FIGURE 13. Mean shuttlebox response latency for groups given 80 tailshocks (tail), 20 min of intermittent footshock (intermittant), 3 min of continuous footshock (brief), restraint, or confinement.

exposure is too brief to lead to such learning but result in opioid SIA. Two stand out. First, conditioned analgesia is often opioid in nature even though very few shocks are required to produce this effect. For example, Fanselow and Baackes[30] have reported opioid conditioned SIA after just two brief shocks. Second, Terman et al.[31] found opioid SIA after brief footshock if the product of the intensity and duration of the footshock was less than 7.5 mA · min.

However, opioid SIA appears to exist in two different forms. One has been labeled hormonal[17] because it requires an intact pituitary-adrenal system for its expression. The other is nonhormonal in that normal pituitary-adrenal activity is not required for it occurrence. It should be noted that both opioid conditioned analgesia and the opioid analgesia after brief footshock is nonhormonal in that they are not disrupted by hypophysectomy.[31-33]

We thus sought to determine the hormonal nature of the SIA produced by 80 inescapable shocks. The reinstated analgesia was completely blocked by hypophysectomy, dexamethasone administration, and adrenalectomy.[34] This analgesia is therefore hormonal in nature and differs from the opioid SIA produced by the shock treatments too brief to lead to the learning of uncontrollability. Moreover, the opioid analgesia produced by the Lewis et al. 20 min footshock procedure is also hormonal.[35] Existing data thus appear consistent with the argument that learning that stressors are uncontrollable is an important factor in activating hormonal opioid SIA.

CONCLUSIONS

The data reviewed in this chapter suggest a relationship between the conditions necessary to produce hormonal opioid SIA and behavioral learned helplessness effects such as poor shuttlebox escape learning. Thus we found opioid SIA only after inescapable but not escapable shocks, and a number of inescapable shocks necessary to produce a shuttlebox deficit were required. Moreover, a variety of procedures that prevent inescapable shock from producing a learned helplessness effect (prior or subsequent experience with escapable shock, passage of 48 hr or more, etc.) also blocked opioid SIA. It might be argued that this correlation occurs because the analgesia actually produces learned helplessness effects! However, this is not so. Hypophysectomy and dexamethasone administration, which block the analgesia, do not mitigate the effects of inescapable shock on shuttlebox escape learning.[36]

More generally, the experiments presented highlight the importance of what the subject learns about the stressor in determining the outcome of SIA experiments. Clearly, a consideration of only the physical aspects of the stressor could not have predicted the outcomes. In addition, it might be necessary to examine the impact of other aspects of experimental procedures on what the subject learns, and of how this can interact with the stressor. For example, Watkins et al.[27] found that prior sham surgery moved the second opioid peak produced by inescapable shock to an earlier than usual number of shocks, just as does prior experience with inescapable shock. Obviously, recovery from sham surgery is a painful experience over which the subject has no control. Similarly, Maier, Ryan, and Kurtz[37] found that injecting formalin into the paw 15 min before a series of inescapable shocks resulted in opioid SIA after a much smaller number of shocks than typically required.

Moreover, the pattern of results suggests that the nature of SIA is not the result of stress, at least not stress conceived of in any simple way. It is difficult to understand how some of the procedures that were able to block the analgesia could have reduced stress. For example, it is not easy to see how an experience with escapable shock after having been exposed to inescapable shock could reduce the stress that had been produced. Escapable shock may well be less stressful than inescapable shock, but it is still stressful to some degree and certainly cannot be negatively stressful. Of course, it is possible to think of stress as being a complex psychological process sensitive to factors such as the organism's expectations about future events. Expectations about the controllability of events would then be one such factor, and there are undoubtedly others. This sort of position moves away from a generalized conception of stress as reflecting some set of simple physical variables and may decrease the usefulness of the concept. The regulation of SIA by these sorts of processes suggests that it is not merely part of a negative feedback loop reflecting a centrifugal pain inhibition system activated by ascending pain input.

REFERENCES

1. BODNAR, R. J., D. D. KELLY, M. BRUTUS & M. GLUSMAN. 1979. Stress-induced analgesia: neural and hormonal determinants. Neurosci. Biobehav. Rev. 4:87–100.
2. LEWIS, J. W., J. T. CANNON & J. C. LIEBESKIND. 1980. Opioid and non-opioid mechanisms of stress analgesia: Assessment of tolerance and cross-tolerance with morphine. Science 208:623–625.

3. WATKINS, L. R., D. A. COBELLI, P. FARIS, M. D. ACETO & D. J. MAYER. 1982. Opiate vs. non-opiate footshock induced analgesia (FSIA): The body region shocked is a critical factor. Brain Res. **242**:299–308.
4. OVERMIER, J. B. & M. E. P. SELIGMAN. 1967. Effects of inescapable shock upon subsequent escape and avoidance learning. J. Comp. Physiol. Psychol. **63**: 23–33.
5. DRUGAN, R. C. & S. F. MAIER. 1982. The nature of the activity deficit produced by inescapable shock. Anim. Learn. Behav. **10**:401–406.
6. RAPAPORT, P. M. & S. F. MAIER. 1978. The effects of inescapable shock on food competition dominance in rats. Anim. Learn. Behav. **6**:160–168.
7. WILLIAMS, J. L. 1982. Influence of shock controllability by dominant rats on subsequent attack and defensive behaviors toward colony intruders. Anim. Learn. Behav. **10**:305–315.
8. MINOR, T. R., R. L. JACKSON & S. F. MAIER. 1984. Effects of task irrelevant cues and reinforcement delay in choice escape learning following inescapable shock. Evidence for a deficit in selective attention. J. Exp. Psychol.: Anim. Behav. Proc. **10**:543–557.
9. MAIER, S. F. & M. E. P. SELIGMAN. 1976. Learned helplessness: Theory and evidence. J. Exp. Psychol.: Gen. **105**:3–46.
10. ANISMAN, H., A. PIZZINO & L. SKLAR. 1980. Coping with stress, norepinephrine depletion and escape performance. Brain Res. **191**:583–588.
11. WEISS, J. M., P. A. GOODMAN, B. A. LOSITO, S. CORRIGAN, J. M. CHARRY & W. H. BAILEY. 1981. Behavioral depression produced by an uncontrollable stressor: Relationship to norepinephrine, dopamine, and serotonin levels in various regions of rat brain. Brain Res. Rev. **3**:167–205.
12. MARGULES, D. L. 1979. Beta-endorphin and endoloxone: Hormones of the autonomic nervous system for the conservation of expenditure of bodily resources and energy in anticipation of famine or feast. Neurosci. Biobehav. Rev. **3**:155–162.
13. JACKSON, R. L., D. J. COON & S. F. MAIER. 1979. Long-term analgesia effects of inescapable shock and learned helplessness. Science **206**:91–94.
14. WILLIAMS, J. L. & S. F. MAIER. 1977. Transitational immunization and therapy of learned helplessness in the rat. J. Exp. Psychol.: Anim. Behav. Proc. **3**:240–253.
15. MOYE, T. B., J. W. GRAU, D. J. COON & S. F. MAIER. 1981. Therapy and immunization of long-term analgesia in the rat. Learn. Motiv. **12**:133–149.
16. MAIER, S. F., D. J. COON, M. A. MCDANIEL & R. L. JACKSON. 1979. The time course of learned helplessness, inactivity, and nociceptive deficits in rats. Learn. Motiv. **10**:467–487.
17. WATKINS, L. R. & D. J. MAYER. 1982. Organization of endogenous opiate and non-opiate pain control systems. Science **216**:1185–1192.
18. MAIER, S. F., S. DAVIES, J. W. GRAU, R. L. JACKSON, D. MORRISON, T. MOYE, J. MADDEN & J. D. BARCHAS. 1980. Opiate antagonists and the long-term analgesia reaction induced by inescapable shock. J. Comp. Physiol. Psychol. **94**:1172–1184.
19. DRUGAN, R. C., J. W. GRAU, S. F. MAIER, J. MADDEN & J. D. BARCHAS. 1981. Cross tolerance between morphine and the long-term analgesic reaction to inescapable shock. Pharm. Biochem. Behav. **14**:677–682.
20. GRAU, J. W., R. L. HYSON, S. F. MAIER, J. MADDEN & J. D. BARCHAS. 1981. Long-term stress-induced analgesia and activation of an opiate system. Science **203**:1409–1412.
21. MOYE, T. B., R. L. HYSON, J. W. GRAU & S. F. MAIER. 1983. Immunization of opioid analgesia: Effects of prior escapable shock on subsequent shock-induced and morphine-induced antinociception. Learn. Motiv. **14**:238–251.
22. HYSON, R. L., L. J. ASHCRAFT, R. C. DRUGAN, J. W. GRAU & S. F. MAIER. 1982. Extent and control of shock affects naltrexone sensitivity of stress-induced analgesia and reactivity to morphine. Pharmacol. Biochem. Behav. **17**:1019–1025.
23. WILLIAMS, J. L., R. C. DRUGAN & S. F. MAIER. 1984. Exposure to uncontrollable stress alters withdrawal from morphine. Behav. Neurosci. **98**:836–846.
24. BASBAUM, A. I. & H. L. FIELDS. 1984. Endogenous pain control systems: Brainstem spinal pathways and endorphin circuitry. Ann. Rev. Neurosci. **7**:309–339.

25. YAKSH, T. L. & T. A. RUDY. 1976. Analgesia mediated by a direct spinal action of narcotics. Science **192**:1357–1358.
26. WATKINS, L. R., D. A. COBELLI & D. J. MAYER. 1982. Classical conditioning of front paw and hind paw footshock induced analgesia (FSIA): Naloxone reversibility and descending pathways. Brain Res. **243**:119–132.
27. WATKINS, L. R., R. C. DRUGAN, R. L. HYSON, T. B. MOYE, S. M. RYAN, D. J. MAYER & S. F. MAIER. 1984. Opiate and nonopiate analgesia induced by inescapable tailshock: Effects of dorsolateral funiculus lesions and decerebration. Brain Res. **291**:325–336.
28. MAIER, S. F., J. E. SHERMAN, J. W. LEWIS, G. W. TERMAN & J. C. LIEBESKIND. 1983. The opioid/nonopioid nature of stress-induced analgesia and learned helplessness. J. Exp. Psychol.: Anim. Behav. Proc. **9**:80–91.
29. DRUGAN, R. C., D. N. ADER & S. F. MAIER. 1985. Shock controllability and the nature of stress-induced analgesia. Behav. Neurosci. (In press.)
30. FANSELOW, M. S. & M. P. BAACKES. 1982. Conditioned fear induced opiate analgesia on the formalin test: Evidence for two aversive motivational systems. Learn. Motiv. **13**:200–222.
31. TERMAN, G. W., Y. SHAVIT, J. W. LEWIS, T. J. CANNON & J. C. LIEBESKIND. 1984. Intrinsic mechanisms of pain inhibition: Activation by stress. Science **221**:1270–1277.
32. FANSELOW, M. S. 1984. Opiate modulation of the active and inactive components of the post-shock reaction: Parallels between naloxone pretreatment and shock intensity. Behav. Neurosci. **98**:269–277.
33. WATKINS, L. R., D. A. COBELLI, H. H. NEWSOME & D. J. MAYER. 1982. Footshock induced analgesia is dependent neither on pituitary nor sympathetic activation. Brain Res. **245**:81–96.
34. MACLENNAN, A. J., R. C. DRUGAN, R. L. HYSON, S. F. MAIER, J. MADDEN & J. D. BARCHAS. 1982. Corticosterone: A critical factor in an opioid form of stress-induced analgesia. Science **215**:1530–1532.
35. LEWIS, J. W., M. G. TORDOFF, J. E. SHERMAN & J. C. LIEBESKIND. 1982. Adrenal medullary enkephalin-like peptides may mediate opioid stress analgesia. Science **217**:557–559.
36. MACLENNAN, A. J., R. C. DRUGAN, R. L. HYSON, S. F. MAIER, J. MADDEN & J. D. BARCHAS. 1982. Hypophysectomy and dexamethasone block the analgesic but not shuttlebox escape learning consequences of inescapable shock. J. Comp. Physiol. Psychol. **96**:904–912.
37. MAIER, S. F., S. M. RYAN & R. KURTZ. 1984. The formalin test and the "opioid" nature of stress-induced analgesia. Behav. Neur. Biol. **41**:54–62.

Hyperalgesia Induced by Emotional Stress in the Rat: An Experimental Animal Model of Human Anxiogenic Hyperalgesia

CATHERINE VIDAL AND JOSEPH JACOB

Laboratory of Pharmacology
Pasteur Institute
75724 Paris, Cedex 15, France

It is well established that many neural and/or hormonal systems are involved in the modulation of pain.[1,2] The existence of such systems was originally revealed in studies of the influence of electrical stimulation of discrete brain regions and pharmacological or neurosurgical procedures on nociception. More recently, attempts have been undertaken to identify the environmental stimuli that may physiologically activate antinociceptive processes. It has become evident that the application of a variety of noxious and/or stressful manipulations results in the development of analgesia.[2-6] Contrasting types of stress analgesia appear to exist; the underlying mechanisms may be opioidergic or non-opioidergic in nature and may or may not be dependent upon hormonal factors derived from the pituitary and/or the adrenal gland. The occurrence of a given type of analgesia depends on a multiplicity of interrelated parameters that are difficult to study independently. The noxious, invasive aspect of a stimulus appears to be sufficient but not necessary to trigger antinociceptive systems. For example, footshock-induced analgesia can be classically conditioned;[2,7] exposure to environmental cues previously paired with noxious electrical shock is associated with an analgesia. Those manipulations eliciting an antinociception would appear to be accompanied by a stress reaction of the body as indicated by an activation of both the pituitary-adrenal axis and sympathetic nervous system. Certain types of stress-induced analgesia may occur independently of the pituitary and/or the adrenals which are not, thus, indispensable for the occurrence of analgesia.[3-6] It must be pointed out that the response of the organism to stress includes not only physiological changes (hormonal, respiratory, cardiovascular, thermoregulatory . . .) but also behavioral shifts in attention, learning, arousal, perception, etc.[8] These reflect the psychological dimension of stress and have their biochemical correlates in alterations in the activity of biogenic amines, GABA, and neuropeptides in those brain areas involved in the control of emotions.[6,9,10] In conceptually elegant studies, Maier *et al.*[11,12] have revealed the importance of the degree to which the organism can exert control over noxious stimuli with regard to the generation of analgesia; rats subjected to inescapable noxious shocks exhibit long-term analgesia whereas rats receiving identical amounts of shocks but which are able to escape do not show analgesia. Thus, the biological significance of environmental events would appear to be a critical factor in the triggering of pain modulatory systems. This is of relevance when one compares the nature of the environmental factors that lead to analgesia with those that produce hyperalgesia.

In animals, electrical foot shock/tail shock, cold-water swim, centrifugal rotation, and immobilization have been shown to elicit an analgesia.[2-6] Certain of these stressors are noxious and/or represent a potential danger to the integrity of the animal; they are also inescapable. In conditioned analgesia,[2,7] the unconditioned stimulus is noxious such that the animal exhibits fear together with analgesia in expectation of punishment. In these situations, analgesia would appear to be the most appropriate adaptative response. In humans, anxiety/fear induced by expectation of an aversive event has also been related to analgesic effects.[13,14] However, other types of anxiety, generally occurring in the absence of knowledge regarding a forthcoming event, produce an overestimation of painful stimuli, i.e. a hyperalgesia.[14] In animals, in certain circumstances, stress can also produce hyperalgesia. Stressors such as ether vapors and horizontal oscillations have been reported by Hayes et al.[7] to induce hyperalgesia. In our laboratory, we have shown that the stress of exposure to a novel environment or gently holding a rat by the nape of the neck induces a clear-cut and reproducible hyperalgesia.[15-17] These manipulations are non-noxious and allow for possible movement of the animal that is not anticipating any identifiable stimulus; that is, the animal does not have sufficient information to elaborate an orientated response. In this case, a higher degree of arousal and a hypersensitivity to sensory stimuli, including noxious stimuli, may appear more beneficial to the organism in the elaboration of behavior. Thus, the hyperalgesia induced by such emotional stress in rats might offer an animal model of anxiogenic hyperalgesia in humans.

In the following sections, the characteristics of the hyperalgesia induced by two models of stress, novelty and holding, will be examined in detail. It will emerge that, dependent upon the nature of the stressor, emotional hyperalgesia may be underlaid by different mechanisms, as with the many contrasting models of stress analgesia that have been discovered.

SELECTION OF AN APPROPRIATE PAIN TEST: METHODOLOGICAL CONSIDERATIONS

As discussed above, the response of the organism to stress includes both physiological and psychological components. The estimation of changes in nociception in stressed animals requires the evaluation not only of the sensory-discriminative dimension of pain but also of its affective, motivational component. The former can be assessed in reflexive pain tests (e.g. tail flick) and the latter in the vocalization test.[18] In our experimental paradigms, both dimensions of pain were examined.[15,16,19] The rats were loosely restrained in cylinders and two sharp needles inserted intracutaneously into the tail. Pain thresholds were determined following the application of incremental electric shocks to the tail: a moderate stimulation produces a tail withdrawal (spinal reflex); a higher intensity induces a single vocalization; and a further increase in intensity elicits additional vocalization components, termed vocalization afterdischarge.[20] The rats were previously accustomed to the testing procedure in order to minimize the stress of testing. Following three days of training, the rats sat quietly in the restraining cylinders and exhibited no reaction to the insertion of the tail needles. Repetitive tail stimulation was associated with the progressive development of a slight degree of analgesia. This analgesia may be due to the prolongation of restraint in cylinders (inescapable) as no changes in nociceptive thresholds were seen in freely moving rats subjected to similar tail stimulation. Our emotional stressors were applied following commencement of restraint in order to avoid interference with analgesia.

HYPERALGESIA INDUCED BY NOVELTY

Following determination of basal pain thresholds, rats were removed from cylinders, placed for 5 min in a novel environment—an observation box—and re-inserted in cylinders for subsequent pain testing. These manipulations induced a pronounced and highly significant decrease in nociceptive thresholds for tail withdrawal and vocalization responses (FIGURE 1). In the observation box, the rats exhibited typical behavioral signs reflecting novelty stress, i.e. exploration, rearing, grooming, and defecation.

Hypophysectomy attenuated the hyperalgesic effects and the behavioral signs concomitant with novelty, indicating the participation of pituitary factors in these phenomena. Dexamethasone, which is known to block the stress-induced release

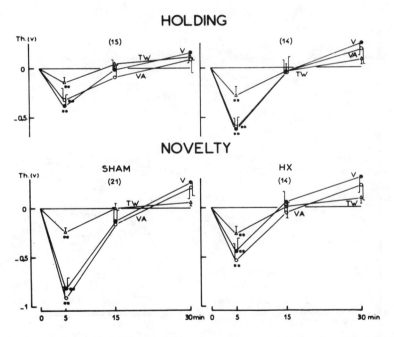

FIGURE 1. Effects of holding and novelty stresses on nociceptive thresholds and modulation by hypophysectomy (HX). Ordinates: mean change (volts ± SEM) from baseline values (= 0) in pain thresholds for tail withdrawal (TW, Δ), vocalization (V, ●), and vocalization afterdischarge (VA, ○). Abscissae: time intervals (min) after exposure to the stressor. The number of subjects is in parentheses. Significantly different from baseline values,* $p < 0.05$,** $p < 0.01$, t-test, paired samples. (From Vidal & Jacob.[16] With permission from *Life Sciences*.)

of ACTH and β-endorphin from the anterior lobe of the pituitary,[21] did not affect novelty hyperalgesia. Thus, hypophyseal factors originating from the intermediate lobe (not affected by dexamethasone) may be involved in the hyperalgesia. The participation of non-pituitary-dependent central mechanisms must also be considered because hypophysectomy reduced but did not totally abolish novelty hyperalgesia. Among putative factors involved, ACTH would be a suitable candidate as it possesses hyperalgesic properties,[22,23] mediates grooming behavior,[24] and evokes fear in a novel environment.[25]

We also investigated the effects of the anxiolytic, diazepam.[26] Diazepam dose dependently produced an increase in basal pain thresholds (FIGURE 2). Novelty hyperalgesia was completely blocked by diazepam, even at low doses that did not induce analgesia. Diazepam also increased exploration and reduced defecation, classical anxiolytic effects. Thus, the blockade by diazepam of novelty hyper-

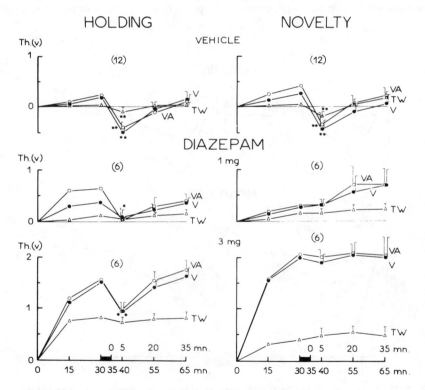

FIGURE 2. Effects of diazepam on emotional hyperalgesia induced by holding and novelty stresses. Ordinates: mean change ± SEM in pain thresholds as in FIGURE 1. Abscissae: time in minutes, lower scale: 0 = commencement of pain testing in restraining cylinders; upper scale: 0 = immediately after exposure to the stressors indicated by a black bar. Significantly different from values prior to exposure to the stressors,* $p < 0.05$,** $p < 0.01$, t-test, paired samples. Diazepam was injected just after 0 time of the lower scale. (From Vidal & Jacob.[16] With permission from *Life Sciences*.)

algesia offers additional evidence for the emotional dimension of hyperalgesia. The action of diazepam is probably GABAergic as the administration of gamma-acetylenic GABA, an irreversible inhibitor of GABA catabolism,[27] behaved similarly to diazepam. Furthermore, we have observed that exposure to a novel environment resulted in hyperthermia, characteristic of emotional stress (FIGURE 3).[17,28] Novelty hyperthermia was also reduced by diazepam.

HYPERALGESIA INDUCED BY HOLDING

Subsequent to measurement of basal pain thresholds, the rats were removed from cylinders and gently held on the bench by the nape of the neck for 5 min. This was evidently not noxious and did not completely impede movements of the head and limbs. The rats periodically exhibited signs of emotional stress, i.e. agitation, vocalization, and defecation but did not behave aggressively. Upon replacement into the cylinders for testing nociception, a clear-cut reduction in pain thresholds was observed both for tail withdrawal and vocalization responses (FIGURE 1).

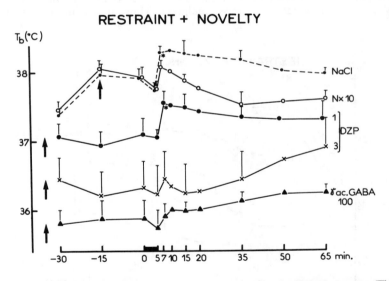

FIGURE 3. Effects of restraint and novelty stresses on body temperature (Tb) and modulations by naloxone (Nx), diazepam (DZP), and gamma-acetylenic GABA. Fifteen min after placing the rats in restraining cylinders a pronounced rise in rectal Tb occurred. After removal of the rats from cylinders, exposure to novelty (black bar), and replacement in cylinders, an additional hyperthermia developed. Ordinates: mean Tb ($°C$) + SEM. Abscissae: time in min. Arrow: time of drug administration. Nx (10 mg/kg, s.c.) was injected in restrained rats 15 min before exposure to novelty. DZP (1–3 mg/kg, s.c.) was injected 30 min prior to placing of the rats in restraining cylinders and gamma-acetylenic GABA (100 mg/kg, i.p.) 6 hr before. Groups of 6 rats were used. *Significantly different from Tb values measured just before novelty, $p < 0.05$, *t*-test, paired samples. (From Vidal *et al.*[28] With permission from *Life Sciences*.)

In contrast to novelty hyperalgesia, hypophysectomy potentiated the hyper-algesia induced by holding. Dexamethasone similarly enhanced this hyper-algesia. Thus, analgesic factors originating in the anterior lobe of the pituitary appear to partially counteract the holding hyperalgesia, which probably reflects CNS-localized mechanisms. Pituitary opioid peptides might be suitable candi-dates in view of their analgesic effects[1,5] and anxiolytic properties.[26]

Neither diazepam nor gamma-acetylenic GABA affected holding hyper-algesia in contrast to their inhibitory effects on novelty hyperalgesia (FIGURE 2).

Moreover, hyperthermia was elicited by novelty, whereas a pronounced hypothermia was associated with holding (FIGURE 4).[17,28]

CONCLUSIONS

As summarized in TABLE 1, the emotional hyperalgesia induced by exposure to novelty or holding are differentially modifiable by hypophysectomy, dexametha-sone, and diazepam. In addition, they are accompanied by opposite changes in body temperature, i.e. hyperthermia is induced by novelty whereas holding results in hypothermia. These contrasting types of emotional hyperalgesia reflect differing mechanisms, dependent on the nature of the stressor, in analogy to the many contrasting models of stress analgesia. Thus, in accordance with its

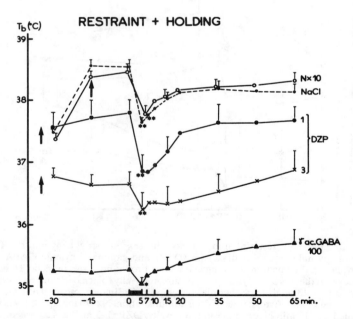

FIGURE 4. Effects of restraint and holding stresses on body temperature and modulations by naloxone, diazepam, and gamma-acetylenic GABA. Holding stress is indicated by a black bar. Other details as legend of FIGURE 3. (From Vidal *et al.*[28] With permission from *Life Sciences*.)

TABLE 1. Summary of the Effects of Experimental Manipulations Upon Stress Hyperalgesia Induced by Novelty or Holding and Associated Change in Body Temperature

	Experimental Manipulations				Associated Change in Body Temperature
	Hypophysectomy	Dexamethasone	Diazepam	γ-Acetylenic GABA	
Novelty Hyperalgesia	↓	O	↓	↓	↑
Holding Hyperalgesia	↑	↑	O	O	↓

NOTE: ↑: potentiation; ↓: attenuation; and O: no effect.

adaptive significance, the response of the organism to a stressor would appear to involve the development not only of analgesia but also of hyperalgesia, depending on the biological relevance of environmental events.

ACKNOWLEDGMENTS

The authors wish to thank Dr. M.J. Millan for helpful discussion and Frau v. Unruh for typing the manuscript.

REFERENCES

1. BASBAUM, A. I. & H. L. FIELDS. 1984. Endogenous pain control systems: Brainstem spinal pathways and endorphin circuitry. Ann. Rev. Neurosci. 7:309–338.
2. WATKINS, L. R. & D. J. MAYER. 1982. Organization of endogenous opiate and non-opiate pain control systems. Science 216:1185–1192.
3. BODNAR, R. J., D. D. KELLY, M. BRUTUS & M. GLUSMAN. 1979. Stress-induced analgesia: neural and hormonal determinants. Neurosci. Biobehav. Rev. 4:87–100.
4. DRUGAN, R. C., T. B. MOYE & S. F. MAIER. 1982. Opioid and non-opioid forms of stress-induced analgesia: some environmental determinants and characteristic. Behav. Neural. Biol. 35:251–264.
5. MAYER, D. J. & L. R. WATKINS. 1981. Role of endorphins in endogenous pain control systems. In Modern Problems of Pharmacopsychiatry: The Role of Endorphins in Neuropsychiatry. H. M. Emrich, Ed. 17:68–96. Karger. Basel.
6. MILLAN, M. J. 1981. Stress and endogenous opioid peptides: A review. In Modern Problems of Pharmacopsychiatry: The Role of Endorphins in Neuropsychiatry. H. M. Emrich, Ed. 17:49–67. Karger. Basel.
7. HAYES, R. L., C. J. BENNETT, P. NEWLON & D. J. MAYER. 1978. Behavioral and physiological studies of non-narcotic analgesia in the rat elicited by certain environmental stimuli. Brain Res. 155:69–90.
8. SELYE, H. 1976. Forty years of stress research: principal remaining problems and misconceptions. Can. Med. Assoc. J. 115(1):53–56.
9. PALKOVITS, N. 1979. Changes in brain amines during stress. In Interaction within the Brain-Pituitary-Adrenocortical System. M. T. Jones, Ed.: 87–95. Academic Press. London.
10. BIGGIO, G., A. CONCAS, M. SERRA, M. SALIS, M. G. CORDA, V. NURCHI, C. CRISPONI & G. L. GESSA. 1984. Stress and β-carbolines decrease the density of low affinity GABA binding sites; an effect reversed by diazepam. Brain Res. 305:13–18.
11. MAIER, S. F., R. C. DRUGAN & J. W. GRAU. 1982. Controllability, coping behavior and stress-induced analgesia. Pain 12:47–56.
12. MAIER, S. F., J. E. SHERMAN, J. W. LEWIS, G. W. TERMAN & J. C. LIEBESKIND. 1983. The opioid/nonopioid nature of stress-induced analgesia and learned helplessness. J. Exp. Psychol.: Anim. Behav. Proc. 9:80–90.
13. WILLER, J. C., H. DEHEN & J. CAMBIER. 1981. Stress-induced analgesia in humans: endogenous opioids and naloxone reversible depression of pain reflexes. Science 212:689–691.
14. BEECHER, H. K. 1969. Anxiety and pain. J. Am. Med. Assoc. 209:1080.
15. VIDAL, C. & J. JACOB. 1982. Hyperalgesia induced by non-noxious stress in the rat. Neurosci. Lett. 32:75–80.
16. VIDAL, C. & J. JACOB. 1982. Stress hyperalgesia in rats: an experimental animal model of anxiogenic hyperalgesia in human. Life Sci. 31:1241–1244.
17. VIDAL, C., C. SUAUDEAU & J. JACOB. 1984. Regulation of body temperature and nociception induced by non-noxious stress in rats. Brain Res. 297:1–10.

18. HOFFMEISTER, F. & G. KRONEBERG. 1966. Experimental studies in animals of the differentiation of analgesic activity. *In* Methods in Drug Evaluation. P. Mantegazza & F. Piccinini, Eds.: 270–277. Elsevier. Amsterdam.

19. VIDAL, C. & J. JACOB. 1980. The effect of medial hypothalamus lesions on pain control. Brain Res. **199**:89–100.

20. CARROLL, M. N. & R. K. S. LIM. 1960. Observations on the neuropharmacology of morphine and morphine-like analgesia. Arch. Int. Pharmacodyn. **125**:383–403.

21. GUILLEMIN, R., T. VARGO, J. ROSSIER, S. MINICK, N. LING, C. RIVIER, W. VALE & F. BLOOM. 1977. β-Endorphin and adrenocorticotropin are secreted concomitantly by the pituitary gland. Science **197**:1367–1369.

22. AMIR, S. 1981. Effects of ACTH on pain responsiveness in mice. Interaction with morphine. Neuropharmacology **20**:959–962.

23. BERTOLINI, A., R. POGGIOLI & W. FERRARI. 1979. ACTH-induced hyperalgesia in rats. Experientia **35**:1216–1217.

24. DUNN, A., E. J. GREEN & R. L. ISAACSON. 1979. Intracerebral adrenocorticotropic hormone mediates novelty-induced grooming in the rat. Science **203**:281–283.

25. CONCANNON, J. T., D. E. RICCIO, R. MALONEY & J. MCKELVEY. 1980. ACTH mediation of learned fear: blockade by naloxone and naltrexone. Physiol. Behav. **25**:977–979.

26. MILLAN, M. J. & T. DUKA. 1981. Anxiolytic properties of opiates and endogenous opioid peptides and their relationship to the actions of benzodiazepines. *In* Modern Problems of Pharmacopsychiatry: The Role of Endorphins in Neuropsychiatry. H. M. Emrich, Ed. **17**:123–141. Karger. Basel.

27. JUNG, M. J., B. W. LIPPERT, B. W. METCALF, P. J. SCHECHTER, P. BÖHLEN & A. SJOERDSMA. 1977. The effect of 4-aminohex-5-yonic acid (gamma-acetylenic GABA, gamma-ethynyl GABA) a catalytic inhibitor of GABA transaminase, on brain GABA metabolism in vivo. J. Neurochem. **28**:717–723.

28. VIDAL, C., C. SUAUDEAU & J. JACOB. 1983. Hyper- and hypothermia induced by non-noxious stress: effects of naloxone, diazepam and gamma-acetylenic GABA. Life Sci. **33** (Suppl. 1): 587–590.

Alterations in Other Sensory Modalities Accompanying Stress Analgesia as Measured by Startle Reflex Modification[a]

DONALD S. LEITNER

Department of Psychology
Saint Joseph's University
Philadelphia, Pennsylvania 19131

The startle reflex in mammals is elicited by intense sensory stimulation that occurs with a rapid onset.[1] It consists of a series of muscular contractions, resulting in an abrupt crouch.[2] In rats, the response is easily elicited by sudden, loud noise.

Originally conceptualized as an all-or-nothing sort of behavior, research over the past two decades has shown that the startle response is quite plastic. Innocuous sensory events (prestimuli), which do not themselves elicit startle or any other overt response, can greatly reduce the amplitude of a subsequently elicited startle response. Any detectable change in the sensory environment can serve as a prestimulus; the onset, offset, or changes in intensity or frequency of a stimulus will reliably inhibit startle amplitude, as long as the change is above sensory threshold and occurs with an appropriate lead interval.[3] In rats, the optimal lead time is between 50 and 150 msec.

Research has shown that a prestimulus need only be at detection threshold for reliable inhibition to occur.[4] Further, reflex inhibition is cross-modal; the prestimulus need not be of the same sensory modality as that used to elicit startle for reflex inhibition to occur.[5,6] Reflex inhibition is also unlearned, being present the very first time that a prestimulus precedes a startle-eliciting stimulus.[7]

Reflex inhibition has proven to be a useful paradigm for studying changes in sensory functioning. The startle reflex is easily elicited and measured and requires no training. Reflex inhibition is also unlearned, and reliable inhibition can be produced by barely perceptible prestimuli. Thus, the paradigm is sensitive, requires no training, and is not dependent upon a motivated operant baseline as are most animal psychophysical procedures. Potential confounding of sensory changes with motor or motivational deficits is minimized, and pretraining large numbers of subjects is unnecessary.

In studies where reflex inhibition has been used to assess sensory acuity, the amplitude of the startle response on trials where a prestimulus precedes a startle-

[a]Supported by Public Health Service Grant R01 NS 18822.

eliciting stimulus is compared to startle amplitude on those trials where the startle-eliciting stimulus is presented alone. Reliable reduction of startle amplitude on those trials where a prestimulus was present is taken as evidence that the subject perceived the prestimulus. The difference between the control trials and prestimulus trials, expressed as a percentage, can be used as an index to monitor changes in the perceived intensity of a prestimulus. The degree to which a reflex is inhibited is solely a function of the characteristics of the prestimulus, most significantly its intensity, and is independent of the characteristics of the startle-eliciting stimulus.

Inhibition of the startle reflex by visual and auditory prestimuli was used by Krauter, Wallace, and Campbell[8] to investigate sensory and motor changes in aging rats. They found that motor ability, as measured by the amplitude of the acoustic startle response, declined steadily with age, beginning as early as the twelfth or thirteenth month of life. Auditory acuity was also assessed with white noise prestimuli of various intensities to inhibit the acoustic startle response. Little change occurred in auditory acuity (measured as percent inhibition) over the first two years of life; this was followed by a steady decline in acuity. Visual acuity, assessed in a similar manner, displayed a sharp, steady decline that began at 10 months of age.

Reflex inhibition has also been used to assess the effects of toxic substances on sensory and motor ability. Fechter and Young[9,10] have shown that by using pure tones of various intensities, auditory thresholds of rats could be assessed using reflex inhibition that closely matched threshold data obtained using operant techniques. Again, percent inhibition of acoustic startle was the measure used to assess auditory sensitivity. Administration of the ototoxin neomycin sulfate produced frequency-specific deficits in reflex inhibition but did not affect control startle amplitude. Administration of the neuromuscular toxin triethyltin bromide produced large decreases in startle amplitude on control trials, but did not affect auditory thresholds for pure tone as measured by reflex inhibition.

Thus, reflex inhibition has proven useful in discriminating between sensory and motor deficits. This is due to the independence of prestimulus inhibition from the startle response itself. In the present experiments, reflex inhibition was used to investigate changes in sensory functioning that may accompany stress-induced analgesia. It has been well-documented that exposure to a severe stressor produces an insensitivity to pain that outlasts the duration of the exposure.[11] It is not normally clear, however, whether the sensory changes induced by an effective analgesic stressor are specific to the modality of somatosensation, or whether some forms of stress analgesia occur as part of a broader sensory deficit or as part of a deficit in motor responsivity. Reflex inhibition was used to investigate what, if any, changes in auditory perception accompanied cold swim stress analgesia. This was compared to the analgesia induced by morphine administration.

METHOD

Subjects

The subjects were nine male Sprague-Dawley rats, all approximately 90 days old at the beginning of the experiment. They were individually housed and allowed ad libitum food and water except while being tested.

Apparatus

The basic apparatus, a small cage fitted with a transducer for measuring startle amplitude, has been described in detail elsewhere.[12] Briefly, a wire mesh cage was suspended from a sheet of Plexiglas to which a piezoelectric film material had been laminated. The abrupt movements characteristic of startle made by a rat in the cage caused the Plexiglas to flex slightly, producing a voltage in the piezoelectric film that bore a linear relationship to the force applied to the floor of the cage. This voltage was fed into a Coulbourn Instruments Peak Detector/Memory (model S76-31), which measured the largest peak of the incoming waveform during the 150 msec immediately following the onset of the startle-eliciting stimulus. The peak voltage was converted into its digital equivalent by a Commodore C-64 microcomputer with a Computer Continuum analog/digital-digital/analog converter board. The computer's printer (Commodore model MPS-801) provided hard copy of the data.

The cage and transducer were housed in a Scientific Prototype chamber (model JP 300), modified with the application of sound-attenuating, anechoic material on the inside surfaces. Two piezoelectric wide-dispersion horns (Realistic 40-1379) wired in parallel were mounted 6 cm from either side of the cage, one on each side. These transducers were used to deliver both the prestimuli and startle-eliciting stimuli. The horns were driven by an ILP power amplifier (model UP7).

All programming, logic, and timing functions were controlled by the Commodore microcomputer, supplemented with Coulbourn Instruments solid-state modules where necessary.

Procedure

In the first phase of the experiment, the subjects were exposed to three different conditions. One of these was a baseline condition consisting of behavioral testing. The subjects were first assessed for nociceptive thresholds in a tail-flick procedure. Each subject was lightly restrained and placed upon an IITC Analgesia Meter (model 33). This device focused a beam of light from a projector bulb upon the subject's tail, 4 cm from the tip. Six trials were presented, with the intensity of the radiant heat varying from trial to trial in the sequence low-medium-high-low-medium-high. Low intensity represented 50% of the full intensity of the device; medium and high represented 70% and 90%, respectively. On each trail, when the light caused the subject's tail to move out of its path, it struck a photocell that previously had been covered by the tail. This stopped a timer that indicated the latency to tail-flick. A 60 sec intertrial interval was used.

Immediately after the completion of the tail-flick test, each subject was placed in the cage used for startle testing. The subject was then presented with a series of 33 startle-eliciting bursts of white noise (intensity: 125 dB SPL; rise-fall time: 1 msec; duration: 25 msec) spaced 20 sec apart. The data for the first three trials were discarded. On 20 of the remaining 30 trials, the startle-eliciting stimulus was preceded at 100 msec by either a 65 or a 75 dB SPL burst of white noise (rise-fall time: 5 msec; duration: 50 msec). The two intensities of prestimuli were presented 10 times each. Thus, there were three types of trials; the startle-eliciting stimulus presented alone, the startle-eliciting stimulus preceded by a 65 dB prestimulus, and the startle-eliciting stimulus preceded by a 75 dB prestimulus, presented 10 times each in a block-randomized sequence. The amplitude of the startle response was recorded on each trial.

Besides the baseline condition, the subjects were exposed to two other experimental conditions. One of these consisted of a forced 3.5 min swim in water maintained at 2°C; the other consisted of a forced 3.5 min swim in water maintained at 28°C. Both cold and warm water swims took place in a cylindrical plastic bucket with tapered sides, 75 cm deep and 37.5 cm at its greatest diameter. The bucket was filled with water to a depth of 35 cm.

Twenty min after exposure to a swim, the subjects were tested in the tail-flick and startle paradigms, as in the baseline condition. All subjects were exposed to all three experimental conditions in sequences determined by a Latin squares matrix. The time between exposure to the conditions was 48 hr.

The second phase of the experiment began two weeks after the termination of the first phase. It was identical to the first and involved the same subjects, except that instead of being exposed to cold and warm water swims, subjects were given injections of morphine. Subjects were exposed to a baseline condition consisting of the behavioral testing only, a condition in which an injection of morphine sulfate in a buffered saline vehicle (5 mg/ml/kg, i.p.) was administered 30 min before behavioral testing, and a condition in which an injection of the vehicle only (1 ml/kg, i. p.) was administered 30 min before behavioral testing.

RESULTS

Means were computed across all trials of a given type in both the startle and tail-flick paradigms for each subject in each condition, and grand means were then computed across subjects in each phase of the experiment. The effects of swim stress upon mean tail-flick latency are depicted in FIGURE 1. It can be seen that, relative to the baseline and warm water swim conditions, the cold water swim condition produced the longest latencies. Also as expected, the highest intensity of radiant heat produced the shortest tail-flick latency, with the low intensity producing the longest and the medium intensity falling between these two.

A 3 (condition) $\times$ 3 (intensity) analysis of variance with repeated measures on both variables was conducted to examine the reliability of these trends. It was found that there was a main effect of condition ($F(2,64) = 12.63, p < .01$), and also a main effect of intensity ($F(2,64) = 76.97, p < .01$); the interaction was not reliable ($F(4,64) = 1.55$, NS).

Post-hoc Newman-Keuls' tests were used to locate the source of these differences. Each intensity of radiant heat produced a tail-flick latency that was reliably different from the others ($p < .05$). Further, the cold swim condition produced latencies that were reliably different from either of the other two conditions ($p < .05$); the baseline and warm swim conditions produced latencies that were not reliably different. These data demonstrate that exposure to cold swim stress did produce reliable analgesia.

FIGURE 2 depicts mean startle amplitude from the reflex inhibition procedure on the control trials, where the startle-eliciting stimulus was presented alone. It can be seen that there was some tendency for startle amplitude to be reduced in the swim conditions compared to the baseline condition, but this trend was not reliable when tested by a one-way analysis of variance with repeated measures ($F(2,16) < 1$, NS). Thus, neither of the swim conditions affected startle amplitude reliably.

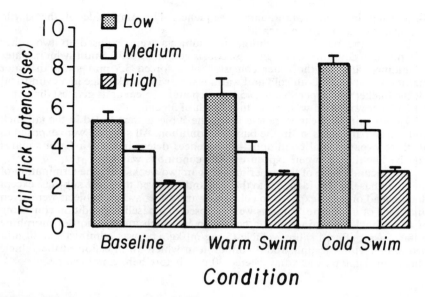

FIGURE 1. Mean tail-flick latency (± SEM) for each intensity of radiant heat in each of the three conditions in the first phase of the experiment.

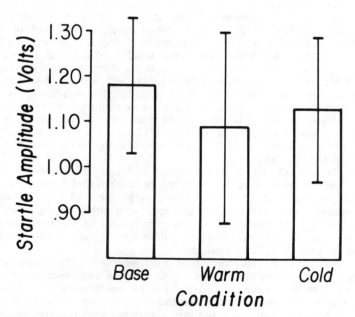

FIGURE 2. Mean startle amplitude (± SEM) on trials where the startle-eliciting stimulus was presented alone in each of the three conditions.

The startle inhibition data were quantified by computing percent inhibition for each subject in each condition for both intensities of prestimuli, and then computing grand means across subjects. The formula used to compute this was: mean startle amplitude on control trials minus mean startle amplitude on pre-stimulus trials divided by mean startle amplitude on control trials. Thus, the larger the percent inhibition, the smaller the size of the startle response (i.e., the more startle was inhibited). These data are depicted in FIGURE 3. It can be seen that, overall, the 65 dB prestimulus engendered less inhibition than did the 75 dB prestimulus, as expected. Also, it can be seen that there was an orderly change in the percent inhibition produced by exposure to the swims. Both swims produced deficits in reflex inhibition, with the greatest interference created by exposure to cold swim stress. The reliability of these trends was examined by a 3 (condition) × 2 (prestimulus intensity) analysis of variance with repeated measures on both variables. A main effect was found for prestimulus intensity (F(1,40) = 11.43, $p < .01$); the more intense prestimulus produced reliably greater inhibition than did the less intense prestimulus, as expected. A main effect was also found for condition (F(2,40) = 4.16, $p < .05$). The interaction was not reliable (F(2,40) < 1, NS).

The main effect found for condition was explored with a post-hoc Newman-Keuls' test. It was found that the cold swim condition produced reliably less startle inhibition than did the baseline condition ($p < .05$); the baseline condition was not reliably different from the warm swim condition, nor was the cold swim condition reliably different from the warm swim condition.

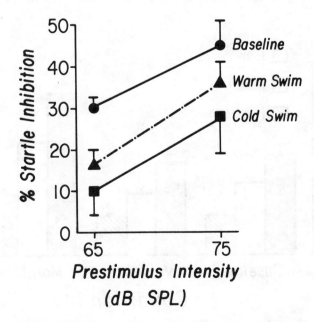

FIGURE 3. Mean percent inhibition of startle (± SEM) for the two intensities of prestimuli in each of the three experimental conditions.

Thus, orderly changes were produced in reflex inhibition by the several experimental conditions. Exposure to a cold swim, a severe stressor which produces analgesia, produced reliable deficits in reflex inhibition. Exposure to a warm swim, a less severe stressor, did not produce reliable analgesia, although there was a trend in this direction. Warm swim exposure did not produce changes in reflex inhibition compared to the baseline condition, but reflex inhibition was not different from that in the cold swim condition, which was reliably different from baseline. Thus, there was again a trend in the appropriate direction.

These data indicate that there was a change in perception produced by exposure to swim stress. For reflex inhibition to decrease, with no change in control startle amplitude, the prestimulus must have been perceived as being less intense, compared to the baseline condition.

A similar approach was used to analyze the data for the second phase of the experiment. FIGURE 4 depicts mean tail-flick latency, computed across subjects for each condition and each intensity of radiant heat. It can be seen that the morphine injection produced a profound analgesia at each of the three intensities of radiant heat used. There was no obvious differences between the baseline and vehicle conditions. The reliability of these trends was tested with a 3 (condition) $\times$ 3 (intensity) analysis of variance with repeated measures on both variables. Main effects were found for intensity $(F(2,64) = 79.88, p < .01)$ and for condition $(F(2,64) = 42.62, p < .01)$, and a reliable interaction was found $(F(4,64) = 3.39, p < .05)$.

Because of the reliable interaction, an analysis of variance for simple main effects with repeated measures was conducted. All possible comparisons proved to be reliable $(p < .01)$. Further analysis with post-hoc Newman-Keuls' tests

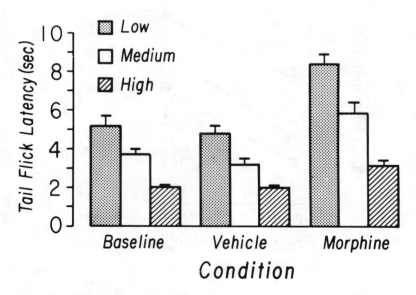

FIGURE 4. Mean tail-flick latency ($\pm$ SEM) for each intensity of radiant heat in each of the three conditions in the second phase of the experiment.

indicated that for each condition, the three intensities of radiant heat produced reliably different tail-flick latencies ($p < .05$). For the low and medium intensities of radiant heat, the vehicle and baseline conditions produced tail-flick latencies that were reliably shorter than in the morphine condition, but not from each other ($p < .05$). For the highest intensity of radiant heat, tail-flick latencies in the vehicle condition were reliably shorter than in the morphine condition ($p < .05$), but there was no reliable difference between the morphine and baseline conditions, nor between the baseline and vehicle conditions. This identifies the source of the interaction.

Overall, then, each of the three intensities of radiant heat produced tail-flick latencies that were reliably different from each other. Morphine administration reliably lengthened tail-flick latencies, compared to vehicle administration or the baseline condition. These data demonstrate that the morphine injections did indeed produce analgesia.

FIGURE 5 depicts mean startle amplitude on the control trials where the startle-eliciting stimulus was presented alone. It can be seen that, compared to the baseline condition, there was some tendency for morphine administration to depress startle amplitude, and for vehicle administration to increase startle amplitude. These trends were not reliable when tested with a one-way analysis of variance with repeated measures, however (F(2,16) < 1, NS). These data demonstrate that neither morphine nor vehicle administration affected startle amplitude reliably.

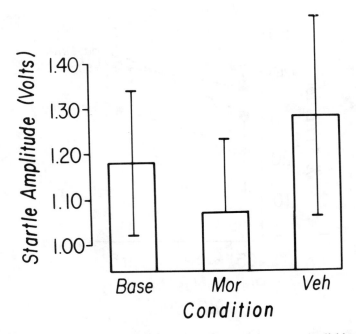

FIGURE 5. Mean startle amplitude (± SEM) on trials where the startle-eliciting stimulus was presented alone in each of the three experimental conditions.

The data from the reflex inhibition procedure were treated in a manner identical to the one used in the first phase of the experiment. Depicted in FIGURE 6 is the mean percent inhibition computed across subjects for the two prestimulus intensities in each condition. It can be seen that there was some tendency for morphine administration to reduce startle inhibition compared to the other two conditions, but this trend was not statistically reliable when tested with a 3 (condition) $\times$ 2 (prestimulus intensity) analysis of variance with repeated measures on both variables ($F(2,40) = 2.78$, NS). There was a reliable effect of prestimulus intensity ($F(1,40) = 4.89$, $p < .05$); the 75 dB prestimulus produced more inhibition than did the 65 dB prestimulus. No reliable interaction was found ($F(2,40) < 1$, NS). Thus, although the more intense prestimulus produced reliably greater inhibition than did the less intense prestimulus, there was no change in the perceived intensity produced by either morphine or vehicle administration.

DISCUSSION

The analgesia induced by cold swim stress has been shown to be non-opioid in nature. It is not reversed by naloxone, and will not develop cross-tolerance with opiates.[13] The present data indicate that there are further differences between the state produced by exposure to cold swim stress and that produced by opiate

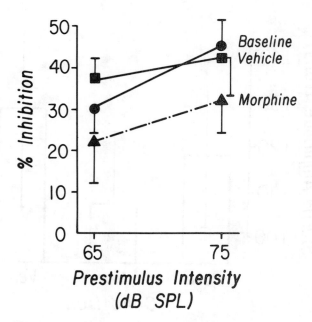

FIGURE 6. Mean percent inhibition of startle ($\pm$ SEM) for the two intensities of prestimuli in each of the three experimental conditions.

administration. Both of these manipulations produced reliable analgesia in the present experiment, but only cold swim stress produced an insensitivity to pain that was accompanied by deficits in auditory perception.

The exact nature of the loss in auditory acuity is not clear. The deficit may be caused by something as simple as a reduction in the motility of the subjects' pinnae as a result of the swim stress, or it may be that such exposure produces changes in the central processing of auditory information. Another possibility is that the loss in sensitivity is not limited to the modality of audition, but is part of a more general deficit in the subjects' sensitivity to environmental stimulation. Research has shown that if human subjects focus their attention on a pre-stimulus, it is more effective in inhibiting startle than if the subjects do not.[14] The opposite may also be true; that is, if attention to the environment is reduced, then reflex inhibition is also reduced. Cold swim stress may produce deficits in attention to environmental stimuli incident to several modalities, audition and somatosensation among them.

If this is the case, then the effects of cold swim stress should be cross-modal, and losses in the other senses should be present. Research currently in progress in this laboratory is examining how reflex inhibition produced by visual prestimuli is affected by exposure to severe stress. If losses in visual sensitivity are found, then the argument that there is a general loss in sensitivity to environmental stimuli produced by exposure to severe stress would be supported.

It is clear that the changes in perception induced by cold swim stress are more general than was previously thought. Therefore, it may be that the state induced by exposure to cold swim stress may not be accurately characterized as analgesia.

REFERENCES

1. FLESHLER, M. 1965. Adequate acoustic stimulus for startle reaction in the rat. J. Comp. Physiol. Psychol. **60**:200–207.
2. LANDIS, C. & W. A. HUNT. 1939. The Startle Pattern. Farrar and Rinehart. New York.
3. HOFFMAN, H. S. & J. R. ISON. 1980. Reflex modification in the domain of startle: I. Some empirical findings and their implications for how the nervous system processes sensory input. Psychol. Rev. **87**:175–189.
4. HOFFMAN, H. S. & B. W. WIBLE. 1970. Role of weak signals in acoustic startle. J. Acoust. Soc. Am. **47**:489–497.
5. SCHWARTZ, G., H. S. HOFFMAN, C. L. STITT & R. MARSH. 1976. Modification of the rat's acoustic startle response by antecedent visual stimulation. J. Exp. Psychol. (Anim. Behav.) **2**:28–37.
6. MARSH, R., H. S. HOFFMAN, C. L. STITT & G. M. SCHWARTZ. 1976. The role of small changes in the acoustic environment in modifying the startle reflex. J. Exp. Psychol. (Anim. Behav.) **20**:248–259.
7. ISON, J. R., G. R. HAMMOND & E. E. KRAUTER. 1973. Effects of experience on stimulus-produced inhibition in the rat. J. Comp. Physiol Psychol. **83**:324–336.
8. KRAUTER, E. E., J. E. WALLACE & B. A. CAMPBELL. 1981. Sensory-motor functioning in the aging rat. Behav. Neural Biol. **31**:367–392.
9. FECHTER, L. D. & J. S. YOUNG. 1983. Discrimination of auditory from nonauditory toxicity by reflex modulation audiometry: effects of triethyltin. Toxicol. Appl. Pharmacol. **70**:216–227.
10. YOUNG, J. S. & L. D. FECHTER. 1983. Reflex inhibition procedures for animal audiometry: A technique for assessing ototoxicity. J. Acoust. Soc. Am. **73**:1686–1693.

11. HAYES, R. L., G. J. BENNET, P. G. NEWLON & D. J. MAYER. 1978. Behavioral and physiological studies of non-narcotic analgesia in the rat elicited by certain environmental stimuli. Brain Res. **155**:69–90.
12. LEITNER, D. S. & M. C. ROSENBERGER. 1983. A simple and inexpensive startle transducer with high output. Behav. Res. Methods Instrumentation **15**:508–510.
13. BODNAR, R. J., D. D. KELLY, M. BRUTUS & M. GLUSMAN. 1980. Stress-induced analgesia: Neural and hormonal determinants. Neurosci. Biobehav. Rev. **4**:87–100.
14. DELPEZZO, E. M. & H. S. HOFFMAN. 1980. Attentional factors in the inhibition of a reflex by a visual stimulus. Science **210**:673–674.

Characteristics of Analgesias Induced by Brief or Prolonged Stress

G. CURZON, P. H. HUTSON, G. A. KENNETT,
AND M. MARCOU

Institute of Neurology
London, England

and

A. GOWER AND M. D. TRICKLEBANK

Centre de Recherche Merrell International
Strasbourg, France

INTRODUCTION

The literature on stress-induced analgesia is replete with data that appear either contradictory or indicative of different mechanisms by which the analgesia is produced. Thus, some workers have found it to be attenuated by small doses of naloxone,[1-4] while others report that even large doses have little or no effect.[5-7] There is also disagreement on the involvement of 5-hydroxytryptamine (5-HT). We have reported experiments in which its availability has been altered by drugs[8-10] indicating that 5-HT decreases the analgesia following brief footshock. However, the analgesia induced by more prolonged shock or immobilization is decreased by antagonists of 5-HT or inhibitors of its synthesis and is enhanced by the precursor of 5-HT, 5-hydroxytryptophan, or the 5-HT agonist, 5-methoxy-N,N-dimethyltryptamine (5MeODMT).[11-15] Results on the role of dopamine (DA) in stress-induced analgesia also appear conflicting. Some studies indicate that it is facilitated by dopamine. Thus, the dopamine antagonist, haloperidol, blocks analgesia induced by both prolonged immobilization and prolonged tail shock.[12,16] In contrast, others report that tail shock analgesia is unaffected by drugs that alter dopaminergic transmission[17] while haloperidol is found to enhance analgesia induced by brief footshock.[18]

These apparently conflicting results can be partly explained by the existence of multiple analgesic mechanisms whose activation depends on such variables as the intensity and duration of stress and the body region to which it is applied.[14,19-22] The present paper summarizes data we have obtained on the contrasting effects of drugs on analgesic responses to brief and prolonged footshock and on the mechanism by which the response to brief shock occurs. These pharmacological experiments alone, while suggestive, do not necessarily indicate the neurochemical changes associated with analgesic responses to stress in the absence of drugs. We have therefore also described a preliminary experiment in which neurochemical and analgesic responses to stress are concurrently monitored in the same drug-free animal by means of one of a group of new (and recently reviewed[23]) techniques for repetitive neurochemical analysis of the conscious brain.

93

METHODS

Methods were as follows except where specifically stated otherwise under RESULTS AND DISCUSSION.

Animals

Male Sprague-Dawley rats were fed ALGH Standard Rodent diet and tap-water ad libitum and housed singly under a 12 hr light-dark (white-red) cycle with white light commencing at 06.00 hr for at least a week before use when they weighed 180–220 g. Experiments were carred out between 14.00 and 17.00 hr.

Stress Procedures

Footshock

This was applied in an aluminum box (240 × 210 × 90 mm high) with a front wall of clear Perspex. The ceiling was too low to permit rearing. The floor was a grid of 4 mm diameter stainless-steel bars, spaced 14 mm between centers, through which a shock of 2 mA intensity (except where otherwise indicated) was delivered via a constant-current source with a scrambler (shock periods of 5 sec, less than 1 sec intervals between shocks).

Immobilization

Rats were taped to a metal grid for 2 hr and released by loosening the tape with acetone. Control rats were left in their home cages.

Analgesia Testing

In the earlier part of the work, responses to noxious heat were monitored using a tail-flick procedure in which the caudal 2 cm of the tail was immersed in a water bath at 51°C and the time taken to withdraw the tail noted. Subsequently, experiments on memory-enhancing drugs or immobilization were made using an Appelex DS20 tail-flick apparatus, which focused heat onto the tail and measured tail-flick latency automatically. A locus 2 cm from the end of the tail was used in all experiments apart from those involving immobilization or putative memory-enhancing drugs, when a locus 10 cm from the end of the tail was used. Heat intensity was adjusted so that control rats gave times of 2–4 sec. Rats were removed from the apparatus if they did not respond within 10 sec.

Monitoring Central Amine Metabolism

In the experiments on immobilization-induced analgesia, central amine metabolism was monitored using 30 µl cisternal CSF samples taken from each rat via a previously implanted catheter at 30 min intervals each sampling being followed by a tail-flick latency measurement as described above at the following times: 75, 45, and 15 min before immobilization; 15, 45, 75, and 105 min after its commencement; 15, 45, 75, and 105 min after the animals were released. The neurochemical procedures and their validation are described in detail elsewhere.[24-27] The 5HT metabolite, 5-hydroxyindoleacetic acid (5HIAA) and the DA metabolites 3,4-dihydroxyphenylacetic acid (DOPAC) and homovanillic acid (HVA) were determined on each CSF sample by HPLC after acid hydrolysis.[25] This is necessary as a large fraction of cisternal DOPAC and HVA occurs in conjugated form.

Experimental Design

The standard procedure used in some experiments included preliminary measurements of tail-flick latency. Values were slightly, but usually not significantly, less (approximately minus 10%, values not given) than subsequent latency values, made after the rat had been returned to its home cage either for 0.5 min (brief shock experiments) or for 30 min (prolonged shock experiments). The latency was then remeasured immediately after applying the shock or at later times as indicated under RESULTS AND DISCUSSION. In the prolonged shock experiments each latency score was obtained from the mean of three values taken at 10 sec intervals. This procedure reduced the variance of the scores without affecting their magnitude. It was also used in the experiments on immobilization stress when tail flick times were measured at 30 min intervals immediately after the withdrawal of CSF samples (see above).

RESULTS AND DISCUSSION

Effects of Drugs on Analgesic Responses to 30 sec and 30 min Footshock

The strikingly different pharmacological profiles of the analgesic responses to 30 sec and 30 min footshock have been described in detail[8,28-30] and will be indicated relatively briefly here. TABLE 1 shows that the increase of tail-flick latency immediately after 30 sec shock is unaffected by naloxone and enhanced by the 5HT synthesis inhibitor parachlorophenylalanine (PCPA) and the DA receptor antagonist, pimozide. In striking contrast to these findings, the increase of latency immediately after 30 min shock is blocked by all three treatments.

The lack of effect of naloxone on the response to 30 sec shock was confirmed at a wide range of doses,[8] while the enhancement of the response by PCPA was consistent with the similar effect of depleting spinal 5HT by injecting the 5HT neurotoxin, 5,7-dihydroxytryptamine, either into the spinal cord or the raphe magnus.[9] Conversely, the response was inhibited by the 5HT releasers *p*-chloroamphetamine and fenfluramine, by the reuptake inhibitor, fluoxetine and by the indolic 5HT agonist, 5MeODMT. The increased response to 30 sec shock after giving pimozide was also shown with another DA agonist haloperidol. It probably involves D_2 receptors as it was decreased by the specific D_2 agonist LY141865, but not by the specific D_1 agonist SKF38393.[29]

The very different characteristics of the responses to 30 sec and 30 min shock

TABLE 1. Effects of Drugs on Changes of Tail-Flick Latency Induced by 30 sec and 30 min Footshock (2 mA)

Shock Time	Drug	Latency of Tail-Flick (sec)	
		L1	L2
Experiment 1			
30 sec	Vehicle	3.2 ± 0.6	7.7 ± 1.7^b
30 sec	Naloxone	3.3 ± 0.9	8.1 ± 2.4^b
30 min	Vehicle	3.3 ± 0.5	5.0 ± 1.0^b
30 min	Naloxone	3.3 ± 0.4	3.7 ± 0.5^d
Experiment 2			
30 sec	Vehicle	4.0 ± 0.7	7.8 ± 0.9^b
30 sec	PCPA	4.1 ± 1.0	$13.4 \pm 2.5^{b,d}$
30 min	Vehicle	2.9 ± 0.3	4.3 ± 0.4^b
30 min	PCPA	3.2 ± 0.7	3.4 ± 0.9^e
Experiment 3			
30 sec	Vehicle	4.8 ± 0.7	9.3 ± 1.5^b
30 sec	Pimozide	4.3 ± 0.5	11.4 ± 2.3^c
30 min	Vehicle	4.2 ± 0.8	7.4 ± 2.9^a
30 min	Pimozide	4.6 ± 0.7	5.0 ± 1.1^c

Values are means $\pm$ SD, 7–10 rats per group. Naloxone (1 mg/kg i.p.) was given 15 min before shock, *p*-chlorophenylalanine (PCPA, 150 mg/kg i.p.) was given 72, 48, and 24 hr before shock and pimozide (1 mg/kg i.p.) was given 30 min before shock.
[a] $p < 0.02$, [b] $p < 0.001$ vs. L1 (Student's *t* test for paired values) [c] $p < 0.05$, [d] $p < 0.01$, [e] $p < 0.001$ vs. L2 of vehicle-treated rats (Student's *t* test for independent groups).
After Tricklebank *et al.*[28,29]

may explain some of the previous conflicts in the literature on the effects of drugs on stress-induced analgesia.

Dependence of the Analgesic Response to 30 sec Footshock: Evidence for Learning

The standard analgesia test procedure we have used included the determination of tail-flick latency on each rat both immediately before and immediately after footshock. We found that 30 sec shock only increased latencies if the animals were previously subjected to the above pre-shock test and that this dependency on pre-shock testing did not occur when the rats were shocked for 30 min (TABLE 2).

The apparent dependency of the analgesia due to brief footshock on the pre-shock determination of latency suggests that the animal responds after shock as if the latter is contingent on exposure to the previous determination of latency. It has thus some similarity with Skinner's "superstition"[31] and with passive avoidance learning. The following drug experiments strengthen this analogy. Thus, TABLE 3 shows that the rapidly acting 5HT agonist, 5MeODMT, attenuated

TABLE 2. Effect of Pre-shock Testing of Tail-Flick Latency on Post-Shock Latency

			Latency of Tail-Flick (sec)	
N	Shock Time	Pre-Shock Test	L1	L2
11	30 sec	+	4.6 ± 1.0	8.9 ± 2.0^b
11	30 sec	−		4.6 ± 1.4^c
7	30 min	+	3.3 ± 0.6	5.7 ± 1.8^a
8	30 min	−		6.6 ± 1.9

Values are means ± SD. 2 mA footshock. L1 and L2 are pre- and post-shock latencies, respectively.
$^a p < 0.01$, $^b p < 0.001$ vs. L1 (Student's *t* test for paired values). $^c p < 0.001$ vs. L2 of pre-shocked test group (Student's *t* test for independent groups).
After Tricklebank *et al.*[28]

the increased tail-flick latency after 30 sec footshock whether the drug was given before shock or 1 min after shock. Although increased latency was still apparent immediately after giving 5MeODMT (presumably because the drug had not yet reached its site of action) the increase that normally was still present 1.5 min later was not evident in the drug-treated rats. This finding is consistent with the reduced retention of conditioned avoidance by drugs that increase 5HT availability.[32-34]

Conversely, two putative memory enhancing drugs,[35,36] physostigmine, the choline esterase inhibitor, and pramiracetam, which (*in vitro* at least) increases choline uptake in hippocampal synaptosomes,[37] prevent the decay with time of the apparent analgesic response to 30 sec of 3 mA footshock.[38] A preliminary

TABLE 3. Effect on Tail-Flick Latency of 5-Methoxy-N,N-Dimethyltryptamine (5MeODMT, 1 mg/kg i.p.) Given Before or After Footshock (2 mA, 30 sec)

	Treatment			Percentage Analgesia Score	
				1 min	2.5 min
N	Pre-Shock	Post-Shock	Pre-Shock	Post-Shock	Post-Shock
18	0.9% NaCl	0.9% NaCl	117 ± 24	148 ± 45^a	155 ± 43^b
7	5MeODMT	0.9% NaCl	113 ± 33	90 ± 29^c	90 ± 42^c
22	0.9% NaCl	5MeODMT	126 ± 27	158 ± 39^b	117 ± 43

Values are means ± SD. In this experiment, pre-shock latency was measured initially (L1), 30 sec after replacement in the home cage (L2), and after shock. Results are given as analgesia scores (pre-shock score = 100 L2/L1, post-shock scores = 100 × latency at time indicated/L2). Pre-shock injections were made immediately after measuring pre-shock latencies. After return to their home cages for 1 min animals were shocked, immediately given the post-shock injections, and returned to their home cages before post-shock latency determination.
$^a p < 0.02$, $^b p < 0.01$ vs. pre-shock controls. $^c p < 0.01$ vs. 0.9% NaCl treated shocked rats (Student's *t* test). The dose of 5MeODMT used had no effect in the absence of footshock.
Data from Hutson *et al.*[10]

experiment (using the standard procedure with tail flick determination both before and after shock) showed that post-shock latency measured immediately after shock was about twice the pre-shock value, and fell to pre-shock values in 2 hr. Results in TABLE 4 show that this decay was completely prevented if the drugs were injected immediately after shock. The drugs did not increase latencies if given either without shock or to rats that were shocked but not subjected to pre-shock latency measurement.

A subsidiary experiment showed that the drugs facilitated retention of a classical passive avoidance response. A two-compartment light-dark apparatus was used with compartments measuring $15 \times 21 \times 22$ cm high and connected by a guillotine door, 6×6 cm. The latency of male albino mice (22–28 g) to enter the dark compartment from one corner of the lighted section was noted. Immediately after entry, the door was lowered, 1.5 sec, 27 V footshock applied and the mouse removed. Twenty-four hours later, the time taken to again enter the dark compartment was measured. These times were significantly increased if physostigmine (0.1–0.4 mg/kg) or pramiracetam (10–40 mg/kg) were injected i.p. immediately after footshock.[38]

Thus, two drugs that prevented the decay of the increase of tail-flick latency after shock also enhanced the retention of a passive avoidance response. As they were without direct analgesic effects and prevented the decay of the apparent analgesia effect only under conditions permitting an association between the tail-flick latency determination and footshock, their effects support the hypothesis

TABLE 4. Effects of Physostigmine and Pramiracetam on Tail-Flick Latency Measured 2 Hours after 30 Sec Footshock (3 mA)

Pre-Shock Tail-Flick Test	Shock	Drug	Latency of Tail-Flick (sec) Pre-Shock	Post-Shock
Experiment 1				
+	+	Vehicle	3.0 ± 1.2	3.3 ± 1.5
+	+	Physostigmine	3.1 ± 1.2	5.8 ± 1.2^a
+	−	Vehicle	3.7 ± 0.3	3.4 ± 1.0
+	−	Physostigmine	3.2 ± 1.2	2.9 ± 1.5
−	+	Vehicle		3.2 ± 1.0
−	+	Physostigmine		3.2 ± 1.7
Experiment 2				
+	+	Vehicle	3.1 ± 1.0	2.6 ± 0.7
+	+	Pramiracetam	2.9 ± 0.7	5.2 ± 1.5^a
+	−	Vehicle	2.9 ± 0.7	2.6 ± 0.7
+	−	Pramiracetam	3.4 ± 1.2	3.8 ± 0.7
−	+	Vehicle		3.7 ± 1.0
−	+	Pramiracetam		3.1 ± 1.7

Values are means $\pm$ SD, 6 rats per group. Physostigmine (0.2 mg/kg s.c.) and pramiracetam (10 mg/kg s.c.) were given immediately after shock.
$^a p < 0.01$ vs. pre-shock latency (Student's t test for paired values).

that the increased latency after 30 sec footshock involves a form of passive avoidance learning. This apparent enhancement of analgesia by drugs that increase (or may tend to increase) cholinergic transmission is to some extent consistent with the blockade by the muscarinic antagonist scopolamine of the reinstatement of analgesia by mild footshock given 24 hr after prolonged footshock.[39]

The results described in this section suggest that the increased tail-flick latency shown under our conditions after brief footshock may reflect a learned inhibition of a motor response to a noxious stimulus but not necessarily a decreased awareness of pain, as strictly implied by the word "analgesia." The dependence of the phenomenon on the pre-stress analgesia test may be of some practical importance, firstly because it might conceivably be used as the basis of a screening test for the ability of drugs to influence memory and secondly, because such test schedules are frequently used in analgesia studies and the diametrically opposite pharmacological spectra of the effects of brief and prolonged stress (TABLE 1) imply that, under some conditions they may oppose or even obliterate each other. Problems of this kind can obviously be avoided by omitting pre-stress analgesia testing and instead using separate control groups. They might also be minimized by considerably increasing the interval between pre-stress testing and shock. These and other methodological questions have recently been discussed.[40]

A New Approach to Stress Analgesia Studies: Concurrent Neurochemical and Behavioral Monitoring

There has recently been considerable interest in new methods by which neurochemical changes can be repeatedly monitored in the conscious rat in parallel with behavioral changes.[23,41] These methods can be applied to stress analgesia studies and we have used one of them in a preliminary experiment on the analgesia that develops when rats are immobilized for relatively long periods (2 hr).[11] Samples of cisternal CSF were withdrawn at 30 min intervals for the determination of transmitter amine metabolites and tail-flick latencies measured on each animal before, during, and after immobilization as described in METHODS, using five immobilized rats and six controls. The latter animals were freely moving (except for the restraint necessary during tail-flick latency measurements). DA and 5HT metabolism are enhanced during immobilization as indicated by increased concentrations of their metabolites in CSF.[27]

All the immobilized rats showed consistent increases in tail-flick latency, but the magnitude and duration of the effect varied greatly between animals. Thus, maximal increases were of the order of 65 to 190% and occurred between 15 and 105 min after the commencement of immobilization. Latencies rapidly returned to approximately control values after the animals were released. CSF DOPAC concentrations rose by between 45 and 105%, 65 to 135 min after initiation of immobilization and 30 to 90 min (average = 66 min) after the corresponding peak tail-flick latency. In four out of five rats the DOPAC concentrations had returned to approximately control levels by 60 min after the normalization of the tail-flick latencies. Time courses of percentage changes of both tail-flick latency and cisternal DOPAC concentration for a representative rat are shown in FIGURE 1. Calculations of the areas under these curves provides measures of the net effects of immobilization on both analgesia and CSF DOPAC concentration. The values for tail-flick latency and DOPAC concentration correlated positively and

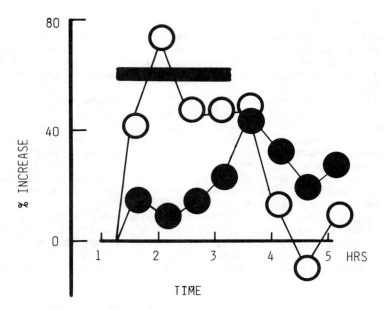

FIGURE 1. Effect of immobilization on tail-flick latency (○) and cisternal CSF DOPAC (●) of a single rat. The period of immobilization is indicated by the bar. Results are given as percentage changes above the means of the values obtained 75, 45, and 15 min before the start of immobilization.

significantly with each other ($r = 0.96$, $N = 5$, $p = 0.01$) for the immobilized rats. The controls showed relatively small changes of tail-flick latency, which were not clearly related to the DOPAC values that tended to rise over the first five to six control sample collections and then to decline. These changes may reflect an initial stress effect due to the tail-flick test followed by habituation: they did not occur in a control group that was not tested.[27] They suggest that preliminary daily tail-flick measurements or handling might have improved the experimental design.

The DOPAC changes on immobilization presumably result from release of DA earlier in the immobilization period. A causal role of this in the increase of tail-flick latency is consistent with the blockade of the analgesia by valine (400 mg/kg i.p.), which (by inhibiting the transport of tyrosine and tryptophan to the brain) would oppose increases of DA, NA, and 5HT metabolism. Although a causal role for DA in immobilization-induced analgesia is suggested by its reported prevention by the DA receptor antagonist, haloperidol[12] and another antagonist pimozide (1 mg/kg i.p.) blocked analgesia due to prolonged footshock (TABLE 1) neither this dose of pimozide nor haloperidol (0.2 mg/kg) blocked the analgesia following immobilization.

These experiments on immobilization analgesia, while of a preliminary nature, illustrate a way of investigating stress-induced analgesia without drug treatment in individual animals that has many potential applications, e.g., in the study of relationships between the time courses of opioid and other peptide changes and analgesia. Also, a similar approach can be used to monitor not only cisternal CSF to give an index of whole brain amine metabolism but also the extracellular fluid of specific brain regions by means of implanted dialysis probes[23,42] or voltammetric electrodes.[23]

Attempts to elucidate neurochemical mechanisms of stress-induced analgesia (or other components of behavior) by any single kind of experiment often lead to results that are not easy to interpret. Thus, studies involving drugs have uncertainties that derive from doubts about their specificity and physiological relevance while neurochemical-behavioral associations found in the absence of drugs are not necessarily of a causal nature. The above experiments indicate the potential utility of combining both experimental approaches.

SUMMARY

Some characteristics of the effects of brief and prolonged stress on tail-flick latency are described. The pharmacological profiles of the latency responses to 30 sec and 30 min footshock are strikingly different. Thus, the increase of tail-flick latency after 30 sec shock is unaffected by naloxone and enhanced by drugs which decrease 5HT or DA-dependent transmission, while the increase after 30 min shock is blocked by naloxone and also by the above drugs. The increased tail-flick latency after 30 sec shock only occurs if tail-flick latency is also determined before shock. This finding, together with the attenuation or enhancement of the post-shock response by drugs that similarly affect conditioned avoidance behavior, suggests that the increased latency after brief shock occurs through a mechanism that is related to passive avoidance learning. Finally, a new approach to the investigation of stress-induced analgesia is described in which neurochemical changes during prolonged immobilization stress are repeatedly monitored using cisternal CSF samples taken in parallel with tail-flick latency measurements.

REFERENCES

1. CHESHER, G. B. & B. CHAN. 1977. Footshock induced analgesia in mice: its reversal by naloxone and cross tolerance with morphine. Life Sci. **21**:1569–1574.
2. AMIR, S. & Z. AMIT. 1978. Endogenous opioid ligands may mediate stress-induced changes in the affective properties of pain related behaviour in rats. Life Sci. **23**:1143–1152.
3. WILLER, J. C. & D. ALBE-FESSARD. 1980. Electrophysiological evidence for a release of endogenous opiates in stress-induced 'analgesia' in man. Brain Res. **198**:419–426.
4. CHATTERJEE, T. K. & G. F. GEBHART. 1984. Failure to produce a non-opioid foot shock-induced antinociception in rats. Brain Res. **323**:380–384.
5. CHANCE, W. T. & J. A. ROSECRANS. 1979. Lack of effect of naloxone on autoanalgesia. Pharmacol. Biochem Behav. **11**:643–646.
6. BODNAR, R. J., D. D. KELLY, A. SPIAGGIA, C. EHRENBERG & M. GLUSMAN. 1978. Dose-dependent reductions by naloxone of analgesia induced by cold-water stress. Pharmacol. Biochem. Behav. **8**:667–672.
7. MILLAN, M. J., R. PRZEWLOCKI, M. JERLICZ, C. H. GRAMSCH, V. HOLT & A. HERZ. 1981. Stress induced release of brain and pituitary endorphin: major role of endorphins in generation of hyperthermia, not analgesia. Brain Res. **208**:325–328.
8. TRICKLEBANK, M. D., P. H. HUTSON & G. CURZON. 1982. Analgesia induced by brief footshock is inhibited by 5-hydroxytryptamine but unaffected by antagonists of 5-hydroxytryptamine or by naloxone. Neuropharmacol. **21**:51–56.

9. HUTSON, P. H., M. D. TRICKLEBANK & G. CURZON. 1982. Enhancement of footshock induced analgesia by spinal 5,7-dihydroxytryptamine lesions. Brain Res. 237:367–372.
10. HUTSON, P. H., M. D. TRICKLEBANK & G. CURZON. 1983. Analgesia induced by brief footshock: blockade by fenfluramine and 5-methoxy-N,N-dimethyl-tryptamine and prevention of blockade by 5HT antagonists. Brain Res. 279:105–110.
11. BHATTACHARYA, S. K., P. R. KESHARY & A. K. SANYAL. 1978. Immobilization stress-induced antinociception in rats: possible role of serotonin and prostaglandins. Eur. J. Pharmacol. 50:83–85.
12. KULKARNI, S. K. 1980. Heat and other physiological stress-induced analgesia: catecholamine mediated and naloxone reversible response. Life Sci. 27:185–188.
13. SHIMIZU, T., T. KOJA, T. FUJISAKI & T. FUKUDA. 1981. Effects of methysergide and naloxone on analgesia induced by the peripheral electric stimulation in mice. Brain Res. 208:463–467.
14. LEWIS, J. W., G. W. TERMAN, L. R. NELSON & J. C. LIEBESKIND. 1984. Opioid and non-opioid stress analgesia. In Stress-induced Analgesia. M. D. Tricklebank & G. Curzon, Eds.:103–133. Wiley. Chichester.
15. CHITOUR, D., A. H. DICKENSON & D. LEBARS. 1982. Pharmacological evidence for the involvement of serotonergic mechanisms in diffuse noxious inhibitory controls (DNIC). Brain Res. 236:329–337.
16. DOI, T. & N. SAWA. 1980. Antagonistic effects of psycholeptic drugs on stress induced analgesia. Arch. Int. Pharmacodyn. 247:264–274.
17. BUCKETT, W. R. 1981. Pharmacological studies on stimulation-produced analgesia in mice. Eur. J. Pharmacol. 69:281–290.
18. SNOW, A. E., S. M. TUCKER & W. L. DEWEY. 1982. The role of neurotransmitters in stress-induced antinociception (SIA). Pharmac. Biochem. Behav. 16:47–50.
19. LEWIS, J. W., J. T. CANNON & J. C. LIEBESKIND. 1980. Opioid and non-opioid mechanisms of stress analgesia. Science 208:623–625.
20. GRAU, J. W., R. L. HYSON, S. F. MAIER, J. MADDEN & J. D. BARCHAS. 1981. Long-term stress-induced analgesia and activation of the opiate system. Science 213:1409–1411.
21. WATKINS, L. R., D. A. COBELLI, P. FARIS, M. D. ACETO & D. J. MAYER. 1982. Opiate vs non-opiate footshock-induced analgesia (FSIA): The body region shocked is a critical factor. Brain Res. 242:299–308.
22. TERMAN, G. W., Y. SHAVIT, J. W. LEWIS, J. T. CANNON & J. C. LIEBESKIND. 1984. Intrinsic mechanisms of pain inhibition: activation by stress. Science 226:1270–1277.
23. MAYERS, R. D. & P. J. KNOTT, Eds. 1986. Neurochemical Analysis of the Conscious Brain: Voltammetry and Push-pull Perfusion. Ann. N.Y. Acad. Sci.
24. SARNA, G. S., P. H. HUTSON, M. D. TRICKLEBANK & G. CURZON. 1983. Determination of brain 5-hydroxytryptamine turnover in freely moving rats using repeated sampling of cerebrospinal fluid. J. Neurochem. 40:383–388.
25. HUTSON, P. H., G. S. SARNA, B. D. KANTAMANENI & G. CURZON. 1984. Concurrent determination of brain dopamine and 5-hydroxytryptamine turnovers in individual freely moving rats using repeated sampling of cerebrospinal fluid. J. Neurochem. 43:151–159.
26. HUTSON, P. H., G. S. SARNA, B. J. SAHAKIAN, C. T. DOURISH & G. CURZON. 1986. Monitoring 5HT metabolism in the brain of the freely moving rat. Ann. N.Y. Acad. Sci. 473. (In press.)
27. CURZON, G., P. H. HUTSON, G. A. KENNETT, M. MARCOU & G. S. SARNA. 1985. Monitoring dopamine metabolism in the brain of the freely moving rat. Ann. N.Y. Acad. Sci. 473. (In press.)
28. TRICKLEBANK, M. D., P. H. HUTSON & G. CURZON. 1984. Analgesia induced by brief or more prolonged stress differs in its dependency on naloxone, 5-hydroxytryptamine and previous analgesia testing. Neuropharmacology 23:417–421.
29. TRICKLEBANK, M. D., P. H. HUTSON & G. CURZON. 1984. Involvement of dopamine in the antinociceptive response to footshock. Psychopharmacol. 82:185–188.

30. HUTSON, P. H., G. CURZON & M. D. TRICKLEBANK. 1984. Anti-nociception induced by brief footshock: characteristics and roles of 5-hydroxytryptamine and dopamine. *In* Stress-induced Analgesia. M. D. Tricklebank & G. Curzon, Eds.:135–164. Wiley. Chichester.

31. SKINNER, B. F. 1948. 'Superstition' in the pigeon. J. Exp. Psychol. **38**:168–172.

32. ESSMAN, W. M. 1978. Serotonin in learning and memory. *In* Serotonin in Health and Disease. The Central Nervous System. W. B. Essman, Ed. **3**:69–143. Spectrum. New York.

33. ARCHER, T. A. 1982. Serotonin and fear retention in the rat. J. Comp. Physiol. **96**:491–516.

34. OGREN, S. O., T. ARCHER & C. JOHANSSON. 1984. Stress-induced analgesia and avoidance behaviour: possible interactions with serotonergic neurotransmission. *In* Stress-induced Analgesia. M. D. Tricklebank & G. Curzon, Eds.:165–183. Wiley. Chichester.

35. BARATTI, C. M., P. HUYGENS, J. MINO, A. MERLO & J. GARDELLA. 1979. Memory facilitation with post trial injection of oxotremorine and physostigmine in mice. Psychopharmacology **64**:85–88.

36. POSCHEL, B. P. H., J. G. MARRIOTT & M. I. GLUCKMAN. 1983. Pharmacology of the cognition activator pramiracetam (CI-879). Drugs Exptl. Clin. Res. **9**:853–871.

37. PUGSLEY, P. A., Y. H. SHIH, L. COUGHENOUR & S. S. STEWART. 1983. Some neurochemical properties of pramiracetam (CI-879) a new cognition enhancing agent. Drugs Dev. Res. **3**:407–420.

38. GOWER, A. J. & M. D. TRICKLEBANK. 1985. Is the analgesia response to footshock a form of passive avoidance learning? Proc. Brit. Pharmacol. Soc. Cardiff Meeting, C89.

39. MACLENNAN, A. J., R. C. DRUGAN & S. F. MAIER. 1983. Long term stress-induced analgesia blocked by scopolamine. Psychopharmacology **80**:267–268.

40. TRICKLEBANK, M. D. & G. CURZON. 1984. Methodological considerations in experiments on stress-induced analgesia. *In* Stress-induced Analgesia. M. D. Tricklebank & G. Curzon, Eds.:185–189. Wiley. Chichester.

41. JOSEPH, M. H., M. FILLENZ & C. A. MARSDEN. 1985. Monitoring neurotransmitter release during behaviour. Ellis. Horwood. In press.

42. HUTSON, P. H., G. S. SARNA, B. D. KANTAMANENI & G. CURZON. 1985. Monitoring the effect of a tryptophan load on brain indole metabolism in freely moving rats by simultaneous cerebrospinal fluid sampling and brain dialysis. J. Neurochem. **44**:1266–1273.

Genetic Modulations of Stress-Induced Analgesia in Mice[a]

JOSEPH J. JACOB, MARIE-ANNE NICOLA,
GÉRARD MICHAUD, CATHERINE VIDAL,
AND NICOLE PRUDHOMME

Laboratory of Pharmacology
Pasteur Institute
F75724 Paris Cédex 15, France

INTRODUCTION

The mechanisms of stress analgesia have been shown to vary according to the nature of the stressor[1,2] and the various features of the applied stimuli, even when a single stressor was used. Footshock analgesia in particular is opioidergic or not according to the parameters of the electrical stimulation,[3,4] the site of application (fore or hind paws),[5] and the controllability of the shocks.[6]

We thought that genetic influences might also modulate stress analgesia as they were shown to modulate various behaviors. In the field of nociception and opioids, genetic differences were indeed already observed for the basal reactivity to pain,[7-9] the number of opioid receptors,[10-13] the analgesic effects of opiates,[7,14-19] and for dependence as assessed by abstinence precipitated by naloxone.[9,19,20] Based on experimental evidence of this type, opioidergic mediation of the analgesia produced by either acupuncture[21] or D-amino acids[22] was shown to vary among different strains of mice. Five strains were selected for this work; two of them are characterized by long latencies before jumping from a hot plate (CXBH: 120 ± 18 sec and C3H/Ou J: 113 ± 4 sec),[9] whereas the other three respond much faster (Swiss OF1:69 ± 4 sec; CXBK: 61 ± 9 sec; and C57BL/6 J: 56 ± 5 sec).[9] Thus pain regulation might be more effective in the first two strains than in the other three. And, further, recombinants CXBH and CXBK have been shown to have very different opioidergic potentialities: levels of cerebral opioidergic sites of the mu type[10,12,13] and responses to morphine are greater in CXBH than in CXBK.[10,13] The other three strains are still under examination. Thus it seemed worth establishing if these strains differed in the amplitude and mechanisms of stress analgesia. We used footshock of short duration as stressor. We also used tail thermic stimulation of given intensity and duration to produce a localized and transient increase of the latency of the tail flick.

MATERIAL AND METHODS

Male mice were used, CXBH and CXBK recombinants were bred in our laboratory. Because CXBK mice reproduce at a low rate few experiments were

[a]This work was supported by the DRET (Direction des Recherches, Etudes et techniques, contract no. 83/1189) and by the INSERM (Institut National de la Santé et de la Recherche Médicale, contract no. 82.3009).

performed with this strain. Swiss 0F1, C3H/Ou J, and C57BL/6 J were purchased from IFFA CREDO (Les Oncins—France).

A modality of the D'Amour and Smith technique[23] was used (Socrel-Apelex Apparatus); the lamp (24 V, 100 W) heated with a current adjusted to 75 μA was at a distance of 40 cm from the tail. The mice were placed in small Plexiglas cylinders 1 hr before the experiments began. The latencies of the tail flick were measured at the same site twice for each mouse, i.e., the first time before and the second time after the footshock or the 7 sec thermic stimulation of the tail. In other words, separate groups of mice were used for each time interval so as to avoid interferences other than those that were actually studied.

The control values were quite reproducible; several groups of 5 to 10 animals were studied; the means ± the S.E. (for a group) were in sec: CXBH, 3.8 ± 0.1 (439 mice); C3H, 3.5 ± 0.2 (265 mice); Swiss 0F1, 3.12 ± 0.08 (958 mice); C57BL/6, 3.03 ± 0.12 (391 mice); and CXBK, 3.03 ± 0.29 (93 mice). When no shock or durable heat was applied, the second reading did not differ from the first by more than 0.5 sec.

Inescapable footshocks (120 scramble stimuli of 0.2 sec duration and 50 Hz internal frequency each; intensity 0.2 or 1 mA) were applied during 1 min through an electrified grid (modified L.E.T.I.C.A. apparatus).

Localized increases of tail-flick latencies were obtained by applying the focused light beam during 7 sec at the site where the latencies were measured before and after the heat treatment (FIGURE 1). The increases developed within 5 min (not illustrated).

They were localized because they did not appear when the tail flick was measured at a site 1 cm distant from that of the heat application (FIGURE 1). They were not due to the manipulations on the animal as these had no effect alone (FIGURE 1). Heat treatment of shorter duration (e.g. 4 sec) or of lesser intensity (e.g. 5 μA) were both ineffective. No apparent tissue damage was observed; tissue damage cannot merely account for the phenomenon because it was, for its greatest part, reversible (50% within 15 min and 75% within 2 hr) (FIGURE 2). The insert of FIGURE 2 also sustains this conception. In this experiment, not only one but two measurements were taken at the same site following each other very closely (less than 1 min): the second reading of each couple always gave a much lower value than the first one, thus indicating that a very fast reflex could be elicited from the very site a few seconds after even large increases in latencies were observed. This phenomenon of sensitization is in a great measure transient (less than 1 min). It is worth noticing that the increases in tail-flick latencies were much smaller when taking the second and not the first reading of each couple into account and that the duration (15 min instead of > 4 hr) of the whole phenomenon then appeared much shorter. For the sake of brevity this phenomenon will be called localized analgesia rather than the more exact but too long expression increases in tail-flick latencies; this term may not be quite correct because this phenomenon might correspond, at least partly, to some kind of local anesthesia.

Spinalectomy was performed under anesthesia with ketamine base (0.1 ml/20 g of a 5 mg/ml solution administered in two injections, the first i.p. the second i.m.) After dissection of muscle and section of the vertebra, the spinal cord was excised between D_5 and D_8. Muscles and skin were sutured and animals warmed till recovery. Some cases of mortality occurred, varying according to the strain. The experiments were performed three days after surgery.

Naloxone hydrochloride or saline (in the controls) was injected subcutaneously 10 min before footshock or 15 min before tail stimulation, i.e., 15 minutes

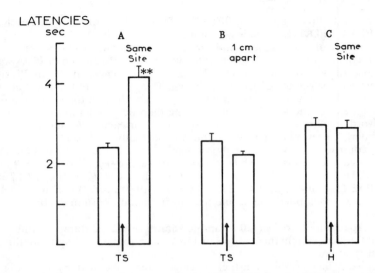

FIGURE 1. Localized tail stimulation analgesia. Tail-flick latencies (in sec) were measured just before and 5 min after a 7 sec stimulation of the tail (TS) with radiant heat. (A) Control, 7 sec stimulation and the second reading on the same site of the tail. (B) Second reading 1 cm away from the site of control and 7 sec stimulation. (C) The two readings on the same site. No 7 sec stimulation but holding (H) and manipulation of the mice. Groups of 15 or 20 mice (Swiss OF1). Bars: standard errors of the mean (S.E.).** Difference between readings before and after TS significant for $p < 0.01$.

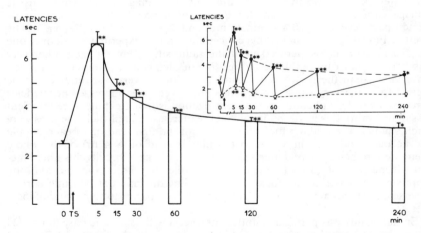

FIGURE 2. Time course of tail stimulation analgesia. Same procedure as in FIGURE 1A. Separate groups of mice were used for each time interval to avoid possible summations of the TS effects. Groups of 18 mice (Swiss OF1). Insert: Couples of two readings following each other as closely as possible on the same site were obtained at each time. The second reading of each couple (O) is systematically lower than the first one (●). This sensitization points to the possibility of a rapid reversing of the analgesia (see text). Separate groups of 18 mice for each time interval. Bars and asterisks as in FIGURE 1 (* for $p < 0.05$).

before the second measurements of the tail-flick latency. Morphine (hydrochloride) effectiveness was determined with the hot plate[24] and radiant heat[23] methods, taking as end point the licking and the tail-flick reaction, respectively. AD50 were calculated according to the Litchfield and Wilcoxon graphical method.[25] The mice whose latency was greater than the mean $\pm$ 2 standard deviations of the corresponding control were regarded as experiencing analgesia. The maximal effect was taken into account, i.e. the effect observed 30 min after the subcutaneous injection of morphine (or sodium chloride in the controls).

The doses are expressed in mg per kg of body weight. Groups of 9 to 25 animals were used. Statistical significance was assessed with the Fisher t test.

RESULTS

Tail-Flick Latencies

Considering the means obtained with several groups of five animals, the five studied strains ranked as follows in normal mice: CXBH (3.8 sec $\pm$ 0.1) > C3H (3.50 $\pm$ 0.20) > Swiss 0F1 (3.12 $\pm$ 0.08) > C57BL/6 (3.03 $\pm$ 0.12) = CXBK (3.03 $\pm$ 0.29). The differences were—thanks to the great number of groups of studied animals—significant between CXBH and the other strains and between C3H and C57BL/6 (too few CXBK having been studied).

Footshock Analgesia

When stimuli of 0.25 mA were applied (FIGURE 3A) analgesia was observed just at the end of the 1 min footshock in the four studied strains; it was statistically significant in the first three strains (CXBH, C3H, Swiss 0F1), but not in the last one (C57BL/6). The strains ranked as follows in the decreasing order of this analgesia (i.e., the differences between the values after and before shock): CXBH (4.2 sec $\pm$ 0.6), C3H (2.5 sec $\pm$ 0.47), Swiss 0F1 (1.75 sec $\pm$ 0.3), and C57BL/6 (1.4 sec $\pm$ 0.78), CXBH was significantly different from the other three strains though these were not from one another. The analgesias partly regressed within 3 min.

When the intensity of the stimuli was increased to 1 mA (FIGURE 3B) the analgesias also increased; the latencies measured just after shock reached the cut-off time value (10 sec) in the three studied strains (CXBH, Swiss 0F1, and CXBK). Significant analgesia still occurred at longer time intervals (5, 15, and 30 min) in CXBH but not in Swiss 0F1 or CXBK.

Naloxone (a classical opiate antagonist) was injected 14 min before footshock. It had no effect on the basal tail-flick latencies. When the intensity of the stimuli was 0.25 mA (FIGURE 4A) clear-cut and highly significant ($p < 0.01$) antagonism was observed in CXBH; it was feeble and not significant in C57BL/6 and Swiss 0F1, absent in C3H. When the intensity was 1 mA (FIGURE 4B) naloxone was ineffective on the analgesia measured in the three strains (CXBH, Swiss 0F1, and CXBK) immediately after footshock (not illustrated); a clear-cut and high statistical significance ($p < 0.01$) was thereafter (15–30 min after shock) observed again in CXBH whereas it was slight and not significant in Swiss OF1 and CXBK.

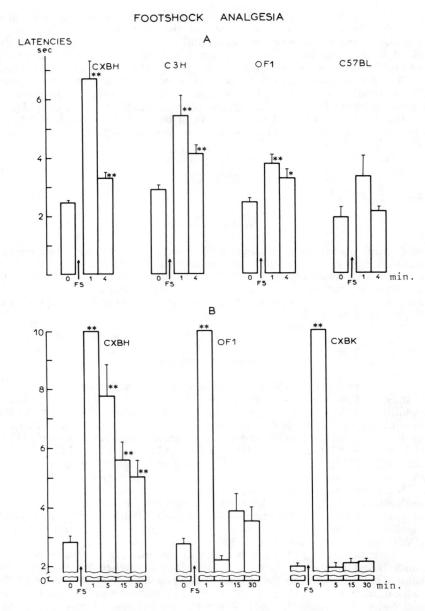

FIGURE 3. Footshock-induced analgesia in various strains of mice. (A) Footshock (FS) of 1 min duration and 0.25 mA intensity were delivered just after the control reading of tail-flick latencies (in sec) and latencies were measured again just after shock and 3 min later. Separate groups of 10 to 20 mice were used for each time interval. (B) The same as in (A) although the intensity of the stimulating current was 1 mA and more time intervals (as indicated in min) were studied, with separate groups of 10 to 20 mice each. Bars and asterisks as in FIGURE 2.

EFFECT OF NALOXONE ON FOOTSHOCK ANALGESIA

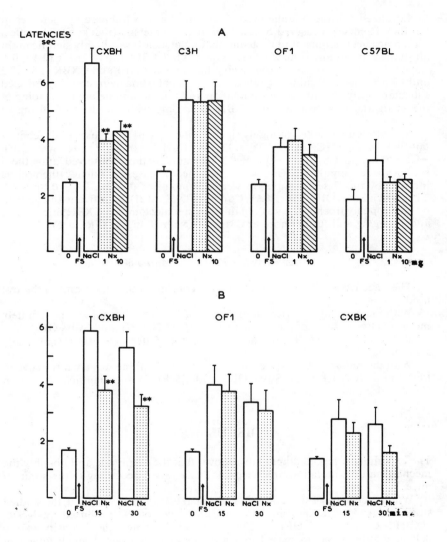

FIGURE 4. Effect of naloxone on footshock analgesia in various strains of mice. (A) Footshock (FS: 1 min at 0.25 mA) was delivered just after the control reading of tail flick latencies (O) and just before the second reading. Blank, dotted, and hatched columns correspond to mice of the various strains that received saline, naloxone HCl (1 mg/kg), or naloxone HCl (10 mg/kg), respectively, 15 min before. Groups of 10 to 20 mice. Bars: S.E. (B) The same as in (A) but the intensity of the footshock was 1 mA and the studied time intervals differed. The time indicated here refers to the beginning of the footshock. Saline or naloxone (1 mg/kg s.c.) was injected 14 min before footshock. Groups of 10 to 20 mice. Bars: S.E. Difference between naloxone-treated and saline controls significant for **$p = 0.01$ and *$p = 0.05$.

Localized Tail Stimulation Analgesia

Localized thermic stimulation of 7 sec duration was followed by increases in tail-flick latencies measured 5 min later at the same site (FIGURE 5). The effect (difference between pre- and post-stimulation latencies) was highly significant in all studied strains and somewhat greater in CXBH, C3H, and C57BL/6 (2.4 ± 0.3, 2.5 ± 0.4, and 2.6 ± 0.3 sec, respectively) than in Swiss OF1 and CXBK (1.8 ± 0.2 and 1.7 ± 0.26 sec). Significant antagonism with naloxone hydrochloride, injected subcutaneously 10 min before stimulation and thus 15 min before the reading of the analgesia, was observed in CXBH mice only with the dose of 10 mg/kg (FIGURE 6).

Spinalectomy resulted in highly significant ($p < 0.01$) decreases of the control tail-flick latencies (CXBH, −1.1 ± 0.135 sec; C3H, −1.09 ± 0.11 sec; Swiss OF1, −0.8 ± 0.1; and C57BL/6, −0.76 ± 0.2 sec) and of those observed after the 7 sec localized stimulation (FIGURE 5) but the increases of latency themselves induced by this 7 sec stimulation were not modified (CXBH, 2.4 ± 0.16; C3H, 2.11 ± 0.25; Swiss OF1, 1.76 ± 0.18; C57BL/6, 1.95 ± 0.21). Significant antagonism by naloxone hydrochloride was obtained in spinalectomized CXBH mice with 1 and 10 mg/kg and furthermore in C3H mice with 10 mg/kg (FIGURE 6).

Antinociceptive Effects of Morphine

The effectiveness of morphine varied according to the strain and to the test used (TABLE 1).

With the hot plate test (reaction: licking of the paw) morphine was definitely more effective in three of the studied strains (CXBH, C3H, and Swiss OF1) than in the other two (C57BL/6 and CXBK), the difference being statistically significant.

With the radiant heat test (reaction: tail flick) morphine was equally active in four strains (CXBH, C3H, Swiss OF1, and C57BL/6) and significantly less in CXBK mice only.

DISCUSSION

The experiments reported here have shown that the amplitude and possibly the mechanism of stimulation-produced analgesia varied according to the strain of mice.

When footshock of short duration (1 min at 0.25 mA) was applied, the studied strains ranked as follows in the decreasing order of the produced analgesia: CXBH > C3H > Swiss OF1 > C57BL/6. Similarly, when the intensity of the delivered stimuli was increased to 1 mA, the analgesia lasted much longer in CXBH than in Swiss OF1. This ranking was that observed for the latencies before jump when mice were placed on a hot plate.[9] It is worth noticing that the site of application of the stimuli (the sole of the feet) was the same in these two tests and under these conditions the relative importance of pain regulation (i.e., of increases in latency) thus appeared to vary similarly. The smaller responses of C57BL/6 and CXBK mice might be connected with a lesser development of the receptors and/or pathways triggered by morphine as these two strains responded less to the alkaloid than the other three strains when the hot plate test was used.

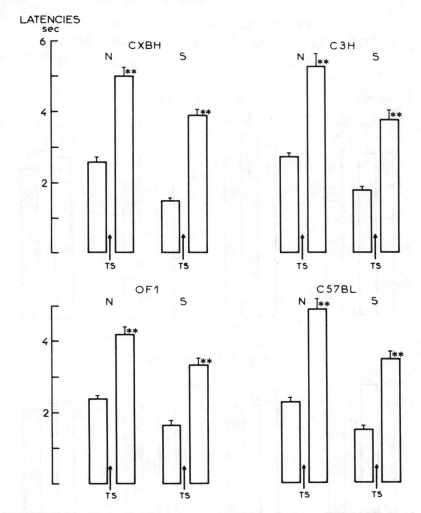

FIGURE 5. Localized tail stimulation analgesia in spinalectomized and non spinalectomized mice of different strains. Tail radiant heat stimulation (TS) was delivered during 7 sec just after control reading and 5 min before the second one. Latencies were measured and TS applied at the same site. N: normal, S: spinalectomized mice. Groups of 9 to 24 mice. Bars and asterisks as in FIGURE 2.

For CXBK mice, the small number of mu receptors might be relevant;[10-13] for C57BL/6 mice, serotoninergic pathways, mediating the morphine analgesia might be absent as it was shown that these mice, in contrast with C3H mice, did not respond to methoxy-5-dimethyl-N,N-tryptamine.[9] Further experiments are necessary to work out these hypotheses.

Clear-cut antagonism of footshock-induced analgesia with a relatively low

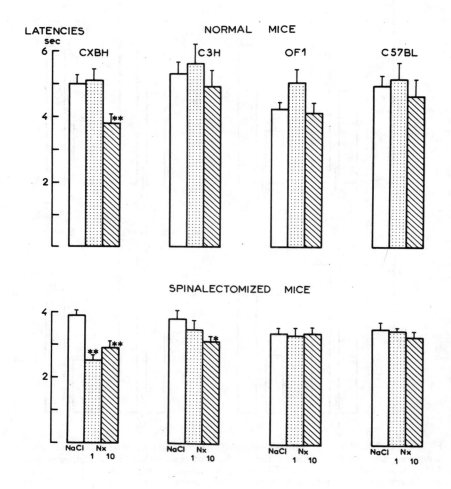

FIGURE 6. Effect of naloxone on tail localized stimulation analgesia (Above) normal mice and (Below) spinalectomized mice. The 7 sec tail radiant heat stimulation was applied 5 min before the determinations of latencies (in sec) at the same site. Blank, dotted, and hatched columns as in FIGURE 4. Saline or naloxone hydrochloride was administered 10 minutes before TS. Groups of 9 to 17 mice. Bars and asterisks as in FIGURE 4.

TABLE 1. AD_{50} (mg/kg s.c.) of Morphine in Various Strains of Mice

	Hot Plate Test	Radiant Heat Test
CXBH	2.25	3
	(1.55–3.3)	(1.8–5.1)
C3H	1.7	3
	(1.1–2.55)	(1.9–4.65)
SWISS OF1	1.3	3.1
	(0.68–2.47)	(2.1–4.65)
C57BL/6	14.2	2.20
	(10.9–18.5)	(1.2–4.1)
CXBK	9.5	> 10
	(6.8–13.3)	

AD_{50} were calculated by considering as under analgesia, each mouse whose latency exceeded the mean ± 2 standard deviations of the controls injected with saline. Nociceptive reactions were licking in the hot plate test and tail flick in the radiant heat test. The maximal effect was taken into account; it was reached 30 minutes after morphine injection; the controls are those measured 30 minutes after saline. Morphine was injected in graded doses to groups of at least 10 mice. Within parentheses: confidence limits for $p = 0.05$.

dose of naloxone (1 mg/kg s.c.) was observed only in CXBH mice whereas even with 10 mg of naloxone antagonisms were small, not statistically significant, or even completely lacking in the other strains. Non-opioidergic components are thus predominant in the footshock-induced analgesia observed in the strains other than CXBH but such a component also exists in this latter strain because 10 mg/kg of naloxone reduced but did not annihilate the footshock analgesia.

A second type of increase in latencies induced by painful stimuli was studied in this work; it can hardly be considered as a stress-induced analgesia because it was localized at the site of the tail where a radiant heat stimulation of 7 sec duration was applied. This characteristic differentiates it from the analgesia produced by the electrical stimulation of the tail in mice, which was not localized at the site of stimulation as it was measured with the hot plate test;[26] further, this latter phenomenon occurred just after stimulation while the one discussed in this work developed in 5 min.

The localized stimulation analgesia is not the mere result of local tissue destruction because it was readily reversible. Its amplitude was strain-dependent again but the genetic differences were not quite the same as those of footshock analgesia: C57BL/6 mice in particular responded as well as CXBH and C3H and OF_1 slightly less. Likewise, the responsiveness of the four strains CXBH, C3H, Swiss and C57BL/6 to morphine was almost the same when using the tail-flick test with radiant heat as stimulus, i.e. the same site of stimulation as for the production of the localized irradiation analgesia. This indicates that, in C57BL/6 mice at least, the pathways triggered by morphine to inhibit the tail-flick reaction are not the same as those involved in the hot plate test. According to the hypothesis suggested above, serotoninergic mediation should not be involved in the tail flick test as it is in the hot plate one. The localized tail stimulation analgesia was not modified by spinalectomy. Thus it is a spinal and (or) a peripheral phenomenon: The similarity between the ranking of the strains according to the analgesia induced by tail stimulation and morphine favors the view that the former is spinal but does not exclude a peripheral component. It should be noted that in normal mice an inhibitory descending tone also exists in all strains for the tail flick reaction as this latter was accelerated in spinalectomized animals.

Clear-cut antagonism of localized stimulation–induced analgesia by naloxone was observed only in CXBH mice, a high dose (10 mg/kg) having a small but statistically significant effect in C3H.

It might be mentioned that this localized analgesia has been searched for because in former experiments we observed that analgesia induced by morphine or other agents, including footshock, appeared to last longer when the same group of mice and not separate groups were used for the different time intervals, without taking care to measure the tail-flick latencies at different sites. The control values did not vary. We believe that the localized analgesia can superimpose itself on the increases of latencies (by drug or footshock), which result in sufficiently long exposure(s) even if a cut-off time prevents a local tissue destruction. A similar phenomenon was observed when the rat tail was completely immersed in hot water, though another interpretation was given.[27]

This localized analgesia might be an experimental model of the therapeutic local physical treatment of pain.

CONCLUSION

Genetic variations of the magnitude of footshock-induced analgesia have been observed using five strains of mice. They were related to their responsiveness to pain and partly to the effectiveness of morphine using the hot plate test, i.e., when the stimulus was also applied on the sole of the feet.

Genetic variations were not quite the same for the localized tail stimulation–induced analgesia. In this latter case, they correlated with the effectiveness of morphine when the method of D'Amour and Smith was used, i.e., when the stimulus was also applied on the same site of the tail. The circuitry is thus different for the two nociceptive testing methods and probably for the two types of stimulation-induced analgesia studied here.

In the two types of analgesia, an opioidergic component (as revealed by the use of naloxone) was clearly and significantly observed in one strain only (CXBH).

ACKNOWLEDGMENTS

We wish to thank Mr. M. Szatanik for his skilled technical assistance, Ms. D. Drouot for typing the manuscript. Naloxone hydrochloride was a generous gift from Du Pont de Nemours ((Dr. V. J. Nickolson).

REFERENCES

1. BODNAR, R. J., D. D. KELLY, M. BRUTUS & M. GLUSMAN. 1979. Stress-induced analgesia: neural and hormonal determinants. Neurosci. Biobehav. Rev. **4:**87–100.
2. VIDAL, C., J. M. GIRAULT & J. JACOB. 1982. The effect of pituitary removal on pain regulation in the rat. Brain Res. **233:**53–64.
3. LEWIS, J. W., J. T. CANNON & J. C. LIEBESKIND. 1980. Opioid and nonopioid mechanisms of stress analgesia. Science **208:**623–625.

4. TERMAN, G. W., Y. SHAVIT, J. W. LEWIS, J. T. CANNON & J. C. LIEBESKIND. 1984. Intrinsic mechanisms of pain inhibition: activation by stress. Science **226**:1270–1277.
5. WATKINS, L. R., D. A. COBELLI, P. FARIS, M. D. ACETO & D. J. MAYER. 1982. Opiate vs non-opiate footshock-induced analgesia (FSIA): the body region shocked is a critical factor. Brain Res. **242**:299–308.
6. MAIER, S. F., R. C. DRUGAN &. J. W. GRAU. 1982. Controllability, coping behavior, and stress-induced analgesia in the rat. Pain **12**:47–56.
7. JACOB, J. & C. BARTHELEMY. 1967. Réactivité nociceptive et sensibilité à la morphine de souris de diverses souches. Thérapie **22**:1435–1448.
8. MICHAUD, G., K. RAMABADRAN, J. C. ROUSSELLE & J. JACOB. 1981. Réactivité nociceptive, sensibilité à la naloxone, dépendance aiguë et récepteurs opioides chez des souris de différentes souches. J. Pharmacol. (Paris) **12**:83.
9. RAMABADRAN, K., G. MICHAUD & J. J. C. JACOB. 1982. Genetic influences on the control of nociceptive responses and precipitated abstinence in mice. Indian J. Exp. Biol. **20**:74–76.
10. BARAN, A., L. SHUSTER, B. E. ELEFTHERIOU & D. W. BAILEY. 1975. Opiate receptors in mice: genetic differences. Life Sci. **17**:633–640.
11. REGGIANI, A., F. BATTAINI, H. KOBAYASHI, P. SPANO & M. TRABUCCHI. 1980. Genotype-dependent sensitivity to morphine: role of different opiate receptor populations. Brain Res. **189**:289–294.
12. REITH, M. E. A., H. SERSHEN, C. VADASZ & A. LAJTHA. 1981. Strain differences in opiate receptors in mouse brain. Eur. J. Pharmacol. **74**:377–380.
13. JACOB, J., G. MICHAUD, M. A. NICOLA & N. PRUDHOMME. 1983. Genetic differences in opioids binding sites and in antinociceptive activities of morphine and ethylketo-cyclazocine. Life Sci. **33**(Suppl. I):645–648.
14. GEBHART, G. F. & C. L. MITCHELL. 1973. Strain differences in the analgesic response to morphine as measured on the hot plate. Arch. Int. Pharmacodyn. **201**:128–140.
15. OLIVERIO, A. & C. CASTELLANO. 1974. Genotype-dependent sensitivity and tolerance to morphine and heroin: dissociation between opiate-induced running and analgesia in the mouse. Psychopharmacologia (Berl.) **39**:13–22.
16. CASTELLANO, C. & A. OLIVERIO. 1975. A genetic analysis of morphine-induced running and analgesia in the mouse. Psychopharmacologia (Berl.) **41**:197–200.
17. SHUSTER, L., G. W. WEBSTER, G. YU & B. E. ELEFTHERIOU. 1975. A genetic analysis of the response to morphine in mice: analgesia and running. Psychopharmacologia (Berl.) **42**:249–254.
18. RACAGNI, G., F. BRUNO, E. JULIANO & R. PAOLETTI. 1979. Differential sensitivity to morphine-induced analgesia and motor activity in two inbred strains of mice: behavioral and biochemical correlations. J. Pharmacol. Exp. Ther. **209**:111–116.
19. HO, I. K., H. H. LOH & E. L. WAY. 1977. Morphine analgesia, tolerance and dependence in mice from different strains and vendors. J. Pharm. Pharmacol. **29**:583–584.
20. BRASE, D. A., H. H. LOH & E. L. WAY. 1977. Comparison of the effects of morphine on locomotor activity, analgesia and primary and protracted physical dependence in six mouse strains. J. Pharmacol. Exp. Ther. **201**:368–374.
21. PEETS, J. M. & B. POMERANZ. 1978. CXBK mice deficient in opiate receptors show poor electroacupuncture analgesia. Nature **273**:675–676.
22. CHENG, R. S. & B. POMERANZ. 1979. Correlation of genetic differences in endorphin systems with analgesic effects of D-aminoacids in mice. Brain Res. **177**:583–587.
23. D'AMOUR, F. E. & D. L. SMITH. 1941. A method for determining loss of pain sensation. J. Pharmacol. Exp. Ther. **72**:74–79.
24. JACOB, J. J. C. & K. RAMABADRAN. 1978. Enhancement of a nociceptive reaction by opioid antagonists in mice. Brit. J. Pharmacol. **64**:91–98.
25. LITCHFIELD, Jr., J. T. & F. WILCOXON. 1949. A simplified method of evaluating DOSE-EFFECT experiments. J. Pharmacol. Exp. Therap. **96**:99–113.
26. BUCKETT, W. R. 1981. Pharmacological studies on stimulation-produced analgesia in mice. Eur. J. Pharmacol. **69**:281–290.
27. COLPAERT, F. C., C. J. E. NIEMEGEERS, P. A. J. JANSSEN & A. N. MAROLI. 1980. The effects of prior fentanyl administration and of pain on fentanyl analgesia: Tolerance to and enhancement of narcotic analgesia. J. Pharmacol. Exp. Ther. **213**:418–424.

Altered Pain and Visual Sensitivity in Humans: The Effects of Acute and Chronic Stress[a]

W. CRAWFORD CLARK, JOSEPH C. YANG,
AND MALVIN N. JANAL

New York State Psychiatric Institute
and
Departments of Psychiatry and Anesthesiology
College of Physicians and Surgeons
Columbia University
New York, New York 10032

INTRODUCTION

Anecdotal evidence concerning the effect of stress on pain sensitivity has a surprisingly long history; James Clark Maxwell, the nineteenth century physicist, dabbled in many diverse subjects and according to Everitt[1] concerned himself with a physiological problem, namely, the athlete's endurance of pain. The physiological mechanisms responsible for stress-induced analgesia are becoming known in animals. However, we are still faced with the problem of discovering these mechanisms in man, an important task since there appear to be significant species differences.

Pain is difficult to define, but stress is even more so. Stress takes many forms and each of these often leads to quite different physiological responses. There is the stress of cognitive activity. There is emotional stress. There is the stress of violent activity, which, furthermore, leads to different psychophysiological responses in the victor and the vanquished. Then there is the stress of pain itself, with acute pain differing from chronic pain. Each of these stresses evokes different patterns of responses including behavioral, cardiovascular, intestinal, immunologic, and endocrinologic changes, any of which may influence the response to noxious stimulation.

The studies to be discussed here involve the effect of various stresses on experimentally contrived ischemic, cold-pressor, and thermal pain, the latter measured by sensory decision theory (SDT) methodology. Experiments on the sensory effects of the following stressors will be discussed: (1) acute exercise stress, (2) acute pain stress produced by electrical stimulation, (3) chronic stress related to clinical pain, (4) chronic stress related to mental illness, and (5) acute stress produced by cold-pressor pain (the last study being on visual, not painful responses).

Various studies have shown that different forms of stress reduce the number of

[a]Supported in part by U.S. Public Health Service Grants NIGM-26461, MH 30906, and NS-09263.

pain reports to calibrated noxious stimulation. It is not clear, however, whether this reflects a true hypoalgesic effect involving an attenuation of neurosensory input or a change in the subjects' expectations and attitude towards reporting pain. Only SDT can answer this question. It alone provides two quantitative measures of perceptual performance: sensory discriminability and psychological report bias. The index of discriminability (d′ or P(A), for the parametric and non-parametric models, respectively) measures the accuracy with which an individual distinguishes amongst stimuli of various intensities. For example, it is possible in the binary decision procedure to score the subjects' responses as right or wrong. No other psychophysical procedure possesses such an accuracy indicator. The discriminability index of sensory performance has been demonstrated to be essentially uninfluenced by changes in nonsensory variables such as the subjects' expectation, mood, motivation, and attitude. The discriminability index is related to the functioning of the neurosensory system: high values (associated with low error rates) suggest that neurosensory functioning is normal and that the information travels unimpeded to higher centers, and low values (associated with high error rates) indicate that the amount of information transmitted has been reduced. Analgesic agents such as morphine, nitrous oxide, and codeine have been shown to lower discriminability and to raise the pain report criterion.

The other measure of perceptual performance, the report criterion, (Lx or B, for the parametric and non-parametric models, respectively) measures response bias, that is, the willingness or reluctance of a subject to use a particular sensory response. The criterion is related to the subject's attitude towards the sensory experience. For pain a high criterion reflects stoicism, while a low criterion indicates that pain is readily reported. The criterion has been shown to be influenced by nonsensory variables such as placebos, direct and indirect suggestion, age, ethnocultural differences, etc. Of the various psychophysical procedures used to study pain, only SDT yields separate quantitative measures that can be so readily identified with the separate neurosensory and emotional components of pain. In contrast, pain thresholds obtained by classical psychophysical procedures have been shown to be unanalyzable mixtures of sensory sensitivity and attitudinal report bias, and thus cannot be trusted as indices of sensory functioning. Clark[2] and McNicol[3] have provided introductions to parametric and non-parametric SDT methods, respectively. Applications of SDT to pain research have been reviewed by Clark and Yang.[4]

EXERCISE STRESS

The effects of intense exercise on pain perception, mood, and plasma endocrine levels in man under naloxone and saline conditions has been described in detail by Janal *et al.*[5] The study involved both chronic and acute exercise stress, since the subjects were in training for the New York City Marathon and regularly ran 40 miles per week.

Methods

Twelve long-distance runners were evaluated by thermal, ischemic, and cold pressor pain tests and on visual analogue mood scales. Blood was drawn for determination of plasma endocrine levels before the pain testing began. These procedures were undertaken before and after a 6.3 mile run at 85% of maximal aerobic capacity. Subjects participated on two occasions in a double-blind procedure counterbalanced for drug order. After the post-run blood was drawn, they received two intravenous (i.v.) injections 20 minutes apart; on one day the injection was naloxone (0.8 mg each dose), on the other day it was normal saline.

Each subject was randomly assigned to a different order of the pain and mood tests. Thus, four separate groups were formed: three subjects received the thermal test first, three received it second, three received it third, and three received it fourth; the same was true of the other pain tests and mood scales. The same order was used pre- and post-run and on each of the two test days. Test lag refers to the time period (20, 30, 40, 50 min) in which a particular test was administered.

Thermal Pain Test

Radiant heat stimuli of 0, 50, 340, and 390 millicalories/sec/cm^2 (mcal) were presented by a subject-held Hardy-Wolff-Goodell dolorimeter. The stimulus duration was 3 sec unless the subject withdrew his arm. The 2 cm diameter heat stimuli, 12 at each intensity, were presented randomly to three patches of India ink applied to the volar surface of each forearm. Subjects rated the intensity of each stimulus on a scale that ranged from nothing through various amounts of heat and pain to withdrawal. Data were treated to yield the non-parametric SDT indices, P(A) and B, and the parametric index, Lx, as described by McNicol.[3]

Thermal discriminability, P(A), was sharply reduced for the noxious (340–390 mcal) stimulus pair, but not for the weaker intensities, when measured within 20 minutes after the run. Thus, there was hypoalgesia without anesthesia, which lasted approximately 20 minutes. The reduction in P(A) represents a relatively strong analgesic effect, equal to that of 10 mg of i.v. morphine.[6] This exercise-induced analgesia was found only within 20 min after the run and failed to appear in those runners whose response to thermal stimulation was tested at 30, 40, and 50 min post-run. No significant changes in the pain report criterion (B and log Lx) were found. Naloxone was without effect on any of the SDT indices.

Ischemic Pain Test

After expressing the venous blood, an automatic tourniquet was inflated to 250 torr and the subject squeezed a hand dynamometer 20 times. The subject then reported his sensory experience every 10 sec using a scale ranging from nothing through strong but not painful sensation to various intensities of pain. Subjects were asked to tolerate the tourniquet for as long as possible, the maximum time being 15 minutes. On the saline day the tourniquet ischemic pain test showed decreased reports of pain—a hypoalgesic effect—20 minutes post-run and increased reports of pain 30 minutes post-run. There were no significant differences between pre-run and post-run values on measures obtained 40 and 50 minutes after the run. Naloxone reversed the exercise-induced hypoalgesia.

Cold-Pressor Test

The subject immersed his hand up to the wrist in an ice water bath and was instructed to tolerate the pain as long as possible, the maximum time allowed being 3 min. During this immersion the subject gave reports of his sensations using a scale ranging from warm through cool, and various amounts of pain. The cold-pressor test failed to show post-run hypoalgesia or naloxone effects.

Mood Tests

Mood was assessed using visual analogue scales (VAS). The three "elation" scales had stems of "Emotionally, I feel _____," followed, respectively, by these poles on the VAS: depressed—euphoric; regretful—joyful; pleasant—miserable. Other scales were designed to measure anxiety, alertness, cooperativeness, etc. The euphoria and joy scales showed an increase in positive affect 30 and 40 min after the run. The improvement in positive mood did not appear on the naloxone day. Scales designed to assess cooperation, e.g., I am pleased that I volunteered for this study, also increased in the positive direction. However, it is worth noting that unlike the elation scales, improvement in cooperativeness was not reversed by naloxone. Ratings of anxiety, energy, and fatigue were not affected by the run.

Endocrine Assays

All plasma endocrine levels were significantly increased by the run: prolactin (PRL), β-endorphin (BEir), and adrenocorticotrophic hormone (ACTH) were approximately doubled, while growth hormone (GH) increased four fold. However, neither of the pre-run pain measures nor post-run change scores correlated with either initial levels or post-run changes in levels of any of the plasma endocrines. The same was true of the mood and cooperativeness measures. Cohen et al.[7] reported that both presurgery and during surgery plasma β-endorphin levels predicted post-operative morphine requirement. Contrary to our results, their findings suggests a close relationship between plasma levels of β-endorphin and the amount of pain experienced. Obviously, the stress and pain encountered differed, but no simple explanation for the discrepancy between the studies is apparent.

Conclusions

Under the saline condition, discriminability of thermal stimuli was reduced post-run. Reduced discriminability is indicative of reduced sensory input and is not caused by a shift in attitude towards reporting pain. The raised pain report criterion usually found with a decrease in sensitivity did not appear; this is probably due to its greater variability relative to P(A) and the small number of subjects. The ischemic tourniquet test also showed post-run hypoalgesia under the saline condition. The duration of both thermal and ischemic hypoalgesic effects was approximately 20 min post-run. This convergence of data from two independent tests of pain sensitivity supports the hypothesis that intense exercise produces hypoalgesia. Two of the findings suggest that surface (thermal) and deep (ischemic) pain sensations are mediated by different mechanisms. First, the post-run hypoalgesia found with saline was reversed by naloxone for ischemic, but not for thermal pain, suggesting that endogenous opioid mechanisms are involved in the modulation of the deep but not the cutaneous pain system. Second, under saline conditions hypoalgesia for the ischemic stimulation was followed by hyperalgesia; no hyperalgesia was observed for the thermal stimuli. This result suggests that a rebound hypersensitivity is present in opioid but not non-opioid antinociceptive systems.

It is not clear why the cold-pressor test failed to show post-run hypoalgesia. The lack of cold pressor effect does, however, argue against attributing post-run changes in pain perception of the heat and ischemic stimuli to changes in thermoregulation and vascular tone. If increased circulation and body temperature were to cause a hypoalgesic effect it would most likely appear on the cold pressor test. Since it did not, it seems unlikely that hypoalgesia was due to vascular or thermoregulatory changes.

Joy, euphoria, and cooperativeness scale ratings were elevated post-run under saline treatment. This effect was reversed by naloxone for the positive affect scales but not for the cooperativeness scales, a result consistent with mediation of mood elevation by an endogenous opioid system. While all subjects were familiar with runner's high, and some with the possibility of a run-induced hypoalgesia, there are a number of reasons for concluding that the results were not due to the effect of expectation. First, neither hypoalgesia nor euphoria were found under the naloxone condition. Since, at the dose used, there are no subjective effects that could break the double-blind control, it is improbable that the subjects could have selectively reduced their pain reports only under the saline condition. Second, an expectation hypothesis would predict a reduced pain report and improved mood at all test lags; this certainly was not found.

ACUTE PAIN STRESS PRODUCED BY ELECTRICAL STIMULATION

Pain itself is stressful and arousing and like exercise could be expected to produce analgesia. The results of two experiments that used SDT to study the effects of electrically induced pain on the perception of thermal stimuli are of interest here. The acupuncture study[8] avoided the stimulation of major nerve trunks, while the transcutaneous electrical nerve stimulation (TENS) study[9] involved stimulation of the median nerve. The dependent measures on both of these studies were thermal discriminability (d') and the pain report criterion (Lx).

Method

In both the acupuncture and TENS studies, 12 thermal stimuli were presented at each of six intensities: 0, 120, 240, 305, 370, and 425 mcal. The rating task and the stimulus conditions were similar to those described earlier. The stimuli were applied to the volar surface of each forearm (acupuncture) or to the palmar aspect of the thumb and lateral two fingers innervated by the median nerve in each hand (TENS). Twelve subjects served in each experiment. SDT measures were obtained before, during, and after the extraneous painful stimulation. The direct comparison of these two procedures has been reported by Clark *et al.*[9]

Acupuncture Study

The acupuncture study has been described in detail by Clark and Yang.[8] The six acupuncture sites and duration of the electrical stimulation were standard for surgery of the arm. The intensity of the electrical stimuli was set to a level of just bearable pain. Thermal testing was done before, during (15–20 min), and after acupuncture; one arm received the acupuncture needles, the other served as a control.

Analysis of variance for thermal discriminability (d') revealed no differences between the acupunctured and control arms, nor between the before, during, and after acupuncture periods (TABLE 1). Thus, the results demonstrated that neither the acupuncture nor the pain associated with it produced hypoalgesia. The subjects did set a significantly higher very faint pain report criterion (Lx = 1.35, fewer reports of pain) in the acupunctured arm during the acupuncture period only. However, the pain report criterion for stimuli applied to the control arm during this time was not altered. Thus, even this possible index of analgesia failed to show a stress effect. Apparently, the subjects' expectation that only the acupunctured arm should show an analgesic effect influenced their pain report. It may be concluded that cutaneous electrical pain does not induce analgesia to thermal simulation. Furthermore, there is no evidence of post-acupuncture hypoalgesia from either the discriminability or the criterion measures. This is important, since the presence of post-stimulation analgesia together with suprasegmental effects from accepted acupuncture sites constitute the two defining characteristics of an acupuncture effect. Comments and replies on various aspects of the study have appeared.[9]

TENS Study

The TENS study has been described in detail by Clark *et al.*[9] Electrode sites at the volar surface of the left wrist (cathode) and the left upper arm (anode) were stimulated until the pain was just bearable and paresthesias and slight muscle

TABLE 1. Effect of Acupuncture on Thermal Discriminability (d') and the Criterion for Reporting Very Faint Pain or Higher (Lvfp)

Period	Pre	During	Post
		Mean d'	
Control arm	1.37	1.40	1.37
Acupunctured arm	1.36	1.35	1.40
		Mean Lvfp	
Control arm	.72	.62	1.49
Acupunctured arm	.99	1.35	1.03

twitching occurred in the region of the hand innervated by the median nerve. After the initial thermal test period, the median nerve was stimulated transcutaneously for 20 minutes while thermal testing continued. The transcutaneous stimulation was then stopped and thermal testing continued for two additional 15 min periods (Post-1 and Post-2). The limb was partially enclosed in a heated electrical blanket to maintain a constant skin temperature, since preliminary observations revealed that the electrical stimulation decreased the temperature of the hand, presumably because sympathetic vasomotor fibers were stimulated.

The TENS stimulation significantly reduced discriminability (d') from 1.58 to 1.23 (TABLE 2). Discriminability on the control hand did not decrease. Thus, the decreased discriminability was segmental, since there was no general loss in sensitivity as might have been caused by distraction. Nor was there any post-stimulus hypoalgesia. An important point is the demonstration that the SDT procedure as used is capable of detecting a sensory loss. This strengthens the conclusion that acupuncture does not induce a sensory loss (i.e., hypoalgesia).

The criterion for reporting very faint pain did not change throughout the experiment for the non-stimulated hand. However, the TENS hand showed a sharply increased pain report criterion (fewer pain reports) during the TENS stimulation. This increase was far greater than that produced by acupuncture. The increase in criterion coupled with the decrease in d' demonstrates an analgesic effect that lasted during, but did not persist after, the TENS stimulation. Thus, in contrast to the exercise study results, which demonstrated the presence of 20 minutes of stress-induced analgesia, neither the pain due to acupuncture nor the pain caused by specific nerve stimulation produced post-stimulation analgesia. The thermal sensory loss during stimulation appears to be due to the direct inhibition of pain fibers by the tetanic stimulation.

EFFECTS OF CHRONIC STRESS AND CHRONIC PAIN

Patients suffering any type of persisting illness may be considered to be under chronic stress. Sensory decision methodology has been used with thermal stimulation to study two such patient populations. Clark and Mehl[11] studied hospitalized psychiatric patients who were suffering mental stress, but not pain, and Yang et al.[12] studied chronic back pain patients who were suffering pain-induced stress as well as considerable mental stress caused by unemployment, family discord, etc.

TABLE 2. Effect of Transcutaneous Electrical Nerve Stimulation on Thermal Discriminability (d') and the Criterion for Reporting Very Faint Pain or Higher (Lvfp)

Period	Pre	During	Post-1	Post-2
	Mean d'			
Control hand	1.68	1.51	1.51	1.63
TENS hand	1.58	1.23	1.55	1.68
		Mean Lvfp		
Control hand	.70	.63	.78	.69
TENS hand	.63	1.38	.80	.85

Psychiatric Patients

Methods

The 64 psychiatric patients were diagnosed as schizophrenic, affective disorders, and other. The age and sex-matched normal volunteers were college students, nurses, and hospital maintenance personnel. As described earlier, the Hardy-Wolff-Goodell dolorimeter was used to present radiant heat stimuli to the volar surface of the nonpreferred forearm. The stimulus intensities were 0, 75, 150, 225, 270, 300, and 330 mcal. There were sixteen stimuli at each intensity, a total of 96. The subjects rated the stimuli along a 10-point scale from "Nothing" through various degrees of "Heat" and "Pain" to "Withdrawal."

Results

ANOVAs for repeated measures with subjects nested within classification, age and sex were performed separately for d' and log Lx. With respect to sensory sensitivity (d'), the analysis revealed a significant interaction for stimulus intensity by group ($F = 3.42$, df $= 4/480$, $p < .01$). Accordingly, separate analyses of variance were performed on data obtained at the noxious intensities of 300 and 330 mcal and the detection intensities of 0 and 75 mcal. As can be seen in TABLE 3, patients were less able to discriminate between the noxious intensities than were the controls ($F = 7.22$, df $= 1/120$, $p < .01$). However, the groups did not differ at the detection of warmth intensities.

Separate analyses of variance for the patient subgroups revealed that discriminability and report criterion were not affected by either medication (no psychotropic drug, $N = 21$; major tranquilizers, $N = 25$; and anti-depressants, $N = 10$) or by diagnosis (schizophrenics, $N = 31$; affective disorders, $N = 24$; and other, $N = 9$).

A separate analysis of variance was performed on the logarithmically transformed likelihood ratio for the criterion very faint pain and above, Lvfp. Since the ANOVA revealed a significant interaction for stimulus intensity by group ($F = 5.11$, df $= 4/480$, $p < .05$) separate analyses were performed for the detection criterion for presence of a stimulus at 0–75 mcal and for the very faint pain criterion at 300–330 mcal (TABLE 3). At the noxious stimulus intensities, patients set a much higher (i.e., more stoical) criterion for pain than controls

TABLE 3. Responses of Psychiatric Patients and Normal Controls to Low and Noxious Intensities of Thermal Stimulation (Ld, Criterion for Detection)

	0–75 mcal		300–330 mcal	
	d'	Ld	d'	Lvfp
Psychiatric patients	1.16	1.32	.80	1.49
Normal controls	1.07	1.09	1.20	.89

(F = 13.58, df = 1/120, p < .01). The patients and normals did not differ with respect to where they located their detection criterion.

Discussion

Patients were less able to discriminate between the noxious stimulus intensities than were controls; this suggests that the emotional stress of psychiatric illness interferes with the sensory systems mediating pain. The possibility that psychotropic medication decreased the patient's ability to discriminate the noxious intensities is eliminated by the fact that no difference was found between patients who received drugs and those who did not. These results are generally supported by Davis and Buchsbaum[13] who, using SDT methodology, found poor discriminability to electrical stimuli and a high pain report criterion in affectively ill (manic and depressed) and schizophrenic patients.

The mechanism(s) causing the sensory losses in both mental illness and chronic pain are complex and not well understood. However, activation of the limbic-hypothalamic-pituitary-adrenal (LHPA) axis appears to be important. The following LHPA axis dysfunctions have been reported in depressed patients: adrenal cortisol hypersecretion, flattened cortisol circadian periodicity, failure of dexamethasone to suppress plasma cortisol concentrations, as well as increased ACTH levels (perhaps mediated by cholinergic mechanisms). Following this line of thought, Risch et al.[14] demonstrated that plasma β-endorphin, like ACTH and cortisol, is elevated in depressed patients.

Chronic Back Pain Patients

The response of chronic back pain patients to thermal stimulation has been studied by Yang et al.[12] by means of SDT. These patients undergo emotional and physical stress in addition to experiencing pain. Chronic back patients, most of whom suffer almost continuous pain, reveal psychological symptomatology (particularly depression) on the Derogatis Brief Symptom Inventory. It seems possible that pain stress might induce analgesia to thermal stimulation similar to that found in the acutely stressed runners and in the continuously stressed depressed patients.

Methods

The subjects were 55 outpatients and 47 healthy volunteers matched for age and sex. The patients suffered chronic low back pain for a period of at least six months caused by herniated lumbar discs, myofascial syndrome, or osteoarthritis. The thermal pain methods were similar to those described previously. Eight stimuli were randomly presented at intensities of 0, 100, 340, and 390 mcal for the patients and at 0, 50, 340, and 390 mcal for the volunteers. It was necessary to use 50 rather than 100 mcal in the volunteer group because of their enormously greater sensitivity to weak stimuli (most detected the 100 mcal stimuli 100% of the time).

Results

The results appear in TABLE 4. Analysis of variance revealed that the chronic pain patients had much poorer discriminability, P(A), than the volunteers for the 340–390 mcal stimulus pair ($F(1,96) = 31.61$, $p < 0.001$). Patients were also markedly poorer discriminators at the lower stimulus intensity pair, since their ability to detect a 100 mcal increment was comparable to the volunteers' ability to detect a 50 mcal increment. The chronic pain patients demonstrated a significantly higher criterion (fewer pain reports) for the 340–390 mcal pair of stimuli ($F(1,96) = 18.45$, $p < 0.001$). The mean value of B was equal to 8.2 for the chronic pain patients, which is in the "Very Faintly Painful" region, while the mean value of B was 6.1 for volunteers, which is in the "Painful" region of the pain scale. Neither the magnitude of the clinical pain of the patients as measured by a visual analogue pain scale nor the type of pain medication (narcotic, psychotropic, nonnarcotic analgesic) taken over the previous two weeks correlated significantly with the thermal SDT indices, P(A) and B.

The chronic pain patients' sensory loss to thermal stimulation was extreme, being greater than that produced by 10 mg of i.v. morphine administered to healthy volunteers, and much greater than that of the psychiatric patients and runners reported earlier. The hypoalgesia found is paradoxical, since one might expect the failure of endogenous mechanisms to control clinical pain to be coupled with a parallel failure to ameliorate experimental pain, that is, high P(A) and low B. The occurrence of experimental pain hypoalgesia in the presence of clinical hyperalgesia suggests that the endogenous analgesic mechanisms have been triggered, but that a segmental failure of mechanisms mediating the clinical pain exists. It is also of interest that those patients who suffered the greatest stress and pain according to the SDT measures at intake had the worst prognosis. The causes of these segmental differences—hyperalgesia at the affected site and hypoalgesia elsewhere—deserves further study at a physiological level.

An interesting difference between the psychiatric patients and the chronic back patients appears in differences in the patterns of discrimination loss at the detection and noxious intensity levels. The psychiatric patients revealed a moderate loss at noxious intensities, but no loss at detection intensities. In contrast, the chronic pain patients showed a marked loss in discriminability at both high and low intensities. Thus the psychiatric patients demonstrated analgesia, that is, a loss in pain sensitivity without a loss in the other somatic sensations, while the chronic pain patients demonstrated anesthesia, that is, a loss

TABLE 4. Mean for Thermal Discriminability, P(A), and Criterion, B, for Chronic Pain Patients and Healthy Volunteers

Thermal Intensity Pair (mcal)	Discriminability P(A) Patients	Volunteers	Criterion B Patients	Volunteers
340–390	0.69	0.83	8.26	6.14
0–100	0.71		12.49	
0–50		0.65		12.32

in sensitivity to the entire spectrum of somatosensory input. Hypoalgesia is often found with centrally acting substances such as morphine, while anesthesia is found with peripheral nerve blocks, e.g. carbocaine.[8] This suggests the possibility that the hypoalgesic mechanisms evoked by the stress of psychiatric illness differs from those evoked by the stress of chronic pain.

Atkinson et al.[15] found chronic pain patients to have the highest plasma levels of β-endorphin; they were followed by a group of psychiatric patients, who in turn had higher levels than healthy controls. Thus, the plasma levels found in these three groups paralleled the amount of thermal hypoalgesia found in our chronic pain, psychiatric illness, and healthy volunteer groups. Accordingly, hypoalgesia appears to reflect levels of central nervous system arousal in response to combinations of stress and pain.

EFFECT OF COLD-PRESSOR PAIN ON VISION AND MEMORY

Is the effect of stress restricted to the somatosensory system, or are other sensory modalities and cognitive functions also affected? To answer these questions Clark et al.[16] studied the effect of painful cold-pressor stress on visual discriminability and short-term memory. Cold-pressor stress produced by immersion of the hand in ice water elicits a complex response of local and general vasoconstriction mediated by sympathetic adrenergic fibers, reflex bradycardia, and the release of catecholamines, vasopressin, angiotensin, adrenocortical hormones, and other substances into the circulation. The purpose of this study was to examine the effect of the cold-pressor response on visual sensitivity and short-term memory.

Method

Measures of visual sensitivity were obtained on 12 healthy college students during and immediately after ice-water immersion and during a control session. The subjects viewed a fixation point with their right eye through a 2 mm artificial pupil to control for stress-induced sympathetic effects on pupil size. The four-alternative spatial forced-choice task used is a type of SDT procedure that yields values of d', but no measure of the report criterion. The task of the subject was to locate the quadrant containing a black dot subtending five seconds of arc, which was presented tachistoscopically against a white background of 10 ft lamberts. Control and experimental sessions were counterbalanced for order effects and separated by a 5 minute recovery period. In the experimental session the subject immersed his hand in ice water and commenced the forced-choice visual detection task. The mean immersion time before withdrawal was 58.4 seconds. The detection task continued without interruption for 30 seconds after the hand was withdrawn (first recovery period). This was followed by a rest period of 60 seconds, and a second visual task period of 30 seconds (second recovery period). The control session followed the same sequence, but with the immersion water at room temperature. Within each session the immersions were repeated, alternating hands, until data had been collected for a total of 10 minutes. Thus, there were approximately 10 immersions. The average number of visual observations was 150 during immersion and 75 during each of the two recovery periods. Pain reports commenced about 10 seconds after the beginning of the immersion. Pain disappeared within 5 to 10 seconds after withdrawal.

Results

The mean percent success rate converted to values of d′ appears in TABLE 5. The values of d′ under the immersion conditions are equivalent to a success rate (corrected for chance) of 68% for control and 56% for the ice-water treatment. A repeated-measure, three-way analysis of variance with subjects nested within order revealed a significant main effect between the stress and the control treatments ($F(1,10) = 33.05$, $p < .001$), as well as amongst the immersion and recovery periods ($F(2,20) = 17.83$, $p < .001$), with sensitivity during immersion being significantly less than either of the two recovery periods, t-critical (20) > .12, $p < .01$. Comparisons between treatments within each period revealed that sensitivity was significantly less under the stress condition, t-critical (40) > .17; $p < .01$. Within the stressed group sensitivity was less during immersion than during either recovery period, and within the control group sensitivity during immersion was slightly less than during the second recovery period, t-critical (30) > .14; $p < .01$. There were no order effects for session, that is, subjects who received the stress condition first did not show a subsequent decline on the control condition 5 minutes later. Thus the reduced visual sensitivity lasted no longer than 8 minutes following ice-water immersion.

Discussion

Cold-pressor stress decreased visual sensitivity for a period of at least 3 but not more than 8 min following the termination of the cold-pressor pain. Mild retinal ischemia following vasoconstriction mediated by sympathetic adrenergic fibers appears to be the most likely mechanism for the sensory loss. Although there is very little sympathetic input to the retinal blood vessels themselves, the central retinal artery has an ample supply of adrenergic fibers. Consideration must also be given to the effect of cold-pressor stress on the sympathetic-adrenal medullary system causing secretion into the circulation of adrenaline and noradrenaline, and on the LHPA axis with the possible increase in the secretion of cortisol and other substances. Henkin[17] has pointed out that patients with Cushing's syndrome exhibit excessive adrenal secretion of carbohydrate-active steroids, and have high olfactory, auditory, and proprioceptive thresholds. Henkin suggests that carbohydrate-active steroids influence neural transmission times and hence sensory thresholds. Sandman et al.[18] studied subjects given an infusion of melanocyte-stimulating hormone and adrenocorticotropic hormone 4-10. They found decreased detection sensitivity for a dot presented tachistoscopically. Thus, stress-induced changes in these or related substances may be responsible for raised visual and perhaps pain thresholds.

TABLE 5. Effect of Cold Pressor Stress on Visual Sensitivity (Mean d′)

	Period		
Condition	Immersion (60 sec)	Recovery-1 (60–90 sec)	Recovery-2 (150–180 sec)
Control session	1.71	1.82	1.88
Stress session	1.34	1.56	1.65

Certain other explanations of the visual loss may be eliminated. Pain causes pupil dilation by inhibiting sphincter tone and possibly slightly relaxing the ciliary muscle controlling accommodation. However, in the present study the artificial pupil controlled for possible changes in pupil size. The slight relaxation towards far vision that may have occurred could have formed a diffusion image; however, because of spatial summation effects (Ricco's Law) blurred diffusion circles from an object subtending only 5 sec of arc would not alter its threshold.[19] It may be concluded that stress-induced changes in the optics of the eye cannot account for the results obtained.

Another possible consequence of cold-pressor response is an alteration in cognitive functioning. On the one hand, one might expect impaired decision-making ability, perhaps brought about by the constriction of cerebral blood vessels, to interfere with visual performance. On the other hand, Weingartner *et al.*[20] have shown that arginine vasopressin (which probably is released by cold-pressor pain) improves human learning and memory. To examine this question, a subsequent short-term memory experiment was conducted. The experimental design just described for the visual study, that is, ice versus warm water conditions and pre, post-1, and post-2 periods, was used. The subjects' task was to memorize a list of 11 random digits. Since it takes three to five repetitions to memorize the list, it places a burden on short-term memory. The supra-digit span memory performance was not affected by the cold-pressor stress. Thus, it may be concluded that the sensory loss is not due to changes in pupil size nor accommodation, nor to centrally mediated cognitive changes. The most likely explanation of the visual loss appears to be stress-induced vasoconstriction of the central retinal artery (and perhaps the arteries of the retina) via sympathetic adrenergic neurons, although changes in the pituitary-adrenal system, including the release of vasopressin cannot be eliminated.

SUMMARY

In the runner study, as measured by tourniquet ischemic pain, exercise stress produced hypoalgesia 20 minutes post-run, followed by hyperalgesia and euphoria at 30 minutes. The hypoalgesia and euphoria were reversed by naloxone. Exercise stress also produced a decrease in P(A), suggesting hypoalgesia to the thermal cutaneous stimulation. However, this analgesia was not naloxone reversible. Nor did exercise stress produce analgesia to cold-pressor pain. In the acupuncture study, noxious electrical stimulation of classical acupuncture sites failed to produce analgesia either during or after stimulation. However, expectation did produce a change in the pain report criterion, but only in the acupunctured arm. Noxious electrical stimulation (TENS) of the median nerve produced no analgesia outside of the related segmental area, that is, acute electrical pain did not produce generalized hypoalgesia. Thus, the effects of the stress produced by noxious electrical stimulation differ from that produced by exercise. In contrast to the results of the acute pain studies, chronic clinical pain, which combines mental stress and pain stress, produced strong hypoalgesia and anesthesia. Again, in contrast to the acute experimental pain studies, the emotional stress of mental illness produces hypoalgesia, but not anesthesia. Finally, the somatosensory system is not the only the sensory system affected by stress. Cold-pressor pain decreases visual sensitivity both during and for a few minutes following stimulation, and does not interfere with short-term (supra-digit span) memory.

REFERENCES

1. EVERITT, C. W. F. 1983. *In* Springs of Scientific Creativity: Essays on Founders of Modern Science. R. Aris, T. Davis & R. H. Stuewer, Eds.: 111. University of Minnesota Press. Minneapolis, MN.

2. CLARK, W. C. 1974. Pain sensitivity and the report of pain: An introduction to sensory decision theory. Anesthesiology **40**:272–287.

3. MCNICOL, D. 1972. A Primer of Signal Detection Theory. George Allen & Unwin. London, England.

4. CLARK, W. C. & J. C. YANG. 1983. Applications of sensory decision theory to problems in laboratory and clinical pain. *In* Pain Measurement and Assessment. R. Melzack, Ed.: 15–25. Raven Press. New York.

5. JANAL, M. N., E. W. D. COLT, W. C. CLARK & M. GLUSMAN. 1984. Pain sensitivity, mood and plasma endocrine levels in man following long-distance running: Effects of naloxone. Pain **19**:13–25.

6. YANG, J. C., W. C. CLARK, S. H. NGAI, B. A. BERKOWITZ & S. SPECTOR. 1979. Analgesic action and pharmacokinetics of morphine and diazepam in man: An evaluation by sensory decision theory. Anesthesiology **51**:495–502.

7. COHEN, M. R., D. PICKAR, M. DUBOIS & W. E. BUNNEY. 1982. Stress-induced plasma beta-endorphin immunoreactivity may predict postoperative morphine usage. Psychiatry Res. **6**:7–12.

8. CLARK, W. C. & J. C. YANG. 1974. Acupunctural analgesia? Evaluation by signal detection theory. Science **184**:1096–1098.

9. CLARK, W. C., W. HALL & J. C. YANG. 1976. Changes in thermal discriminability and pain report criterion after acupunctural or transcutaneous electrical stimulation. *In* Advances in Pain Research and Therapy. J. J. Bonica & D. Albe-Fessard, Eds. **1**:769–773. Raven Press. New York.

10. CLARK, W. C., J. C. YANG & W. HALL. 1975. Acupuncture, pain and signal detection theory. Science **189**:66–68.

11. CLARK, W. C. & L. MEHL. 1976. Thermal pain: Sensory (d') and criterion (Lx) differences between psychiatric patients and normals. 21st International Congress of Psychology. Paris, France.

12. YANG, J. C., D. RICHLIN, L. BRAND, J. WAGNER & W. C. CLARK. 1985. Thermal sensory decision theory indices and pain threshold in chronic pain patients and healthy volunteers. Psychosomatic Med. **47**:461–468.

13. DAVIS, G. C. & M. S. BUCHSBAUM. 1981. Pain sensitivity and endorphins in functional psychoses. Modern Problems Pharmacopsych. **17**:97–108.

14. RISCH, S. C., D. S. JANOWSKY, L. L. JUDD, J. C. GILLAN & S. F. MCCLURE. 1983. The role of endogenous opioid systems in neuroendocrine regulation. Psychiatric Clinics North America **6**:429–441.

15. ATKINSON, J. H., E. F. KREMER, S. C. RISCH, C. D. MORGAN, R. F. AZAD, C. L. EHLERS & F. E. BLOOM. 1983. Plasma measures of beta-endorphin/beta-lipotropin-like immunoreactivity in chronic pain syndrome and psychiatric subjects. Psychiatry Res. **9**:319–327.

16. CLARK, W. C., D. SCHIMMEL, D. BLENDINGER & M. N. JANAL. 1981. Effect of cold-pressor stress on visual sensitivity, d' in man. Soc. Neurosci. **7**:869.

17. HENKIN, R. I. 1970. The neuroendocrine control of perception. *In* Perception and its Disorders. Proceedings of the Association for Research in Nervous and Mental Diseases. D. A. Hamburg, K. H. Pribram & A. J. Stunkard, Eds.:54–107. Williams & Wilkins. Baltimore, MD.

18. SANDMAN, C. A., J. GEORGE, T. R. MCCANNE, J. D. NOLAN, J. KASEWAN & A. J. KASTIN. 1977. MSH/ACTH 4-10 influences behavioral and physiological measures of attention. J. Clin. Endocrinol. Metab. **44**:884–890.

19. ADLER, F. H. 1953. Physiology of the Eye: Clinical Application. C. V. Mosby. St. Louis, MO.

20. WEINGARTNER, H., P. GOLD, J. C. BALLENGER, S. A. SMALLBERG, R. SUMMERS, D. R. RUBINOW, R. M. POST & F. K. GOODWIN. 1981. Effects of vasopressin on human memory functions. Science **211**:601–603.

Multiple Morphine and Enkephalin Receptors: Biochemical and Pharmacological Aspects

GAVRIL W. PASTERNAK[a]

The Cotzias Laboratory of Neuro-Oncology
Memorial Sloan-Kettering Cancer Center
and
Departments of Neurology and Pharmacology
Cornell University Medical College
New York, New York 10021

INTRODUCTION

The past decade has seen enormous advances in our understanding of opiate action. Like most hormones and neurotransmitters, opiates produce their actions through specific recognition sites, or receptors. One of the most important concepts in opiate research to emerge over the past few years has been the presence of multiple classes of these sites. Martin and co-workers[1] proposed three classes of opiates based upon studies on the chronic spinal dog and named them according to prototypic drugs: mu (morphine), kappa (ketocyclazocine), and sigma (SKF10,047). Shortly after the isolation and identification of the enkephalins, receptors selective for these (delta) peptides were proposed.[2-4] Since then, a major effort has been made to identify, localize, and characterize these proposed selective binding sites (TABLE 1). The two most extensively studied types include the mu (morphine) and delta (enkephalin) receptors.

MORPHINE AND ENKEPHALIN: MU AND DELTA RECEPTORS

The pharmacological properties of opiates, including their rigid structure-activity relationships, their strict stereospecificity, and the existence of highly specific antagonists such as naloxone, led pharmacologists to suggest the existence of specific opiate recognition sites, or receptors, long before their biochemical demonstration in binding assays. The demonstration of these opiate binding sites quickly prompted a search for naturally occurring opioid substances. These studies soon led to the discovery of the enkephalins, pentapeptides differing only in their last amino acid (try-gly-gly-phe-leu and tyr-gly-gly-phe-met). These two peptides have many pharmacological characteristics similar to those of the classical opiate alkaloids. Like morphine, the intracerebroventricular administration of the enkephalins and some of their more stable derivatives produced

---

[a]Address correspondence to: Dr. G. W. Pasternak, Dept. of Neurology, Memorial Sloan-Kettering Cancer Center, 1275 York Avenue, New York, NY 10021.

TABLE 1. Tentative Classification of Opioid Receptors

Subtype	Ligand Selectivity
Mu	
Mu$_1$	Opiates and enkephalins
Mu$_2$	Morphine
Delta	Enkephalin
Kappa	Ketocyclazocine
Sigma	SKF10, 047 (N-allylnormetazocine)
Epsilon	β-Endorphin

naloxone-reversible analgesia in several different types of animal antinociceptive assays, demonstrating the similarities between these endogenous peptides and morphine, the classic opiate analgesic.[5]

However, a number of important differences soon became apparent. The ability of opiates to inhibit the contractions of the electrically stimulated guinea pig ileum had long been used as a screening test. As expected, early experiments with the enkephalins demonstrated a similar inhibition of these contractions, which was effectively antagonized by naloxone. Similar results were seen in another peripheral bioassay system, the mouse vas deferens. However, detailed studies comparing the potency of the enkephalins to morphine in these two peripheral bioassay systems demonstrated different rank orders of potency.[2] In the guinea pig ileum assay morphine was more than seven fold more effective than the enkephalins, while the reverse was found in the mouse vas deferens. In addition, unlike analgesia, the actions of morphine and the enkephalins did not show extensive cross-tolerance in these peripheral bioassays.[6] Based upon these findings, receptors selective for either morphine (mu) or the enkephalins (delta) were proposed.[2]

Binding studies in rat brain homogenates confirmed the existence of selective morphine (mu) and enkephalin (delta) sites.[3,4] Although the binding of opiate alkaloids, such as radiolabeled dihydromorphine and naloxone, could be displaced by the enkephalins, the peptides were far less potent than classical opiates such as morphine. On the other hand, radiolabeled enkephalin binding was inhibited far more easily by enkephalins than by opiates such as morphine, suggesting sites selective for either morphine or the enkephalins. Regional differences in the distribution of these morphine-selective and enkephalin-selective sites were also described.[2] Detailed autoradiographic studies permitting a far more accurate localization of the various binding sites strongly supported these regional differences.[7]

MULTIPLE MU RECEPTORS

Recently, we proposed that in addition to their selective sites, morphine and the enkephalins also interact with very high affinity to a common site, which we termed mu$_1$ in distinction to the morphine-selective (mu$_2$) and enkephalin (delta)-selective sites (FIGURE 1).[8] Evidence for the existence of this site, first described in 1975 as the "high affinity" binding site,[9] comes from a variety of experimental approaches.

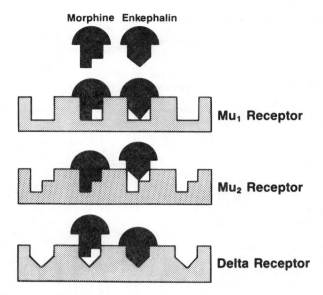

FIGURE 1. Schematic of morphine and enkephalin binding sites. (From Goodman and Pasternak.[22] With permission from the *Proceedings of the National Academy of Sciences*.)

Analysis of saturation studies of radiolabeled opiates and enkephalins revealed high ($K_D < 1$ nM) and low affinity (K_D 1–15 nM) binding components.[3,8-14] At first, it was thought that these binding components might represent mu and delta sites; that is, the higher affinity enkephalin component, representing delta sites, corresponded to the lower affinity morphine component and vice versa. However, other binding studies implied that this was not the case. Naloxazone, a long-acting antagonist, selectively inhibited the high affinity binding component of a large series of radiolabeled mu (morphine and dihydromorphine), kappa (ethylketocyclazocine and Mr2034), sigma (SKF10,047) opiates, enkephalins (met-enkephalin, leu-enkephalin, D-ala-met-enkephalinamide, and D-ala-D-leu-enkephalin), β-endorphin, and antagonists (naloxone and naltrexone), suggesting a common high affinity binding component for these various classes of opiates and opioid peptides.[8,12-18] Furthermore, the loss of the high affinity component of both agonist and antagonist binding implied that this high affinity component did not simply represent conformational shifts between agonist and antagonist forms of a single binding site.

Competition studies provided another approach to this question. As noted above, comparisons of the overall potency of morphine-like compounds and the enkephalins in the inhibition of radiolabeled opiates and enkephalins demonstrated selective sites for the enkephalins and morphine. However, detailed competition studies revealed multiphasic competition curves, suggesting that both types of radiolabeled drugs were binding to more than one class of site. For example, Chang and Cuatrecasas reported that a portion of radiolabeled enkephalin binding was potently displaced by low morphine concentrations

(IC$_{50}$ value 0.31 ± 0.14 nM) while the remainder of the enkephalin binding required far higher morphine concentrations (IC$_{50}$ value 47 ± 12 nm).[3] These results implied that the enkephalins bound to both mu and delta sites. In similar studies, naloxazone-treatment eliminated the morphine-sensitive binding of radiolabeled enkephalins (FIGURE 2), implying that the high affinity binding component of radiolabeled enkephalins corresponds to a mu binding site.[8,13]

These findings were supported by saturation studies performed with radiolabeled enkephalins in which the higher affinity component of binding was more potently inhibited by low morphine concentrations (FIGURE 3). Similarly, saturation studies of the mu compound [^{3}H]dihydromorphine showed that it was inhibited more potently by the enkephalins that its lower affinity sites.[13] Together, these results were most easily explained by a common high affinity binding site for both opiate and opioid peptides.

The evidence for selective sites for morphine and enkephalins was quite strong. How did the concept of a common high affinity binding site for both opiates and enkephalin fit with these selective sites? The lower affinity binding components of [^{3}H]morphine (K_D 8–11 nM) and [^{3}H][D-ala^2,-D-leu^5]enkephalin (K_D 4–8 nM) were relatively resistant to naloxazone's actions. Could these lower affinity sites correspond to the selective sites? In tissue whose high affinity sites had been blocked with naloxazone, opiates selectively inhibited the binding of the mu ligand [^{3}H]dihydromorphine while the enkephalins preferentially in-

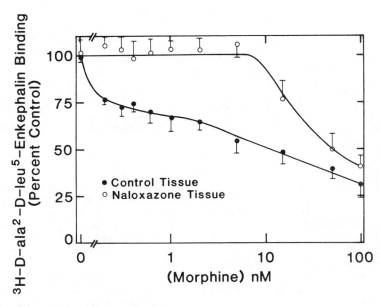

FIGURE 2. Competition of radiolabeled enkephalin binding by morphine. Rat brain homogenates were prepared and treated with either nothing (closed circles) or naloxazone (open circles) and assayed with [^{3}H][D-ala^2,D-leu^5]enkephalin at 1 nM and the stated concentrations of morphine. (From Wolozin and Pasternak.[8] With permission from the *Proceedings of the National Academy of Sciences.*)

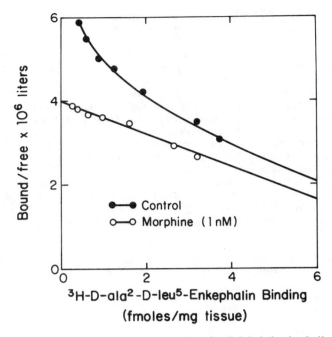

FIGURE 3. Scatchard analysis of saturation studies of radiolabeled enkephalin binding in the absence and presence of morphine. Rat brain homogenates were prepared and incubated with [^{3}H][D-ala^2,D-leu^5]enkephalin (0.04 to 2.7 nM) in the absence and presence of morphine (1 nM). Computer analysis of the binding curves revealed two components for the control curve: (1) K_D 0.6 nM with a B_{max} of 1.9 fmoles/mg tissue and (2) K_D 3.2 nM with a B_{max} of 9.2 fmoles/mg tissue. In the presence of morphine the curve was best fit as a single line with an apparent K_D 2.5 nM and B_{max} 9.9 fmoles/mg tissue. Note that as a competitive inhibitor, morphine does not eliminate sites; it merely lowers the apparent affinity of those sites which bind the morphine. (From Nishimura et al.[13] With permission from *Molecular Pharmacology*.)

hibited [^{3}H][D-ala^2,-D-leu^5]enkephalin (delta) binding. For example, morphine lowered the binding of the radiolabeled mu ligand (IC$_{50}$ 11 ± 0.7 nM) far better than the delta one (IC$_{50}$ 89 ± 32 nM). The reversed selectivity was observed for D-ala-D-leu-enkephalin displacements of [^{3}H]dihydromorphine (IC$_{50}$ 64 ± 7.4 nM) and [^{3}H][D-ala^2,D-leu^5]enkephalin (IC$_{50}$ 10 ± 1.2 nM). Thus, the lower affinity binding components (K_D < 10 nM) possessed the same selectivity towards opiates or peptides as previously described.

Together, these results suggested three classes of morphine and enkephalin binding sites.[8,13] We proposed naming the common high affinity site for opiates and enkephalins mu$_1$, since many of mu characteristics of the enkephalins might be explained by this site. The morphine-selective site was termed mu$_2$ while the enkephalin-selective site corresponded to the previously defined delta site.

The essential difference between this hypothesis and previous ones rested upon the existence of a distinct high affinity, or mu$_1$, binding site in addition to the selective sites. Additional binding studies examining the developmental appearance of the various sites,[19] their phylogenetic distribution,[20] their biochemical properties,[13] and their regional distribution within the brain by both homogenate binding assays[21] and autoradiography[22] supported the existence of mu_1 sites.

ANALGESIA

The selectivity of the peripheral bioassays for various classes of compounds provided a powerful tool in the demonstration of multiple populations of opioid receptors. Correlating receptor subtypes with pharmacological actions in the central nervous system (CNS) have proven far more difficult due to its vast complexity and the lack of highly selective ligands. On the basis of early studies, Martin proposed that mu receptors mediated analgesia.[1] Studies from our laboratory now implicate mu_1, not mu_2, sites in these analgesic actions.[12,14-18,23] Blockade of the mu_1 (high affinity) sites in vivo with naloxazone markedly lowered the analgesic potency of mu (morphine), kappa (ketocyclazocine and ethylketocyclazocine), and sigma (SKF10,047) opiates, as well as several enkephalins, [D-ala^2,met^5]enkephalin, [D-ala^2,met^5]enkephalinamide, and [D-ala^2,D-leu^5]enkephalin) and β-endorphin. Naloxonazine produced similar decreases in morphine's analgesic potency in the tail-flick assay in rats, shifting the dose-response curve four fold to the right (FIGURE 4). Thus, the mu_1 sites clearly played a role in opiate and opioid peptide analgesia.

The above studies strongly suggested a role for the mu_1 sites in opioid analgesia, but could another opioid receptor also be involved with analgesia? Based upon several studies investigating the interactions of nalorphine and morphine, Martin suggested a number of years ago that opioid analgesia was mediated by two types of receptors, a concept he termed "receptor dualism."[24] Much evidence now supports an analgesic role for delta sites,[25,26] including studies with naloxazone.[27] Although mu_1 blockade lowered the analgesic potency of opiates and opioid peptides, compounds potent at delta receptors were affected far less than drugs less active at delta sites. Delta analgesia appears to be particularly important at the level of the spinal cord. Direct administration of opiates and opioid peptides intrathecally elicited analgesia. However, delta compounds were far more active than mu drugs. Similar results were reported using a spinal transection model.[27] Kappa sites in the spinal cord have also been shown in rats to mediate analgesia.[28]

RESPIRATORY DEPRESSION

Respiratory depression is a serious side-effect of narcotic use.[24] It remains the primary cause of mortality in overdosed patients and results from a decrease in the medullary center's ability to respond to increasing CO_2 levels.[29] Obviously, a major question is whether the receptor mediating this serious adverse side-effect also mediates analgesia or whether different receptor subtypes are involved. A number of groups have suggested different receptor mechanisms.[30-32] More detailed studies have ruled out a role of mu_1 sites in respiratory depression (FIGURE 4) and have suggested that mu_2 sites might mediate this action.[33,34] Developmental studies also dissociated analgesic and respiratory depression, demonstrating a much later development of analgesic response to morphine, β-endorphin, and enkephalins than their respiratory depressant actions.[19]

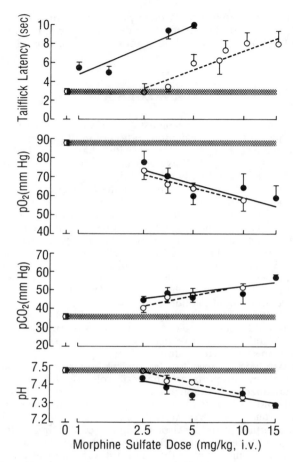

FIGURE 4. Effects of naloxonazine on morphine analgesia and respiratory depression. Rats were treated with either saline (closed circles) or naloxonazine (10 mg/kg, i.v.; open circles) and then tested for analgesia with the tailflick assay (top) or respiratory depression using arterial blood gases (bottom three). Peak values ± S.E.M. are given. The dose response curve for morphine analgesia is shifted four-fold by the naloxonazine treatment ($p < 0.001$) while the blood gas curves were not shifted at all. Hatched areas are the baseline values. (From Ling *et al.*[34] With permission from the *Journal of Pharmacology and Experimental Therapeutics.*)

OTHER OPIOID ACTIONS

The role of mu_1 receptors have also been studied in other systems (TABLE 2).[35-40] Opioids also have a number of actions on the endocrine system, particularly prolactin and growth hormone release. Morphine releases both hormones, but through different opiate receptors. Studies using mu_1-selective antagonists clearly

TABLE 2. Tentative Classification of Mu$_1$ Receptor Actions

Mu$_1$ Mediated	Not Mu$_1$ Mediated
Supraspinal analgesia	Spinal analgesia (delta/kappa)
Catalepsy	Respiratory depression (mu$_2$)
Prolactin release	Growth hormone release
Acetylcholine turnover	Dopamine turnover
Feeding (free and food	Deoxyglucose-induced feeding
deprivation)	Sedation (kappa)
	Guinea pig ileum bioassay
	Most signs of physical dependence

demonstrated the role of mu$_1$ sites in prolactin but not growth hormone release.[35] The further classification of other opiate receptor subtypes in the hormonal control needs to be explored more fully.

Work in rats and mice suggested mu and kappa site involvement in opioid inhibition of gastrointestinal motility, an important clinical side-effect of opioid use.[35] At the level of the gut, mu$_2$ rather than mu$_1$ sites appear to be important.[36] Also, recent work has demonstrated the lack of mu$_1$ involvement in the development of many of the signs of physical dependence in the rat.[37] The contribution of other receptor subtypes has not yet been fully investigated.

CONCLUSION

The discovery of multiple opiate receptor subtypes has had major implications in all aspects of opiate pharmacology. The demonstration that analgesia is probably mediated by more than one receptor type, for example, illustrates the complexity of the opioid system. The understanding of these alternative opioid analgesic systems will almost certainly have a major impact on the development and use of analgesics.

Multiple opiate receptors will also be important in other opiate actions. Pharmacologists have long attempted to synthesize analgesics lacking undesirable actions, such as respiratory depression and dependence. The existence of multiple classes of opiate receptors has brought this possibility closer to reality.

Many questions remain, including such basic ones as the identification of the endogenous ligand for the mu$_2$ site. Much work remains before we will completely understand the full physiological and pharmacological implications of opioid receptors.

REFERENCES

1. MARTIN, W. R., C. G. EADES, J. A. THOMPSON, R. E. HUPPLER & P. E. GILBERT. 1976. The effects of morphine- and nalorphine-like drugs in the nondependent and morphine-dependent chronic spinal dog. J. Pharmacol. Exp. Therap. 197:517–532.
2. LORD, J. H., A. A. WATERFIELD, J. HUGHES & H. W. KOSTERLITZ. 1977. Endogenous opioid peptides: multiple agonists and receptors. Nature 267:495–499.

3. CHANG, K. -J. & P. CUATRECASAS. 1979. Multiple opiate receptors: enkephalins and morphine bind to receptors of different specificity. J. Biol. Chem. **254**:2610–2618.
4. CHANG, K. -J., B. R. COOPER, E. HAZUM & P. CUATRECASAS. 1979. Multiple opiate receptors: different regional distribution in the brain and differential binding of opiates and opioid peptides. Molec. Pharmacol. **16**:91–104.
5. BELLUZZI, J. D., N. GRANT, V. GARSKY, D. SARANTAKES, C. D. WISE & L. STEIN. 1976. Analgesia induced in vivo by central administration of enkephalin in the rat. Nature **260**:625–626.
6. SCHULZ, R., M. WUSTER, H. KRENS & A. HERZ. 1980. Selective development of tolerance without dependence in multiple opiate receptors of mouse vas deferens. Nature **285**:242–243.
7. GOODMAN, R. R., S. H. SNYDER, M. J. KUHAR & W. S. YOUNG. 1980. Differentiation of delta and mu opiate receptor localizations by light microscopic autoradiography. Proc. Natl. Acad. Sci. USA **77**:6239–6243.
8. WOLOZIN, B. L. & G. W. PASTERNAK. 1981. Classification of multiple morphine and enkephalin binding sites in the central nervous system. Proc. Natl. Acad. Sci. USA **78**:6181–6185.
9. PASTERNAK, G. W. & S. H. SNYDER. 1975. Identification of novel high affinity opiate receptor binding in rat brain. Nature **253**:563–565.
10. LUTZ, R. A., R. A. CRUCIANI, T. COSTA, P. J. MUNSON & D. RODBARD. 1984. Biochem. Biophys. Res. Commun. **12**:265–269.
11. TOLL, L., C. KEYS, W. POLGAR & G. LOEW. 1984. Neuropeptides **5**:205–208.
12. HAZUM, E., K.-J. CHANG, P. CUATRECASAS & G. W. PASTERNAK. 1981. Naloxazone irreversibly inhibits the high affinity binding of $[^{125}I]$D-ala^2-D-leu^5-enkephalin. Life Sci. **28**:2973–2979.
13. NISHIMURA, S. L., L. D. RECHT & G. W. PASTERNAK. 1984. Biochemical characterization of high affinty ^{3}H-opioid binding: further evidence for mu$_1$ sites. Mol. Pharmacol. **25**:29–37.
14. PASTERNAK, G. W. 1980. Multiple opiate receptors: [^{3}H]Ethylketocyclazocine receptor binding and ketocyclazocine analgesia. Proc. Natl. Acad. Sci. USA **77**:3691–3694.
15. PASTERNAK, G. W., S. R. CHILDERS & S. H. SNYDER. 1980. Naloxazone, a long-acting opiate antagonist: effects in intact animals and on opiate receptor binding in vitro. J. Pharmacol. Exp. Ther. **214**:455–462.
16. PASTERNAK, G. W., S. R. CHILDERS & S. H. SNYDER. 1980. Opiate analgesia: evidence for mediation by a subpopulation of opiate receptors. Science **208**:514–516.
17. ZHANG, A. - Z. & G. W. PASTERNAK. 1981. Opiates and enkephalins: a common binding site mediates their analgesic actions in rats. Life Sci. **29**:843–851.
18. PASTERNAK, G. W., M. CARROL-BUATTI & K. SPIEGEL. 1981. The binding and analgesic properties of sigma opiate, SKF 10, 047. J. Pharmacol. Exp. Therap. **219**:192–198.
19. ZHANG, A. - Z. & G. W. PASTERNAK. 1981. Ontogeny of opioid pharmacology and receptors: high and low affinity site differences. Eur. J. Pharmacol. **73**:29–40.
20. BUATTI, M. C. & G. W. PASTERNAK. 1981. Multiple opiate receptors: phylogenetic differences. Brain Res. **218**:400–405.
21. ZHANG, A. -Z. & G. W. PASTERNAK. 1980. Mu and delta- opiate receptors: correlation with high and low affinity opiate binding sites. Eur. J. Pharmacol. **67**:323–324.
22. GOODMAN, R. R. & G. W. PASTERNAK. 1985. Visualization of mu$_1$ opiate receptors in rat brain using a computerized autoradiographic subtraction technique. Proc. Natl. Acad. Sci. USA **82**:6667–6671.
23. PASTERNAK, G. W. 1981. Opiate, enkephalin and endorphin analgesia: relations to a single subpopulation of opiate receptors. Neurology **31**:1311–1315.
24. MARTIN, W. R. 1967. Opioid antagonists. Pharmacol. Rev. **19**:463–521.
25. FREDERICKSON, R. C. A., E. L. SMITHWICK, R. SHUMAN & K. G. BEMIS. 1981. Metkephamid, a systematically active analog of methionine enkephalin with potent opioid delta receptor activity. Science **211**:603–605.
26. YAKSH, T. L., S. P. HUANG, T. A. RUDY & R. C. A. FREDERICKSON. 1977. The direct and specific opiate-like effect of met-enkephalin and analogs on the spinal cord. Neuroscience **2**:593–596.
27. LING, G. S. F. & G. W. PASTERNAK. 1983. Spinal and supraspinal analgesia in the

mouse: the role of subpopulations of opioid binding sites. Brain Res. **271**:152–156.

28. WOOD, P. L., A. RACKHAM & J. RICHARD. 1981. Spinal analgesia: Comparison of mu agonist morphine and the kappa agonist ethylketocyclazocine. Life Sci. **28**:2119–2125.

29. BORISON, H. 1971. The nervous system. *In* Narcotic Drugs: Biochemical Pharmacology. D. H. Clouet, Ed.:342–365. Plenum Press. New York.

30. SMITH, A., R. ALBIN & M. CROFFORD. 1976. Heterogeneity of receptors for analgesia, respiration, and lenticular effect. *In* Opiate and Endogenous Opioid Peptides. H. W. Kosterlitz, Ed.:289–294. Elsevier/North Holland Biomedical Press. Amersterdam.

31. MCGILLIARD, K. L. & A. E. TAKEMORI. 1978. Antagonism by naloxone of narcotic-induced respiratory depression and analgesia. J. Pharmacol. Exp. Therap. **207a**:494–503.

32. PAZOS, A. & J. FLOREZ. 1983. Interaction of naloxazone with mu and delta opioid agonists on the respiration of rats. Eur. J. Pharmacol. **87**:309–314.

33. LING, G. S. F., K. SPIEGEL, S. NISHIMURA & G. W. PASTERNAK. 1983. Dissociation of morphine's analgesic and respiratory depressant actions. Eur. J. Pharmacol. **86**:487–488.

34. LING, G. S. F., K. SPIEGEL, S. H. LOCKHART & G. W. PASTERNAK. 1985. Separation of opioid analgesia from respiratory depression: evidence for different receptor mechanisms. J. Pharmacol. Exp. Ther. **232**:149–155.

35. SPIEGEL, K., I. KOURIDES & G. W. PASTERNAK. 1982. Prolactin and growth hormone release by morphine in the rat: different mechanisms. Science **217**:745–747.

36. GINTZLER, A. R. & G. W. PASTERNAK. 1983. Multiple mu receptors: evidence for mu_2 sites in the guinea pig ileum. Neurosci. Lett. **9**:51–56.

37. LING, G. S. F., J. M. MCLEOD, S. LEE, S. LOCKHART & G. W. PASTERNAK. 1984. Separation of morphine analgesia from physical dependence. Science **226**:462–464.

38. WOOD, P. L., J. W. RICHARD & M. THAKUR. 1982. Mu opiate isoreceptors: differentiation with kappa agonists. Life Sci. **31**:2313–2317.

39. WOOD, P. L. & G. W. PASTERNAK. 1983. Specific mu_1 opioid isoreceptor regulation of nigrostriatal neurons: in vivo evidence with naloxonazine. Neuroscience Lett. **37**:291–293.

40. HOLADAY, J. W. & G. W. PASTERNAK. 1983. Naloxazone pretreatment modifies cardiorespiratory and behavioral effects of morphine. Neurosci. Lett. **37**:199–204.

The Many Possible Roles of Opioids and Related Peptides in Stress-Induced Analgesia[a]

HUDA AKIL, ELIZABETH YOUNG,
J. MICHAEL WALKER,[b] AND STANLEY J. WATSON

Mental Health Research Institute
Department of Psychiatry
University of Michigan
Ann Arbor, Michigan 48109

[b]*Psychology Department*
Brown University
Providence, Rhode Island 02912

The potential role of opioids in analgesic brain mechanisms has consistently been a matter of debate. In the last decade, the debate has shifted from whether there are opioid mechanisms of analgesia to the exact nature of these opioid mechanisms. In this, as in many other cases of biology meeting psychology, the task is made more arduous by the intrinsic and well known difficulties inherent in studying pain on the one hand, and by the newly discovered complexities of opioid biology on the other.

We shall discuss the role of opioids in pain regulation in general, and then report on some specific effects of stress on pituitary and brain opioids. In the first section, we shall briefly describe the potential role of two endogenous opioid families in pain modulation. The two families, pro-opiomelanocortin and pro-dynorphin, produce distinctly different effects on pain responsiveness, may interact with varying opioid and non-opioid receptors in brain, have unique hormonal roles of potential importance to stress and coping, and contain non-opioid peptides also capable of modulating pain. In contrasting them, we hope to reveal to the reader the range of possible roles that these two families may play in pain regulation in general and in stress-induced analgesia in particular. This is not to say that pro-enkephalin products are not relevant to this discussion. We are not considering them here primarily because they are likely to be even more complex in their roles, in view of their widespread anatomy and of the presence of seven distinct opioid cores within their precursor.

The second section of the paper will be concerned with the actual effect of stress on β-endorphin and related peptides in pituitary and in brain. In this section, we shall not attempt to prove that β-endorphin is the key to opioid stress–induced analgesia. Rather, we hope to convey to the reader the importance of understanding the cell biology and its regulatory dynamics in attempting to link

[a]Supported by National Institute of Drug Abuse Grants DA02265 and DA00254, and by the Theophile Raphael Fund. E. Young is the recipient of Research Career Development Award #MH00427.

this or any opioid peptide to the production of stress-induced analgesia. Our efforts to understand the β-endorphin stress interface have led to some insights into regulatory strategies of peptidergic systems, and point to possible new approaches in studying the problem. The discussion, therefore, is more specu-lative and future oriented as it focuses on these possible directions.

PRO-OPIOMELANOCORTIN AND PRO-DYNORPHIN PRODUCTS: OPIOID AND NON-OPIOID EFFECTS ON PAIN RESPONSIVENESS

The existence of three opioid precursors was fully established in 1982, when the full sequences of the pro-hormones for pro-opiomelanocortin, the enkephalins, and dynorphins/alpha neo-endorphin were established using recombinant DNA tools that elucidated the messenger RNA structure.[1,2] The first precursor that had been elucidated was pro-ACTH/β-endorphin otherwise known as pro-opiomelanocortin or POMC.[3] The structures of the precursors, their homologies, detailed anatomy, and post-translational processing have been recently re-viewed.[4]

For the purposes of the present discussion, we remind the reader that POMC contains the full sequence of ACTH (adrenocorticotropin hormone), as well as that of β-endorphin 1–31, and three repeats of the ACTH 4–10 core. POMC is present in the pituitary anterior lobe corticotrophs, in every cell of the pituitary intermediate lobe, and in two distinct cells in the brain. The major cell group is in the hypothalamic arcuate nucleus, projecting rostrally to the septal area and caudally through medial thalamus to the midbrain central grey. The smaller cell group, found in the nucleus tractus solitarius (NTS), was first described by Schwartzberg and Nakane[5] and confirmed by a number of groups.[6] Its projectional pathways rostrally and caudally are yet to be fully described.

Pro-dynorphin contains three active opioid cores all beginning with the leucine-enkephalin sequence followed by unique carboxy-terminal extensions. The three opioid sequences are known as neo-endorphin,[7] dynorphin A,[8] and dynorphin B or rimorphin.[9,10] Pro-dynorphin is expressed in multiple cell groups in the brain including several associated with pain-modulating structures, such as the dorsal horn of the spinal cord, the periaqueductal grey area, and cortex. Pro-dynorphin is also found in the magnocellular hypothalamic groups that synthesize vasopressin, project to the posterior lobe of the pituitary, and modulate anterior lobe corticotrophs (those same cells that make and release POMC). The anatomy of pro-dynorphin and its comparison to pro-enkephalin were also summarized.[6]

Pro-Opiomelanocortin and Analgesia

Electrical Stimulation of Brain POMC Systems

Of the numerous naturally including opioids (over twelve identified forms in brain), β-endorphin produces the most clear-cut and longest lasting opiate analgesia. Its analgesic potency is evident with the unmodified peptide, requiring no efforts to stabilize it against enzymatic degradation *in vivo*. This observation, coupled with the fact that POMC pathways course along classical limbic and pain-modulating structures (e.g. medial thalamus and periaqueductal grey area), has led us and others to focus on the potential role of β-endorphin in endogenous analgesia.

One of the most obvious questions is whether electrical stimulation of β-endorphin systems in the brain produces analgesia. The results are interestingly mixed. Electrical stimulation along the midbrain POMC bundle produces profound analgesia, which is partially reversible by naloxone. Indeed, the overlap between that bundle and the independently described sites for stimulation-produced analgesia is quite remarkable.[11] However, stimulation of the arcuate cell group does not produce analgesia, a finding that remains unexplained. More recently, we have found that electrical stimulation of the nucleus tractus solitarius, a structure which expresses all three opioid precursors, produces clear-cut, naloxone-reversible analgesia (Lewis et al., in preparation). Whether this is due to the sole action of POMC products or to a combination of opioids released from this structure remains to be determined.

The Many POMC-Derived Peptides in Brain

While a potential role for β-endorphin in modulating nociception is easy to accept, the question arises as to the possible functions of the peptides that are co-synthesized with β-endorphin. As mentioned above, the precursor codes for ACTH and for a 16,000 dalton amino-terminal peptide that contains a structural homology with ACTH 4–10. The region of the N-terminal peptide that contains this homology has been termed gamma-MSH. Do ACTH and gamma-MSH play a role in nociception? While apparently simple, this question is closely related to the issue of post-translational processing of POMC in brain. It is well known that the same precursor, POMC, gives rise to distinctly different peptide products depending on the cells that express it. Thus, in the anterior lobe, the precursor yields β-endorphin 1–31, ACTH, and the full N-terminal protein. In the intermediate lobe, however, these products are further modified to yield shorter, more processed peptides with unique biological activities, such as the opiate-inactive N-acetyl-β-endorphin 1–27, and the ACTH product alpha-MSH, which is devoid of steroidogenic activity.[4]

Thus, the issue of the potential role of brain POMC products in brain is closely intertwined with the question of what is really made in the brain by the POMC neurons. Unfortunately, the answers are not all in on this question. It is becoming clear that N-acetylation of β-endorphin occurs only to a small extent in the hypothalamus and along the arcuate projection pathway (H. Akil, unpublished data). On the other hand, β-endorphin 1–31 becomes converted to β-endorphin 1–27 quite actively, with more conversion becoming evident as one proceeds from hypothalamus to central grey regions. In the midbrain, there are almost equal parts of β-endorphin 1–31 to β-endorphin 1–27 (H. Akil, unpublished data).[12,13] It should be noted that β-endorphin 1–27 is still an active opioid although its affinity at the mu and delta opiate receptors is appoximately ten times lower than is seen with β-endorphin 1–31.[14] Furthermore, its analgesic activity is also substantially decreased relative to β-endorphin 1–31.[15]

Within the arcuate system, one can detect small amounts of ACTH, but the predominant product from this region is ACTH 1–13 amide (or non-acetylated alpha-MSH).[16] The fate of the N-terminal peptide is not well delineated in rat brain.

The second POMC-producing cell group is found in the NTS; it produces the same peptides as the arcuate system, plus their N-acetylated counterparts. Thus one can find significant amounts of N-acetylated forms of β-endorphin 1–31 and β-endorphin 1–27, which are not active at the opioid receptor, along with their non-acetylated opioid active counterparts.[37] Similarly, one can find both alpha-MSH and its non-acetylated form.

It is unclear at this point whether brain cells release all these peptides in proportions identical to their stored levels. Our results to date (see below) argue that this may not be the case. It is entirely conceivable that a given POMC cell would release β-endorphin 1–27 under some circumstances, and β-endorphin 1–31 under others. It is also quite likely that it would co-release ACTH, alpha-MSH, or des-acetyl-alpha-MSH alongside the opioids. Finally some form of the N-terminal gamma MSH region may also be liberated. The exact conditions that may lead to a particular combination of peptide products at the synapse are yet to be explored. It is clear however, that the cell has a great deal more latitude than previously anticipated, and that its output may change as a function of recent or long term history (see below). Thus, the following description of the pharmacological actions of POMC products should be seen as exploring the possibilities, rather than revealing an ultimate truth about POMC products modulating nociception.

Modulation of Pain by Non-Opioid Products of POMC

We can now return to our question as to the possible role of other POMC products in modulating nociception. The exact role of N-acetylated and shorter forms of β-endorphin in pain control has scarcely been addressed, possibly because the nature of β-endorphin forms in brain has been, until recently, a matter of debate. Interestingly, C. H. Li and his colleagues[38] have suggested that the less active forms of β-endorphin might act as antagonists to analgesia. A likely explanation is that they may act as weak partial agonists, which are recognized by the relevant opioid receptor or receptors, producing long-lasting occupancy because of their hydrophobicity, with little efficacy. These notions are clearly worthy of being pursued at the physiological level, since the idea that two products derived from the same neuron may exhibit checks and balances between them is unusual and appealing.

The potential role of ACTH and its products in nociception is also likely to be complex. While there are several reports that intraventricular injection of ACTH can diminish opiate analgesia or produce hyperalgesia, we have found that, within the central grey, ACTH can be an analgesic with a potency equivalent to morphine.[17] Furthermore, ACTH-derived products, such as alpha-MSH and ACTH 1–13 amine (the predominant ACTH-like peptide in hypothalamus) also produce reliable analgesia when micro-injected in the midbrain central grey.

Finally, gamma-MSH, the potential peptide derived from the N-terminal domain of POMC, does not produce analgesia, but produces substantial potentiation of the ACTH-induced analgesia.[17,39] These observations, coupled with several more on the additivity of sub-analgesic doses of β-endorphin and ACTH peptides, have suggested to us that POMC products, when released into the periaqueductal grey, may exhibit co-ordinate actions all leading to pain inhibition.[40] This is not to say however that these actions may not be self-limiting; indeed antagonistic or partially agonistic effects may play a critical physiological role against the potentially long-lasting effects of β-endorphin 1–31–induced analgesia.

It is evident from the above overview that POMC in brain can give rise to numerous peptides with both opioid and non-opioid properties and analgesic and non-analgesic properties. It is therefore not surprising that stimulation of POMC cells does not always produce analgesia and that the analgesia elicited from stimulating POMC systems in the brain is not always fully naloxone reversible.

Pro-Dynorphin and Analgesia

Pro-Dynorphin–derived products provide an interesting contrast with β-endorphin *vis-a-vis* analgetic profiles. While β-endorphin micro-injections yielded readily recognizable, potent opiate analgesia, the administration of dynorphin A has resulted in a much more complex pattern of results. In our own hands, and in those of other investigators, initial attempts to demonstrate analgesia with dynorphin A were largely negative, regardless of whether the peptide was administered intracerebroventricularly or within the central grey.[18] On the other hand, investigators have obtained analgesia by intrathecal injection.[19] The lack of supraspinal analgesia was surprising in view of the great potency of dynorphin *in vitro*. The most obvious interpretations were either in terms of rapid breakdown of dynorphin A, or in terms of its possible interactions with a unique receptor subtype, the kappa receptor. Since there was a suggestion in the literature that kappa-induced analgesia may be more evident at the level of the spinal cord rather than supraspinally, a number of groups have given dynorphin A intrathecally, at the level of the spinal cord, and have observed very long-lasting inhibition of withdrawal reflexes, sometimes likened to a paralysis.[19] Meanwhile, Lee and her colleagues[20] showed that dynorphin-induced analgesia can in fact antagonize morphine analgesia, and suggested possible interactions between multiple opioid receptor subtypes.

Our own work led us to propose a somewhat different interpretation for the same observation, and for a number of other behavioral paradoxes seen with dynorphin A. We [21,22] showed that when the amino-terminal tyrosine is removed from dynorphin A (yielding dynorphin 2–17 or des-tyrosine dynorphin), it loses, as expected, its ability to interact with opioid receptors. However, dynorphin 2–17 continues to exhibit a number of behavioral and electrophysiological effects, identical to those seen with dynorphin A 1–17, and is, of course, not naloxone reversible. Most relevant to this discussion, dynorphin A 2–17 can also produce an antagonism of morphine analgesia, shifting the dose-response curve to the right.[23] We therefore suggested that dynorphin A may contain two active cores, the classic opioid core encoded by the leucine-enkephalin sequence followed by a carboxy-terminal extension, and a second, non-opioid core, which we believe resides primarily at the amino terminus, beyond position 9. (This conclusion is based on some preliminary structure-activity studies). Interestingly, Herz's group[24] at the Max Planck Institute has shown that the spinal cord analgesia induced by dynorphin A can be mimicked by the non-opioid dynorphin 2–17.

Recent work in our laboratory[25] using coupled reverse-phase HPLC with radioimmunoassay, has demonstrated that dynorphin A 1–17, when micro-injected into the central grey, is rapidly converted to dynorphin A 2–17. This latter product is then stable enough to be detected by radioimmunoassay following sacrifice, dissection, and extraction of the peptides. This finding suggests that the unique and non-naloxone reversible effects seen upon dynorphin A administration are not due to interaction with the kappa receptor, but rather with a unique non-opioid receptor that recognizes dynorphin A 2-17. Whether dynorphin A 2-17 occurs naturally and is stored in synaptic vesicles is currently under study. We also do not know whether dynorphin A, when released naturally, is accorded sufficient protection within the synapse to interact with the opioid receptors at that junction.

We should mention that dynorphin A 1-17 is not always the dominant form of that peptide in brain. Weber and co-workers[26] have reported that dynorphin A 1-8, previously identified by Seizinger *et al.*[27] is the more dominant form in rat brain. Our findings suggest that there is a great deal of regional and species differences in the ratios of dynorphin A 1-17 and dynorphin A 1-8.[28] Thus, within rat brain the substantia nigra stores almost exclusively dynorphin A 1-8 whereas the nucleus tractus solitarius has a predominance of dynorphin A 1-17. Since dynorphin A 1-17 and dynorphin A 1-8 exhibit differences in their opioid profiles[29] and since the former may contain the non-opioid core while the latter may not, it becomes important to understand which peptide form is released in which regions.

Thus, while there is little work on the other opioid and non-opioid regions of pro-dynorphin with regard to pain regulation, the study of the dynorphin A region reveals the same range of complexities seen with POMC. While we are dealing with two different families, with different anatomies, with opioid products that have different opioid receptor preferences, we are struck with the same overall pattern: In both cases, we can have opioid and non-opioid peptide products, both capable of modulating pain in a complex fashion, sometimes leading to analgesia, and sometimes counteracting that analgesia.

The study of POMC and pro-dynorphin products and their role in pain modulation does not allow one to pre-select a system most likely to be implicated in stress-induced analgesia—or any other endogenous pain regulatory response. We suspect that consideration of pro-enkephalin peptides and their role in nociception would lead to very similar conclusions. However, the behavioral studies, in conjunction with the information on multiple peptide forms, have given us a sense of the richness of these systems, and their capacity to fine-tune pain responsiveness in ways not previously suspected by us. The opioid systems are apparently capable of bringing to bear the actions of multiple co-synthesized products on pain inhibition, as well as producing and releasing peptides that may terminate, reverse, or prevent this analgesia.

We cannot overemphasize, however, that such pharmacological and metabolic studies only give us a glimpse of "possible scenarios." A true understanding of what happens in brain when analgesia is produced requires a more complete knowledge of which systems are activated, which combinations and forms of peptides are release, their eventual fate at the synapse, and the array of opioid and non-opioid receptors they encounter and activate. This is clearly a tall order, rendered more discouraging by the fact that most of us have been unable to discern consistent changes in brain opioid peptide contents following various stressors. Thus, the answer to even the first and most basic of questions—which systems are activated—is not at hand. The following section describes our efforts to show that β-endorphin systems are activated by a stressor that activates opioid analgetic mechanisms.

THE EFFECT OF FOOTSHOCK STRESS ON
β-ENDORPHIN IN PITUITARY AND IN BRAIN

The initial studies on changes in opioid levels following various stressors emphasized measurements of steady-state levels following the first stressor. The results were generally variable across laboratories, substances, and assays, although a number of groups suggested a change in opioid levels following stress-induced analgesia.[4] Even within our own laboratory, we have occasionally found increases in β-endorphin content or decreases, depending on the exact timing of the measurements following the stressors. It became evident that measurement of peptide content in a particular brain region was not sufficient to implicate a particular opioid in stress-induced analgesia. Even if one found a change, its interpretation would be problematic. Does an eventual increase in content signify overall activation of the system, leading to increases in the stores of peptides, or does it point to the opposite explanation, i.e., a decrease in activation and release? Such practical and conceptual problems indicated to us the need to address the issue of opioid changes that accompany stress in a more dynamic framework. It became apparent that we needed to understand the regulatory biology of opioid cells in order to evolve strategies for measuring dynamic changes following stress or any other environmental manipulation.

Thus, we undertook a series of studies that focused on the effect of acute and repeated footshock on the cell biology of the β-endorphin/ACTH system in both pituitary and brain. We focused on β-endorphin for a number of reasons, including the fact that it is likely to be involved in stress responsiveness given its close association with ACTH, the fact that it may play a role in analgesia given its pharmacological potency in regulating pain, and the fact that its brain anatomy is relatively simpler than that of the other two families, allowing more discrete dissection of cell groups and target areas. We studied the pituitary for two reasons: it is a tissue particularly rich in POMC, which could be more easily subjected to biosynthetic studies and some researchers had suggested that stress-induced analgesia may in fact be mediated, at least partially, by activation of pituitary endorphins.[30] Furthermore the pituitary of rat contains two distinct tissues that express POMC, the anterior lobe and the intermediate lobe. Since the anterior lobe corticotrophs are classically thought to be responsive to stress, while the role of the intermediate lobe in stress is unclear, this would permit us to study two POMC cell types with unique POMC processing, with possibly varying degrees of stress responsiveness. It was our hope that we could learn from the pituitary studies in order to generalize to brain.

In all the studies to be described below the same stress paradigm was employed in male, adult, Sprague-Dawley rats. The conditions of the footshock are similar to those previously shown to produce opioid analgesia.[31-33] Each study included four groups of animals: (1) a control group, unstressed and unhandled; (2) an acute stress group that receives a 30 minute session of intermittent footshock immediately prior to sacrifice; (3) a chronically stressed/rested group that was subjected to a daily, 30 minute session of footshock for 14 days followed by 24 hours of rest prior to sacrifice; and (4) a chronically stressed/acutely stressed group that was repeatedly stressed for 14 days and stressed immediately prior to sacrifice. It should be noted that, while acute stress resulted in analgesia, repeated stress appears to engender a tolerance such that a chronically stressed/acutely stressed animal exhibits no analgesia.[31,32]

Stress Effects on Anterior Lobe POMC

As expected, acute footshock stress leads to substantial elevations of ACTH, β-endorphin, and corticosteroids in the plasma of the stressed rats.[34] Simultaneously, the content of the anterior lobe decreases by approximately 20–25% relative to control values. Repeated stress, as given to the chronically stressed/rested group, leads to a substantial increase in the content of β-endorphin in the anterior lobe (approximately 300% of control). Yet the resting plasma levels in that group are indistinguishable from controls. When this chronically stressed group is re-challenged with acute stress, there is a substantial drop in anterior lobe content relative to the chronically stressed/rested levels. However, the plasma peptide and steroid levels appear very similar to the acutely stressed group. Thus, there is an apparent discrepancy between what the plasma levels indicate and what is happening at the level of the anterior lobe. Measurement of the circulating hormones alone would have led us to conclude that the system responds in an identical fashion after the fifteenth stressor as it did after the first—normal resting levels, similar stress responses. Yet, the results of measurement of gland content suggest that this is being achieved in dramatically different ways as function of the animal's history.

The most evident change is that the stored levels are substantially higher in the chronically stressed rats. This suggests a change in the long-term steady-state levels of POMC. The most likely explanation for such a change in stores, in the face of repeated activation and release, is an increase in biosynthesis at the level of transcription and translation. Indeed, measurement of the messenger RNA (mRNA) specific to POMC using a specific mouse cDNA probe (courtesy of Dr. James Roberts, Columbia University) has demonstrated a 50% elevation in anterior lobe POMC message following chronic stress.[40] Thus, the anterior lobe corticotrophs appear to have responded to the repeated demand by having more of the POMC message available for translation. Whether this was achieved by an increase in the rate of gene transcription or a change in the stability of the mRNA is not yet determined. Regardless, more peptides are made and stored. Furthermore release studies in these animals show that in chronically stressed rats ACTH and POMC are highly releasable.[34] Thus, chronic stress appears to lead to a specific increase in stores and in the releasable pool of POMC products.

The question remains, what happens following the first acute stress? Why does the depletion in anterior lobe stores appear minimal, even though the same levels of hormones are achieved in plasma? A possible answer to these questions were derived from work on the biosynthesis of POMC in short-term cultures immediately following stress.[35,40] In these studies, the anterior lobe was dissected away from the neurointermediate lobe and a cell suspension was produced that was maintained for a few hours to obtain an index of biosynthetic rates. This was done by using a pulse-chase paradigm followed by purification of POMC products on immunoaffinity columns. The results of these studies can be summarized as follows: In a control rat, approximately 15 minutes are required to synthesize POMC de novo in these cultures. This POMC is converted to its products (β-lipotropin and β-endorphin for the COOH-terminal domain) with an apparent $t_{1/2}$ of approximately 32 minutes. Following acute stress, the rate of conversion of POMC to its products becomes accelerated, with an apparent $t_{1/2}$ of approximately 16 minutes. Furthermore, after 15 minutes of labeling, 50% more POMC is made in the acutely stressed lobes as compared to the controls. Note that this latter increase cannot be due to an increase in mRNA since that remains unchanged after acute stress (the time is too short for a significant change in the message pool). One must presume that whatever mRNA is available to these cells has become translated more efficiently. In turn, the POMC thus formed is more rapidly processed into its products. The net effect is an acceleration in biosynthesis after acute stress that relies on increased efficiency of co-translational and post-translational mechanisms. Interestingly, in the chronically stressed/rested animals, which had a threefold increase in stored POMC products, the rate of POMC conversion to its products was not elevated. On the contrary, it was somewhat slower than control, with an apparent $t_{1/2}$ of 40 minutes.[35,40]

Thus, there appears to be two mechanisms of regulation of anterior lobe POMC that become evident following our stress paradigm: a short term mechanism that is apparently triggered by release of the peptide hormones and involves more efficient handling of the precursor/product conversion, and a longer term mechanism that involves an increase in mRNA for POMC. The two appear to occur at different times for the organism and result in differences in rates of biosynthesis and releasability of the stores. It should be noted here that the short-term effect (i.e., increase in biosynthesis immediately following release) would tend to replenish the stores of peptides as they become depleted by stimulation. Thus, it is not uncommon that with mild stress, no change in content of anterior lobe ACTH/β-endorphin can be detected, in spite of substantial elevation in plasma hormone levels. It is likely that a similar mechanism may operate in brain and mask changes in peptide levels following stimulation of a peptidergic pathway.

Stress Effects on Intermediate Lobe POMC

The effects of the stress paradigm on the intermediate lobe have recently been described[36] and will only be summarized here. Our studies in the intermediate lobe have led us to the following conclusions. (1) Following acute stress there is a small but reliable response from the intermediate lobe as evidenced by an increase in plasma α-MSH and N-acetyl-β-endorphin, which are exclusively intermediate lobe products. Interestingly, content of POMC products in the intermediate lobe remains unchanged. (2) Following chronic stress, the intermediate lobe becomes induced, exhibiting more POMC-specific mRNA, (unpublished data), more stored POMC products, and more releasable stores.[36] (3) There is evidence of an increase in processing coupled to release, as was seen in the anterior lobe. However, since the material in the intermediate lobe becomes increasingly more releasable with repetition, the change in $t_{1/2}$ is more evident in chronically stressed rats.

Studies in the intermediate lobe generally confirm the general conclusions drawn from the anterior lobe results—that these cells have multiple mechanisms of regulation, triggered by changes in demand, resulting in changes in post-translational events as well as changes in the overall biosynthetic capacity of the system as marked by the amount of mRNA and the total stores.

Which is the Real Product?

A main issue that the pituitary studies have allowed us to address is that of a strategy for determining "the" products that are released among a host of possibilities. As mentioned earlier in this chapter, the anterior lobe stores more β-lipotropin (β-LPH) than it does β-endorphin. Which of these is released? Are they released in ratios equivalent to what is stored? Similarly, the intermediate lobe contains at least five different forms of β-endorphin, the most dominant form being N-acetyl-β-endorphin 1–27. Is this the most important product of the intermediate lobe? Such questions are intrinsically important and relevant to the question of a potential role of peripheral β-endorphin-like peptides in mediating stress-induced analgesia. Further, they have implications for the brain studies, since multiple peptide forms exist in the brain. However, release studies in brain tissue are substantially more difficult.

It was thus our hope to derive a criterion by which a peptide form could be construed as the major releasable product of a given cell. Is this determined by stored ratios? Is the most processed form the most readily releasable? Is the most biologically active peptide the one to focus on, while the others can be seen as metabolites? These issues were addressed within the context of the above studies by examining which peptide forms were specifically altered by stress, were released into the blood stream, or were changed the most obviously by the regulatory mechanisms we have described.

We have learned that a product is not necessarily the most abundantly stored peptide form. For instance, we see a higher release of β-endorphin than β-LPH in plasma,[41] in spite of the fact that β-LPH is more abundant in the anterior lobe.[13] Similarly, we have observed a selective release of N-Acetyl-β-endorphin 1–31 following chronic stress, in spite of the fact that it is not, normally, the most abundant form in the intermediate lobe.[36] Nor does opioid potency appear to be a relevant criterion, since the N-acetylated peptides are not opioid active. Finally, while β-endorphin is more processed than β-LPH and appears more releasable, N-acetyl-β-endorphin 1–31 is not the most processed form in the intermediate lobe. Thus, none of the criteria stated above appeared to allow us to predict which of the many sizes and forms of β-endorphin-like peptides would be selectively treated as the cell's major product.

However, we have been able to derive a correlate of releasability. To date, it appears that the more releasable products are more clearly regulated by the parent cells. For example, if we compare changes in β-endorphin to the simultaneous changes in POMC as we move through the stress paradigm, it is apparent that β-endorphin is more clearly depleted following acute stress, most clearly enriched in the chronically stressed/rested animal, and again more clearly depleted upon re-challenge. A similar situation holds for N-acetyl-β-endorphin 1–31 in intermediate lobe. Hence, a possible criterion for a highly releasable product is that it be selectively regulated as a function of changing cellular demands, particularly being selectively enriched and sequestered upon a chronic increase in demand.

A note of caution, however: It is conceivable that the product is different as a function of the animal's recent history, e.g., we have preliminary evidence suggesting that this may be the case in anterior lobe, when the ratio of β-LPH: β-endorphin released rises following chronic stress—possibly because of the deceleration of processing noted above (Young & Akil, unpublished data).

The pituitary studies let to some insight in the regulatory mechanisms employed by endocrine POMC cells, revealing both short-term and long-term strategies available to these systems. Furthermore, they suggested an index for focusing on a particular peptide form as likely to be highly releasable. Interestingly, they did not lend strong support to the idea of pituitary β-endorphin playing an important role in stress-induced analgesia. While we have clear evidence of an elevation in circulating β-endorphin following acute stress, β-endorphin levels are at least equally high in the chronically stressed/acutely stressed rats, which exhibit a tolerance to the analgetic property of footshock stress.

The Effect of Footshock Stress on Brain/β-Endorphin

As mentioned above, acute footshock does not lead to reliable changes in midbrain β-endorphin levels. On the other hand, repeated footshock followed by a 24 hour rest resulted in a 30–50% elevation in β-endorphin immunoreactivity, a finding that parallels what we have observed in the two pituitary lobes. This suggests to us that the system has been induced to form more mRNA as we observed in the gland, but this hypothesis awaits confirmation. Finally, when the chronically stressed rat is re-stressed acutely, there is a measurable decrease in the midbrain β-endorphin total levels.

Since we were unable to carry out pulse-labeling studies in the brain because of their technical difficulties, we studied the forms of β-endorphin like material under the four conditions. It should be stated here that in the control rat midbrain we observe a ratio of 1:0.6 in materials the size of β-endorphin 1–31 and β-endorphin 1–27 + 1–26, respectively, which shows that most of the material is full sized but a substantial proportion is cleaved at the COOH-terminal.

Following acute stress, the proportions are not substantially altered. However, following chronic stress shorter, more processed forms accumulate selectively (β-endorphin 1–31:β-endorphin 1–27+1−26 is 1:1.5).

It appears as though the system is not simply generally induced, but that there is a shift in the overall profile leading to greater accumulation of these highly processed products. Upon re-challenge with acute stress, the chronically stressed rats show a return to normal profile of ratios as if the smaller peptides (β-endorphins 1–27 and 1–26) have become selectively released (β-endorphin 1–31:β-endorphin 1–27 is 1:0.6 in the chronic/acute group).

Our data lead us to a number of tentative conclusions. (1) Even though we cannot see the effect of footshock stress using acute stress, it is likely to have an impact on brain POMC, since it results in an induction of the system upon repetition. It is likely that the content does not change acutely because of an acceleration of biosynthetic efficiency as seen in the pituitary. (2) The composition of stored products is significantly altered in the chronically stressed rat as compared to the control (more processed opioid peptides are stored). (3) It is quite likely that the chronically stressed rat when re-challenged releases the shorter peptides. These are clearly relatively inactive as compared to β-endorphin 1–31. They have 10–20-fold lower analgesic potency if not acetylated and no analgesic potency if acetylated.[15] (4) The main open question is this: Does β-endorphin 1–31 ever get released in the midbrain? Is it released upon the first stressor but not the fifteenth (where the less active products may be liberated)? If this were the case, we would have a possible mechanism for the behavioral tolerance we observe, as we would be releasing different products on different occasions.

CONCLUSIONS AND FUTURE DIRECTIONS

The studies outlined above suggest a richer and more complex role of endogenous opioids in the regulation of pain in general, and in stress-induced analgesia in particular. They also point to the importance of determining what is released in brain and which opioid and non-opioid receptors are occupied and activated. To this end, it may be critical to devise strategies for determining occupancy of specific receptors after a particular treatment. Preliminary results from our group[42] suggest the feasibility of such an approach. This, coupled with the study of these peptides at the cell biological and anatomical levels, should enable us to answer our original question: Which opioid systems become activated by stress and are responsible for opioid analgesia?

ACKNOWLEDGMENT

The authors would like to thank Ms. Adele Henry for manuscript preparation.

REFERENCES

1. KAKIDANI, H., Y. FURUTANI, H. TAKAHASHI, M. NODA, Y. MORIMOTO, T. HIROSE, M. ASAI, S. INAYAMA, S. NAKANISHI & S. NUMA. 1982. Cloning and sequence analysis of cDNA for porcine beta-neo-endorphin dynorphin precursor. Nature **289**:245.
2. NODA, M., Y. FURUTANI, H. TAKAHASHI, M. TOYOSATA, T. HIROSE, S. INAYAMA, S. NAKANISHI & S. NUMA. 1982. Cloning and sequence analysis of cDNA for bovine adrenal proenkephalin. Nature **29**:202–206.
3. NAKANISHI, S., A. INOUE, T. KITA, M. NAKUMURA, A. C. Y. CHANG, S. N. COHEN & S. NUMA. 1979. Nucleotide sequence of coned cDNA for bovine corticotropin-beta lipotropin precursor. Nature **274**:423–427.
4. AKIL, H., S. J. WATSON, E. YOUNG, M. E. LEWIS, H. KHACHATURIAN & J. M. WALKER. 1984. Endogenous opioids: Biology and function. Ann. Rev. Neurosci. **7**:223–255.
5. SCHWARTSBERG, D. G. & P. K. NAKANE. 1983. ACTH-related peptide containing neurons within the medulla oblongata of the rat. Brain Res. **276**:351–356.
6. KHACHATURIAN, H., M. E. LEWIS, M. R-H. SCHAFER & S. J. WATSON. 1985. Anatomy of CNS opioid systems. Trends Neurosci. **8**:111–119.
7. KARGOWA, K., N. MIROMIRO, N. CHINO, S. SAKAKIBARA & MATSUO. 1981. The complete amino acid sequence of alpha-neo-endorphin. Biochem. Biophys. Res. Commun. **99**:111–117.
8. GOLDSTEIN, A., S. TACHIBANA, L. E. LOWNEY, M. HUNKAPILLER & L. HOOD. 1979. Dynorphin-(1-3), an extraordinarily potent opioid peptide. Proc. Natl. Acad. Sci. USA **76**:666.
9. FISCHLI, W., A. GOLDSTEIN, M. HUNKAPILLER & L. E. HOOD. 1981. Two "big" dynorphins from porcine pituitary. Life Sci. **31**:1769.
10. KILPATRICK, D. L., A. WAHLSTROM, H. W. LAHM, R. BLACKER & S. UDENFRIEND. 1982. Rimorphin, a unique, naturally occurring (Leu)enkephalin containing peptide found in association with dynorphin and alpha-neo-endorphin. Proc. Natl. Acad. Sci. USA **79**:6480.
11. WATSON, S. J., H. AKIL & J. D. BARCHAS. 1979. Immunohistochemical and biochemical studies of the enkephalins, beta-endorphin and related peptides. *In* Endorphins in Mental Health Research. E. Usdin, W. M. Bunney & N. S. Kline, Eds.:30–44.
12. ZAKARIAN, S. & D. SMYTH. 1982. Beta-endorphin is processed differently in specific regions of rat pituitary and brain. Nature **296**:250–252.
13. ZAKARIAN, S. & D. G. SMYTH. 1982. Review article: Distribution of beta-endorphin related peptides in rat pituitary and brain. Biochem. J. **202**:561–571.
14. AKIL, H., E. YOUNG, S. J. WATSON & D. COY. 1981. Opiate binding properties of naturally occurring N and C terminus modified beta-endorphins. Peptides **2**:289–292.

15. DEAKIN, J. F., J. O. DOSTROVSKY & D. G. SMYTH. 1980. Influence of N-terminal acetylation and C-terminal proteolysis on the analgesic activity of beta-endorphin. Biochem J. **189**:501–506.

16. EVANS, C. J., R. LORENZ, E. WEBER & J. D. BARCHAS. 1982. Variants of alpha-melanocyte stimulating hormone in rat brain and pituitary: evidence that acetylated a-MSH exists only in the intermediate lobe of pituitary. Biochem. Biophys. Res. Commun. **106**:910–919.

17. WALKER, J. M., H. AKIL & S. J. WATSON. 1980. Evidence for homologous action of pro-opiocortin products. Science **210**:1247–1249.

18. WALKER, J. M., R. J. KATZ & H. AKIL. 1980. Behavioral effects of dynorphin (1-13) in monkey and rat: Initial observations. Peptides **1**:341–345.

19. HERMAN, B. H. & A. GOLDSTEIN. 1985. Antinociception and paralysis induced by intrathecal Dyn-A. J. Pharm. Exp. Ther. **232**(1):27–32.

20. FRIEDMAN, H. H., M. F. JEN, J. K. CHANG, N. M. LEE & H. H. LOH. 1981. Dynorphin-A possible modulatory peptide on morphine or B-endorphin analgesia in mouse. Eur. J. Pharmacol. **69**:53–57.

21. WALKER, J. M., H. MOISES, D. COY, G. BALDRIGHI & H. AKIL. 1982. Non-opiate effects of dynorphin and Des-tyr-dynorphin. Science **218**:1136–1138.

22. WALKER, J. M., H. MOISES, D. COY, E. YOUNG, S. WATSON & H. AKIL. 1982. Dynorphin-(1-17): lack of analgesia but evidence for non-opiate electrophysiological and motor effects. Life Sci. **31**:1821–1824.

23. WALKER, J. M., D. E. TUCKER, D. H. COY, B. B. WALKER & H. AKIL. 1982. Des-Tyrosine-dynorphin antagonizes morphine and analgesia. Eur. J. Pharmacol. **85**:121–122.

24. PRZEWLOCKI, R., G. T. SHEARMAN & A. HERZ. 1983. Mixed opioid/nonopioid effects of dynorphin and dynorphin-related peptides after their intrathecal injection in rats. Neuropeptides **3**:233.

25. YOUNG, E. A., J. M. WALKER, R. HOUGHTEN & H. AKIL. 1985. The breakdown of ^{3}H dynorphin A *in vivo* and *in vitro*. INRC Abstracts.

26. WEBER, E., C. EVANS & J. D. BARCHAS. 1982. Predominance of aminoterminal octapeptide fragment of dynorphin in rat brain. Nature **299**:77.

27. SEIZINGER, B., V. HOLLT & A. HERZ. 1981. Evidence for the occurrence of the opioid octapeptide dynorphin(1-8) in the neurointermediate pituitary of rats. Biochem. Biophys. Res. Commun. **102**:197–205.

28. DORES, R. M. & H. AKIL. 1985. Steady state levels of pro-dynorphin-related end products in the striatum and substantia nigra of the adult rhesus monkey. Peptides. (In press.)

29. CORBETT, A., A. J. PATTERSON, A. T. MCKNIGHT, J. MAGNAN & E. W. KOSTERLITZ. 1982. Dynorphin (1-8) and dynorphin (1-9) are ligands for the kappa subtype of opiate receptor. Nature **229**:79.

30. LEWIS, J. W., E. H. CHADLER, J. T. CANNON & J. C. LIEBESKIND. 1981. Hypophysectomy differentially affects morphine and stress analgesia. Proc. West. Pharmacol. Soc. **24**:323–326.

31. AKIL, H., J. MADDEN, R. L. PATRICK & J. D. BARCHAS. 1976. Stress-induced increase in endogenous opiate peptides: Concurrent analgesia and its partial reversal by naloxone. *In* Opiates and Endogenous Opioid Peptides. H. W. Kosterlitz, Ed.:63–70. North Holland Publishing Co. Amsterdam.

32. MADDEN, J., H. AKIL & J. D. BARCHAS. 1977. Stress-induced parallel changes in central opioid levels and pain responsiveness in the rat. Nature **266**:358–360.

33. LEWIS, J. W., J. T. CANNON & J. C. LIEBESKIND, 1980. Opioid and nonopioid mechanisms of stress analgesia. Science **208**:623–625.

34. YOUNG, E. A. & H. AKIL. 1985. CRF stimulation of ACTH/Beta-endorphin release: Effects of acute and chronic stress. Endocrinology **117**:23–30.

35. SHIOMI, H. & H. AKIL. 1982. Pulse chase studies of POMC/beta-endorphin system in the pituitary of acutely and chronically stressed rats. Life Sci. **31**:2185–2188.

36. AKIL, H., H. SHIOMI & J. MATTHEWS. 1985. Induction of the intermediate pituitary by stress: Synthesis and release of a nonopioid form of beta-endorphin. Science **227**:424–426.

37. Dores, R. M., M. Jain & H. Akil. 1986. Characterization of the forms of β-endorphin and α-MSH in the caudal medulla of the rat and guinea pig. Brain Research. (In press.)
38. Li, C. H. *et al.* 1985. Fed. Proc.
39. Walker, J. M., A. Ghessari, B. A. Peters, S. J. Watson, N. Seidah, M. Chretien & H. Akil. 1986. Interactions among pro-opiomelanocortin products: modulation of pain sensitivity. *In* Neutrotransmitters and Pain. H. Akil & J. Lewis, Eds. S. Karger-Verlag. Basel. (In press.)
40. Shiomi, H., S. J. Watson, G. Kelsey & H. Akil. 1986. A pre-translational and a post-translational mechanism for regulating β-endorphin/ACTH cells: Studies in anterior lobe. Endocrinology. (Submitted for publication.)
41. Young, E., J. W. Lewis & H. Akil. 1986. The preferential release of β-endorphin from the anterior lobe by corticotropin releasing factor. Peptides. (Submitted for publication.)
42. Lewis, J. W., M. E. Lewis, D. J. Loomus & H. Akil. 1985. Acute systemic administration of morphine selectively increases mu opioid receptor binding in rat brain. Neuropeptides **5**:117–120.

Hyperalgesic Functions of Peripheral Opiate Receptors[a]

DEREK VAN DER KOOY

Department of Anatomy
University of Toronto
Toronto, Canada M5S 1A8

STATEMENT OF THE PROBLEM

Opiates have paradoxical motivational effects.[1,2] The euphoric or positive reinforcing effects of opiates are well known to human addicts and recreational drug users, yet patients receiving opiates as analgesics often report nauseous reactions. In rats, morphine produces positive reinforcing effects when paired with visual and textural environmental stimuli.[3,4] Yet, at similar doses over the same routes of administration, morphine produces aversive effects as shown when paired with taste stimuli.[5] Until recently, there was no evidence that differentiated the neural substrates mediating these opposite motivational effects.

The realization that opiate receptors are not only localized to the brain, but also prevalent throughout the peripheral nervous system,[6,7] has led to the hypothesis that opioids produce positive reinforcing effects through an action on brain opiate receptors and aversive effects through an action on peripheral opiate receptors.[8] The hypothesis has recently received support from a number of experiments, especially those involving local, low dose application of opiates and the administration of opiate antagonists that do or do not cross the blood-brain barrier.[8,9] The existence of a peripheral opioid system producing hyperalgesia and aversion and a central opioid system mediating analgesia and euphoria would have important implications for the evolution and function of motivation and pain perception systems in the body. Stress may be the process that allows us to understand the organization of these opioid pain perception and motivational systems, which apparently function in opposite ways in the central versus peripheral nervous systems.

OPIATE RECEPTORS ARE LOCALIZED
IN PRIMARY SENSORY NEURONS

Autoradiographic receptor binding techniques have revealed that a subpopulation of neuronal cell bodies in primary sensory ganglia from rodents and primates bind radiolabeled opiates (FIGURE 1).[7,10] This opiate receptor subpopulation comprises approximately 10% of cervical dorsal root ganglion neuronal cell bodies[7] but over 50% of the nodose (vagal) ganglion neuronal cell bodies.[10] Given that two populations of primary sensory cell bodies (big and

[a]Supported by Medical Research Council of Canada.

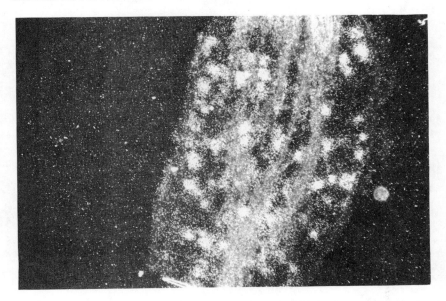

FIGURE 1. Opiate binding in a section through a rat dorsal root ganglion that was incubated in 1 nM [³H]etorphine. This dark-field autoradiograph of a colchicine-treated (covered with a swab soaked in 200 µg/µl colchicine for 24 hr prior to sacrifice), low cervical dorsal root ganglion demonstrates dense clusters of silver grains scattered over a subpopulation of the neuronal cell bodies. (Prepared in collaboration with Mary Ninkovic and Stephen P. Hunt).

small) can be recognized in Nissl section,[11] it is the smaller cells that have opiate receptors.[7] Many of the cells that have opiate receptors were also shown to have histamine H1 receptors[7] and some contain substance P.[12]

Perhaps the localization of opiate receptors to primary sensory perikarya is not surprising in light of evidence suggesting that opiate receptors are present on primary afferent terminals in the spinal cord. Dorsal rhizotomies have been shown to produce significant depletions of opiate receptor binding in the substantia gelatinosa of the dorsal horn of the spinal cord.[13,14] However, the occurrence of opiate receptors in the peripheral processes of primary sensory neurons has not been similarly emphasized. The transport of opiate receptors peripherally in viscero-sensory[10] and somatosensory nerves has recently been observed (FIGURE 2). Ligation of both the vagal and sciatic nerves results in the proximal build-up of opiate receptors 24 hr later as measured autoradiographically in sections along the long axis of the nerves (FIGURE 2). A much higher density of receptors can be seen to build-up at vagal than sciatic ligations, reflecting in part the greater proportion of vagal than spinal ganglion cell bodies synthesizing opiate receptor protein (see above). It is assumed that the opiate receptors are transported in sensory rather than motor components of the nerves because receptor binding is seen in the appropriate sensory ganglia but is not prevalent in the dorsal motor nucleus of the vagus nor the spinal anterior horn.[15,16]

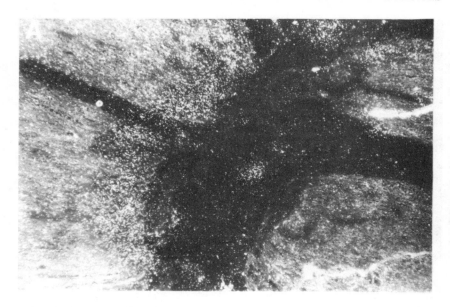

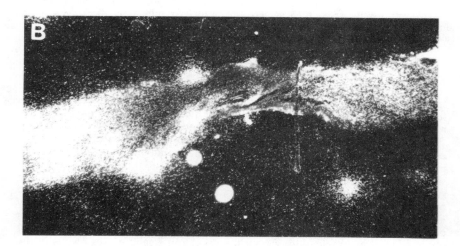

FIGURE 2. Dark-field autoradiograph demonstrating build up of silver grains to the proximal (left) side of the ligated sciatic (A) and vagus (B) nerves. The proximal pile up as well as the distal (right side) binding is much greater in the vagus (B) nerve. When the [³H]etorphine binding is done in the presence of cold levorphanol very few silver grain are seen over the nerves. (Prepared in collaboration with Mary Ninkovic and Stephen P. Hunt).

The relatively poor resolution of the autoradiographic opiate receptor binding technique (in the absence of irreversible ligands) has prevented the localization of receptors to individual nerve ending in the skin or viscera. For the same reason, it is not possible to determine whether the opiate receptors localized to the various parts of primary sensory neurons are actually imbedded in the membrane on the cell surface or internalized and non-functional binding sites simply undergoing processing or transport. This question may be more appropriately answered through physiological and behavioral experiments.

One electrophysiological study[17] failed to show morphine actions on isolated dorsal root ganglion cell bodies, however another study demonstrated an enkephalin-produced inhibition of substance P release from cultured dorsal root ganglion neurons.[18] These discrepancies may be resolved by a detailed analysis of the opiate receptor subtypes present on primary sensory neurons. Recently, specific electrophysiological effects of dynorphin (a kappa receptor agonist) were observed on many cultured dorsal root ganglion neurons.[19]

A great deal of physiological work has been done on opiate actions near the peripheral terminals of vagal neurons in the gut. A potent inhibitory effect of opiates on contraction of isolated strips of guinea pig ileum has clearly been shown to be mediated by mu type opiate receptors.[20] Interestingly, a similar effect in rabbit and mouse ileum seems to be due to delta type opiate receptors.[6] None of these *in vitro* effects on ileum seem to be opiate effects on the presumed kappa receptors prevalent at the distal ends of vagal axons in the gut. The ileum opiate effects are apparently actions on receptors located on postganglionic, acetyl-choline-containing myenteric plexus neurons.[6] Opiates might also be acting in the ileum on receptors shown autoradiographically to be present on various elements of the enteric nervous system,[21] but opiates are probably not acting directly on the smooth muscle cells themselves.[6] In spite of the presence of many opiate receptors in the periphery, the determination of the site of opiate action in whole animals is not trivial. For example, the major portion of opiate effects on bladder contraction in whole animals has recently been shown to be mediated by receptors located in the central nervous system.[22,23]

It is important to ask about the source of endogenous opioids that could have access to and physiologically activate opiate receptors on primary afferent neurons. There are a number of possibilities. Perhaps most importantly, dynorphin has been localized to approximately 2% of dorsal root ganglion neurons themselves when analyzed in culture.[24] A population of spinal cord dorsal horn enkephalin immunoreactive neurons[25] could innervate the central branches of dorsal root ganglion neurons, although synaptic contacts between the intrinsic enkephalin-staining processes and primary afferent terminals have not been found.[26] Blood-borne endogenous opioids affecting all portions of the primary sensory neurons could arise from the pituitary[27] or adrenal medulla.[28,29] Some portions of certain primary sensory neurons could conceivably also be exposed to endogenous opioids normally contained in post-ganglionic sympa-thetic neurons[28] or pre-ganglionic parasympathetic neurons.[30] Indeed in sympa-thetic ganglia themselves it has been suggested that enkephalin-containing preganglionic terminals may be presynaptic to some primary afferent terminals that are present there.[31,32] The presence of opioids in Merkel cells[33,34] and possibly in mast cells[35] might provide an endogenous source for the physiological stimulation of opiate receptors on neurons in the skin. Finally, the widespread localization of endogenous opiate peptides in the cell bodies and processes of enteric neurons provides a source for stimulating opiate receptors in the gut.[36,37]

It should be noted that although most opiate receptors in the periphery are thought to be present on neurons,[6] some localization to other peripheral tissues has not been ruled out. For example β-endorphin binds to lymphocytes and glioblastoma cells, although this binding is not blocked by other opiates but is rather binding of the C-terminal (non-opioid) end of the β-endorphin molecule.[38,39]

OPIATE EFFECTS ON THE PERIPHERAL SIDE OF THE BLOOD-BRAIN BARRIER ARE AVERSIVE

The microinjection of morphine directly into certain specific central nervous system sites can produce positive reinforcing and analgesic effects similar to those seen after systemically administered drug.[40–42] The central dose required to produce these effects is lower than that needed to produce similar effects after systemic administration.[3,40–42] These results suggest that the primary population of receptors mediating the positive reinforcing and analgesic effects may be localized to the central nervous system. The localization of opiate receptors to primary afferent neurons in the periphery prompted the hypothesis that the paradoxical aversive effects of opiates are mediated through an action on these peripheral receptors. To test this hypothesis we studied the motivational effects of specific opioid receptor antagonists that do or do not cross the blood-brain barrier.

Employing a place preference paradigm,[3,8] separate groups of drug naive rats were administered various doses (subcutaneously or intraperitoneally) of naltrexone or its quaternary derivative, methylnaltrexone, which does not cross the blood-brain barrier effectively.[43] Briefly, each rat received four drug injections spaced equally over 8 days, and was immediately confined after each injection to a visually and texturally distinctive environment for 30 minutes. On the four alternating days when no opiate antagonist injection was given, each rat was injected with saline vehicle and confined for 30 minutes to another separate and different distinctive environment.[3,8] Order of injections and drug-paired environment were counterbalanced within groups. On the ninth day, each uninjected rat was tested by recording the amount of time the rat spent in each of the two previously paired distinctive environments, when given a 10 minute period to freely explore both environments.

FIGURE 3 shows that, regardless of the route of administration, increasing doses of naltrexone were aversive whereas increasing doses of methylnaltrexone were positively reinforcing.[8] The results suggest that the place aversions observed were due to an antagonism by the antagonist of endogenous opioid peptides acting on central opiate receptors. This suggestion is based on the fact that the majority of opiate receptors are located in the brain, and therefore the net effects of naltrexone (which can cross the blood-brain barrier) are mainly due to their binding to central receptors. Similar results have been reported previously using another opiate antagonist, naloxone.[3] The preferences produced by methylnaltrexone, which does not effectively cross the blood-brain barrier, must be due primarily to its binding to peripheral opiate receptors and its blockade of peripheral endogenous opioid actions.

Interestingly, one anomalous result occurred with an intraperitoneal injection 0.1 mg/kg of naltrexone, but not with a subcutaneous injection, which produced a place preference (FIGURE 3). We hypothesized that this was due to a local block of

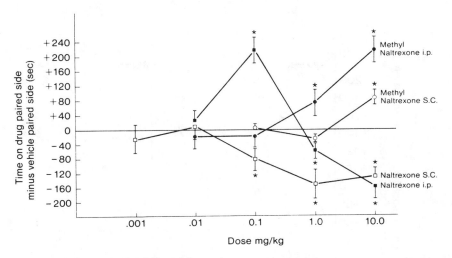

FIGURE 3. The effects of various doses of naltrexone and methylnaltrexone (s.c. and i.p.) in the place conditioning paradigm. *$p < .05$. (From Bechara and van der Kooy.[8] With permission from *Nature*.)

aversive opiate effects in the gut without significant central action at this low dose. This implies that the majority of the peripheral aversive effects of opiates are mediated by receptors in the gut. Based on this hypothesis we predicted that a low dose of morphine, given intraperitoneally, should produce aversions. FIGURE 4 shows that a dose of .05 mg/kg of morphine intraperitoneally produced significant place aversions. The same dose administered subcutaneously had no effect. Higher doses of morphine (subcutaneously and intraperitoneally) were positively reinforcing in the place preference paradigm; doses lower than .05 mg/kg had no effects. Because the vagus nerve carries sensory information from the gut to the brain (as well as itself displaying opiate receptors) we further predicted that subdiaphragmatic vagotomies should abolish the observed effects at the low doses of i.p. morphine and naltrexone (.05 mg/kg morphine place aversions and 0.1 mg/kg naltrexone place preferences), but not abolish the opposite motivational effects seen at higher i.p. doses (1.25 mg/kg morphine place preferences and 10.0 mg/kg naltrexone place aversions). These predictions were confirmed.[8] Vagotomy (verified at sacrifice by measuring food retention in the stomach)[44] blocked the .05 mg/kg morphine-induced place aversions and the 0.1 mg/kg naltrexone-induced place preferences. No significant effects of vagotomies were observed on the 1.25 mg/kg morphine place preferences nor on the 10.0 mg/kg naltrexone place aversions. These data support the hypothesis that the aversive properties of opiates are mediated primarily by means of gut opiate receptors.

Finally, as a further test of this hypothesis, we investigated the effects of vagotomy on the aversive effects of opiates in the conditioned taste aversion paradigm,[5] where only aversive effects are seen even with higher doses of morphine. Control rats demonstrated an aversion for the saccharin flavor previously paired with 15 mg/kg i.p. morphine, whereas vagotomized and morphine-injected rats showed the normal preference for saccharin that is seen

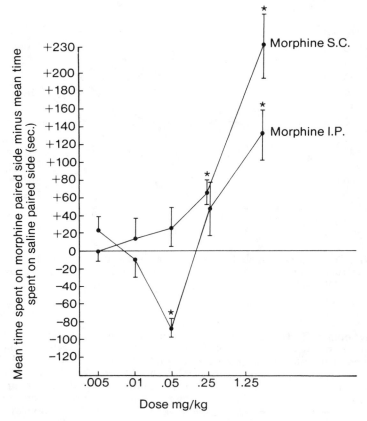

FIGURE 4. The effects of various doses of morphine (s.c. and i.p.) in the place conditioning paradigm. *$p < .05$. (From Bechara and van der Kooy.[8] With permission from *Nature*.)

in uninjected animals.[8] These results show that the aversive effects of even high doses of systemically administered opiates are mediated through an action on peripheral opiate receptors. Moreover, the majority of the peripheral receptors responsible for these systemic aversive effects are located in the gut rather that the skin, as might be predicted from the much greater transport of opiate receptors seen in the vagus nerve than in the sciatic nerve.

Recent evidence suggests that there may be a pharmacological as well as an anatomical specificity to the aversive effects of opiates. A specific kappa receptor agonist (U50,488)[45] produced conditioned place aversions at lower i.p. doses than morphine (Bechara and van der Kooy, in preparation), although morphine is more than four times more potent than U50,488 in producing analgesia as measured in hot-plate and tail-flick tests.[46] In addition, even at high doses the kappa receptor agonist never produced conditioned place preferences[46] (Bechara and van der Kooy, in preparation). These results imply that peripheral kappa receptors, which are prevalent in primary sensory neurons,[19] mediate the aversive effects of opiates, whereas central nervous system opiate receptors (probably mu receptors[46]) mediate the positive reinforcing and analgesic effects of opiates.

HYPERALGESIA RESULTS FROM STIMULATING OPIATE RECEPTORS IN THE SKIN

Many more opiate receptors seem present in visceral (vagal) peripheral nerves than somatosensory nerves, and these visceral receptors are most important in mediating the systemic aversive effects of opiates. Nevertheless, the function of the smaller population of opiate receptors transported out to the peripheral process of a somatosensory nerve in the skin remains to be investigated. Our initial hypothesis (before the work with opiate antagonists that do not cross the blood-brain barrier) was that opiate receptors on nerve endings in the skin might play a role in the analgesic effects of opiates. Although the major site where opiates act to produce analgesia has always been considered to be in the brain, later studies employing intrathecal drug administration suggested that there may also be a spinal locus of action in opiate analgesia.[42] We originally envisioned that opiate receptors on the primary afferent neurons themselves would provide an even more peripheral locus for opiate analgesic effects. However, our experiments with local application of opiates to the skin supported the opposite conclusion: opiate receptors on primary afferent neurons in the skin mediate hyperalgesic responses.

The algesic effects of the local application of the opiate etorphine (a highly lipophilic drug that acts on all of the kappa, delta, and mu opiate receptor subtypes[47]) to the skin were studied in an ear-scratch test. Jancso[48] and Jancso and Jancso-Gabor[49] have previously reported that a 0.5% capsaicin solution, or a dilute 0.05% capsaicin solution applied to the ear in combination with exposure to a heat lamp, elicits ear scratching. We found that 0.1% capsaicin was the lowest topical dose to produce scratching in the absence of exposure to radiant heat. Significant ear scratching generally began 3–7 min after application of capsaicin, lasted for approximately 6–10 minutes, and was usually over by 15–20 min, after which time the rats appeared to rest quietly.[9]

FIGURE 5 shows the effects of topical application of capsaicin, preceded by various doses of etorphine or its vehicle control, on numbers of ear scratches. The application of capsaicin to both ears (preceded 5 min earlier by administration of the alcohol vehicle to both ears) elicited considerable scratching of both ears. There was no significant difference in the number of scratches to the left compared with the right ear. Other baseline control groups (not shown) demonstrated that there was no appreciable ear scratching elicited by 0.05% or 0.5% etorphine followed by application of the alcohol vehicle. FIGURE 5 shows the dose-dependent effects of etorphine on capsaicin-elicited ear scratching. Statistical analysis revealed that at 0.005% and 0.05% etorphine there was significantly more scratching of the etorphine compared with the vehicle-treated ear, whereas in the 0.5% etorphine group there was significantly more scratching of the alcohol vehicle compared with etorphine-treated ear.[9] There was very little scratching of either ear in the 5.0% etorphine group due to the systemic cataleptic effect of the drug.

Thus, lower doses of etorphine (0.005% and 0.05%) produced a local

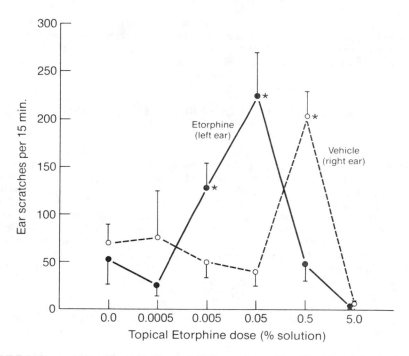

FIGURE 5. Ear scratches observed after various doses of etorphine (●—●) and the alcohol vehicle (O--O) applied topically to the ear. Etorphine was always applied to the rat's left ear and the alcohol vehicle to the right. Ear scratches were counted for the 15 min immediately following capsaicin application to both ears. Capsaicin application followed the etorphine and alcohol vehicle applications by 5 min. A volume of 40 µl of each drug (dissolved in alcohol) was applied to each ear. *$p < .05$ left and right ear scratch counts compared. (From van der Kooy and Nagy.[9] With permission from *Behavior and Brain Research*.)

hyperalgesic response. This lower dose hyperalgesia response was blocked by systemic pretreatment with naloxone.[9] Moreover, the effect was also blocked by systemic pretreatment with methylnaltrexone (which does not cross the blood-brain barrier effectively[43]), suggesting that this local hyperalgesia was mediated by peripheral opiate receptors.[9] A high dose of topical etorphine (0.5%) produced what seemed to be a local analgesic effect, more scratching of the contralateral vehicle-treated ear. Perhaps there is a local anesthetic effect of high doses of etorphine, which produces a relative shift in the scratching to the vehicle-treated ear. At any rate, the local high dose analgesic effect of etorphine is not relevant to the function of the opiate receptor on primary sensory neurons in the skin, because this analgesic effect was not blocked by systemic naloxone pretreatment.[9]

We concluded that primary afferent neuron opiate receptors mediate hyperalgesic functions. However, it should be noted that relevant opiate receptors might possibly be located on other non-neural cutaneous tissue elements. For example, mast cells are purported to contain opiate receptors.[50,51] Preliminary unpublished observations indicate that mast cell depletion produced by repeated treatments with compound 48/80[52] does not block the local hyperalgesic effects of etorphine in the ear-scratch test. Perhaps the most striking test of the hypothesis that primary afferent neuron opiate receptors mediate hyperalgesia comes from experiments asking whether neonatal destruction and adult depletion of the small dorsal root ganglion cells, which presumably bear opiate receptors, would modify the systemic effects of opiates.[9] After removal of the peripheral hyperalgesic primary sensory population of opiate receptors, then the primarily central analgesic population of opiate receptors would be left to act unopposed, and potentiated analgesic effects to systemic morphine might be expected. Neonatal and adult systemic treatments with capsaicin were shown to potentiate the analgesic effects of morphine.[9] These systemic capsaicin treatments are known to destroy specifically or disrupt small dorsal root ganglia cell bodies and their central and peripheral processes.[53-57] A subpopulation of these same primary sensory neurons[11] bear opiate receptors.[7] Indeed, systemic neonatal capsaicin treatment depletes opiate receptor binding in the spinal cord[56] to an extent similar to that produced by dorsal rhizotomies.[13,14] Neonatal and adult systemic capsaicin treatment potentiated the analgesic effect of 5.0 mg/kg of systemic morphine in the tail-flick test,[9] as would be predicted if the well known central analgesic actions of opiates were no longer counteracted by more peripheral hyperalgesic opiate actions.

Several additional lines of evidence support the contention that activation of primary afferent neuron opiate receptors produces hyperalgesia. First, there are both animal[58,59] and human[60] reports that systemic opiate injections produce irritative itching and scratching responses of the skin. Second, local application of morphine to scarified human skin produces irritative itching.[61] Third, the local skin injection of naloxone produces analgesia effects against local prostaglandin-induced hyperalgesia.[62] Fourth, the peripheral administration a quaternary analogue of naloxone (which does not cross the blood-brain barrier) has recently been reported to produce analgesia to inflammatory pain.[63] Finally, it has recently been shown that removal of two sources of endogenous opioids that might normally stimulate peripheral opiate receptors, the pituitary or the adrenal, results in potentiated analgesic responses to opiate and other treatments.[64] This result is conceptually similar to the capsaicin lesion experiment mentioned above in that disruption of the supposed peripheral opiate hyperalgesia system in both cases may permit the central opiate analgesia system to act unencumbered.

The demonstration of the hyperalgesic function of opiate receptors probably located on primary sensory neurons outlines only one example of the complex processing that "creates" sensory information for the brain and spinal cord. Primary sensory neurons are not simply passive conductors of information from the periphery to the spinal cord and brainstem. Different dorsal root ganglion neurons appear to contain substance P, somatostatin, vasoactive intestinal peptide, cholecystokinin, angiotensin II,[65] and histamine.[66] Some of these substances are probably released from the peripheral terminals of primary sensory neurons and participate in local irritative and inflammatory reactions.[48,67,68] Somatostatin, for example, can induce histamine secretion from mast cells.[69] The sensory messages received by the spinal cord and brainstem are probably partially defined by the interaction of peripheral primary afferent neurotransmitters with other chemical mediators in the skin. Such chemical mediators may include substances contained in and released from discrete tissue compartments (such as the endogenous opioids discussed above or mast cell histamine and serotonin), in addition to more ubiquitous substances such as bradykinin and prostaglandins.[70-72] Almost all of these substances, as well as other peripherally localized substances such as acetycholine, have been shown to cause pain and itch in the cantharadin blister base test.[73]

STRESS AND THE ORGANIZATION OF MOTIVATION AND PAIN PERCEPTION SYSTEMS

Recent evidence has suggested that the biochemical elements of intracellular communication arose very early in evolution and have been highly conserved.[74] In line with this we would suggest that the complexity of opiate mechanisms is the result of the evolution of specialized systems in the body that used the highly conserved opioids for different functions. In the present case opioids acting on peripheral sensory nerves appear to function in signalling pain, irritation, and nausea, whereas the central opiate system apparently evolved a pain-inhibition and euphoric role. The fact that both opiate systems are involved in mediating the effects of aversive stimuli may mean only that pain-facilitating and pain-inhibiting systems had a common ancestral origin. Perhaps stress, in the sense originally used by Selye[75]—a non-specific alarm signal eliciting specific responses—provided the selective evolutionary pressure for the divergence of the endogenous opioid systems into a central analgesic and euphoric one and a peripheral hyperalgesic and aversive one.

We have classified two general opioid systems in the body, with analgesia and euphoria grouped together as central effects, and cutaneous hyperalgesia and irritation and visceral nausea grouped together as peripheral effects. However it is clear that various effects within each of these two compartments are actions on receptors in different anatomical subsystems. The aversive or nauseating effects produced by stimulation of the major population opiate receptors in the viscera are separate from the hyperalgesic and irritating effects produced by local, cutaneous application of opiates. Similarly, experiments involving the brain microinjection of morphine have partially dissociated the sites mediating analgesic versus positive reinforcing effects.[41] We are speculating here only on the initial evolutionary divergence and organization of central and peripheral pain perception and motivational systems.

Perhaps what seem to be opposite central and peripheral roles for opioid systems can be shown to function now as adaptive responses of the whole animal to stress. For example, animals must make at least two responses to stressful injuries (injuries which it should be noted are potent releasers of the opioid β-endorphin from the pituitary[76]). First, animals must pay attention to the local hyperalgesic peripheral site of injury in order to stop the external source of the pain and remember it so it can be avoided in the future. Second, animals must stop the pain so that they can get away and engage in other important species-specific behaviors such as eating and drinking. It is clear that the endogenous opioid sytems could mediate both of these types of responses—the local hyperalgesic or aversive response and the central responses of analgesia and partaking of other positive reinforcers. Psychological theorists have noticed many examples of apparently opposite responses in motivation or pain perception that occur in cycles one after the other. These examples have been codified into an opponent process theory of motivation,[77,78] which in some ways is a restatement of the phenomenon of homeostasis. Opioid-based pain perception and motivation systems may provide a single biochemical substrate (and point to a common ancestral origin) for the adaptive but opposite responses seen in the central versus peripheral nervous systems.

ACKNOWLEDGMENTS

Thanks to my collaborators in the experiments mentioned here: Mary Ninkovic, Stephen P. Hunt, Antione Bechara, and James I. Nagy.

REFERENCES

1. CAPPEL, H. & A. E. LeBLANE. 1975. Conditioned aversion by psychoactive drugs: Does it have significance for an understanding of drug dependence? Addictive Behav. **1**:55–64.
2. WISE, R. A., R. A. YOKEL & H. DeWIT. 1976. Both positive reinforcement and conditioned aversion from amphetamine and apomorphine in rats. Science **191**:1273–1275.
3. MUCHA, R. F., D. VAN DER KOOY, M. O'SHAUGHNESSY & P. BUCENIEKS. 1982. Drug reinforcement studied by the use of place conditioning in rat. Brain Res. **243**:91–105.
4. WEEKS, J. R. 1962. Experimental morphine addiction: Method for automatic intravenous injections in unrestrained rats. Science **138**:143–144.
5. VAN DER KOOY, D. & A. G. PHILLIPS. 1977. Temporal analysis of naloxone attenuation of morphine-induced taste aversions. Pharmac. Biochem. Behav. **6**:637–641.
6. HUGHES, J. 1981. Peripheral opiate receptor mechanisms. Trends Pharmac. Sci. **3**:21–24.
7. NINKOVIC, M., S. P. HUNT & J. R. W. GLEAVE. 1982. Localization of opiate and histamine H_1 - receptors in the primate sensory ganglia and spinal cord. Brain Res. **241**:197–206.
8. BECHARA, A. & D. VAN DER KOOY. 1985. Opposite motivational effects of endogenous opioids in brain and periphery. Nature **314**:533–534.
9. VAN DER KOOY, D. & J. I. NAGY. 1985. Hyperalgesia mediated by peripheral opiate receptors in the rat. Behav. Brain Res. **17**:203–211.
10. YOUNG III, W. S., J. K. WAMSLEY, M. A. ZARBIN & M. J. KUHAR. 1980. Opioid receptors undergo axonal flow. Science **210**:76–78.
11. LAWSON, S. N. 1979. The postnatal development of large light and small dark neurons in mouse dorsal root ganglia: a statistical analysis of cell numbers and size. J. Neurocytol. **8**:275–294.
12. NINKOVIC, M. & S. P. HUNT. 1985. Opiate and histamine H1 receptors are present on some substance P-containing dorsal root ganglion cells. Neurosci. Lett. **53**:133–137.
13. LaMOTTE, C., C. B. PERT & S. H. SYNDER. 1976. Opiate receptor binding in primate spinal cord: distribution and changes after dorsal root section. Brain Res. **112**:407–412.
14. NINKOVIC, M., S. P. HUNT & J. S. KELLY. 1981. Effect of dorsal rhizotomy on the autoradiographic distribution of opiate and neurotensin-like immunoreactivity within the rat spinal cord. Brain Res. **230**:111–119.
15. ATWEH, S. F. & M. J. KUHAR. 1977. Autoradiographic localization of opiate receptors in rat brain. I. Spinal cord and lower medulla. Brain Res. **124**:53–67.
16. HERKENHAM, M. & C. P. PERT. 1982. Light microscopic localization of brain opiate receptors: a general autoradiographic method which preserves tissue quality. J. Neurosci. **2**:1129–1149.
17. WILLIAMS, J. & W. ZIEGLGANSBERGER. 1981. Mature spinal ganglion cells are not sensitive to opiate receptor mediated actions. Neurosci. Lett. **21**:211–216.
18. MUDGE, A. W., S. E. LEEMAN & G. D. FISCHBACH. 1979. Enkephalin inhibits release of

substance P from sensory neurons in culture and decreases action potential duration. Proc. Natl. Acad. Sci. USA **76**:526–530.

19. WERZ, M. A. & R. L. MACDONALD. 1984. Dynorphin reduces calcium-dependent action potential duration by decreasing voltage-dependent calcium conductance. Neurosci. Lett. **46**:185–190.

20. LORD, J. A. H., A. A. WATERFIELD, J. HUGHES & H. W. KOSTERLITZ. 1977. Endogenous opioid peptides: multiple agonists and receptors. Nature **267**:495–499.

21. JESSEN, K. R., M. NINKOVIC & S. P. HUNT. 1981. Autoradiographic localization of receptors for putative peptide neurotransmitters in the gastrointestinal tract. Neurosci. Lett. **57**:5452.

22. DRAY, A. & I. NUNAN. 1984. Evidence that naloxonizine produces prolonged antagonism of central delta opioid activity in vivo. Brain Res. **323**:123–127.

23. HISAMITSU, T. & W. C. DE GROOT. 1984. The inhibitory effect of opioid peptides and morphine applied intrathecally and intracerebroventricularly on the micturition reflex in the cat. Brain Res. **198**:51–65.

24. SWEETNAM, P. M., J. H. NEALE, J. L. BARKER & A. GOLDSTEIN. 1982. Localization of immunoreactive dynorphin in neurons cultured from spinal cord and dorsal root ganglia. Proc. Natl. Acad. Sci. USA **79**:6742–6746.

25. HUNT, S. P., J. S. KELLY, P. C. EMSON, J. R. KIMMEL, R. J. MILLER & J. Y. YU. 1981. An immunohistochemical study of neuronal populations containing neuropeptides or γ-aminobutyrate within the superficial layers of the rat dorsal horn. Neurosci. **6**:1883–1898.

26. HUNT, S. P., J. S. KELLY & P. C. EMSON. 1980. The electron microscopic localization of methionine-enkephalin within the superficial layers (I and II) of the spinal cord. Neurosci. **5**:1871–1890.

27. GOLDSTEIN, A. 1976. Opioid peptides (endorphins) in pituitary and brain. Science **193**:1081–1086.

28. SCHULTZBERG, M., T. HOKFELT, L. TERENIUS, L. G. ELFIRN, J. M. LUNDBERG, J. BRANDT, R. P. ELDE & M. GOLDSTEIN. 1979. Enkephalin immunoreactive nerve fibers and cell bodies in sympathetic ganglia of the guinea pig and rat. Neurosci. **4**:249–270.

29. YANG, H. Y. T., T. HEXUM & E. COSTA. 1980. Opioid peptides in adrenal gland. Life Sci. **27**:1119–1125.

30. GLAZER, E. J. & A. I. BASBAUM. 1980. Leucine enkaphalin: localization in and axonal transport by sacral parasympathetic preganglionic neurons. Science **208**:1479–1481.

31. DALSGAARD, C.-J., T. HOKFELT, L.-G. ELFIN & L. TERENIUS. 1982. Enkephalin-containing sympathetic preganglionic neurons projecting to the inferior mesenteric ganglion: evidence from combined retrograde tracing and immunohistochemistry. Neurosci. **7**:2039–2050.

32. KONDO, H. & R. YUI. 1982. An electron microscopic study on enkephalin-like immunoreactive nerve fibers in the celiac ganglion of guinea pig. Brain Res. **252**:142–145.

33. HARTSCHUCK, W., E. WEICKE, M. BUCHLER, V. HELMSTAEDTER, G. E. FEURLE & W. G. FORSSMANN. 1979. Met-enkephalin-like immunoreactivity in Merkel cells. Cell Tissue Res. **201**:343–348.

34. WEBER, U., W. HARTSCHUH, G. E. FEURLE & E. HEIHE. 1980. Met-enkephalin-like immuno- and bioreactivity in extracts from skin containing Merkel cells. Neurosci. Lett. **2**:201–240.

35. DIAUGUSTINE, R. P., L. H. LAZARUS, G. JAHNKE, M. N. KHAN, M. D. ERISMAN & R. I. LINNOILA. 1980. Corticotrophin/β-endorphin immunoreactivity in rat mast cells. Peptide or protease? Life Sci. **27**:2663–2668.

36. DALSGAARD, C. J., S. R. VINCENT, T. HOKFELT, I. CHRISTENSSON & L. TERENIUS. 1983. Separate origins for the dynorphin and enkephalin immunoreactive fibers in the inferior mesenteric ganglion of guinea pig. J. Comp. Neurol. **221**:482–489.

37. FURNESS, J. B., M. COSTA & R. J. MILLER. 1983. Distribution and projections of nerves with enkephalin-like immunoreactivity in the guinea-pig small intestine. Neurosci. **8**:653–664.
38. HAZUM, E., K. J. CHANG & P. CUATRECASAS. 1979. Specific nonopiate receptors for β-endorphin. Science **205**:1033–1035.
39. WESTPHAL, M. & C. H. LI. 1984. B-Endorphin: characterization of binding sites specific for the human hormone in human glioblastoma SF 126 cells. Proc. Natl. Acad. Sci. USA **81**:2921–2923.
40. HERZ, A. & H. TESCHEMACHER. 1971. Activities and sites of antinocicpetive action of morphine-like analgesics. Adv. Drug Res. **6**:79–119.
41. VAN DER KOOY, D., R. F. MUCHA, M. O'SHAUGHNESSY & P. BUCENIEKS. 1982. Reinforcing effects of brain microinjections of morphine revealed by conditioned place preference. Brain Res. **243**:107–117.
42. YAKSH, T. L. & T. A. RUDY. 1977. Studies on the direct spinal action of narcotics in the production of analgesia in the rat. J. Pharmacol. Exp. Therap. **202**:411–428.
43. VALENTINO, R. J., S. HERLING, J. H. WOODS, F. MEDZIHRADSKY & H. MERZ. 1981. Quaternary naltrexone: evidence for the central mediation of discriminative stimulus effects of narcotic agonists and antagonists. J. Pharmac. Exp. Ther. **217**:652–659.
44. MARTIN, J. R., R. C. ROGERS, D. NOVIN & D. A. VAN DER WEELE. 1977. Excessive gastric retention by vagotomized rats and rabbits given a solid diet. Bull. Psychonom. Soc. **10**:291–294.
45. VONVOIGTLANDER, P. F., R. A. LAHTI & J. H. LUDENS. 1983. U-50,488: A selective and structurally novel non-mu (kappa) opioid agonist. J. Pharmac. Exp. Therap. **224**:7–12.
46. MUCHA, R. F. & A. HERZ. 1985. Motivational properties of kappa and mu opioid receptor agonists studied with place and taste preference conditioning. Psychopharmacology **86**:274–280.
47. PATTERSON, S. J., L. E. ROBSON & H. W. KOSTERLITZ. 1983. Classification of opioid receptors. Br. Med. Bull. **39**:31–36.
48. JANCSO, N. 1960. Role of the nerve terminals in the mechanism of inflammatory reactions. Bull. Millard Fillmore Hospital, Buffalo **7**:53–57.
49. JANCSO, N. & A. JANCSO-GABOR. 1959. Dauerausschaltung der chemischen schmerzempfindlichkeit durch capsaicin. Arch. Exp. Path. Pharmakol. **236**:142–145.
50. ELLIS, III, H. L., A. R. JOHNSON & N. C. MORAN. 1970. Selective release of histamine from rat mast cells by several drugs. J. Pharmac. Exp. Therap. **175**:627–631.
51. YAMASAKI, Y., O. SHIMAMURA & H. IJICHI. 1981. Opioid receptors on rat mast cells. Intl. Narcotic Club Conf., Abst. 58.
52. KIERNAN, J. A. 1977. A study of chemically induced acute inflammation in the skin of the rat. Q. J. Exp. Physiol. **62**:151–161.
53. JANCSO, G., E. KIRALY & A. JANCSO-GABOR. 1977. Pharmacologically induced selective degeneration of chemosensitive primary sensory neurons. Nature **270**:741–743.
54. JESSEL, T. M., L. L. IVERSEN & A. C. CUELLO. 1978. Capsaicin-induced depletion of substance P from primary sensory neurons. Brain Res. **152**:183–188.
55. NAGY, J. I. 1982. Capsaicin: a chemical probe for sensory neuron mechanisms. *In* Handbook of Psychopharmacology. L. L. Iversen, S. D. Iversen & S. H. Snyder, Eds. **15**:185–235. Plenum Press. New York.
56. NAGY, J. I., S. R. VINCENT, W. A. STAINES, H. C. FIBIGER, T. D. REISINE & H. I. YAMAMURA. 1980. Neurotoxic action of capsaicin on spinal substance P neurons. Brain Res. **86**:435–444.
57. NAGY, J. I., S. P. HUNT, L. L. IVERSEN & P. C. EMSON. 1981. Biochemical and anatomical observations on the degeneration of peptide-containing primary afferent neurons after neonatal capsaicin. Neurosci. **6**:1923–1934.

58. Fog, R. 1970. Behavioural effects in rats of morphine and amphetamine and a combination of the two drugs. Psychopharmacologia 16:305–312.
59. Norton, S. 1977. The structure of behaviour of rats during morphine-induced hyperactivity. Commun. Psychopharm. 1:333–341.
60. Mansky, P. A. 1978. Opiates: human psychopharmacology. In Handbook of Psychopharmacology. L. L. Iversen, S. D. Iversen & S. H. Snyder, Eds. 12:95–185. Plenum Press. New York.
61. Sollmann, T. & J. D. Pilcher. 1917. Endermic reaction. J. Pharmac. Exp. Therap. 9:309–340.
62. Ferreira, S. H. & M. Nakamura. 1979. Prostaglandin hyperalgesia: the peripheral analgesic activity of morphine, enkephalins and opioid antagonists. Prostaglandins 18:191–200.
63. Rios, L. & J. Jacob. 1983. Local inhibition of inflammatory pain by naloxone and its n-methyl quaternary analogue. J. Pharmac. 96:277–283.
64. Watkins, L. R. & D. J. Mayer. 1982. Organization of endogenous opiate and nonopiate pain control systems. Science 216:1185–1192.
65. Hokfelt, T., O. Johansson, A. Ljungdahl, J. M. Lundberg & M. Schultzberg. 1980. Peptidergic neurons. Nature 284:515–521.
66. MacDonald, S. M., M. Mezei & C. Mezei. 1981. Effect of Wallerian degeneration on histamine concentration of the peripheral nerve. J. Neurochem. 36:9–16.
67. Jancso, N., A. Jancso-Gabor & J. Szolcsanyi. 1967. Direct evidence for neurogenic inflammation and its prevention by denervation and by pretreatment with capsaicin. Br. J. Pharmacol. Chemother. 31:138–151.
68. Lembeck, F., R. Gamse & H. Juan. 1977. Substance P and sensory nerve endings. In Substance P. U.S. von Euler & B. Pernow, Eds.:169–181. Raven Press. New York.
69. Theoharides, T. C., T. Betchaku & W. W. Douglas. 1981. Somatostatin-induced histamine secretion in mast cells. Characterization of the effect. Eur. J. Pharm. 69:127–137.
70. Kuehl, F. A. & R. W. Egan. 1980. Prostaglandins, arachidonic acid, and inflammation. Science 210:978–984.
71. Ferreira, S. H. 1977. Prostaglandins, aspirin-like drugs and analgesia. Nature 240:200–203.
72. Collier, H. O. J. & C. Schneider. 1972. Nociceptive response to prostaglandins and analgesic actions of aspirin and morphine. Nature 236:141–143.
73. Keele, C. A. & D. Armstrong. 1964. Substances Producing Pain and Itch. Williams and Wilkins Co. Baltimore, MD.
74. Roth, J., D. Le Roith, J. Schiloach, L. Rosenzweig, M. A. Lesniak & J. Havrankova. 1982. The evolutionary origins of hormones, neurotransmitters, and other extracellular chemical messengers. Implications for mammalian biology. N. Eng. J. Med. 306:523–527.
75. Selye, H. 1956. The Stress of Life. McGraw Hill. New York.
76. Guillemin, R., T. Vargo, J. Rossier, S. Minick, H. Ling, C. Rivier, W. Vale & F. Bloom. 1977. B-endorphin and adrenocorticotropin are secreted concomitantly by the pituitary gland. Science 197:1367–1368.
77. Solomon, R. L. & J. D. Corbit. 1974. An opponent-process theory of motivation: I. Temporal dynamics of affect. Psych. Rev. 81: 119–145.
78. Bolles, R. C. & M. S. Fanselou. 1982. A perceptual-defensive-recuperative model of fear and pain. Behav. Brain Sci. 3:291–323.

Role of Circulating Opioids in the Modulation of Pain[a]

JAMES L. HENRY

Departments of Physiology and Psychiatry
McGill University
Montreal, Quebec
H3G 1Y6
Canada

INTRODUCTION

In this paper I shall present some earlier data[1-3] that led to the suggestion that endogenous opioids circulating in the blood may participate in the suppression of nociceptive transmission at the spinal level. To support this suggestion, further evidence is presented in the discussion that nociceptive transmission is likely under a homeostatic type of control, that this type of control functions under normal physiological conditions and that the set point, in this case pain threshold, can be modified by clearly identifiable physiological conditions.

Stress, the focus of this volume, is clearly one of the physiological perturbations that alter this set point. However, there is also ample evidence to support a belief that stress is only one of a number of such perturbations, perturbations that are all components of normal daily life.

METHODS

Experiments were done on adult cats. After induction with halothane/oxygen they were anesthetized with alpha-chloralose (60 mg/kg) intravenously. Spinal segments L5–L7 were exposed for recording and covered with warm mineral oil to prevent drying. To eliminate the influence of supraspinal structures on the excitability of the units studied and to ensure that changes in the discharge rate of these units upon the administration of naloxone were not due to actions on supraspinal structures, the cords were transected at the level of the first lumbar vertebra. Core temperture was maintained at 38°C. Carotid arterial pressure was monitored on a Grass polygraph and mean pressure was always above 100 mm Hg. Spinal circulation was checked periodically throughout the experiment using a Carl Zeiss zoom stereomicroscope.

Extracellular single unit spikes were recorded with multibarrelled micropipettes. The central barrel was filled with 2.7 M NaCl and was used for recording. One additional barrel was filled with Na L-glutamate (1 M, pH 7.4, Sigma) and one with Pontamine Sky Blue 6BX (2% in 0.5 M sodium acetate, Gurr) for histological identification of sites of recording, using a method described elsewhere.[4]

[a]Supported by the Medical Research Council of Canada.

169

All units were classified carefully according to their responses to natural stimulation of the cutaneous receptive field: blowing with an air stream, gentle to heavy pressure with a blunt glass probe, pinching with forceps or clamps, burning with an infrared bulb. Proprioceptive units were identified as such by passive movements of the limb.

Naloxone was administered via a catheter in the jugular vein. In most cases a dose of 0.1 mg/kg was given, but with units that were unaffected by this dose, 0.3– 0.4 mg/kg were given.

RESULTS

As the route of administration of naloxone was intravenous, only one unit was studied in each experimental animal; this was done to avoid the possibility of persisting effects of earlier doses, which might modify the response to naloxone. In all cases, carotid arterial pressure was unaffected by the intravenous administration of naloxone.

Character of Response to Intravenous Naloxone

Intravenous administration of naloxone caused excitation of approximately two-thirds of the single spinal units tested. Typically, this excitation began within one min of administration and reached its maximum after two to five min. The discharge rate remained elevated usually for more than one hour, and occasionally failed to return to its original level even after two hours.

FIGURE 1 shows a typical response, in which a clear increase in ongoing activity occurred. While a dose of 0.1 mg/kg was used in most cases, a similar increase in activity was seen with as little as 0.05 mg/kg. In the cases where this excitation did not occur additional doses of naloxone were given, up to 0.3–0.4 mg/kg; in all these cases, excitation still failed to occur.

Correlation of Naloxone Excitation with Adequate Stimulus

All nociceptive units were excited by naloxone. These neurons included the so-called wide dynamic range units[5] as well as nociceptive units. The non-nociceptive units responding to cutaneous stimuli were all unaffected by naloxone administration. Two proprioceptive units were studied: one was excited by naloxone, the other was unaffected.

Effects of Naloxone on Responses to Noxious Heat

In view of this preferential effect of naloxone on nociceptive neurons, the response to automatically controlled, periodic applications of heat was compared before and after the intravenous administration of naloxone. With 13 of 15 neurons studied, naloxone enhanced the magnitude of this nociceptive response. A typical effect is illustrated in FIGURE 2. This enhancement consisted of an increase in the peak discharge rate in the response to the noxious stimulus and also an increase in the duration of the after-discharge of this response. The time

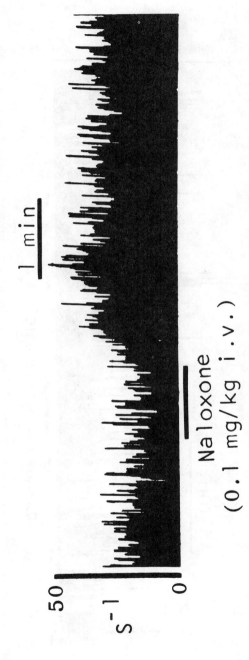

FIGURE 1. Ratemeter record of a single nociceptive unit in the dorsal horn showing an increase in ongoing spike activity upon the intravenous administration of naloxone. The period of drug administration is indicated by the horizontal bar below the records. The ordinate shows the rate of discharge in spikes per second.

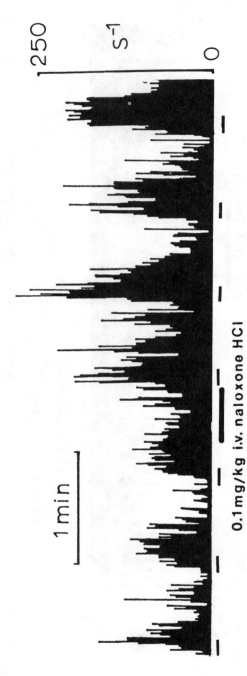

FIGURE 2. Ratemeter record of a single nociceptive unit in the dorsal horn showing a naloxone-induced increase in the magnitude of the response to automatically controlled regular applications of noxious radiant heat (indicated by the short horizontal bars) to the cutaneous receptive field. The thick horizontal bar represents the period of administration of naloxone.

course of this effect on the heat response was similar to the increase in ongoing discharge rate described above.

Effects of Dorsal Rhizotomy on Response to Naloxone

To determine whether the responses to naloxone were due to actions on afferent neurons peripherally or to actions in the spinal cord, the effects of cutting the ipsilateral dorsal roots on the excitatory response to naloxone were studied in five cats. During surgical preparation of each cat a fine silk thread was looped around the dorsal roots of segments L4–S2 on the side of recording. Later, while recording, when a unit was found that responded to noxious cutaneous stimulation, an initial dose 0.1 mg/kg of naloxone was given to confirm the excitatory effect seen in the earlier experiments. Once this had been achieved the looped roots were cut and, once the level of activity was considered to be stable, a second dose of 0.1 mg/kg of naloxone caused a prolonged increase in the rate of activity, and the time course of this increase was similar to the excitation reported above and illustrated in FIGURES 1 and 2.

Results from Experiments Done at Night

It was considered that endogenous opioid mechanisms might underlie the responses to naloxone and, in view of the observation that pain threshold varies on a diurnal cycle, the initial experiments with intravenous administration of naloxone were repeated, but the experiments were done at night rather than during the day. Thus, instead of starting the experiments at 09:00 h, they were started approximately twelve hours later, at 21:00 h.

Of the eight units studied at night only one was excited by intravenous administration of naloxone, even when doses up to 0.6 mg/kg were used. In the seven experiments in which excitation did not occur, the cats used were fully conditioned to the time schedule of the animal quarters. The one experiment in which excitation was seen was done on a cat that had been delivered to the animal quarters early in the day of the experiment.

Effects of Hypophysectomy on Responses to Naloxone

During the course of the experiments it became apparent that a circulating opioid factor might be having a tonic inhibitory effect on nociceptive neurons in the dorsal horn, at least during the day. Therefore experiments were done on hypophysectomized cats in an effort to identify the origin of this factor. The pituitary glands were removed via a trans-buccal approach. After survival times of 7 to 26 days, blood samples were taken from each cat and measured for cortisol by the method of Murphy.[6] Five cats were found to be without detectable basal levels of cortisol. In each of these five cats, naloxone administered in doses up to 0.5 mg/kg failed to alter the ongoing rate of discharge or the response to noxious cutaneous stimulation. On the other hand, in an experiment on a sixth hypophysectomized cat, in which basal levels of 10 ng/kg of cortisol were detected, naloxone at 0.1 mg/kg increased both the ongoing rate of discharge and the response to noxious cutaneous stimuli. Similar excitatory effects of naloxone were observed in four surgical control cats done during the same sequence of experiments.

Correlation of Naloxone Effects with Depth in Grey Matter

Attempts were made to sample neurons throughout the various laminae of the dorsal horn equally in the daytime and in the nighttime experiments. Thus, neurons were studied in Rexed's laminae I, IV, and V.

DISCUSSION

These results suggest that the intravenous administration of naloxone has a preferential excitatory effect on nociceptive neurons in the spinal cord. It is probable that this excitatory effect is not an excitation per se, but rather is a disinhibition, due to the withdrawal of a tonic inhibition imposed by the action of an endogenous chemical agent with morphine-like properties. The results also suggest that this effect of naloxone occurs by an action within the spinal cord, because all experiments were done on spinal-transected animals and because the effect was still seen after the sensory axons were cut. The variable effectiveness of naloxone, depending on the time of day during which it was administered, suggests that the endogenous opioid factor varies in its concentration on a diurnal cycle, with the highest concentrations occurring during the day and the lowest during the night, at least under the conditions of the present experiments. It is difficult to visualize a mechanism within the spinal cord that could account for the diurnal variation of the effects observed in the study. It seems more plausible that the endogenous opioid factor comes from the circulation, and that its origin is from an endocrine gland whose output varies on a diurnal cycle. The experiments on hypophysectomized cats demonstrate that an intact pituitary gland is necessary for the expression of the excitatory effects of naloxone on spinal nociceptive units. Therefore it is proposed that naloxone causes excitation, strictly speaking a disinhibition, by its antagonism of an endogenous opioid agent, that this peptide reaches the spinal cord from the circulation and that it is present in the circulation only when the pituitary gland is functioning. Whether the origin of this agent is the pituitary gland itself or another endocrine gland regulated by pituitary output remains to be determined.

Several features in this proposal go against conventional thought in terms of control of central nervous function. Therefore the rest of this discussion will be devoted to the citation of some of the evidence in the literature that suggests that circulating peptides cross the blood-brain barrier, perhaps especially at the spinal level, that there is a large number of different factors in the circulation with opioid properties and that several physiological conditions exist that trigger the release of opioid peptides into the circulation and also produce an increase in the pain threshold.

Peptides and the Blood-Brain Barrier

The possibility that the blood-brain barrier is even mildly permeable to peptides has been an unpopular topic among physiologists, because the physical properties of the CNS capillaries do not suggest such a penetration and perhaps also because the generalized action of peptide hormones, which one might visualize if they indeed did have access to the CNS, stands in marked contrast to the hard-wired neural pathways and the specificity of function that neuro-anatomists and neurophysiologists have uncovered for us. However, the facts that peripheral administration of peptides leads to CNS effects and that many peptides are found both in the CNS and in the circulation force us to re-examine this possibility. We find there is a growing body of evidence suggesting that there is some permeability of the blood-brain barrier to peptides. Some of the most relevant experimental evidence will now be reviewed briefly. To begin with, an interesting and thorough review of this topic has recently been published by Meisenberg and Simmons.[7]

Evidence on the passage of enkephalins into CNS tissue is varied: some papers report little or no such passage[8] while others report significant levels of enkephalins or enkephalin analogues in brain regions after systemic ad-ministration.[9-11] Beta-endorphin seems to cross into the CSF but not into brain tissue[12] although an analogue of beta-endorphin has been reported to cross the blood-brain barrier.[10] Alpha-MSH, a member of the opiocortin family, has only limited entry into brain tissue.[13] Behavioral effects, reported to occur after peripheral administration of endorphins,[14] also lend support to the possibility that circulating opioids cross the blood-brain barrier.

Angiotensin II given systemically induces drinking behavior due to an action on the subfornical organ[15] and induces an increase in arterial pressure due to an action on the area postrema and on the subfornical organ.[16] This evidence raises the further possibility that circulating opioid peptides may alter CNS activity through their actions on circumventricular organs where the blood-brain barrier is thin or absent. Continuing with angiotensin II, though, it may also pass into brain tissue besides or beyond the circumventricular organs.[17,18]

Besides opioid peptides and angiotensin II, delta sleep–inducing peptide has also been found in brain tissue after systemic administration[19] and others have been reported to cross the blood-CSF barrier, including an angiotensin analogue,[20] vasopressin and oxytocin,[21] an oxytocin fragment,[17] alpha-MSH,[14] and prolactin.[22]

While on the subject of the blood-brain barrier and peptides, it should also be pointed out that the permeability of this barrier may be modified by circulating hormones, among which are melanotropic peptides, which increase perme-ability,[23] and a melanotropin-related peptide[24] and corticosterone,[25] which decrease permeability.

It cannot go unsaid that the evidence on passage of peptides through the blood-brain barrier is still contradictory and controversial. Methods of assaying quantities that might pass may lack the sensitivity to detect the trace amounts required to produce physiological effects. It is important to know the specific peptide or fragment that may be eliciting the physiological effect. It is important to consider circumventricular organs or structures in their immediate vicinity as possible mediators of the physiological effects seen. Further information is needed on the possible differences between the blood-brain and the blood-spinal barrier.

Opioid Factors in the Circulation

A number of different peptides with opioid properties has been reported in the blood. Of course, one of the principal groups of opioid peptides is that derived from opiocortin. Beta-endorphin was reported in the circulation as early as 1977.[26,27] Its source is believed to be the anterior and intermediate lobes of the pituitary[28] and recent evidence suggests that it is localized in two compartments in the blood, viz. the plasma and associated with erythrocytes.[29]

Met-enkephalin is found in the circulation and its probable source is the adrenal medulla.[30]

Several different forms of dynorphin have been reported to circulate in the blood and the source is speculated to be the neural lobe of the pituitary.[28]

Several as yet unidentified peptides besides beta-endorphin, enkephalin, and dynorphin have also been identified in the blood. In one report, two opioid factors were found that caused a naloxone-antagonizable inhibition of the electrically induced twitch of guinea pig myenteric plexus-longitudinal muscle.[31] In another, relatively large quantities of opioid peptides were found, and these were thought to originate in the adrenal medulla and sympathetic nerve terminals.[28]

In the context of the present manuscript, beta-endorphin and enkephalin are unlikely candidates for the circulating factor proposed to be involved in the experiments reported here, beta-endorphin because of its poor penetrability into the CNS and enkephalin because of its rapid degradation in the blood.[30] In addition, in one study, naloxone administration failed to alter pain sensitivity in patients with high plasma levels of beta-endorphin.[32] However, the remaining opioid peptides must remain candidates, and it will be interesting when the structures of other circulating opioids become know because then they may become available for physiological experiments and can be studied for their possible penetration of the blood-brain barrier.

Surprisingly, little has been done on the effects of circulating opioid peptides on central nervous function, especially as they may affect nociception and pain. In an early study sytemic administration of beta-endorphin was reported to produce analgesia,[33-35] but the amounts required to produce analgesia were unphysiologically high[36] and this early initiative has not been followed either with beta-endorphin or with other opioid peptides.

Conditions that Increase Plasma Opioids and Produce Analgesia

Stress

As this volume is on stress and analgesia, it is redundant to go into detail to establish that stress induces the release of opioid peptides into the circulation and also produces analgesia. It is worth noting, however, that these effects on circulating opioid peptides[36] have been know since 1977.

Excessive Physical Exertion

While they may be considered as forms of stress, long distance running[37] and excessive exercise[38] have been reported to increase plasma levels of beta-endorphin as well as other circulating hormones in humans[39-41] and in experimental animals.[42,43] Among athletes extreme physical exertion is well known for its analgesic effects.

Acupuncture

Acupuncture is best known as a procedure for the alleviation of pain and its analgesic properties therefore do not need to be substantiated. In a search for the mechanisms of this analgesia several studies have reported that plasma levels of circulating opioids and other opiocortin peptides are increased by acupuncture,[44,45] although one report observed increases in brain but not plasma beta-endorphin.[46]

Copulation

This increases plasma levels of beta-endorphin[47,48] and increases pain threshold in animals,[48] and naloxone changes sexual behavior in experimental animals.[49] The possible role of circulating opioids in sexual behavior has been explored in a previous paper. [50]

While it is not a noticeable physiological condition like the others, there is a diurnal variation in circulating levels of opioid peptides[51-54] as well as in pain threshold.[53,55,56] Interestingly, a diurnal variation has even been noted in a nociceptive reflex in the spinal rat.[57]

Several other conditions have been shown to increase circulating levels of opioid factors, including food deprivation,[58] menstruation,[59] conditioned fear,[60] and even caffeine.[61] Factors that increase pain threshold include food deprivation,[58,62] pain,[50] menstruation,[59] pregnancy,[63] vaginal and cervical probing,[64] social conflict, crowding or isolation,[65-67] hibernation,[68] suggestion,[69-73] hypertension,[74-77] and a number of other conditions.

CONCLUSION

We are still far from knowing which circulating opioid factors are participating in the effects observed in my experiments. One can be reasonably optimistic that this information will become available as there is evidence in the literature that conditions exist that raise pain threshold and increase plasma levels of opioid peptides, that a substantial number of opioid peptides circulate in the blood, and that at lease some peptides have access to central nervous tissue from the circulation.

REFERENCES

1. HENRY, J. L. 1979. Naloxone excites nociceptive units in the lumbar dorsal horn of the spinal cat. Neuroscience **4**:1485–1491.
2. HENRY, J. L. 1981. Diurnal variation in naloxone excitation of dorsal horn units in the spinal cat suggests a circulating opioid factor. Neuroscience **10**:1935–1942.
3. HENRY, J. L. 1981. Naloxone excitation of spinal nociceptive units fails to occur in hypophysectomized cats. Br. J. Pharmacol. **72**:157P–158P.
4. HENRY, J. L. 1976. Effects of substance P on functionally identified units in cat spinal cord. Brain Res. **114**:439–452.
5. PRICE, D. D. & R. DUBNER. 1977. Neurons that subserve the sensory-discriminative aspects of pain. Pain **3**:307–338.

6. MURPHY, B. E. P. 1967. Some studies of the protein-binding of steroids and their application to the routine micro and utramicro measurements of various steroids in body fluids by competitive protein binding radioassay. J. Clin. Endocrinol. Metab. 27:973–990.

7. MEISENBERG, G. & W. H. SIMMONS. 1983. Peptides and the blood-brain barrier. Life Sci. 32:P2611–2623.

8. CORNFORD, E. M., L. D. BRAUN, P. D. CRANE & W. H. OLENDORF. 1978. Blood brain barrier restriction of peptides and low uptake of enkephalins. Endocrinology 103:1297–1303.

9. KASTIN, A. J., C. NISSEN, A. V. SCHALLY & D. H. COY. 1976. Blood brain barrier, half time disappearance, and brain distribution for labeled enkephalin and a potent analog. Brain Res. Bull. 1:583–589.

10. RAPOPORT, S. T., W. A. KLEE, K. D. PETTIGREW & K. OHNO. 1980. Entry of opioid peptides into the central nervous system. Science 207:84–86.

11. DUBEY, A. K., J. HERBERT, N. D. MARTENSZ, U. BECKFORD & M. T. JONES. 1983. Differential penetration of three anterior pituitary peptide hormones into the cerebrospinal fluid of Rhesus monkeys. Life Sci. 32:1857–1864.

12. PEZALLA, P. D., M. LIS, N. G. SEIDAH & M. CHRETIEN. 1978. Lipotropin, melanotropin and endorphin in vivo catabolism and entry into cerebrospinal fluid. Can. J. Neurol. Sci. 3:183–188.

13. WILSON, J. F., S. ANDERSON, G. SNOOK & K. D. LLEWELLYN. 1984. Quantification of the permeability of the blood-CSF barrier to alpha-MSH in the rat. Peptides 5:681–685.

14. KASTIN, A. J., D. H. COY, A. V. SCHALLY & L. H. MILLER. 1978. Peripheral administration of hypothalamic peptides results in CNS changes. Pharmacol. Res. Commun. 10:293–312.

15. PHILLIPS, M. I. 1978. Angiotensin in the brain. Neuroendocrinology 2501:354–377.

16. SIMPSON, J. B. 1981. The circumventricular organs and the central actions of angiotensin. Neuroendocrinology 32:248–256.

17. HOFFMAN, P. L., R. WALTER & M. BULAT. 1977. An enzymatically stable peptide with activity in the central nervous sytem: its penetration through the blood-CSF barrier. Brain Res. 122:87–94.

18. VAN HOUTEN, M., E. L. SCHIFFRIN, J. F. E. MANN, B. I. POSNER & R. BOUCHER. 1980. Radioautographic localization of specific binding sites for blood-borne angiotensin II in the rat brain. Brain Res. 186:480–485.

19. BANKS, W. A., A. J. KASTIN & D. H. COY. 1984. Evidence that [^{125}I]N-Tyr-delta sleep-inducing peptide crosses the blood-brain barrier by a non-competitive mechanism. Brain Res. 301:201–207.

20. HOFFMAN, W. E. & M. I. PHILLIPS. 1976. Evidence for sar^1-ala^8-angiotensin crossing the blood cerebrospinal fluid barrier to antagonize central effects of angiotensin II. Brain Res. 109:541–552.

21. MENS, W. B. J., A. WITTER & T. B. VAN WIMERSMA GREIDANUS. 1983. Penetration of neurohypophyseal hormones from plasma into cerebrospinal fluid (CSF): half-times of disappearance of these neuropeptides from CSF. Brain Res. 262:143–149.

22. BELCHETZ, P. E., R. M. RIDLEY & H. F. BAKER. 1982. Studies on the accessibility of prolactin and growth hormone to brain: effect of opiate agonists on hormone levels in serial, simultaneous plasma and cerebrospinal fluid samples in the rhesus monkey. Brain Res. 239:310–314.

23. RUDMAN, D. & M. H. KUTNER. 1978. Melanotropic peptides increase permeability of plasma/cerebrospinal fluid barrier. Am. J. Physiol. 234:E327–E332.

24. GOLDMAN, H. & S. MURPHY. 1981. An analog of ACTH/MSH/4-9 Org-2766, reduces permeability of the blood brain barrier. Pharmacol. Biochem. Behav. 14:845–848.

25. LONG, J. B. & J. W. HOLADAY. 1985. Blood-brain barrier: endogenous modulation by adrenal-cortical function. Science 227:1580–1583.

26. GUILLEMIN, R., T. VARGO, J. ROSSIER, S. MINICK, N. LING, C. RIVIER, W. VALE & F. BLOOM. 1977. Beta-endorphin and adrenocorticotropin are secreted concomitantly by the pituitary gland. Science 197:1367–1369.

27. AKIL, H., S. J. WATSON, J. D. BARCHAS & C. H. LI. 1979. Beta-endorphin immuno-reactivity in rat and human blood—radioimmunoassay, comparative levels and physiological alterations. Life Sci. 24:1659–1666.

28. BOARDER, M. R., E. ERDELYI & J. D. BARCHAS. 1982. Forms of opioid peptides circulating in human blood—investigation with multiple radioimmunoassays and radioreceptor assay. In Regulatory Peptides: From Molecular Biology To Function. Advances in Biochemical Psychopharmacology. E. Costa & M. Trabucchi, Eds. 33:117–122. Raven Press. New York.

29. FISHER, A., R. DO, L. TAMARKIN, A. F. GHAZANFARI & A. B. MUKHERJEE. 1984. Two pools of beta-endorphin-like immunoreactivity in blood: plasma and erythrocytes. Life Sci. 34:1839–1846.

30. CLEMENT-JONES, V., P. J. LOWRY, L. H. REES & G. M. BESSER. 1980. Metenkephalin circulates in human plasma. Nature 283:295–297.

31. SCHULZ, R., M. WUSTER & A. HERZ. 1977. Detection of a long acting endogenous opioid in blood and small intestine. Life Sci. 21:105–116.

32. MOHS, R. C., B. M. DAVIS, G. S. ROSENBERG, K. L. DAVIS & D. T. KRIEGER. 1982. Naloxone does not affect pain sensitivity, mood or cognition in patients with high levels of beta endorphin in plasma. Life Sci. 30:1827–1833.

33. LING, N. & R. GUILLEMIN. 1976. Morphinomimetic activity of synthetic fragments of beta-lipotropin and analogs. Proc. Natl. Acad. Sci. USA 73:3308–3310.

34. GRAF, L., E. BARAT & A. PATTHY. 1976. Isolation of a COOH-terminal beta-lipotropin fragment (residues 61-91) with morphine-like analgesic activity from porcine pituitary glands. Acta Biochem. Biophys. Acad. Sci. Hung. 11:121–122.

35. TSENG, L.-F., H. H. LOH & C. H. LI. 1976. Beta-endorphin as a potent analgesic by intravenous injection. Nature 263:239–240.

36. ROSSIER, J., E. D. FRENCH, C. RIVIER, N. LING, R. GUILLEMIN & F. E. BLOOM. 1977. Foot-shock induced stress increases beta-endorphin levels in blood but not brain. Nature 270:618–620.

37. COLT, E. W. D., S. L. WARDLAW & A. G. FRANTZ. 1981. The effect of running on plasma beta-endorphin. Life Sci. 28:1637–1640.

38. FRAIOLI, F., C. MORETTI, D. PALUCCI, E. ALICICCO, F. CRESCENZI & G. FORTUNIO. 1980. Physical exercise stimulates marked concomitant release of beta-endorphin and adrenocorticotrophic hormone (ACTH) in peripheral blood in man. Experientia 36:987–989.

39. PERTOVAARA, A., T. HUOPANIEMI, A. VIRTANEN & G. JOHANSSON. 1984. The influence of exercise on dental pain thresholds and the release of stress hormones. Physiol. Behav. 33:923–926.

40. JANAL, M. N., E. W. D. COLT, W. C. CLARK & M. GLUSMAN. 1984. Pain sensitivity, mood and plasma endocrine levels in man following long-distance running: effects of naloxone. Pain 19:13–25.

41. BLAKE, M. J., E. A. STEIN & A. J. VOMACHKA. 1984. Effects of exercise training on brain opioid peptides and serum LH in female rats. Peptides 5:953–958.

42. WARDLAW, S. L. & A. G. FRANTZ. 1980. Effect of swimming stress on brain beta-endorphin and ACTH. Clin. Res. 28:482A.

43. SHYU, B. C., S. A. ANDERSSON & P. THOREN. 1982. Endorphin mediated increase in pain threshold induced by long-lasting exercise in rats. Life Sci. 30:833–839.

44. MALIZIA, E., G. ANDREUCCI, D. PAOLUCCI, F. CRESCENZI, A. FABBRI & F. FRAIOLI. 1979. Electroacupuncture and peripheral beta-endorphin and ACTH levels. The Lancet 2:535.

45. SZCZUDLIK, A. & A. LYSKA. 1981. Acupuncture-induced changes in endorphin and insulin levels in human blood. Pain Suppl. 1:281.

46. WEN, H. L., W. K. K. HO, N. LING, L. MA & G. H. CHOA. 1979. The influence pf electro-acupunture on naloxone-induced morphine withdrawal. II. Elevation of immuno-assayable beta-endorphin activity in the brain but not the blood. Am. J. Chinese Med. 7:237–240.

47. MURPHY, M. R., D. L. BOWIE & C. B. PERT. 1979. Copulation elevates plasma beta-endorphin in the male hamster. Neurosci. Abs. 5:470.

48. SZECHTMAN, H., M. HERSHKOWITZ & R. SIMANTOV. 1981. Sexual behavior decreases pain sensitivity and stimulates endogenous opioids in male rats. eur. J. Pharmacol. **70**:279–285.

49. MCCONNELL, S. K., M. J. BAUM & T. M. BADGER. 1981. Lack of correlation between naloxone-induced changes in sexual behavior and serum LH in male rats. Hormones Behav. **15**:16–35.

50. HENRY, J. L. 1982. Circulating opioids: possible physiological roles in central nervous function. Neurosci. Biobehav. Rev. **6**:229–245.

51. FOLKARD, S., C. J. GLYNN & J. W. LLYOD. 1976. Diurnal variation and individual differences in the perception of intractable pain. J. Psychosom. Res. **20**:289–301.

52. DENT, R. R. M., C. GUILLEMINAULT, L. H. ALBERT, B. I. POSNER, B. M. COX & A. GOLDSTEIN. 1981. Diurnal rhythm of plasma immunoreactive beta-endorphin and its relationship to sleep stages and plasma rhythms of cortisol and prolactin. J. Clin. Endocrinol. Metab. **52**:942–947.

53. WESCHE, D. L. & R. C. A. FREDERICKSON. 1980. Diurnal differences in enkephalin levels correlated with nociceptive sensitivity. In Endogenous and Exogenous Opiate Agonists and Antagonists. E. L. Way, Ed.:463–466. Pergamon Press. Toronto.

54. GIBSON, M. J., G. L. COLURSO, L. APPLEBAUM & D. T. KRIEGER. 1983. Circadian variation of beta-endorphin-like immunoreactivity in neurointermediate pituitary. Peptides **4**:305–307.

55. KAVALIERS, M. & M. HIRST. 1983. Daily rhythms of analgesia in mice: effects of age and photoperiod. Brain Res. **279**:387–393.

56. KAVALIERS, M., M. HIRST & G. C. TESKEY. 1984. Aging and daily rhythms of analgesia in mice: effects of natural illumination and twilight. Neurobiol. Aging **5**:111–114.

57. WRIGHT, D. M. 1981. Diurnal rhythm in sensitivity of a nociceptive spinal reflex. Eur. J. Pharmacol. **69**:385–388.

58. DAVIS, J. M., M. T. LOWY, G. K. W. YIM, D. R. LAMB & P. V. MALVEN. 1983. Relationship between plasma concentrations of immunoreactive beta-endorphin and food intake in rats. Peptides **4**:79–83.

59. VEITH, J. L., J. ANDERSON, S. A. SLADE, P. THOMPSON, A. R. LANGEL & S. GETZLEF. 1984. Plasma beta-endorphin, pain thresholds and anxiety levels across the human menstrual cycle. Physiol. Behav. **32**:31–34.

60. SCALLET, A. C. 1982. Effect of conditioned fear and environmental novelty on plasma beta-endorphin in the rat. Peptides **3**:203–206.

61. ARNOLD, M. A., D. B. CARR, D. M. TOGASAKI, M. C. PIAN & J. B. MARTIN. 1982. Caffeine stimulates beta-endorphin release in blood but not in cerebrospinal fluid. Life Sci. **31**:1017–1024.

62. HAMM, R. J. & B. G. LYETH. 1984. Nociceptive thresholds following food restriction and return to free-feeding. Physiol. Behav. **33**:499–501.

63. BARON, S. A. & A. R. GINTZLER. 1984. Pregnancy-induced analgesia: effects of adrenalectomy and glucocorticoid replacement. Brain Res. **321**:341–346.

64. BODNAR, R. J. & B. R. KOMISARUK. 1984. Reduction in cervical probing analgesia by repeated prior exposure to cold-water swims. Physiol. Behav. **32**:653–655.

65. TESKEY, G. C., M. KAVALIERS & M. HIRST. 1984. Social conflict activates opioid analgesic and ingestive behaviors in male mice. Life Sci. **35**:303–315.

66. PILCHER, C. W. T. & S. M. JONES. 1981. Social crowding enhances aversiveness of naloxone in rats. Pharmacol. Biochem. Behav. **14**:299–303.

67. PULISI-ALLEGRA, S. & A. OLIVERIO. 1983. Social isolation: effects on pain threshold and stress-induced analgesia. Pharmacol. Biochem. Behav. **19**:679–681.

68. BECKMAN, A. L., C. LLADOS-ECKMAN, T. L. STANTON & M. W. ADLER. 1981. Physical dependence on morphine fails to develop during the hibernating state. Science **212**:1527–1529.

69. LEVINE, J. D., N. C. GORDON, R. SMITH & H. L. FIELDS. 1981. Analgesic responses to morphine and placebo in individuals with postoperative pain. Pain **10**:379–389.

70. GREVERT, P., L. H. ALBERT & A. GOLDSTEIN. 1983. Partial antagonism of placebo analgesia by naloxone. Pain **16**:129–143.

71. MELAZCK, R., A. Z. WEISZ & L. T. SPRAGUE. 1963. Stratagems for controlling pain: contributions of auditory stimulation and suggestion. Exp. Neurol. **8**:239–247.
72. BEECHER, H. K. 1956. Evidence for increased effectiveness of placebos with increased stress. Am. J. Physiol. **187**:163–169.
73. LASAGNA, L., F. MOSTELLER, J. M. VON FELSINGER & H. K. BEECHER. 1954. A study of the placebo response. Am. J. Med. **16**:770–779.
74. ZAMIR, N. & E. SHUBER. 1980. Altered pain perception in hypertensive humans. Brain Res. **201**:471–474.
75. SAAVEDRA, J. M. 1981. Naloxone reversible decrease in pain sensitivity in young and adult spontaneously hypertensive rats. Brain Res. **209**:245–249.
76. MAIXNER, W., K. B. TOUW, M. J. BRODY, G. F. GEBHART, & J. P. LONG. 1982. Factors influencing the altered pain perception in the spontaneously hypertensive rat. Brain Res. **237**:137–145.
77. FRIEDMAN, R., D. MURPHY, W. PERSONS & J. A. MCCAUGHRAN. 1984. Genetic predisposition to hypertension, elevated blood pressure and pain sensitivity: a functional analysis. Behav. Brain Res. **12**:75–79.

Functional Response of Multiple Opioid Systems to Chronic Arthritic Pain in the Rat[a]

M. J. MILLAN,[a] M. H. MILLAN,[a] A. CZŁONKOWSKI,[a]
C. W. T. PILCHER,[a] V. HÖLLT,[a] F. C. COLPAERT,[b] AND
A. HERZ[a]

[a]Max Planck Institute for Psychiatry
Department of Neuropharmacology
D-8033 Planegg-Martinsried
Federal Republic of Germany

[b]Janssen Pharmaceutical Research Laboratories
B-2340 Beerse, Belgium

INTRODUCTION

In view of the antinociceptive properties of the endogenous opioid peptides and their localization in regions of the brain and spinal cord involved in nociceptive processing, it is not surprising that many studies have examined their response to noxious stimulation. However, attention has generally been focused on the effects of acute imposition of noxious stimuli and regrettably few investigations have been conducted concerning chronic/long-term exposure. This is particularly unfortunate considering the possible clinical relevance of such information.

In evaluating the relationship between opioid systems and nociceptive processing, it is imperative to take into account their multiplicity. Currently, three families of endogenous opioid peptides may be recognized, corresponding to three independent precursors encoded by their three respective genes.[1] Pro-opiomelanocortin (POMC), processing of which yields β-endorphin; pro-enkephalin A, which is split to met-enkephalin and related peptides; and pro-enkephalin B, the precursor for dynorphin and α-neo-endorphin. There is evidence for contrasting roles of opioids of each family in the control of nociception. In addition, there is a multiplicity of opioid receptor types, of which the three most comprehensively characterized are μ-, δ-, and κ-receptors, which appear to fulfill differing roles in the control of nociception.[2-4] There is no straightforward correspondence between the multiplicity of opioid ligands and that of receptors, with the exception that there is acceptable evidence that dynorphin (and α-neo-endorphin) represents endogenous ligand(s) of the κ-receptor.[5]

There is, thus, a multiplicity of opioid ligands and opioid receptors that display a differential distribution and modulation and appear to subserve

[a]Supported by the Deutsche Forschungsgemeinschaft.

contrasting functional roles.[1,2,6] In addition, there are many independently localized pools of the respective opioid peptides and opioid receptors. Consequently, the often-formulated question as to the role of opioid systems in pain control may be a misleading oversimplification. It is necessary to examine these questions within the perspective of the multiplicity of these opioid systems. The present paper summarizes the findings of our recent work in which such an approach was adopted for an evaluation of the functional response of particular opioid systems to a model of chronic pain in the rat—adjuvant-induced arthritis. A detailed account can be found elsewhere.[7-10]

CHARACTERISTICS OF ADJUVANT-INDUCED ARTHRITIS IN THE RAT

Rats were inoculated intradermally at the root of the tail with Freunds adjuvant, which leads to a swelling and inflammation of the limbs and upper tail and is most accentuated on the hind limbs. These symptoms commence around day 10, peak at 3 weeks, and largely disappear by 10 weeks post-inoculation (FIGURE 1). Arthritic rats present a constellation of symptoms indicative of chronic pain and reminiscent of chronic pain conditions in man. These include a progressive loss of body weight, depression of appetite, irritability, and hyperreactivity.[11-13] In addition, they self-administer both anti-inflammatory agents and opiates.[12,14] The paws display a pronounced hypersensitivity to mechanical stimuli (FIGURE 1). Such a hyperalgesia to pressure has also been seen in electrophysiological studies of neurons in the dorsal horn of the spinal cord and the ventrobasal thalamus of arthritic rats: these reveal an enhanced spontaneous rate of firing, a lowered threshold, and heightened response to mechanical stimuli.[15,16] However, as summarized in TABLE 1, in distinction to pressure, arthritic rats manifest an increased latency to respond to noxious heat. This observation likewise corresponds to electrophysiological data according to which dorsal horn and thalamic neurons in arthritic rats display an elevated threshold for responding to noxious heat.[15,16] The differential influence of arthritic pain upon thresholds to noxious pressure, heat, and electrical stimulation (TABLE 1) exemplifies the important and general point that one cannot simply designate an animal to be either hyperalgesic or analgesic without reference to the nature of the noxious stimulus applied. In addition, it is necessary to specify the site of application of the stimulus, as indicated by the fact that inoculation of rats in a single paw leads to changes in nociceptive thresholds restricted to this affected region.[17]

INFLUENCE OF CHRONIC ARTHRITIC PAIN UPON MULTIPLE OPIOID SYSTEMS

We evaluated the levels of β-endorphin, dynorphin, α-neo-endorphin, and met-enkephalin, representatives of the three respective families, by use of specific radioimmunoassays at 1, 3, and 10 weeks following inoculation. The changes detailed below were observed at 3 weeks, coinciding with peak arthritic symptoms. No such alterations were apparent at either 1 or 10 weeks. Thus, the biochemical changes are reversible and parallel the time-course for the development and subsidence of arthritic symptoms.

Whereas in discrete tissues of brain no alterations in levels of immunoreactive

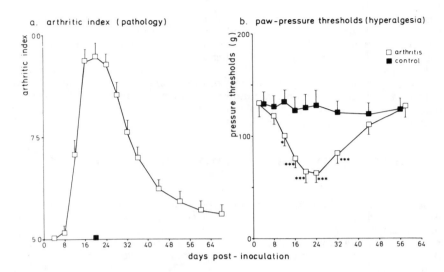

FIGURE 1. Time-course for the development of adjuvant-induced arthritis in the rat. The Arthritic Index comprises the sum of hind-paw weight and tibiotorsal joint diameter. The paw-pressure thresholds relate to the pressure applied by a wedge to the hind-paw, which elicits withdrawal. Mean ± S.E.M. depicted. N as follows: arthritis = 21, control = 10. Significance of arthritis versus control values indicated by asteriks. $*p \leqslant 0.05$, $***p \leqslant 0.001$ (Student's two-tailed test).

β-endorphin were detected, there was a pronounced rise in this in the anterior pituitary. This was accompanied by an elevation in immunoreactive β-endorphin in the systemic circulation together with an increase in anterior lobe levels of messenger ribonucleic acid (mRNA) encoding POMC. Thus, there is a selective facilitation of the generation of β-endorphin in, and its liberation from, the anterior pituitary. In individual regions of brain, no changes were seen in levels of immunoreactive met-enkephalin whereas a modest rise was observed in lumbo-sacral spinal cord (FIGURE 2). This increase is consistent with previous results in arthritic rats.[18]

TABLE 1. The Influence of Chronic Arthritic Pain Upon Nociceptive Thresholds in the Rat

	Withdrawal Response		Vocalization Response	
	Heat	Pressure	Electrical Stimulation	Pressure
Tail	↑	↓	–	?
Hind paw	↑↑	↓↓	?	↓↓

↑, increase; ↓, decrease; –, no change; and ?, not determined.

As regards immunoreactive dynorphin, an increase in levels was observed in the anterior pituitary but not in its neurointermediate counterpart. Of numerous structures of brain, only the thalamus displayed a rise in content. This is of note since electrophysiological studies have shown thalamic neurons to display alterations in their response to stimulation of the inflamed joints.[15] In addition, an extremely pronounced elevation was seen in the lumbosacral spinal cord (FIGURE 2) and a lesser rise in thoracic and cervical cord. (A very comparable pattern of changes was detected with immunoreactive α-neo-endorphin.) The shift in the spinal cord was greatest in the lumbosacral section that receives nociceptive input from the hind limbs, the region showing the most severe arthritic symptoms. It was previously found that inoculation of rats in fore paws or hind paws leads to a rise in levels of immunoreactive met-enkephalin and dynorphin in, respectively, cervical or lumbosacral cord[17] (R. Przewłocki, personal communication). Thus, there may be a regional specificity in the effects. Further, the lack of alteration in levels of immunoreactive vasopressin and oxytocin in the spinal cord of arthritic rats is suggestive of a neurochemical selectivity.[19] Moreover, the fact that the rise in immunoreactive ME in lumbo-

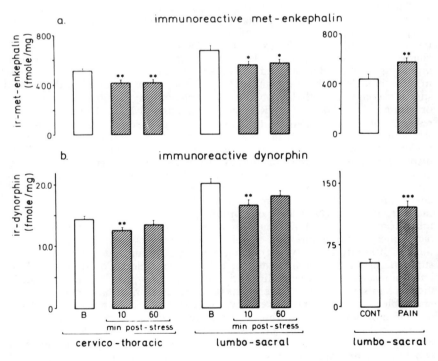

FIGURE 2. The influence of acute foot-shock or chronic arthritic pain upon spinal pools of immunoreactive met-enkephalin and immunoreactive dynorphin. Mean ± S.E.M. depicted. $N \geqslant 8$ per column. Significance of post-stress versus basal and pain versus control values indicated by asteriks. $*p \leqslant 0.05$, $**p \leqslant 0.01$, $***p \leqslant 0.001$ (Student's two-tailed t-test).

sacral cord is prevented by transsection of the sciatic nerve is evidence that the changes are dependent on the integrity of pathways conveying afferent noxious information.[17]

We detected no change in the binding of a universal ligand to all opioid receptors in various regions of the brain and spinal cord (affinity constant and binding density were unaffected). However, in addition, we exploited the technique of sequential blocking to allow for an evaluation of the effects upon multiple opioid receptor types. In the spinal cord, a fall in the density of κ-receptors was seen together with a relative rise in μ-receptors but no change in δ-receptors. A similar pattern of changes was seen in the thalamus but no alteration in the midbrain. Thus, in those tissues in which levels of immunoreactive dynorphin were elevated, a comparative loss of κ-receptors was apparent. Since dynorphin is considered an endogenous ligand of the κ-receptor,[5] this parallelism is of especial note. It is conceivable that a rise in dynorphin activity results in a down-regulation of κ-receptors, in analogy to the effects upon opioid receptors of long-term exposure of neuroblastoma cells to opioid agonists.[20] Although this interpretation must be regarded as speculative, it is of pertinence to mention the concomitant down-regulation of β-adrenoceptors and increased release of noradrenaline displayed by rats subjected to chronic stress.[21]

Thus, chronic arthritic pain in the rat is associated with pronounced, selective, and reversible effects upon multiple opioid peptide networks and multiple opioid receptors. It is appropriate to question whether the changes reflect a response to the pain of arthritis rather than other symptoms. Certain evidence that the changes in the spinal cord are related to an increase in primary afferent noxious input was mentioned above and one might expect to see a comparable response in other models of chronic pain. In TABLE 2, the results acquired in the present study are compared with data obtained in our laboratory as concerns either acute or chronic foot-shock[1,6,22-24] (R. Przewłocki, unpublished). The fact that the response of opioid systems to the quite different model of chronic foot-shock resembles the response to arthritis supports the contention that the effects reflect a response to the pain. In addition, those pools modified under arthritis similarly display a response to acute foot-shock, with the rapid depletion possibly reflecting an accelerated release of the opioids. In FIGURE 2, the data for the influence of acute foot-shock or chronic arthritis upon spinal pools of immunoreactive met-enkephalin and dynorphin are presented. These data and those of TABLE 2 indicate, interestingly, effects of chronic pain are comparatively greater on immunoreactive dynorphin than on met-enkephalin. Importantly, by use of techniques for the monitoring of opioid peptide levels *in vivo* in cerebrospinal fluid (CSF) perfusates, a variety of acute noxious stimuli, such as sciatic nerve stimulation, have been indicated to enhance the release of spinal pools of immunoreactive met-enkephalin and probably dynorphin.[25-28] Unfortunately, the mechanisms underlying alterations in tissue levels in chronic models are less amenable to intepretation. However, we found that elevations in circulating levels of immunoreactive β-endorphin and adenohypophyseal levels of mRNA encoding POMC accompany the rise in immunoreactive β-endorphin in the anterior pituitary of rats suffering from arthritis or subjected to chronic foot-shock; these findings are demonstrative of an activation of these pools of β-endorphin. In the case of spinal dynorphin, there are indications for an increase rather than a decrease in activity that relates to the rise in its levels. Firstly, the long-term pharmacological deactivation of opioid receptors leads to their up-regulation,[29] whereas no such a rise was seen in arthritic rats: on the contrary, a

TABLE 2. Comparison of Changes in Immunoreactive Opioid Peptide Levels in Arthritic Rats to those in Chronic and Acute Foot Shock

		Chronic Arthritis	Chronic Foot Shock[a]	Acute Foot Shock
Dynorphin	Spinal cord	↑	↑	↓
	Thalamus	↑	↑	–
	Anterior pituitary	↑	?	↓
Met-enkephalin	Spinal cord	↑	?	↓
β-Endorphin	Anterior pituitary	↑	↑	↓
	Plasma	↑	↑	↑

↑, increase; ↓, decrease; –, no change; and ?, not determined.
[a]Data acquired by R. Przewłocki.

fall in density, more consistent with a down-regulation due to an enhanced activation, was observed. Further, as discussed below, there is behavioral evidence for an activation of spinal dynorphin neurons in the control of nociception in arthritic rats. Moreover, the extremely large magnitude of the rise would be difficult to reconcile with a depression in activity resulting in such an accumulation of unreleased immunoreactive dynorphin.

However, in the cases of the other changes observed it has not been possible to acquire any concrete data. Indeed, *in vitro* and *in vivo* studies of the release of immunoreactive met-enkephalin from the spinal cord of arthritic rats have not provided unambiguous support for the notion of an enhanced activity.[18]

Moreover, a comparison with the data obtained in clinical studies of chronic pain is instructive in this regard. Atkinson *et al.* evaluated levels of immunoreactive β-endorphin in the systemic circulation of patients in which psychological factors were considered to contribute to the nature and severity of the pain experienced. They observed that plasma levels were elevated and that this rise could only partly be related to psychological variables and could also be attributed to the pain suffered.[30] Such data are consistent with the present findings in arthritic rats but, in other studies of arthritic patients, either a depression in circulating immunoreactive β-endorphin[31] or no change (C. Jones, personal communication) was observed. Indeed, in numerous studies of a variety of pain conditions, including intractable cancer, recurrent trigeminal pain, and chronic primary headache conditions, either a decrease or no alteration in levels of immunoreactive β-endorphin has been detected in the plasma or CSF.[32-38] Further, there is no evidence available for an elevation in levels of immunoreactive met-enkephalin in the circulation or CSF of patients undergoing various types of chronic pain.[34,35] Data pertaining to immunoreactive dynorphin are not, unfortunately, presently available. Nevertheless, in the studies of Knorring *et al.* employing a radioreceptor assay for opioids, fraction I has been tentatively attributed to dynorphin.[40] As compared to pain-free control subjects, lower and higher levels were seen in, respectively, organic and psychogenic pain. The significance of levels of opioids in human tissue fluids is of course no less refractory to interpretation than animal tissue levels and factors such as differential precursor-processing, metabolism, or clearance rather than synthesis or release may explain any changes seen. Nevertheless, overall, they do not offer any compelling evidence for an enhancement in the activity of endogenous opioid systems under chronic pain in man.

OPIOIDS IN THE CONTROL OF NOCICEPTION IN CHRONIC ARTHRITIC PAIN

Arthritic rats exhibit both alterations in nociceptive thresholds and changes in multiple opioid peptide and receptor systems. It is, thus, reasonable to question whether there may be a direct relationship between the influence upon opioid systems and the alterations in nociception. In addition, it is of interest to determine whether there may be changes in the antinociceptive response to exogenously applied opioids.

In TABLE 3, the drugs that we employed as highly preferential agonists or moderately preferential antagonists at particular types of opioid receptors are specified. TABLE 4 presents the effects of administration of antagonists moderately preferential for either μ-, δ-, or κ-receptors upon withdrawal thresholds to noxious heat or pressure applied to the paw or tail. Since, in no case, was the response to heat affected, opioids presumably do not mediate the elevated latencies to heat. The mechanisms underlying this are unknown, but appear to reflect a central mechanism rather than peripheral pathological changes for the following reasons. First, chronic treatment with opiates abolishes this rise without influencing the pathology.[11,12] Second, arthritic rats show a rise in latencies to heat at the tip of the tail where no pathological damage is seen. Third, chronic, noxious mechanical stimulation of the paws likewise results in a rise in tail-flick latencies to heat.[41]

In distinction to naloxone and ICI 154,129, the preferential κ-antagonist, MR 2266, (but not its inactive isomer, MR 2267) stereospecifically decreased latencies to respond to pressure: thus, it potentiated the hyperalgesia. It was inactive in control rats. As mentioned above, dynorphin is a probable endogenous ligand of the κ-receptor. Pharmacological studies have indicated that the role of κ-receptors in the control of nociception is expressed primarily at the spinal level and predominantly against non-thermal as opposed to thermal stimuli.[2,4,42] In view of these observations and that intrathecally applied dynorphin acts antinociceptively against non-thermal noxious stimuli,[2,4,42] it may be suggested that spinal pools of dynorphin, via an action on spinal κ-receptors, play a role in the suppression of reflex hyperalgesia to pressure in arthritic rats.

In other studies, it has been the vocalization threshold, for example, to noxious pressure applied to the paw, that has been determined; this response

TABLE 3. Preferential Agonists and Antagonists for Particular Opioid Receptor Types

	μ	δ	κ
Agonist	Morphine	–	U-50,488H
Antagonist	Naloxone	ICI 154,129	MR 2266[a]

[a]MR 2267 is the inactive stereoisomer of MR 2266.

TABLE 4. Influence of Preferential Antagonists at Particular Receptor Types upon Nociception in Arthritic Rats

	Naloxone	MR 2266	MR 2267	ICI 154,129
Paw pressure	–	↓	–	–
heat	–	–	–	–
Tail pressure	–	↓	–	–
heat	–	–	–	–

–, no effect and ↓, decrease in withdrawal latency.

reflects the affective/emotional dimension of pain and is integrated in the brain. High or moderate doses of naloxone have been found to decrease vocalization thresholds to noxious pressure applied to the paw in arthritic as compared to control rats.[43] In line with this finding, naloxone also elicited a hyperalgesia in the vocalization response to electrical tail stimulation and this was more pronounced and longer-lasting in arthritic as compared to control rats.[44] Thus, a naloxone-sensitive action of an opioid, possibly via the μ-receptor, may act to modulate the affective experience of this pain in arthritic rats. In addition, a paradoxical analgesia, or increase in vocalization thresholds to pressure applied to the paw, has been reported with extremely low doses of naloxone.[43] Studies of the effects of opioid antagonists in acute inflammation suggest that this effect reflects an extra-CNS action, probably in the paw itself.[22,45–47] Thus, in acutely inflamed paws, tiny doses similarly produce analgesia: such doses are effective upon intraplantar injection but not if administered into the brain. Further, systemically applied naloxone analogues that fail to penetrate the blood-brain barrier are similarly active. It appears that these actions reflect a direct interaction with peripheral nerve fibers but the nature of the opioid receptors involved and the mechanisms underlying such peripheral analgesia remain unclear in the case of both acute and chronic inflammation.

To summarize, in contrast to normal rats, in arthritic rats, there is evidence for the following. First, that opioids in the brain, probably via μ-receptors, act in the control of the emotional/conscious dimension of the intensity of chronic pain. Second, in the spinal cord, dynorphin acts via κ-receptors in the control of the sensory reflexive response to noxious mechanical stimuli. In addition, actions on peripheral nerve endings at the site of inflammation, via an as yet uncertain mechanism, may also be apparent.

However, it must be pointed out that in clinical studies naloxone has consistently failed to modify either the appreciation of pain or pain thresholds in human patients suffering from chronic pain.[48,49] The doses applied are small and we know very little concerning the ability to block the effects of endogenous opioid receptors in man. Further, this lack of action does not imply that an action mediated at δ- or κ-receptors can be discounted. Nevertheless, this lack of effect of naloxone together with the biochemical data mentioned above hardly constitute compelling evidence for a role of endogenous opioids in the modulation of chronic pain in man.

Arthritic rats also manifest alterations in their antinociceptive response to morphine. Indeed, they reveal a pronounced potentiation of the actions of morphine against noxious pressure or heat applied to the tail or paw. In addition, it has been documented that the antinociceptive potency of morphine is enhanced as regards the vocalization response to noxious stimulation of the paw.[50] In analogy, rats either subjected to repetitive foot-shock or noxious mechanical stimulation of the paws likewise display an enhanced antinociceptive potency of morphine.[41,51] The mechanism underlying this potentiation is unclear though for spinally coordinated reflexes, it is possible that the comparative rise in μ-receptors may be of relevance. Alternatively, the potentiation may reflect an augmented activity of a network involved in the expression of the antinociceptive actions or morphine. In this respect, serotonin is of interest since it has been implicated in the mediation of the antinociceptive properties of morphine.[22,52] An increased turnover/release of serotonin and an enhanced ability of morphine to increase serotoninergic activity has been found in the spinal cord, forebrain, and brainstem of arthritic rats.[53] Moreover, acute stress has been suggested to facilitate the antinociceptive actions of morphine via a mobilization of CNS pools of serotonin.[54]

Other studies have indicated that arthritic pain may interfere with the development of tolerance to morphine-induced antinociception (R. Przewłocki, personal communication[11,12]). Similar observations have been obtained in rats subjects to chronic noxious mechanical stimulation or the paws.[41] We may mention here the numerous occasions on which the development of tolerance to the pain-relieving actions of morphine in man has been reported to be slower and less extensive than expected.

The studies of acute and chronic morphine administration discussed above collectively suggest that the ability of opioids to exert an antinociception via μ-receptors is exaggerated in arthritic rats.

GENERAL DISCUSSION

In conclusion, chronic adjuvant-induced arthritis is accompanied by pronounced effects upon particular opioid systems. As we previously observed with acute pain, the pattern ot changes is complex with the three opioid peptide families, represented by β-endorphin, met-enkephalin, and dynorphin/α-neo-endorphin, respectively, and the three opioid receptor types, μ, δ, and κ, exhibiting contrasting responses. The pattern of changes was also characteristic for each individual tissue examined. In addition, a recovery was seen upon disappearance of arthritic symptoms. The response of multiple opioid systems to chronic pain is thus both selective and reversible.

Parallel behavioral investigations indicated that there are functional correlates of these alterations, as revealed in the influence of opioid agonists and antagonists preferential for particular receptor types upon nociception. Of particular note was the indication that an action of dynorphin via κ-receptors in the spinal cord may play a role in the control of the reflex hyperalgesia of the limbs to mechanical stimuli. This observation is consistent with pharmacological observations of the effects of acute intrathecal application of dynorphin and synthetic κ-agonists in rodents.[2,4,42] In fact, the spinal route of administration has been the subject of considerable attention in recent years as regards the employment of opiates in the management of severe and/or chronic pain in man.[55] In analogy to the rat, the human spinal cord possesses populations of μ-, δ-, and κ-receptors.[56] In the rat, a functionally independent population of each receptor type can mediate antinociception at the spinal level, in the absence of the development of mutual cross-tolerance upon long-term administration.[2,4,42] In contrast, the respective roles of the receptor types have not been evaluated in man. In the majority of cases, it has been μ-acting opioids that have been applied. Nevertheless, in subjects tolerant to the pain-relieving actions of morphine, a δ-agonist was shown to be still effective, evidence of an independent functional population.[57,58] As yet, no attempt has been made to assess the potential utility of κ-agonists at the spinal level in man. The present data indicate that it may be a κ-like action that constitutes an endogenous opioidergic mechanism for the modulation of chronic pain at the segmental level. This finding raises important questions concerning the possible value of spinal application of κ-like opioids in the therapy of chronic pain in man.

In general, nevertheless, one must be circumspect in extrapolating from animal models of pain to the clinical situation. A number of apparent differences between the present findings in arthritic rats and those of studies of chronic pain in man were specified above. Further, there are problems of comparability in view of the very long duration of pain in the subjects of clinical studies ($\geqslant 6$ months), that they undergo therapy for alleviation of pain, and the fact that there are major psychological and social factors contributing to the clinical picture of chronic pain. It would be desirable to more comprehensively characterize other models of chronic pain as regards multiple opioid systems. As such, it is encouraging to the note the similarities between chronic arthritis and foot-shock presented in TABLE 2.

As regards the significance of opioids in chronic pain (and in functional studies in general), it is now clear that this can only be adequately understood within the light of the multiplicity of opioid systems that appear to subserve a diversity of roles. In addition, in addressing these questions, it appears that it is a complementary biochemical and behavioral approach that proves most informative in elucidating the physiological importance of multiple opioid systems in the modulation of nociception.

CONCLUDING COMMENTS

In concluding this article, it may be instructive, for the sake of balance, to introduce a few theoretical arguments that actually tend not to favor the hypothesis of a role of endogenous opioid (or other) systems in the alleviation of chronic pain. (1) Pain fulfills an alerting function to actual or potential tissue damage. (2) Chronic pain may constitute a pathological state entailing neuronal dysfunction and damage such that mechanisms for its relief may not exist. (3) The causes, nature, and conditions of occurrence of chronic pain do not tend to promote genetic evolution of mechanisms specifically for its control. Thus, it is often associated with some severe, incapacitating damage such that the sufferer is unlikely to survive and reproduce. Further, it is often an affliction of older individuals, which are low in frequency in a population and low in reproductive activity. Thus, an individual with chronic pain is unlikely to significantly contribute to the gene pool of the succeeding generation. Indeed, even if the pain were eliminated, its causes would be so crippling (or rapidly fatal) that little improvement in individual fitness would be incurred.

Thus, although the data discussed above facilitate our understanding of chronic pain conditions and may promote the development of improved methods for its therapy in man, we should not automatically assume that they offer convincing evidence for the existence of endogenous mechanisms specifically for the control of chronic pain in man.

REFERENCES

1. MILLAN, M. J. & A. HERZ. 1985. Int. Rev. Neurobiol. **26**:1-84.
2. PRZEWLOCKI, R., L. STALA, M. GRECZEK, G. T. SHEARMAN, B. PRZEWŁOCKA & A. HERZ. 1983. Life Sci. **33** (Suppl. I):649-652.
3. ROBSON, L. E., S. J. PATERSON & H. W. KOSTERLITZ. 1983. Opiate receptors. *In* Handbook of Psychopharmacology. S. Iverson, L. L. Iverson & S. Snyder, Eds. **14**:13-80. Plenum Press. New York.
4. SCHMAUSS, C. & T. L. YAKSH. 1984. J. Pharmacol. Exp. Ther. **228**:7-14.
5. WÜSTER, M., R. SCHULZ & A. HERZ. 1981. Biochem. Pharmacol. **30**:1883-1887.
6. MILLAN, M. J. 1981. Mod. Probl. Pharmacopsychiatry **17**:49-67.
7. MILLAN, M. J., M. H. MILLAN, A. CZŁONKOWSKI, V. HÖLLT, C. W. T. PILCHER, F. C. COLPAERT & A. HERZ. 1986. J. Neuroscience. (In press.)
8. MILLAN, M. J., M. H. MILLAN, C. W. T. PILCHER, F. C. COLPAERT & A. HERZ. 1985. Neuropeptides **5**:423-424.
9. MILLAN, M. J., M. H. MILLAN, C. W. T. PILCHER, A. CZŁONKOWSKI, F. C. COLPAERT & A. HERZ. 1985. Brain Res. **340**:156-159.
10. MILLAN, M. J., M. H. MILLAN, F. C. COLPAERT & A. HERZ. 1985. Neurosci. Lett. **54**:33-37.
11. COLPAERT, F. C. 1979. Life Sci. **24**:1201-1210.
12. COLPAERT, F. C., TH. MEERT, P. DE WITTE & P. SCHMITT. 1982. Life Sci. **31**:67-75.
13. COLPAERT, F. C. & R. H. W. M. VAN DEN HOOGEN. 1983. Life Sci. **32**:957-963.
14. COLPAERT, F. C., P. DE WITTE, A. N. MAROLI, F. AWOUTERS, C. J. E. NIEMEGEERS & P. J. A. JANSSEN. 1980. Life Sci. **27**:921-928.
15. GAUTRON, M. & G. GUILBAUD. 1982. Brain Res. **237**:459-471.
16. MENETREY, D. & J. M. BESSON. 1982. Pain **13**:243-264.
17. FACCINI, E., H. UZUMAKE, S. GOVONI, C. MISSALE, P. F. SPANO, V. COVELLI & M. TRABUCCHI. 1984. Pain **18**:25-31.
18. CESSELIN, F., S. BOURGOIN, F. ARTAUD & M. HAMON. 1984. J. Neurochem. **43**:763-773.
19. MILLAN, M. J., C. SCHMAUSS, M. H. MILLAN & A. HERZ. 1984. Brain Res. **309**:384-388.
20. LAW, P. Y., D. S. HOM & H. H. LOH. 1982. Molec. Pharmacol. **22**:1-4.
21. STONE, E. A. & J. E. PLATT. 1982. Brain Res. **237**:405-414.
22. MILLAN, M. J. 1982. Meth. Find. Exptl. Clin. Pharmacol. **4**:445-462.
23. MILLAN, M. J., R. PRZEWŁOCKI, M. H. JERLICZ, C. GRAMSCH, V. HÖLLT & A. HERZ. 1981. Brain Res. **208**:325-328.
24. MILLAN, M. J., Y. TSANG, R. PRZEWŁOCKI, V. HÖLLT & A. HERZ. 1981. Neurosci. Lett. **24**:75-79.
25. IADORALA, M. J., J. TANG, H-Y-T. YANG & E. COSTA. 1984. Fed. Proc. **43**:841.
26. NYBERG, F., T. L. YAKSH & L. TERENIUS. 1983. Life Sci. **33** (Suppl. I):17-20.
27. YAKSH, T. L. & R. P. ELDE. 1981. J. Neurophysiol. **46**:1056-1075.
28. YAKSH, T. L., L. TERENIUS, F. NYBERG, K. JHAMANDAS & J-L. WANG. 1983. Brain Res. **268**:119-128.
29. SCHULZ, R., M. WÜSTER & A. HERZ. 1979. Naunyn-Schmiedeberg's Arch. Pharmacol. **306**:93-96.
30. ATKINSON, J. H., E. F. KREMER, S. C. RISCH, C. D. MORGAN, R. F. AZAD, C. L. EHLERS & F. E. BLOOM. 1983. Psychiat. Res. **9**:319-327.
31. DENKO, C. W., J. APONTE, P. GABRIEL & M. PETRICEVIC. 1982. J. Rheumatol. **9**:827-833.
32. ANSELMI, B., E. BALDI, F. CASACCI & S. SALMON. 1980. Headache **20**:294-299.
33. BALDI, E., S. SALMON, B. ANSELMI, M. G. SPILLANTINI, G. CAPPELLI, A. BROCCHI & F. SICUTERI. 1982. Cephalagia **2**:77-81.
34. CLEMENT-JONES, V., S. TOMLIN, L. H. REES, N. L. McLOUGH, G. M. BESSER & H. L. WEN. 1980. Lancet i:946-949.
35. FACCHINETTI, F., G. NAPPI, F. SAVOLDI & A. R. GENAZZANI. 1981. Cephalagia **1**:195-201.

36. GENAZZANI, A. R., G. NAPPI, F. FACCHINETTI, G. MICIELI, F. PETRAGLIA, G. BONO, C. MONITTOLA & F. SAVOLDI. 1984. Pain **18**:127–133.
37. PANERAI, A. E., A. MARTINI, A. DE ROSA, F. SALERNO, A. M. DI GUILIO & P. MANTEGAZZA. 1982. Plasma β-endorphin and met-enkephalin in physiological and pathological conditions. *In* Regulatory Peptides: From Molecular Biology to Function. E. Costa & M. Trabucchi, Eds.:139–149. Raven Press. New York.
38. TSUBOKAWA, T., T. YAMAMOTO, Y. KATAYAMA, T. HIRAYAMA & H. SIBUYA. 1984. Pain **18**:115–126.
39. KISER, R. S., R. S. GATCHEL, K. BHATIA, M. KHATAMI, X. A. HUANG & K. Z. ALTSCHULER. 1983. Lancet i:1394–1396.
40. VON KNORRING, L., F. JOHANSSON & B. G. L. ALMAY. 1982. The importance of the endorphin systems in chronic pain patients. *In* Endorphins and Opiate Antagonists in Psychiatric Research. N. S. Shah & A. G. Donald, Eds.:407–426. Plenum Press. New York.
41. COLPAERT, F. C., C. J. E. NIEMEGEERS, P. J. A. JANSSEN & A. N. MAROLI. 1980. J. Pharmacol. Exp. Ther. **213**:418–424.
42. HAN, J-S., G. X. XIE & A. GOLDSTEIN. 1984. Life Sci. **34**:1573–1579.
43. KAYER, V. & G. GUILBARD. 1981. Brain Res. **226**:344–348.
44. OLIVERAS, J. L., J. BRUXELLE, A. M. CLOT & J. M. BESSON. 1979. Neurosci. Lett (Suppl. 3):S263.
45. FERREIRA, S. H. & M. NAKAMURA. 1979. Prostaglandins **18**:191–200.
46. FERREIRA, S. H. & M. NAKAMURA. 1979. Prostaglandins **18**:201–211.
47. RIOS, L. & J. J. C. JACOB. 1983. Eur. J. Pharmacol. **96**:277–283.
48. LINDBLOM, U. & R. TEGNER. 1979. Pain **7**:65–68.
49. WALKER, J. B. & R. L. KATZ. 1981. Pain **11**:347–354.
50. KAYER, V. & G. GUILBAUD. 1983. Brain Res. **267**:131–138.
51. LEWIS, J. W., J. E. SHERMAN & J. C. LIEBESKIND. 1981. J. Neurosci. **1**:358–363.
52. MESSING, R. B. & L. D. LYTLE. 1977. Pain **4**:1–21.
53. WEIL-FUGAZZA, J., F. GODEFROY & J. M. BESSON. 1979. Brain Res. **175**:291–301.
54. KELLY, S. J. & K. B. J. FRANKLIN. 1984. Neurosci. Lett. **44**:305–310.
55. COUSINS, M. J. & L. E. MATHER. 1984. Anesthesiology **61**:276–310.
56. CZŁONKOWSKI, A., T. COSTA, R. PRZEWŁOCKI, A. PASI & A. HERZ. 1983. Brain Res. **267**:392–396.
57. MOULIN, D., M. MAX, R. KAIKO, C. INTURRISI, J. MAGGARD & K. FOLEY. 1984. Pain (Suppl. 2):S343.
58. ONOFRIO, B. M. & T. L. YAKSH. 1983. Lancet i:1386–1387.

Multiple Neurochemical and Hormonal Mechanisms of Stress-Induced Analgesia[a]

JAMES W. LEWIS

Mental Health Research Institute
University of Michigan
Ann Arbor, Michigan 48109

The principal theme of our work on the phenomenon of stress-induced analgesia has been that multiple neurochemically and neurohormonally discrete pain-inhibitory systems exist and that these systems can be selectively activated by a single stressor, inescapable footshock. Some of these stress-activated endogenous mechanisms of analgesia involve opioid peptides, others do not. Similarly, some forms of stress analgesia rely principally on central nervous system substrates, but others are dependent upon hormonal factors, possibly opioid peptides, as well. This chapter describes our initial investigations identifying these various forms of stress analgesia, highlights some of the evidence indicating the independence of these multiple forms, and attempts to integrate some of our findings with those reported by others.

EVIDENCE FOR MULTIPLE ENDOGENOUS ANALGESIA SYSTEMS

That portions of the central nervous system have, as their normal function, the inhibition of pain was clearly indicated by the observations of Reynolds[1] and Mayer et al.[2] that electrical stimulation of the periaqueductal gray region of the medial brainstem causes profound analgesia. Subsequently, the report of Akil et al.[3] that this analgesia is blocked by administration of an opiate antagonist drug provided compelling evidence for the existence of an endogenous, opioid-mediated analgesia system. More recently, Cannon et al.[4] have demonstrated the existence of neuroanatomically distinct, nonopioid pain-inhibitory systems. They confirmed the finding of Akil et al.[3] that stimulation of particular brain loci can cause opioid-mediated analgesia and also showed that stimulation of anatomically adjacent sites can elicit an equally potent, non-opioid-mediated analgesia.

In 1976, Hayes et al.[5] and Akil et al.[6] found that exposure to environmental stressors could activate endogenous mechanisms of antinociception. Both groups entertained the hypothesis that stress-induced analgesia may be mediated by the recently discovered opioid peptides. Their conclusions, however, were quite

[a]This work was supported by grants NS07628 from National Institutes of Health and DA0254 from National Institute on Drug Abuse. J.W.L. is the recipient of a NIDA postdoctoral fellowship #DA05221.

different. Akil *et al.*[6] found that the analgesia induced by exposure to 30–60 minutes of intermittent footshock was prevented by an opiate antagonist drug, suggesting the involvement of opioids. Hayes *et al.*[5,7] using a variety of stressors, including footshock of brief duration, observed no effect of opiate antagonist drugs and concluded that stress analgesia was mediated by non-narcotic systems. Subsequently, several investigators confirmed the finding that exposure to stress can elicit analgesia in laboratory animals,[8-11] although taken together, their results were inconclusive regarding the activation of opioid systems by environmental stimuli. The use of qualitatively different stressors, or quantitatively different applications of the same stressor, in these studies, however, made a general reconciliation of the data difficult.

SELECTIVE ACTIVATION OF OPIOID AND NON-OPIOID PAIN-INHIBITORY SYSTEMS BY FOOTSHOCK STRESS

When we began our investigations of stress analgesia in 1979, our goals were to clarify what role, if any, was played by the opioid peptides in this phenomenon, and to identify and characterize non-opioid-mediated forms of stress analgesia. To accomplish this, we chose to employ a single stressor, inescapable footshock. Using modifications of the intermittent footshock procedure described by Akil *et al.*[6] and the continuous footshock paradigm of Hayes *et al.*,[7] we demonstrated that a single stressor could elicit either an opioid-mediated or a non-opioid-mediated analgesic response depending upon the parameters of its application. The analgesia induced by intermittent footshock was antagonized by pretreatment with low doses of naloxone,[12,13] suggesting opioid involvement. The analgesia following exposure to continuous footshock was equipotent, but refractory to even high doses of naloxone.[12] To explore further the opioid and non-opioid characteristics of these two forms of stress analgesia, experiments were conducted to test for (1) the development of tolerance upon repeated stress exposure; (2) cross-tolerance between stress analgesia and morphine analgesia; and (3) cross-tolerance between these two forms of stress analgesia. Consistent with the hypothesis that intermittent footshock-induced analgesia is mediated by opioid systems, we found that tolerance develops to this form of footshock after 14 daily exposures,[14,15] and that this form of stress analgesia is nearly absent in animals rendered tolerant to morphine.[14] By contrast, there was no evidence of the development of tolerance to the continuous footshock stressor, nor was this form of stress analgesia affected in morphine-tolerant rats.[14] Finally, further testifying to the independence of the pain-inhibitory systems subserving these two forms of stress analgesia was the finding of no cross-tolerance between these stressors.[16] Thus, multiple endogenous pain-inhibitory systems exist and they can be selectively activated by different parameters of footshock administration.

Continuous Footshock-Induced Analgesia

In our early work, we reported that the analgesia following exposure to 3 minutes of continuous footshock (2.5 mA) was non-opioid in nature.[12] Subsequently, work of Terman *et al.*[17] has extended these observations and indicated that the analgesic response to continuous footshock is not unitary, rather its neurochemical basis is very dependent upon both the intensity and duration of the footshock stimulus. If footshock duration is fixed (e.g., 3 minutes), low current intensities (1–2 mA) elicit an opioid analgesia, whereas exposure to higher intensities (2.5–3.5 mA) results in a non-opioid response. Similarly, if current intensity is held constant (e.g. 2.5 mA), sessions of brief duration (1–2 minutes) produce opioid analgesia, and those of longer duration (4–5 minutes) activate non-opioid mechanisms. The opioid and non-opioid nature of these two forms of stress analgesia was inferred using the same criteria as before (e.g. antagonism by naloxone, development of tolerance, and manifestation of cross-tolerance with morphine analgesia). Thus, once again, the opioid or non-opioid basis of stress analgesia is critically dependent upon the parameters of the stressor. In the case of continuous footshock, it is the interaction of intensity and duration that appears to define which pain-inhibitory systems are accessed.

Although neurochemically different, these two forms of stress analgesia depend on similar anatomical substrates. Both forms are reliant on brainstem and descending neural systems; they are blocked by spinal transection and are unaffected by decerebration.[18,19] Moreover, both forms of stress analgesia appear to be mediated principally by neural systems since they are affected neither by hypophysectomy nor adrenalectomy.[17,20,21] Interestingly, Terman et al.[17] have found that it is possible to elicit opioid and non-opioid stress analgesia in pentobarbital-anesthetized rats. That is, the analgesic response to 1 or 4 minutes of continuous footshock displayed by anesthetized rats is indistinguishable, in magnitude or duration, from the behavior emitted by awake animals. This observation attests to the importance of lower brain structures, those not affected by pentobarbital, in the organization of these forms of stress analgesia, and opens the possibility of studying these behaviors in anesthetized animals to technical and ethical advantage.

Intermittent Footshock-Induced Analgesia

As we[12] and Akil et al.[6] have shown, the analgesic response to intermittent footshock stress appears to be dependent upon opioid systems. This analgesia is similar to the opioid analgesia elicited by continuous footshock in that these two forms of stress analgesia manifest cross-tolerance with each other, but not with the non-opioid form.[18] This form of stress analgesia also shares a common neuroanatomy, the dorsolateral funiculus of the spinal cord, with both forms induced by continuous footshock.[18,22]

The neurochemical and hormonal mediation of this opioid stress analgesia, however, is distinct from the other forms. For example, acetylcholine has long been thought to be involved in central mechanisms of antinociception.[24] We have found that the opioid analgesia caused by intermittent footshock, but not the opioid or non-opioid analgesic responses to continuous footshock, is reduced by scopolamine, a muscarinic cholinergic antagonist drug.[18,24] Importantly, methyl-scopolamine, a muscarinic cholinergic antagonist with only peripheral activity, failed to affect the analgesic response to intermittent footshock. That acetylcholine serves to stimulate the release of opioid peptides involved in pain inhibition is suggested by the finding that oxotremorine, a potent muscarinic agonist, causes analgesia sensitive to opiate antagonist blockade.[23–25] We therefore conclude that a muscarinic cholinergic synapse exists in the central pathway mediating some, but not all, forms of opioid stress analgesia.

Role of Pituitary-Adrenal and Sympatho-Adrenal Hormones

Regarding the hormonal mediators of stress analgesia, several groups have identified a key role for pituitary factors. Hypophysectomy has been shown to markedly reduce many forms of stress analgesia,[26-29] particularly those forms sensitive to naloxone blockade. This surgical manipulation, however, has been found ineffective in attenuating some opioid[17,30] and most non-opioid[17,30,31] forms of stress analgesia. Consistent with such findings, we have reported that hypophysectomy reduces intermittent footshock-induced analgesia, but enhances non-opioid stress analgesia.[20]

In our original report[12] we found that administration of the synthetic glucocorticoid, dexamethasone, powerfully antagonized the analgesic response to intermittent footshock stress. At that time, the elimination of the analgesia was attributed to inhibition of the release of pituitary β-endorphin. Since this time, however, several findings have caused us to re-evaluate this hypothesis. First, since the magnitude of the reduction in opioid stress analgesia caused by hypophysectomy is modest compared to that due to dexamethasone treatment, it is possible that steroids exert their antagonistic effects at other, extra-pituitary, loci. Second, there is considerable evidence to suggest that corticosteroids can interact with opioid systems,[32] and we have shown that chronic treatment with dexamethasone sensitizes rats to the analgesic effects of morphine (unpublished observations). Finally, Chatterjee et al.[33] demonstrated that glucocorticoids can have opposite effects on opiate action. Depending upon the dose given and time of administration relative to morphine challenge, low doses can potentiate and high doses can antagonize morphine analgesia. It may be that the effect of hypophysectomy, in our experiments, is due to the reduction in stress-induced release of steroids, not opioids.

To test the hypothesis that adrenal steroids can interact with opioid pain-inhibitory systems, we assessed the effects of corticosterone administration on opioid analgesia induced by continuous footshock.[34] We chose this form of stress analgesia since it shares common mechanisms (i.e. is cross-tolerant with) that opioid form induced by intermittent footshock, but it is not dependent upon pituitary or adrenal factors.[17] Opioid stress analgesia was enhanced by pretreatment with low doses of corticosterone and antagonized by high doses. That these effects are mediated by corticosteroid action in the brain, not the pituitary, is indicated by the finding that hypophysectomy affected neither the analgesic response to continuous footshock nor the potentiating or antagonizing effects of corticosterone. Thus, it appears likely that adrenal steroid hormones serve either as critical mediators[29] or modulators[12,34] of opioid forms of stress analgesia.

Another peripheral source of opioid peptides is the adrenal medulla. The adrenal medulla contains enkephalin-like peptides that are stored and co-released with catecholamines.[35] Although the precise physiological function of these peptides remains to be determined, we have suggested that they are importantly involved in the analgesic response to certain forms of stress. Intermittent, but not continuous, footshock-induced stress analgesia is markedly reduced by adrenalectomy, adrenal demedullation, or denervation of the adrenal medulla via celiac ganglionectomy.[21] Because demedullation and ganglionectomy have as great an effect as removal of the entire adrenal gland, and because both basal and stressed adrenocortical functions were unimpaired in the adrenal denervated animals yet these rats failed to manifest opioid stress analgesia, we concluded that this form of stress analgesia depends specifically upon adrenal medullary, not cortical, function. Moreover, enkephalin-like peptides but not catecholamines, appear to be involved in this response. A dose of reserpine, known to increase the adrenal content of enkephalins and their stimulation-induced release,[36] significantly augments opioid stress analgesia. This enhanced analgesia appears to reflect increased release of enkephalin-like peptides by stress rather than a nonspecific drug effect in that the analgesia is still virtually eliminated by an opiate antagonist drug.

Biochemical correlates of these behavioral observations have been measured in a collaborative study with Dr. O.H. Viveros.[37] The amount of opiate-like material in adrenal medulla was significantly reduced by intermittent, but not by continuous, footshock, suggesting that acute exposure to this stressor results in the release of enkephalin-like peptides. Medullary enkephalin content was dramatically increased in reserpine-treated rats. This new elevated content was also reduced by exposure to intermittent footshock. Finally, rats made tolerant to intermittent footshock analgesia no longer showed a depletion of adrenal enkephalin-like peptides after stress. These several converging lines of evidence strongly implicate adrenal enkephalin-like peptides in opioid stress analgesia.

Possible Involvement of the Nucleus Tractus Solitarius in Opioid Stress Analgesia

Although we have provided clear evidence for involvement of adrenal opioids in intermittent footshock-induced analgesia, several important questions, such as the locus of the opiate receptor mediating this analgesia, remain to be answered. It may be that enkephalins of adrenal origin are transported to the central nervous system and act upon opioid pain-inhibitory systems. While this hypothesis cannot be discounted, it is unlikely due to the relatively short half-life of these peptides in plasma. An alternate mechanism, based upon peripheral activity of enkephalins, has been suggested by the work of Maixner and Randich.[38,39] They have shown that analgesia elicited either by intermittent footshock or systemic administration of enkephalins is attenuated by unilateral vagotomy. These findings imply that enkephalin-like peptides, secreted by the adrenal medulla, cause peripheral effects, possibly alterations in hemodynamics, and that information regarding these perturbations is sent to the central nervous system via the vagus.

A recent finding in our laboratory may extend this neural circuitry to the brain. One of the principal central nervous system projections of the vagus is the nucleus tractus solitarius (NTS), a nucleus located in the lower brainstem well known to be involved in autonomic control.[40] Several lines of evidence suggest that the NTS may be an integral part of endogenous pain-inhibitory systems. Biochemically, this region is rich in opioid peptides and their receptors,[41,42] and anatomically it has extensive projections to, or receives afferents from, several brain loci thought to be important for pain inhibition.[43] We have recently found that electrical stimulation of the nucleus tractus solitarius causes opioid-mediated analgesia in rats.[44] Thus, since exposure to stress is accompanied by a host of autonomic sequelae, and because the NTS is involved in these responses and NTS stimulation causes analgesia, it is reasonable to hypothesize that an important linkage between stressful stimuli and endogenous analgesia systems occurs via the nucleus tractus solitarius.

FIGURE 1 provides a schematic diagram detailing several of the neural and

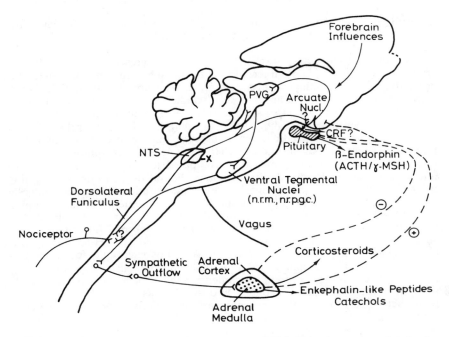

FIGURE 1. This schematic diagram illustrates several of the neural systems and endocrine factors thought to be involved in some forms of opioid-mediated stress analgesia. Abbreviations: ACTH, adrenocorticotropic hormone; CRF, corticotropin releasing factor; MSH, melanocyte stimulating hormone; NRM, nucleus raphe magnus; NRPGC, nucleus reticularis paragigantocellularis; NTS, nucleus tractus solitarius; PVG, periventricular/periaqueducatal gray matter; X, nucleus of the vagus.

endocrine structures and factors thought to contribute to the various forms of footshock-induced analgesia.

Involvement of Central Nervous System Opioids

That adrenal opioids are critical to intermittent footshock-induced analgesia by no means precludes the involvement of central opioids as well. In fact, many investigators have shown alterations in brain opioid content following exposure to stress.[15,45–47,69] One experimental strategy that has been employed in an attempt to quantify stress-induced release of opioids in the brain involves either *in vivo* administration of radioactive opiate drugs or submission of brain homogenates of normal and stressed rats to *in vitro* opiate receptor binding procedures. The predicted outcome of such experiments is that opioids released by stress will occupy receptor sites in the brains of stressed animals and inhibit the binding of exogenously applied radioactive opiates. Using these procedures, several investigators have observed decreased radioactive ligand binding in stressed brains, and have inferred that exposure to stressors, such as footshock, forced swimming, or conditioned fear, causes occupation of opioid receptors by endogenous ligands.[48-51]

Over the past few years, however, it has become increasingly clear that there are multiple subtypes of opioid receptors.[52] Since each of the previous stress and occupancy studies employed only a single, usually non-discriminating, radio-active ligand, we have conducted several studies to extend their findings by quantification of occupation of specific subtypes of opioid receptors following exposure to intermittent footshock stress or administration of morphine.[53,54] To measure occupancy of specific receptor subtypes, we have used two approaches. First, using subcutaneous injections of [³H]naloxone or [³H]etorphine to label mu receptors *in vivo*, we have shown that, compared to controls, rats exposed to intermittent footshock have decreased opiates bound in the brain. In fact, this decrease is comparable to that obtained by administration of a supra-analgesic dose of morphine (10 mg/kg). In a second series of experiments, we have coupled *in vitro* binding assays with *in vivo* manipulations. Rats were either subjected to intermittent footshock stress or served as non-stressed controls. Immediately after stress, brain homogenates were prepared and incubated with ³H-labeled ligands of mu, delta, or kappa receptor selectivity. With this technique, footshock was found to cause an occupation of principally mu, but also delta and kappa receptors. These findings support the contention that exposure to stress can cause synaptic release of opioid peptides and suggest, as others have based on pharmacological data,[55] that mu receptors are particularly important in analgesic mechanisms.

COMPARISON OF CONTINUOUS AND INTERMITTENT FOOTSHOCK-INDUCED ANALGESIA TO OTHER FORMS OF STRESS ANALGESIA

Although it is often difficult to reconcile seemingly disparate findings between laboratories, parsimony would dictate that the numerous forms of stress analgesia characterized to date, ultimately will represent the activation of a finite number of analgesia systems. Toward this end, we have engaged in collaborative endeavors and conducted studies aimed at integration of findings between laboratories.

Importance of Stressor Intensity

As Terman et al.[17] have shown, the opioid or non-opioid basis of the analgesic response to continuous footshock stress is dependent upon the intensity and duration of the stimulus. This conclusion is similar to that presented by Fanselow[56] in studies of conditioned fear-induced analgesia. Moreover, Terman[18] has extended this intensity × duration principle to analgesia induced by another stressor, forced swimming. He has found that manipulation of the intensity of this stimulus (i.e. water temperature) can also determine the opioid or non-opioid nature of the resultant analgesia. Animals forced to swim in low temperature water display analgesia that is relatively refractory to naloxone, whereas the analgesic response to warm water swims is readily antagonized by this drug. This observation is consistent with those of Bodnar et al.[9] using cold water swims, and Christie et al.,[57] using warm water swims.

In 1982, Watkins and Mayer[30] published a series of studies suggesting that the body region shocked (i.e. front paws versus hind paws) can critically define the neurochemical basis of stress analgesia. We conducted an experiment to assess the role that stimulus intensity may play in their footshock paradigm.[58] We were able to reproduce their findings that shock applied to the front paws causes opioid-mediated analgesia and shocking the hind paws resulted in a non-opioid response. When the intensity of the stimulus was varied, however, opioid analgesia was obtained following low intensity shock, and non-opioid analgesia following higher intensities, independent of the body region shocked. These results suggest that in the work of Watkins and Mayer, in which similar current intensities were used to stimulate the front and hind paws, that footshock delivered to the hind paws had, for whatever reason, a sufficiently greater impact on the animal such that a non-opioid analgesia was evoked. These data are not meant to imply that the opioid and non-opioid forms of footshock analgesia elicited by continuous footshock are identical to those evoked by front and hind paw shock since other differences have been reported.[18,59] Nevertheless, it is our conclusion that shock intensity is a more critical determinant of stress analgesia neurochemistry than is the body region shocked.

Importance of Stress Controllability

A question that often arises is: What is different about intermittent versus continuous footshock that should lead to such dramatically different effects? Both of these stimuli are equal in intensity, are noxious as indicated by the animals' behavioral response, and both cause a nearly equivalent pituitary-adrenal stress response indexed by increases in plasma corticosterone.[60] The critical dimension on which they may vary is psychological. There is considerable evidence, beginning with the work of Maier and Seligman,[61] to suggest that equivalent amounts of stressful stimuli can have dramatically different impact on the animal depending upon whether or not the aversive stimulus is controllable.

The important role of stress controllability in the elicitation of stress analgesia has been demonstrated by Maier and colleagues. They showed that rats exposed to 80 inescapable tail-shocks, and tested 24 hr later following a reminder shock, displayed an opioid-mediated analgesia. Exposure to an equivalent amount of escapable shock, by contrast, was either without effect or caused a non-opioid analgesia.[62,63] This opioid-mediated form of analgesia shares several properties with that elicited by intermittent footshock; both forms are blocked by dexamethasone, hypophysectomy, and adrenalectomy.[29] Furthermore, if pain sensitivity is assessed immediately after the tail-shock procedure, 80 inescapable tail-shocks cause analgesia that is blocked by naltrexone, whereas 20 tail-shocks elicit analgesia insensitive to antagonist blockade.[64] This finding is quite parallel with our observations on the analgesic effects of intermittent and 4–5 minute continuous footshock, respectively.

Although all of the footshock stress procedures employed in our work are technically inescapable, it may be that only in the intermittent footshock condition do rats learn this contingency. To test this hypothesis, we engaged in a collaborative experiment with Maier and co-workers.[65] We showed that a single exposure to intermittent, but not continuous, footshock caused behavioral deficits in a shock-escape task. These deficits are termed "learned helplessness" and are similar to those disruptions induced by the inescapable, but not escapable, tail-shock procedure used in Maier's work. Recently, we have confirmed and extended this observation by demonstrating that repeated exposure to intermittent, but not continuous, footshock causes behavioral deficits in a forced swimming model of "behavioral despair."[66,70] In further support of the contention that these opioid forms of analgesia are similar and dependent upon learning, are findings that both forms of analgesia are antagonized by scopolamine[24,67] and that this anti-cholinergic drug has previously been shown to disrupt learning, including learned helplessness.[68] Thus, taken together, these findings provided striking parallels between the analgesia due to intermittent footshock and that caused by inescapable shock, indicating that controllability or coping factors, and not simply exposure to stress per se, may dictate the impact of stressors on endogenous mechanisms of analgesia.

ACKNOWLEDGMENTS

I would like to thank my collaborators on the work described in this paper including John Liebeskind, J. Timothy Cannon, Gregory Terman, Jack Sherman, Michael Tordoff, O. Humberto Viveros, and Huda Akil.

REFERENCES

1. REYNOLDS, D. V. 1969. Science **164**:444–445.
2. MAYER, D. J., T. L. WOLFLE, H. AKIL, B. CARDER & J. C. LIEBESKIND. 1971. Science **174**:1351–1354.
3. AKIL, H., D. J. MAYER & J. C. LIEBESKIND. 1976. Science **191**:961–962.
4. CANNON, J. T., G. J. PRIETO, A. LEE & J. C. LIEBESKIND. 1982. Brain Res. **243**:315–321.
5. HAYES, R. L., G. J. BENNET, P. G. NEWLON & D. J. MAYER. 1976. Soc. Neurosci. Abstr. **2**:939.
6. AKIL, H., J. MADDEN, R. L. PATRICK & J. D. BARCHAS. 1976. In Opiates and Endogenous Opioid Peptides. H. W. Kosterlitz, Ed.:63–70. Elsevier. Amsterdam.
7. HAYES, R. L., G. J. BENNETT, P. G. NEWLON & D. J. MAYER. 1978. Brain Res. **155**:69–90.
8. AMIR, S. & Z. AMIT. 1978. Life Sci. **23**:1143–1152.
9. BODNAR, R. J., D. D. KELLY, A. SPIAGGIA, C. EHRENBERG & M. GLUSMAN. 1978. Pharmacol. Biochem. Behav. **8**:667–672.
10. CHANCE, W. T. 1980. Neurosci. Biobehav. Rev. **4**:55–67.
11. CHESHER, G. B. & B. CHAN. 1977. Life Sci. **21**:1569–1574.
12. LEWIS, J. W., J. T. CANNON & J. C. LIEBESKIND. 1980. Science **208**:623–625.
13. LEWIS, J. W., J. T. CANNON, J. M. STAPLETON & J. C. LIEBESKIND. 1980. Proc. West. Pharmacol. Soc. **23**:85–88.
14. LEWIS, J. W., J. E SHERMAN & J. C. LIEBESKIND. 1981. J. Neurosci. **1**:358–363.
15. MADDEN, J., H. AKIL, R. L. PATRICK & J. D. BARCHAS. 1977. Nature **265**:358–360.
16. TERMAN, G. W., J. W. LEWIS & J. C. LIEBESKIND. 1983. Brain Res. **260**:147–150.
17. TERMAN, G. W., Y. SHAVIT, J. W. LEWIS, J. T. CANNON & J. C. LIEBESKIND. 1984. Science **226**:1270–1277.
18. TERMAN, G. W. 1985. Doctoral Dissertation. University of California. Los Angeles.
19. KLEIN, M. V., G. W. TERMAN, K. M. LOVAAS & J. C. LIEBESKIND. 1983. Soc. Neurosci. Abstr. **9**:795.
20. LEWIS, J. W., E. H. CHUDLER, J. T. CANNON & J. C. LIEBESKIND. 1981. Proc. West. Pharmacol. Soc. **24**:323–326.
21. LEWIS, J. W., M. C. TORDOFF, J. E. SHERMAN & J. C. LIEBESKIND. 1982. Science **217**:557–559.

22. LEWIS, J. W., G. W. TERMAN, L. R. WATKINS, D. J. MAYER & J. C. LIEBESKIND. 1983. Brain Res. **267**:139–144.
23. PEDIGO, N. W. & W. L. DEWEY. 1981. Adv. Behav. Biol. **25**:795–807.
24. LEWIS, J. W., J. T. CANNON & J. C. LIEBESKIND. 1983. Brain Res. **270**:289–293.
25. HOWES, J. F., L. S. HARRIS, W. L. DEWEY & C. VOYDA. 1969. J. Pharmacol. Exp. Ther. **169**:23–28.
26. AMIR, S. & Z. AMIT. 1979. Life Sci. **24**:439–448.
27. BODNAR, R. J., M. GLUSMAN, M. BRUTUS, A. SPIAGGIA & D. D. KELLY. 1979. Physiol. Behav. **23**:53–62.
28. MILLAN, M. J., R. PRZEWLOCKI & A. HERZ. 1980. Pain **8**:343–353.
29. MACLENNAN, A. J., R. C. DRUGAN, R. L. HYSON, S. F. MAIER, J. MADDEN & J. D. BARCHAS. 1982. Science **215**:1530–1532.
30. WATKINS, L. R. & D. J. MAYER. 1982. Science **216**:1185–1192.
31. CHANCE, W. T., G. M. KRYNOCK & J. A. ROSENCRANS. 1979. Psychoneuroendocrinol. **4**:199–205.
32. HOLADAY, J. W. & H. H. LOH. 1979. Adv. Biochem. Psychopharmacol. **20**:227–258. Raven Press. New York.
33. CHATTERJEE, B., S. DAS, P. BANERJEE & J. J. GHOSH. 1982. Eur. J. Pharmacol. **77**:119–123.
34. TERMAN, G. W., J. W. LEWIS & J. C. LIEBESKIND. 1984. Proc. West. Pharmacol. Soc. **27**:447–450.
35. VIVEROS, O. H. & S. P. WILSON. 1983. J. Autonom. Nerv. Sys. **7**:41–58.
36. VIVEROS, O. H., E. J. DILIBERTO JR., E. HAZUM & K.-J. CHANG. 1979. Molec. Pharmacol. **16**:1101–1108.
37. LEWIS, J. W., M. G. TORDOFF, J. C. LIEBESKIND & O. H. VIVEROS. 1982. Soc. Neurosci. Abstr. **8**:778.
38. MAIXNER, W. & A. RANDICH. 1984. Brain Res. **298**:374–377.
39. RANDICH, A. & W. MAIXNER. 1984. Pharmacol. Biochem. Behav. **21**:441–448.
40. KORNER, P. 1979. *In* Handbook of Physiology, Sect. 2, Vol. 1. R. M. Berne, N. Sperelakis & S. R. Geiger, Eds.:691–739. American Physiology Society. Baltimore, MD.
41. KHACHATURIAN, H., M. E. LEWIS, M. SHAFER & S. J. WATSON. 1985. Trends Neurosci. **8**:111–119.
42. LEWIS, M. E., H. KHACHATURIAN & S. J. WATSON. 1985. Peptides. (In press.)
43. RICARDO, J. A. & E. T. KOH. 1978. Brain Res. **153**:1–26.
44. LEWIS, J. W., G. BALDRIGHI, S. J. WATSON & H. AKIL. 1985. Soc. Neurosci. Abstr. (In press.)
45. ROSSIER, J., E. D. FRENCH, C. RIVIER, N. LING, F. E. BLOOM & R. GUILLEMIN. 1977. Nature **270**:618–620.
46. ROSSIER, J., R. GUILLEMIN & F. E. BLOOM. 1978. Eur. J. Pharmacol. **48**:465–456.
47. MILLAN, M. J., Y. F. TSANG, R. PRZEWLOCKI, V. HOLLT & A. HERZ. 1981. Neurosci. Lett. **24**:75–79.
48. CHANCE, W. T., A. C. WHITE, G. M. KRYNOCK & J. A. ROSECRANS. 1978. Brain Res. **141**:371–374.
49. CHRISTIE, M. J. 1982. Neurosci. Lett. **33**:197–202.
50. PERT, C. B. & D. L. BOWIE. 1979. *In* Endorphins and Mental Health Research. E. Usdin, Ed.:93–104. MacMillan Press. New York.
51. SEEGER, T. F., G. A. SFORZO, C. B. PERT & A. PERT. 1984. Brain Res. **305**:303–311.
52. CHANG, K.-J. & P. CUATRECASAS. 1979. J. Biol. Chem. **254**:2610–2618.
53. LEWIS, J. W., M. E. LEWIS, D. J. LOOMUS & H. AKIL. 1984. Neuropeptides **5**:117–120.
54. LEWIS, J. W., M. E. LEWIS & H. AKIL. 1985. Presented at International Narcotics Research Conference. Seacrest, MA.
55. PASTERNAK, G. W., S. R. CHILDER & S. H. SNYDER. 1980. Science **208**:514–516.
56. FANSELOW, M. 1984. Behav. Neurosci. **98**:79–95.
57. CHRISTIE, M. J., G. B. CHESHER & P. TRISDIKOON. 1982. Life Sci. **31**:839–845.
58. CANNON, J. T., G. W. TERMAN, J. W. LEWIS & J. C. LIEBESKIND. 1984. Brain Res. **323**:316–319.

59. WATKINS, L. R., Y KATAYAMA, I. B. KINSCHECK, D. J. MAYER & R. L. HAYES. 1984. Brain Res. **300**:231–242.
60. NELSON, L. R. 1985. Doctoral Dissertation. University of California. Los Angeles.
61. MAIER, S. F. & M. E. P. SELIGMAN. 1976. J. Exp. Psychol.: Gen. **105**:3–46.
62. JACKSON, R. L., S. F. MAIER & D. J. COON. 1979. Science **206**:91–93.
63. MAIER, S. F., S. DAVIES, J. W. GRAU, R. L. JACKSON, D. H. MORRISON, T. MOYE, J. MADDEN & J. D. BARCHAS. 1980. J. Comp. Physiol. Psychol. **94**:1172–1183.
64. GRAU, J. W., R. L. HYSON, S. F. MAIER, J. MADDEN & J. D. BARCHAS. 1981. Science **213**:1409–1410.
65. MAIER, S. F., J. E. SHERMAN, J. W. LEWIS, G. W. TERMAN & J. C. LIEBESKIND. 1983. J. Exp. Psych.: Animal Behav. Proc. **9**:80–90.
66. PORSOLT, R. D., G. ANTON, N. BLAVET & M. JALFRE. 1978. Eur. J. Pharmacol. **47**:379–391.
67. MACLENNAN, A. J., R. C. DRUGAN & S. F. MAIER. 1983. Psychopharmacology **80**:267–268.
68. ANISMAN, H., G. REMINGTON & L. S. SKLAR. 1979. Psychopharmacol. **61**:107–124.
69. AKIL, H., E. YOUNG, J. M. WALKER & S. J. WATSON. 1986. Ann. N.Y. Acad. Sci. This volume.
70. LEWIS, J. W. & L. R. NELSON. 1985. (Unpublished data.)

Behavioral and Neurochemical Consequences Associated with Stressors[a]

HYMIE ANISMAN AND ROBERT M. ZACHARKO

Department of Psychology
Carleton University
Ottawa, Ontario K1S 5B6
Canada

The view has repeatedly been expressed that aversive events may increase vulnerability to a wide range of psychological disturbances, including clinical depression. While not dismissing the contribution of cognitive alterations in the provocation of affective disorders, it has been maintained that the neurochemical consequences associated with aversive events are responsible for the depressive symptomatology.[1,2] Specifically, it was proposed that when an organism is confronted with a stressor, it will adopt any of a number of behavioral styles in order to escape from the insult or to diminish its impact. Concurrently, a series of neurochemical changes may occur, whose function may be one of either blunting the physical or psychological impact of the stressor or enabling the organism to emit appropriate responses to deal effectively with the stressor. Failure of these adaptive mechanisms may render the organism more vulnerable to behavioral depression. In the present report we document both transient and persistent neurochemical sequelae of stressors and relate these to the behavioral consequences associated with psychological and physical insults.

ADAPTIVE NEUROCHEMICAL CHANGES IN RESPONSE TO AVERSIVE STIMULI

Although stressful events provoke several neurochemical and hormonal variations, the present report will focus on only two of these, specifically norepinephrine (NE) and dopamine (DA). Omission of other transmitters and hormones does not imply that they are of lesser importance. Indeed, as will be seen later, the very great number of behavioral alterations associated with stressors, and their potential modification by various types of pharmacological manipulations, provide *prima facie* evidence that transmitters other than the catecholamines are also associated with the behavioral effects of uncontrollable aversive events.

[a]Supported by Grants A9845 and A1087 from the Natural Sciences and Engineering Research Council of Canada and Grants MT-6486 and MA-8130 from the Medical Research Council of Canada.

Norepinephrine

FIGURE 1 provides a schematic representation of the presumed NE variations that occur under various aversive conditions. Upon presentation of a mild or controllable stressor the release of brain NE is increased, as is the rate of synthesis,[3,4] and concentrations of the amine are unaltered. If the stressor is sufficiently severe and protracted, then the rate of amine utilization may exceed synthesis, resulting in a net reduction of the transmitter concentration.[3-5] While reductions of NE have been detected in numerous brain regions, it appears that the increased release and consequent decline of the transmitter levels are more readily provoked in some areas than in others.[6]

The organism's ability to cope behaviorally with the stressors is a major determinant of the central NE variations. Several investigators[5,7] have, indeed,

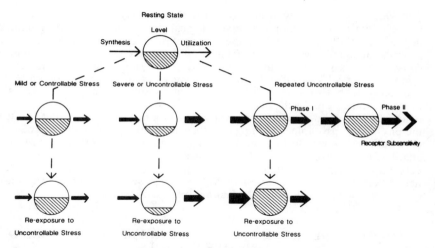

FIGURE 1. Schematic representation of the norepinephrine variations that occur under various aversive conditions. From left to right: Under conditions of mild or controllable aversive stimulation norepinephrine utilization is increased, and this is met by increased synthesis. Consequently amine concentrations remain stable. If the stressor is uncontrollable, then amine utilization increases further, and if the rate of synthesis is exceeded, then amine reductions occur. With repeated stressor application a compensatory increase in synthesis is provoked, and consequently concentrations of the amine will equal or exceed control values. Following repeated stressor application subsensitivity of β-norepinephrine receptors may occur, and in addition norepinephrine-stimulated adenylate cyclase activity may be reduced. From left to right, the lower portion of the figure displays the effects of re-exposure to a stressor as a function of the organism's previous stress history. In mildly stressed animals re-exposure to the stressor provokes a modest increase of amine turnover; however, in animals previously exposed to an uncontrollable stressor, subsequent re-exposure to even a limited amount of aversive stimulation leads to a rapid amine release, which may exceed synthesis, hence resulting in reduced amine levels. In animals that had been exposed to a chronic stressor such that neurochemical adaptation had occurred, re-exposure to the stressor subsequently provokes elevated norepinephrine concentrations presumably as a result of a rapid and marked increase of norepinephrine synthesis.

demonstrated that the NE reduction is not readily apparent in animals that were exposed to escapable shock, whereas an identical amount of inescapable shock applied in a yoked paradigm elicits the amine reduction (FIGURE 2). It has been argued that in the absence of behavioral methods of dealing with the stressor greater demands are placed on endogenous mechanisms. Thus, utilization of the amine may become excessive, hence leading to the NE reduction (FIGURE 1). It has been maintained that conditions that favor the amine reduction will also increase vulnerability to psychological and physical pathologies.[2,3,8,9]

In addition to stressor controllability, it has been reported that organismic variables, such as the age and strain of the animal, may influence both the magnitude and the time course of the NE variations associated with stressors. Likewise, the background conditions upon which the stressor is applied (e.g., social housing conditions) will influence NE turnover and concentrations.[3,8] Inasmuch as these variables also influence vulnerability to physical pathologies,[10] as well as behavioral disturbances,[8] the possibility was considered that these effects may have been a consequence of the stressor-induced amine variations.

In considering the potential impact of stressors on pathology, it might not only be important to assess the magnitude of the neurochemical changes, but also the time course for these changes. Although stressor-induced NE reductions may be short-lived, it was reported that under some conditions[9] the amine reductions may be fairly persistent. Moreover, data are available that indicate that the course of the amine depletion varies with organismic variables that are associated with increased vulnerability to illness.[8] In effect, the magnitude of the neurochemical change may be indicative of lability of the neurotransmitter system in response to the environmental insult, whereas the course of the amine variations may be a better index of the adaptability of such systems.

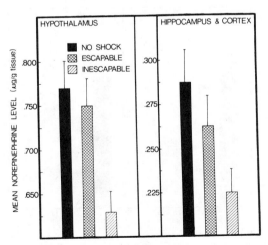

FIGURE 2. Mean norepinephrine (NE) concentrations (±S.E.M) in mice that were exposed to 60 escapable shocks, an equivalent amount of inescapable shock (yoked) or no shock. (From Anisman & Sklar.[11] With permission from *Journal of Comparative and Physiological Psychology.*)

In addition to the immediate neurochemical and behavioral repercussions associated with traumatic events, it appears that stressors may also influence the response of the organism to subsequently encountered aversive stimuli. Specifically, although the NE alterations associated with stressors of moderate severity may be relatively transient, aversive stimulation may result in the conditioning or sensitization of the mechanisms subserving the NE alterations (FIGURE 1). Accordingly, upon subsequent encounters with aversive stimuli, or cues that had been previously paired with the stressors, the amine variations may be reinduced. As seen in FIGURE 3, NE concentrations determined 24 hr after inescapable shock were approximately equal to those of nonstressed mice. Likewise, immediately after a limited amount of footshock, NE concentrations were not appreciably affected. Interestingly, however, in mice that had previously been exposed to the more traumatic stressor, subsequent re-exposure to mild shock resulted in a decline of hypothalamic and hippocampal NE.[11] We subsequently observed that such an effect was evident even when a two week period intervened between the original shock and re-exposure sessions.[12] Moreover, in mice that had received inescapable shock subsequent application of a different form of aversive stimulation (restraint) provoked a more pronounced NE reduction.[13] While such findings were taken to support the view that stressors resulted in the sensitization of the mechanisms responsible for the NE alterations, data have been reported that suggest that the neurochemical alterations were subject to conditioning processes. In particular, it was observed[14] that in rats treated with inescapable shock, subsequent re-exposure to cues that had been associated with the primary stressor effectively increased the accumulation of the NE metabolite, 3-methoxy-4-hydroxyphenylglycol sulfate (MHPG). In light of these findings it was

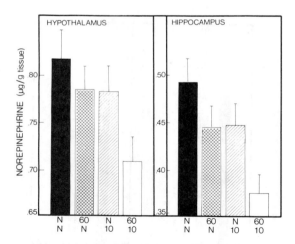

FIGURE 3. Mean norepinephrine (NE) concentrations (±S.E.M) in mice that received no shock treatment on each of two consecutive days, 60 shocks on one day followed by no shock on the next day, no shock on the initial day followed by 10 shocks on the next day, or 60 shocks on the first day and 10 shocks on the second day. (From Anisman et al.[3] With permission from Academic Press.)

suggested that long-term behavioral effects of stressors may stem from the amine alterations that are re-induced upon stressor re-exposure.[11] Indeed, it has been demonstrated that several behavioral consequences of stressors that ordinarily persist for brief periods may be reinstated by a mild stressor.[15] Likewise, re-exposure to aversive stimuli may exacerbate the persistent behavioral deficits associated with uncontrollable stressors.[11]

The reduction of NE produced by stressors persists for only a brief period of time, during which vulnerability to behavioral pathology is thought to be increased. With repeated exposure to aversive stimulation adaptive changes occur, such that the NE reductions are prevented (FIGURE 1) and resistance to pathology may be increased. It seems that with repeated aversive stimulation activity of the synthetic enzymes tyrosine hydroxylase and dopamine-β-hydroxylase are enhanced, enabling the rate of amine synthesis to keep pace with utilization, thereby preventing amine depletion.[16,17] The increased synthesis may persist over a 24 hr period following termination of the chronic stress regimen,[17] and there is some indication that utilization rates may drop below control values.[18] As a result, NE concentrations may exceed those of nonstressed animals (FIGURE 4). In effect, it seems that upon presentation of a stressor in chronically shocked animals the synthesis and utilization of NE increase, presumably as an adaptive response to deal with immediate environmental demands. It is thought that following stressor termination the sustained increase of amine synthesis,

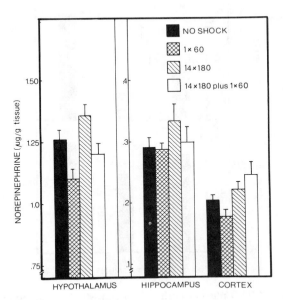

FIGURE 4. Mean (±S.E.M) norepinephrine (NE) concentrations in mice that received no shock, a single session of 60 shocks (6 sec duration, 150 µA) and decapitated immediately thereafter, 14 sessions of 180 shocks on successive days and decapitated 24 hr afterward, or 14 sessions of 180 shocks followed by a single session of 60 shocks immediately prior to decapitation. (From Irwin et al.[18] With permission from Society for Neuroscience Abstracts.)

coupled with the decline of utilization, represents an ideal way of conserving amine supplies in the event that the stressor is again encountered.[8]

We recently observed that chronic stressor application may have relatively long-term repercussions on neurochemical changes elicited upon subsequent stressor application.[18] In particular, it was found that 14 days following acute shock (a single session of 360 shocks of 2 sec duration, 150 μA) or chronic shock (15 sessions of shock applied on consecutive days) NE levels and utilization were comparable to those of nonstressed mice. As seen in FIGURE 5, in naive mice a limited amount of shock (60 shocks of 2 sec) did not appreciably influence hypothalamic NE concentrations. However, in acutely stressed mice re-exposure to the stressor 14 days later reinduced the amine depletion, indicating that the sensitization effect persists even when a relatively long period intervenes between the initial shock and reexposure session. When 60 shocks were applied to mice that had received the chronic shock treatment 14 days earlier, NE concentrations were markedly elevated. The fact that utilization was also increased (as gauged by the increased MHPG accumulation) suggests that the elevated NE concentrations induced by chronic shock resulted from accelerated NE synthesis. Thus, it appears that just as acute stress may sensitize neurochemical mechanisms so that reductions of NE are engendered upon re-exposure to a stressor, chronic shock

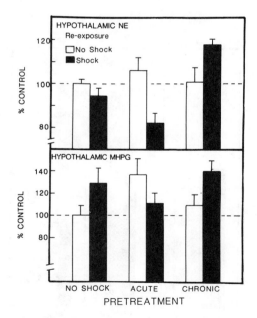

FIGURE 5. Mean (±S.E.M) norepinephrine (NE) and MHPG concentrations in hypothalamus of mice that received either no shock, a single session of 360 shocks of 2 sec duration (acute), or 14 sessions of 360 shocks on consecutive days (chronic). Fourteen days afterward mice of these groups were either placed in the apparatus and not shocked (open bars) or were exposed to 60 shocks of 2 sec duration (closed bars). (From Irwin & Anisman.[12] With permission from *Society for Neuroscience Abstracts*.)

may result in sensitization, whereby re-exposure to a stressor increases NE turnover and levels. It is thought that such a sequence of neurochemical changes may render the organism better prepared to deal with environmental insults.

There appeared to be regional differences with respect to the variations of amine activity and concentrations. As shown in FIGURE 6, in the hippocampus elevated NE concentrations were apparent in chronically shocked animals that were subsequently reexposed only to the cues associated with shock. It seems as if NE activity in the hippocampus was subject to conditioning processes, whereas the hypothalamic NE alterations were subject to a sensitization effect. Since this study was not conducted to assess conditioning versus sensitization processes, the necessary control conditions were not included. Accordingly, the conclusion advanced here should be considered as being provisional.

In addition to variations of amine synthesis and utilization, Stone[19,20] reported that chronic stressor application may result in a transient subsensitivity of β-NE receptors and a more persistent reduction in the magnitude of the cAMP response. Inasmuch as chronic antidepressant treatment has been shown to provoke down-regulation of the β-NE system,[21] it was suggested that the development of the β-NE receptor subsensitivity following chronic stressor application may be responsible for behavioral adaptation associated with such a

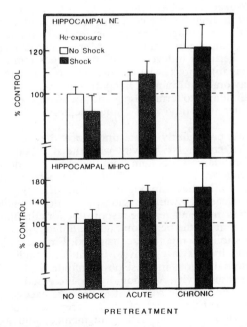

FIGURE 6. Mean (±S.E.M) norepinephrine (NE) and MHPG concentrations in hippocampus of mice that received either no shock, a single session of 360 shocks of 2 sec duration (acute), or 14 sessions of 360 shocks on consecutive days (chronic). Fourteen days afterward mice of these groups were either placed in the apparatus and not shocked (open bars) or were exposed to 60 shocks of 2 sec duration (closed bars). (From Irwin & Anisman.[12] With permission from *Society for Neuroscience Abstracts*.)

treatment. Pathology was hypothesized to follow when down regulation failed to occur, and pharmacological intervention would be necessary to engender the down-regulation of the β-NE coupled adenylate cyclase system. In accordance with such a view, it was demonstrated that the disappearance of some of the behavioral and physiological effects associated with stressors, such as ulceration and anorexia, corresponded with the variations of β-NE receptor sensitivity.[22]

It might be noted at this juncture that the variations associated with repeated stressors are not restricted to β-NE receptors, nor is it the case that the cyclic AMP change is a consequence of the β-NE alterations. For instance, the β-NE receptor alterations are not apparent 24 hr after stressor termination, while the down-regulation of cAMP persists at this interval.[23,24] Furthermore, it appears that chronic stressor application may result in an increase in α-2 receptor density,[25] and if the effects of chronic stressors actually parallel those of chronic antidepressant treatment, then up-regulation of α-1 receptors might be expected as well.[26]

In their analysis of the neurochemical processes governing stressor-related behavioral disturbances, Weiss and Goodman[9] emphasized the importance of locus coeruleus NE variations in eliciting the behavioral deficits associated with acute shock. Specifically, it was suggested that the reduction of releasable NE from the locus coeruleus resulted in diminished autoreceptor stimulation. Consequently, increased NE release was induced in forebrain terminal regions, which ultimately provoked the behavioral disturbances. Support for this position was derived from the finding that the course of the NE reductions in the locus coeruleus paralleled the time course for the behavioral disturbances, whereas NE reductions in other brain regions did not.[27] Moreover, α-2 receptor blockers applied to the locus coeruleus induced behavioral deficits reminiscent of those engendered by inescapable shock, whereas α-2 receptor stimulants eliminated shock-provoked behavioral disturbances. In contrast, intracerebral application of α-1 and β-receptor stimulants to terminal regions (an effect similar to that which would be induced after inhibition of α-2 autoreceptors) provoked behavioral impairments.[9]

These findings are particularly interesting since they reconcile the data concerning stressor effects on NE activity with the data suggesting that the therapeutic effects of antidepressants stem from their ability to down-regulate the β-NE coupled adenylate cyclase system. That is, the behavioral impairments associated with stressors, like the symptoms associated with depression, may stem from heightened NE release at terminal regions, while down-regulation of β-NE receptors by antidepressant agents may be responsible for eliminating the effects of the stressor. To account for the behavioral adaptation associated with chronic shock two related possibilities might be considered. First, the chronic stressor may increase tyrosine hydroxylase activity in the cell bodies, which when transported to the terminal regions increase post-synaptic NE activity sufficiently to engender receptor subsensitivity. Additionally, the increased availability of NE within the locus coeruleus may be sufficient to provoke excessive autoreceptor stimulation, and hence subsensitivity of these receptors. Consequently, NE activity in terminal regions will be further augmented, and as a result the likelihood of β-NE receptor subsensitivity increases.

Dopamine

The data concerning the effects of stressors on dopamine (DA) concentrations and turnover are less extensive than those involving NE. Most early studies that assessed the effects of stressors on DA activity indicated that stressors were without effect.[3] Analyses of discrete brain regions, however, revealed pronounced DA variations that were restricted to a few regions. For instance, it was reported that stressors will provoke reductions of DA in the arcuate nucleus of the hypothalamus[28] and in the lateral septum.[29] Moreover, release of DA is increased in the nucleus accumbens and mesolimbic frontal cortex (as determined from increased accumulation of the metabolite dihydroxyphenylacetic acid; DOPAC), and in some studies reduction of DA concentrations were evident as well.[30-35] In other DA-rich regions, such as the substantia nigra, stressors tended not to influence DA concentrations or turnover appreciably, although exceptions have been reported in this respect.[36] In these studies the stressor involved cold exposure (e.g., cold water immersion), and it is possible that the DA variations were secondary to motoric factors associated with the stressor or were related to thermoregulatory effects.

Consistent with earlier reports, as yet unpublished data collected in our laboratory revealed region-specific DA alterations in response to stressors. As shown in FIGURE 7, footshock did not affect DA concentrations appreciably in the hypothalamus or substantia nigra, although accumulation of hypothalamic DA metabolites was increased. In contrast, in the mesolimbic cortex shock produced a marked increase of DOPAC accumulation and greatly reduced DA concentrations. The DA alterations were less pronounced in the nucleus accumbens than in the mesolimbic cortex, although DOPAC accumulation was increased. Subsequent studies involving shock of greater severity revealed marked DA reductions

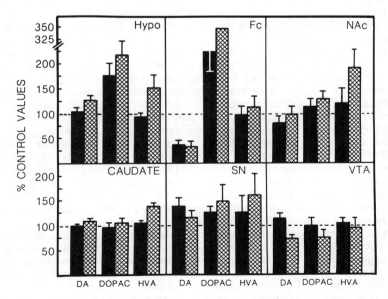

FIGURE 7. Dopamine (DA), DOPAC, and homovanillic acid (HVA) as a percent of control values (±S.E.M) in hypothalamus (Hypo), frontal cortex (Fc), nucleus accumbens (NAc), caudate, substantia nigra (SN), and ventral tegmentum (VTA) of mice that received either 30 or 360 shocks of 2 sec duration (150 μA).

in the nucleus accumbens. Moreover, it appears that the DA alterations associated with stressors, like those of NE, are dependent upon the background conditions upon which the stressor was applied[30] and also varied with the strain of animal employed.[37]

Limited data are available concerning the contribution of stressor controllability to the DA variations. It was reported that controllable and uncontrollable shock differentially influenced DA receptor binding in mesocortical regions.[38] In this particular study the shock treatment was applied over the course of an 8 hr period on each of four successive days, and thus it is not certain whether stressor chronicity interacted with controllability to determine the observed outcome. Preliminary data collected in this laboratory have also revealed that both controllable and uncontrollable shock reduced DA concentrations in the nucleus accumbens. Unfortunately, a large number of shock trials of long duration were employed, and it is not certain whether DA variations would be more readily attained after uncontrollable shock if a lesser number of trials had been applied. There is, however, reason to believe that the DA alterations associated with stressors in limbic regions may be a reflection of anxiety or arousal associated with the stressor. In fact, it has been demonstrated that the DA variations induced by aversive stimuli are prevented in animals that had been pretreated with a benzodiazepine.[31]

As in the case of NE, there is reason to believe that variations of DA neuronal activity induced by stressors are subject to sensitization or conditioning effects. It was demonstrated[32] that acute footshock increased DOPAC concentrations in the anteromedial and frontal cortices, olfactory tubercle, nucleus accumbens, and amygdala. Upon subsequent re-exposure to the stimulus array in which the shock had previously been delivered, DOPAC accumulation in the frontal cortex was substantially increased, while the concentrations of DOPAC were unaffected in other regions. These data are not only consistent with the proposition that the DA variations are influenced by the organism's stress history, but also suggest regional specificity concerning the potential for conditioning of DA neuronal alterations. Of course, it may simply be the case that the frontal cortex is more sensitive to stressor effects, and hence the consequences of exposing animals to cues associated with a stressor would be more detectable in this brain region than in others. Further evidence suggesting sensitization or conditioning of DA neuronal activity is derived from studies demonstrating that stressors enhance the behavioral response to subsequent amphetamine treatment. In particular, it was demonstrated that stereotypy elicited by amphetamine, a behavior which is largely subserved by DA activity, was greatly exaggerated in rats that had been exposed to a stressor several days earlier.[39] Moreover, such an effect was evident if the stressor involved inescapable shock, but not escapable shock.[40] Thus, the possibility needs to be considered that some of the long-term behavioral alterations associated with stressors may be related to the proactive changes of DA, as well as those of NE described earlier.

With repeated exposure to a stressor, adaptation appears to occur with respect to DA activity. It has been reported,[41] for instance, that the reduction of forebrain DA engendered by 2 hr of restraint was absent in rats that received such a treatment on five consecutive days. Indeed, in the rats that received the repeated restraint treatment DA concentrations significantly exceeded those of non-stressed animals. In assessing the consequences of acute and chronic footshock on DA activity it was observed that DA synthesis and utilization were enhanced in the frontal cortex by exposure to a single session of shock.[42] Curiously, following exposure to shock for five days, increased DA synthesis did not occur and in fact was slightly reduced. Since concentrations of DA and its catabolites were not monitored, there is no way of knowing what mechanisms might have been operative in provoking the increased DA concentrations reported by Richardson.[41] Given that chronic shock enhanced NE synthesis in the studies of Kramarcy et al.[42] and the previously cited reports,[16,17] it appears that the mechanisms responsible for DA and NE activation are different from one another.

BEHAVIORAL DEFICITS INDUCED BY UNCONTROLLABLE STRESSORS

Considerable effort has been expended in the development of an animal model of depression. The most oft studied behavior in this respect has been the shuttle escape deficits typically observed in animals after exposure to inescapable shock. These deficits, which are characterized by passivity in the face of a stressor, are not evident in animals that had been exposed to escapable shock, indicating that control over the stressor was fundamental in determining the behavioral impairment. It had been proposed that during inescapable shock animals learned that their responses were independent of shock offset, leading to the development of helplessness. Accordingly, upon subsequent encounters with the stressor animals ceased attempts to escape.[43] As an alternative to this position it was suggested that inescapable shock may result in either learned or unconditioned motor variations (e.g., inactivity) that are incompatible with the active response necessary for successful performance.[44] It was further argued[45] that inescapable shock may result in disturbances in the animal's ability to initiate active responses in the face of weak stimuli (e.g., a CS) and in maintaining active responses in the presence of strong stimuli (e.g., shock). Indeed, it was demonstrated that altering the motoric demands of the task or modifying the organism's ability to initiate or maintain a response influenced the magnitude of the escape disturbances introduced by inescapable shock.[44,45]

According to a related position, the interference was attributed to neurochemical variations elicited by the stressor. While some investigators focused primarily on NE variations,[5] others also attributed a role for DA and acetylcholine in subserving the interference effect.[8,11,45] Commensurate with these views it was shown that pharmacological compounds that reduced NE concentrations (e.g., the dopamine-β-hydroxylase inhibitor, FLA-63), reduced both NE and DA concentrations (e.g., the tyrosine hydroxylase inhibitor, α-MpT), blocked DA receptors (e.g., haloperidol or pimozide), or increased acetylcholine concentrations (e.g., by inhibiting acetylcholinesterase by physostigmine), provoked behavioral deficits reminiscent of those elicited by inescapable shock (FIGURE 8).[45] In particular, these compounds disrupted performance only when the task necessitated sustained active responding.

As might be expected, catecholamine stimulants (e.g., l-DOPA) or anticholinergics (e.g., scopolamine) eliminated the effects of inescapable shock (FIGURE 9). It should be underscored that the effects of these compounds were behaviorally distinguishable from one another. Specifically, whether administered prior to testing or prior to inescapable shock, l-DOPA eliminated the escape interference. That is, the compound was effective as either a treatment for previously

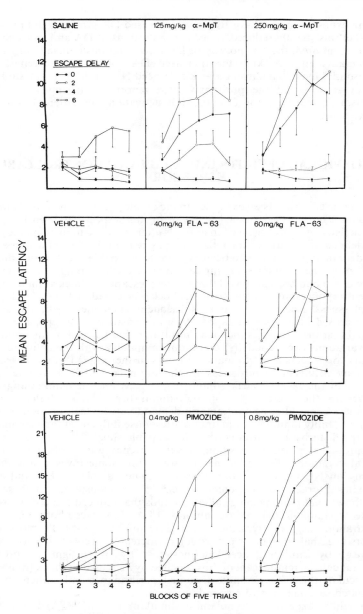

FIGURE 8. Mean (±S.E.M) escape latencies in a shuttle escape test where escape was possible either immediately upon shock onset or after a delay of 2, 4, or 6 sec. In independent experiments mice received either α-MpT, FLA-63, or pimozide (or their respective vehicles) prior to the test session. (From Anisman et al.[45] With permission from *Psychopharmacology*.)

administered inescapable shock or as a prophylactic in preventing the effects of to-be-administered shock. The anticholinergic, in contrast, was only effective when administered prior to the test session.[11,45,46] More recently, we have also observed that release of serotonin (5-HT) by acute administration of *p*-chloro-amphetamine (PCA) prior to escape testing eliminated the effects of previously applied inescapable shock, but was ineffective as a prophylactic. Thus, while alterations of NE, DA, 5-HT, and acetylcholine influence the behavioral disturbance associated with previously administered shock, reductions of NE and/or DA activity may be fundamental in the induction of the interference effect. In a similar fashion, it has been reported that although benzodiazepines and opiate antagonists did not influence escape performance in previously stressed animals, when applied prior to inescapable shock these treatments prevented the appearance of the escape interference.[47,48] Thus, alterations of endogenous opioids or alleviation of anxiety may be requisite for the development of an interference effect.

Further evidence favoring the hypothesis that the stressor related behavioral disturbances are due to neurotransmitter variations is derived from studies that assessed the behavioral effects of repeated shock exposure. It will be recalled that following chronic shock the activity of tyrosine hydroxylase is increased and NE concentrations are elevated. Paralleling these findings, the escape deficit ordinarily elicited by acute shock was absent following repeated shock.[5] Thus, it was

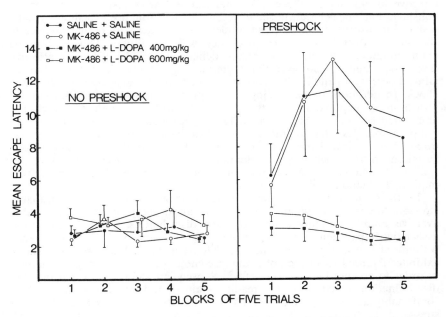

FIGURE 9. Mean (±S.E.M) escape latencies in mice that received inescapable shock or no shock 24 hr prior to shuttle escape testing. Prior to the test session mice received l-DOPA or vehicle. (From Anisman *et al.*[45] With permission from *Psychopharmacology*.)

suggested that the increased NE activity limited the behavioral impairment. Inasmuch as chronic stressors also induce subsensitivity of β-NE receptors, the possibility exists that the elimination of the escape interference was related to the down regulation of the β-NE system, as opposed to alterations of transmitter levels or synthesis. Indeed, correspondence was detected between the development of β-NE subsensitivity and adaptation to stressor-provoked anorexia and disturbances in a swim test.[22,49] It will be noted, however, that these studies were correlational in nature, and it is certainly possible that other amine variations that occur following repeated stressor application, such as altered DA activity or variations of α-1 or α-2 NE receptors, may have been responsible for the behavioral adaptation.

PERSEVERATION AND ANXIETY

In formulating animal models for human disorders it is, of course, essential that the behaviors examined in animals are similar to the symptoms associated with the human disorder. Furthermore, it would be expected that treatments effective in eliminating the illness in humans would also reduce the behavioral impairments in animals. With respect to the latter considerations, it was demonstrated that repeated treatment with compounds that alleviate depression in humans (e.g., desmethylimipramine) also eliminated the escape interference in animals.[50] Yet, compounds such as l-DOPA, which are not effective antidepressants, are also effective in eliminating the escape interference.[45] With respect to the former consideration, one is hard pressed to accept that performance in a shuttle escape task is reminiscent of the symptoms of depression, other than perhaps reflecting the motoric disturbances often associated with the illness. Thus, it may be counterproductive to rely on the escape deficits as a model of human affective disorders. It appears, however, that there are other similarities between human clinical depression and the behavior of animals exposed to acute uncontrollable shock. In addition to the finding that coping failure may contribute to the induction of depression and the escape disturbances, both of which are eliminated by comparable pharmacological treatments, the two share similar symptom profiles. Besides the motoric disturbances, uncontrollable aversive events, like clinical depression, are associated with anorexia and weight loss, variations in social behaviors and dominance hierarchies, sleep disturbances, as well as disruptions of general exploratory patterns and responding in appetitively motivated situations.[8,9,15,51,52]

In their analysis of the performance deficits provoked by inescapable stressors, Maier and Seligman[43] suggested that animals exposed to uncontrollable aversive events not only suffer cognitive disturbances, but also encounter associative impairments involving response-outcome associations. In accordance with this view it was shown that rats that had been exposed to inescapable shock exhibited retarded acquisition of a response-choice discrimination (i.e., turn right in order to escape) in a Y-maze task.[53] Subsequent studies indicated that the discrimination deficits were not readily attained, and when present could be comfortably accounted for on the basis of attentional deficits elicited by the stressor.[54]

Recent experiments conducted in our laboratory[55] provided further insights concerning the effects of stressors on discrimination performance. Although discrimination deficits were not detected in either cue or response-choice discrimination paradigms, inescapable shock was found to disrupt reversal performance in one form of the response-choice task. It did not appear that the performance disruption was due to an associative deficit, but rather may have stemmed from a perseverative tendency engendered by the inescapable shock treatment. It is thought that inescapable shock results in the restriction of the animal's problem-solving strategy such that it persists in adopting previously acquired (or highly prepared) strategies even though more appropriate response patterns may be available.

In addition to the response perseveration tendency, stressors were shown to elicit stimulus perseveration. For instance, when placed in a water-filled maze or arena where one area was illuminated, mice tended to remain in the vicinity of the light. This tendency was further enhanced in animals exposed to inescapable shock. It was suggested that the perseverative response pattern represents a narrowing of the animal's defensive style, arising because of anxiety or panic provoked by the aversive situation. Indeed, when tested in a forced-swim task soon after exposure to escapable or inescapable shock mice exhibited a pronounced response excitation (reduced time engaged in passive floating). The excitation diminished with time following shock, and in mice that received uncontrollable shock increased floating was apparent relative to mice that had received either no shock or escapable shock.[57] Subsequent experiments revealed that both the response excitation and the perseveration were eliminated by diazepam.[78] It was posited that the initial arousal or panic may enable the organism to adopt highly prepared defensive postures or strategies. If the response requirements of the task are fairly simple, then the rudimentary response tendencies (motor excitation coupled with the stereotyped response strategy) may benefit the animal (viz. the absence or diminishes shuttle escape deficit evident soon after inescapable shock relative to that seen after longer intervals).[44,45] However, the fact that the organism's defensive repertoire is restricted may render it less well prepared to deal with novel environmental insults, particularly when the response required of the animal is a fairly complex one.

In view of the finding that a component of the behavioral profile associated with stressors may involve anxiety, it might be postulated that the animal model provided is most closely aligned with depression where anxiety is an associated feature. This view is similar to that advanced by Weiss and Goodman,[9] as well as that of Foote et al.[59] The latter investigators suggested that activation of the locus coeruleus blunts the neuronal response to stimuli that appear irrelevant with respect to environmental demands, while enhancing attention or responsivity to cues that may be of value for behavioral coping. The feature extraction might be manifested behaviorally as heightened vigilance[9] and may be associated with characteristics reminiscent of anxiety. It is conceivable that the stressor-provoked perseverative tendencies we observed, which may be subserved by NE alterations,[60,61] are related to increased vigilance and anxiety.

MOTIVATION AND REWARD

Although there appear to be similarities between the behavioral profile associated with uncontrollable stressors and that of clinical depression, limited attention has been devoted to the analysis of stressor effects on motivational state, despite the fact that anhedonia is a fundamental symptom of depression. To be sure, it has been maintained that uncontrollable shock will result in reduced motivation,[43] but this conclusion is based on findings such as those obtained from shuttle escape performance, a behavior that is largely influenced by the motoric consequences of the inescapable shock treatment.

In view of the finding that stressors may influence DA neuronal activity, coupled with the proposition that DA may be involved in reward processes,[62] it would not be unreasonable to suppose that stressors may come to affect responding for rewarding brain stimulation. Inasmuch as the effects of stressors on DA neuronal activity vary across brain regions, it was expected that responding for brain stimulation would be unaffected from those regions where stressors do not influence DA activity (e.g., substantia nigra), whereas a reduction in responding would be expected from regions where stressors affect DA (e.g., nucleus accumbens) or through which DA fibers traverse (medial forebrain bundle). Following the establishment of stable rates of baseline responding (head-dip) for intracranial stimulation, mice were matched for response rate and exposed to 60 escapable shocks, yoked inescapable shock, or no shock. Immediately thereafter, and again 24 and 168 hr later mice were tested in the self-stimulation paradigm.

As shown in FIGURE 10, responding in nonstressed and escapably shocked animals remained fairly stable over the various test sessions. In contrast, in mice that had been exposed to inescapable shock a marked response reduction was evident from both the nucleus accumbens and medial forebrain bundle. Responding for electrical stimulation from the substantia nigra was hardly affected by inescapable shock. It was thought that the differential effects of inescapable shock on response from the substantia nigra and nucleus accumbens may have stemmed from the fact that in the former case mice were self-stimulating from cell bodies, while in the latter case stimulation was activating terminal regions.[63] Accordingly, an additional experiment assessed the effects of uncontrollable shock on response from the ventral tegmentum, which contains the cell bodies of neurons projecting to the nucleus accumbens. As in the case of the nucleus accumbens, the shock treatment was found to produce a rapid and marked reduction of responding for stimulation from the ventral tegmentum.[64]

It is unlikely that the observed results were a consequence of stressor-induced variations of general arousal or variations of motor activity. Aside from the fact that measurements of activity did not reveal differences as a function of the shock condition, it would have been expected that effects of arousal or anxiety would have influenced responding from the substantia nigra, as well as from the other sites. We provisionally maintained that uncontrollable stressors influence the mechanisms subserving reward processes, and that the effectiveness of stressors in producing alterations in reward mechanisms vary with the specific brain region examined. While the present data are consistent with the suggestion that DA alterations are related to variations in reward, it is certainly possible that this relationship is not a causal one, and that other neurochemical events that covary with DA are actually responsible for the alterations in performance.

As in the case of the DA variations associated with inescapable shock, it seems that the reduction in self-stimulation associated with an acute shock session is absent in mice that had received repeated exposure to the stressor. Specifically, it was observed[65] that in mice responding for brain stimulation from the nucleus accumbens a single shock session produced a decline of responding which exceeded 50%. In contrast, in mice that received five sessions of inescapable shock the reduction was less than 30%, and in the same animals shock applied for five more days was associated with a reduction of response of less than 10%. It might

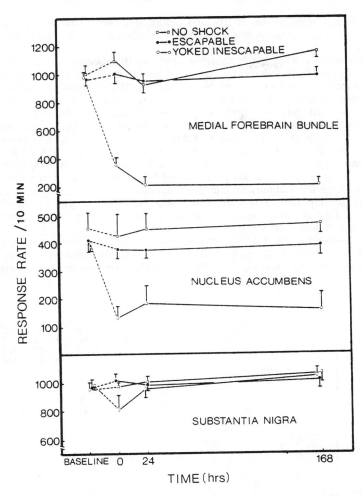

FIGURE 10. Mean (±S.E.M) rates of responding for brain stimulation from either the medial forebrain bundle, nucleus accumbens, or substantia nigra. Following the establishment of baseline rates of responding mice received escapable shock, yoked inescapable shock, or no shock and then tested in the self-stimulation task immediately thereafter and again 24 and 168 hr afterwards. (From Zacharko et al.[63] With permission from *Behavioral Brain Research*.)

be noted at this juncture that in parallel with this particular study we conducted several additional studies that assessed the effects of acute and repeated shock on shuttle escape and forced swim performance. Contrary to the results of studies where behavioral adaptation was evident,[5,22,49] the stressor parameters we employed did not lead to an adaptation in these tasks. Inasmuch as shuttle escape and swim performance are largely influenced by motoric variations, these data support our contention that the behavioral change seen in the self-stimulation paradigm was independent of motor factors associated with the shock treatment employed.

In accordance with the proposition that the disruption of self-stimulation performance might be suitable as a model of human depression, it was found that repeated treatment with desmethylimipramine (DMI) effectively eliminated the stressor-provoked reduction of self-stimulation response.[66] As seen in FIGURE 11, in saline-treated mice a single session of inescapable shock provoked a progressive deterioration of performance over test sessions. In contrast, in mice that had been repeatedly treated with DMI only a small decline of response was evident immediately after the test session, and at the 24 and 168 hr intervals performance was comparable to that of nonstressed mice. It might be noted that although DMI is thought to act primarily on NE neuronal functioning, the view has been expressed that the antidepressant actions of the drugs may stem, in part, from the development of DA autoreceptor subsensitivity.[67] The fact that DMI antagonized the effects of the inescapable shock treatment on a behavior thought to involve DA activity is consistent with this suggestion.

Taken together, the findings concerning the effects of stressors on self-stimulation performance suggest that uncontrollable aversive events alter motivational/reward processes. As such, these data are commensurate with the

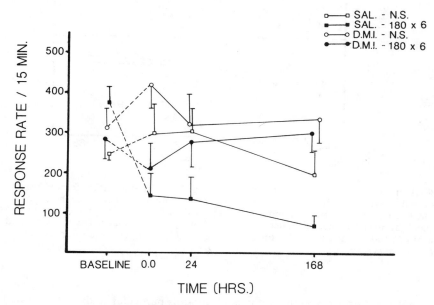

FIGURE 11. Mean (±S.E.M) response rates for electrical stimulation from the nucleus accumbens at three intervals following a single session of inescapable shock (180 shocks of 6 sec duration) or no shock (NS). Prior to the shock session mice had received administration of desmethylimipramine on 15 consecutive days (5.0 mg/kg twice per day) or were treated with saline. (From Zacharko et al.[66] With permission from *Brain Research*.)

view that stressors elicit a depressive-like state. This proposition is further supported by the fact that DMI antagonized the effects of inescapable shock. In effect, affective disturbances engendered by stressors are viewed as being subserved by several different neurotransmitters, including DA. The fact that disturbances in self-stimulation are brain region–specific raises the possibility that interindividual differences in the symptom profile associated with depression may be related to regional variations of stressor-induced transmitter alterations.

SUMMARY

A series of neurochemical changes occur in response to stressors that may permit the organism to contend with environmental demands. When the organism is exposed to a stressor the utilization and synthesis of brain NE and DA increases. Under conditions where utilization exceeds synthesis, owing either to the nature of the stressor (uncontrollability), experiential factors (e.g., prior exposure to acute stressors), or organismic variables (e.g., strain, age), reductions of the amine may be incurred. It is suggested that the reduced amine concentrations leave the organism less well prepared to deal with the demands placed upon it, and ultimately increase vulnerability to psychological disturbances. It follows that the more persistent the amine reduction, the greater the probability of pathology being engendered. In effect, in our analyses of stressor effects it is not sufficient merely to determine whether amine reductions occur, but also to assess the ability of the system to re-establish adequate levels and turnover. Additionally, since stressors may result in the conditioning or sensitization of neurochemical processes, it is essential not only to assess the immediate impact of the stressor, but also the neurochemical variations that occur upon re-exposure to stressors or cues associated with the stressor.

In considering the consequences of stressors and the potential implications for human pathology, it is important to consider the impact of chronic stressors. After all, many stressors encountered by humans are chronic in nature, particularly if one considers ruminations associated with the aversive event. It seems that with repeated stressor application a further series of adaptive neurochemical changes occur. The activity of tyrosine hydroxylase is increased, and concentrations of NE and DA approach those of nonstressed animals. Indeed, it appears that after stressor termination the increased amine synthesis may persist for some time leading to a further increase of amine concentrations, which may enable the organism to deal with environmental demands. In addition, receptor variations may occur, including down-regulation of β-NE receptors, and possibly alterations of α-1 and α-2 receptors as well. It is believed that the receptor variations may be the essential element in maintaining the integrity of the organism. It is our contention that where such adaptive changes do not occur or are slow in occurring, pharmacological intervention may be necessary to engender such neuronal variations.

ACKNOWLEDGMENT

Appreciation is extended to Jill Irwin and Pardeep Ahluwalia for their helpful comments.

REFERENCES

1. ANISMAN, H. & R. M. ZACHARKO. 1982. Behav. Brain Sci. **5**:89–137.
2. WEISS, J. M., H. I. GLAZER, L. A. POHORECKY, W. H. BAILEY & L. H. SCHNEIDER. 1979. *In* The Psychobiology of Depressive Disorders. R. A. Depue, Ed.:141–173. Academic Press. New York.
3. ANISMAN, H., L. KOKKINIDIS & L. S. SKLAR. 1981. *In* Theory in Psychopharmacology. S. J. Cooper, Ed. **1**:65–102. Academic Press. London.
4. STONE, E. A. 1975. *In* Catecholamines and Behavior. A. J. Friedhoff, Ed.:31–72. Plenum Press. New York.
5. WEISS, J. M., H. I. GLAZER & L. A. POHORECKY. 1976. *In* Animal Models in Human Psychobiology. G. Serban & A. Kling, Eds.:141–173. Plenum Press. New York.
6. NAKAGAWA, R., M. TANAKA, Y. KOHNO, Y. NODA & N. NAGASAKI. 1981. Pharmacol. Biochem. Behav. **14**:729–732.
7. ANISMAN, H., A. PIZZINO & L. S. SKLAR. 1980. Brain Res. **191**:583–588.
8. ANISMAN, H. 1984. *In* Neurobiology of Mood Disorders. R. M. Post & J. C. Ballenger, Eds.:407–431. William & Wilkins. Baltimore.
9. WEISS, J. M. & P. A. GOODMAN. 1984. *In* Stress and Coping. T. Field, P. McCabe & N. Schneiderman, Eds. Lawrence-Erlbaum Associates. Hillsdale, NJ.
10. SKLAR, L. S. & H. ANISMAN. 1981. Psychol. Bull. **89**:369–406.
11. ANISMAN, H. & L. S. SKLAR. 1979. J. Comp. Physiol. Psychol. **93**:610–625.
12. IRWIN, J. & H. ANISMAN. Soc. Neurosci. Abstr. **10**:1173.
13. IRWIN, J., W. BOWERS, R. M. ZACHARKO & H. ANISMAN. Soc. Neurosci. Abst. **8**:359.
14. CASSENS, G., M. ROFFMAN, A. KURUC, P. J. URSULAK & J. J. SCHILDKRAUT. 1980. Science **209**:1138–1140.
15. BRUTO, V. & H. ANISMAN. 1983. Behav. Neur. Biol. **37**:302–316.
16. WEISS, J. M., H. I. GLAZER, L. A. POHORECKY, J. BRICK & N. E. MILLER. 1975. Psychosom. Med. **37**:522–534.
17. THIERRY, A. M., F. JAVOY, J. GLOWINSKI & S. S. KETY. 1968. J. Pharmacol. Exp. Therap. **163**:163–171.
18. IRWIN. J. & H. ANISMAN. 1983. Soc. Neurosci. Abst. **9**:563.
19. STONE, E. A. 1979. Res. Commun. Psychol. Psychiat. Behav. **4**:241–255.
20. STONE, E. A. 1983. Behav. Brain Sci. **6**:535–578.
21. SULSER, F. 1982. *In* Typical and Atypical Antidepressants: Molecular Mechanisms. E. Costa & G. Racagni, Eds.:1–20. Raven Press. New York.
22. STONE, E. A. & J. E. PLATT. 1982. Brain Res. **237**:405–414.
23. STONE, E. A., J. E. PLATT, R. TRULLAS & A. V. SLUCKY. 1984. Psychopharmacology **82**:403–405.
24. U'PRICHARD, D. C. & R. KVETNANSKY. 1980. *In* Catecholamines and Stress: Recent Advances. E. Usdin, R. Kevtnansky & I. J. Kopin, Eds.:299–308. Elsevier. New York.
25. U'PRICHARD, D. C. 1981. *In* Psychopharmacology of Clonidine. H. Lal & S. Fielding, Eds.:53–74. Alan R. Liss, Inc. New York.
26. VETULANI, J. 1983. Behav. Brain Sci. **4**:560–561.
27. WEISS, J. M., P. A. GOODMAN, B. G. LOSITO, S. CORRIGAN, J. M. CHARRY & W. H. BAILEY. 1981. Brain Res. Rev. **3**:167–205.
28. KVETNANSKY, R., A. MITRO, M. PALKOVITS, M. BROWNSTEIN, T. TORDA, M. VIGAS & L. MIKULAJ. 1976. *In* Catecholamines and Stress. E. Usdin, R. Kvetnansky & I. J. Kopin, Eds.:39–50. Pergamon Press. Oxford.
29. SAAVEDRA, J. M. 1982. Neuroendocrinology **35**:396–401.
30. BLANC, G., D. HERVE, H. SIMON, A. LISOPRAWSKI, J. GLOWINSKI & J. P. TASSIN. 1982. Nature **284**:265–267.
31. FEKETE, M. I. K., T. SZENTENDREI, B. KANYICSKA & M. PALKOVITS. 1981. Psychoneuro-endocrinology **6**:113–120.
32. HERMAN, J. P., D. GUILLONNEAU, R. DANTZER, B. SCATTON, L. SEMERDJIAN-ROUQUIER & M. LE MOAL. 1982. Life Sci. **30**:2207–2214.
33. THIERRY, A. M., J. P. TASSIN, G. BLANC & J. GLOWINSKI. 1976. Nature **263**:242–244.

34. TISSARI, A. H., A. ARGIOLAS, F. FADDA, G. SERRA & G. L. GESSA. 1979. Arch. Pharmacol. **308**:155-158.
35. FADDA, F., A. ARGIOLAS, M. R. MELIS, A. H. TISSARI, P. L. ONALI & G. L. GESSA. 1978. Life Sci. **23**:2219-2224.
36. DUNN, A. J. & N. R. KRAMARCY. 1984. *In* Handbook of Psychopharmacology. L. L. Iversen, S. D. Iversen & S. H. Snyder, Eds. **18**:455-515. Plenum Press. New York.
37. HERVE, D., P. TASSIN, C. BARTHELEMY, G. BLANC, S. LAVIELLE & J. GLOWINSKI. 1979. Life Sci. **25**:1659-1664.
38. CHEREK, D. R., J. D. LANE, M. E. FREEMAN & J. E. SMITH. 1980. Soc. Neurosci. Abst. **6**:543.
39. ANTELMAN, S. M., A. J. EICHLER, C. A. BLACK & D. KOCAN. 1980. Science **207**:329-331.
40. MACLENNAN, A. J. & S. F. MAIER. 1983. Science **219**:1091-1093.
41. RICHARDSON, J. S. 1984. Int. J. Neurosci. **23**:57-68.
42. KRAMARCY, N. R., R. L. DELANOY & A. J. DUNN. 1984. Brain Res. **290**:311-319.
43. MAIER, S. F. & M. E. P. SELIGMAN. 1976. J. Exp. Psychol: Gen. **105**:3-46.
44. GLAZER, H. I. & J. M. WEISS. 1976. J. Exp. Psychol.: Anim. Behav. Proc. **2**:202-223.
45. ANISMAN, H., G. REMINGTON & L. S. SKLAR. 1979. Psychopharmacology **61**:107-124.
46. ANISMAN, H., S. J. GLAZIER & L. S. SKLAR. 1981. Psychopharmacology **74**:81-87.
47. DRUGAN, R. C., S. M. RYAN, T. R. MINOR & S. F. MAIER. 1984. Pharm. Biochem. Behav. **21**:749-754.
48. MAIER, S. F., S. DAVIES, J. W. GRAU, R. L. JACKSON, D. H. MORRISON, T. MOYE, J. MADDEN & J. D. BARCHAS. 1980. J. Comp. Physiol. Psychol. **94**:1172-1183.
49. PLATT, J. E. & E. A STONE. 1982. Eur. J. Pharmacol. **82**:179-181.
50. SHERMAN, A. D., J. L. SACQUITNE & F. PETTY. 1982. Pharm. Biochem. Behav. **16**:449-454.
51. ROSELLINI, R. A. 1976. Anim. Learn. Behav. **6**:155-159.
52. WILLIAMS, J. L. 1982. Anim. Learn. Behav. **10**:305-313.
53. JACKSON, R. L., S. F. MAIER & P. M. RAPAPORT. 1980. J. Exp. Psychol.: Anim. Behav. Proc. **6**:1-20.
54. MINOR, T. R., R. L. JACKSON & S. F. MAIER. 1984. J. Exp. Psychol. Anim. Behav. Proc. **10**:543-556.
55. ANISMAN, H., M. HAMILTON & R. M. ZACHARKO. 1984. J. Exp. Psychol.: Anim. Behav. Proc. **10**:229-243.
56. SZOSTAK, C. & H. ANISMAN. 1985. Behav. Neur. Bio. **43**:178-198.
57. PRINCE, C. R. & H. ANISMAN. 1984. Behav. Neur. Biol. **42**:99-119.
58. PRINCE, C. R., C. COLLINS & H. ANISMAN. 1984. Meeting of the Canadian Psychological Association. Ottawa.
59. FOOTE, S. L., F. E. BLOOM & G. ASTON-JONES. 1983. Physiol. Rev. **63**:844-914.
60. KOKKINIDIS, L. & H. ANISMAN. 1980. Psychol. Bull. **88**:551-579.
61. ANISMAN, H., B. HAHN, D. HOFFMAN & R. M. ZACHARKO. 1985. Pharm. Biochem. Behav. (In press.)
62. WISE, R. A. 1982. Behav. Brain Sci. **5**:39-87.
63. ZACHARKO, R. M., W. J. BOWERS, L. KOKKINIDIS & H. ANISMAN. 1983. Behav. Brain Res. **9**:129-141.
64. ZACHARKO, R. M., W. J. BOWERS, C. PRINCE & H. ANISMAN. 1983. Soc. Neurosci. Abst. **9**:561.
65. ZACHARKO, R. M., W. J. BOWERS & H. ANISMAN. 1984. Prog. Neuro-Psychopharmacol. Biol. Psychiat. **8**:601-606.
66. ZACHARKO, R. M., W. J. BOWERS, M. S. KELLEY & H. ANISMAN. 1984. Brain Res. **321**:175-179.
67. ANTELMAN, S. M. & L. A. CHIODO. 1984. *In* Handbook of Psychopharmacology. L. L. Iversen, S. D. Iversen & S. H. Snyder, Eds. **18**:279-342. Plenum Press. New York.

Catalepsy Induced by Body Pinch: Relation to Stress-Induced Analgesia

SHIMON AMIR

Department of Isotope Research
The Weizmann Institute of Science
76100 Rehovot, Israel

INTRODUCTION

It is now well established that exposure to stressful stimuli such as electric foot shock, immobilization, or cold water swim can profoundly suppress responsiveness to pain in experimental animals.[1-4] This phenomenon, termed stress-induced analgesia, is thought to involve activation of intrinsic pain inhibitory systems located in the brain and spinal cord.[5] It has been suggested that both opiate as well as non-opiate mechanisms function as mediators in these pain inhibitory systems.[4-6] Recently, I have demonstrated together with colleagues that exposure to a mild stressor—pinching to the scruff of the neck—elicits in drug-free mice powerful, long lasting catalepsy in addition to analgesia.[7,8] In subsequent studies it was observed that the development of this pinch-induced catalepsy is markedly attenuated by pretreatment with the opiate antagonist naloxone.[7,9] This suggested that the elaboration of pinch-induced catalepsy involves activation of endogenous opiate (endorphin) systems. Other studies have implicated the involvement of cholinergic mechanisms in pinch-induced catalepsy.[10,11] The functional relationship of this endorphin-mediated cholinergic-dependent cataleptic response and the concomitant analgesia as well as the mechanisms subserving the pinch-induced analgesic effect have not been elucidated. Earlier studies have shown that exposure to brief physical restraint induces in some animal species (e.g. rabbits) a state of marked motor inhibition resembling catalepsy or catatonia that can be potentiated by nociceptive stimuli.[12,13] Moreover, it has been demonstrated that painful stimuli facilitate the cataleptic response elicited by the administration of drugs such as morphine or the dopamine receptor antagonist haloperidol.[14-16] In the present investigation I have explored potential links between the neurochemical processes mediating pinch-induced catalepsy and analgesia. In the first series of experiments I have analyzed the role of endorphin and dopamine in the development and maintenance of pinch-induced catalepsy. In subsequent studies I evaluated the relationship of catalepsy to the analgesic response using a testing procedure that allowed the simultaneous evaluation of these responses and their underlying neurochemical mechanisms within the same animal.

PINCH-INDUCED CATALEPSY

Catalepsy was studied in male C_3Heb mice, 12 weeks old, as previously described.[7] Briefly, the mice were held by the tail and the scruff of the neck was firmly pinched using the thumb and the index finger as shown in FIGURE 1(A). The pinch was terminated gently after 5 sec as the mice were positioned head up on circular parallel bars spaced 5 cm apart and having a 5 cm difference in height (FIGURE 1, B). Each animal was given eight pinching trials. A trial ended when either the animal moved or after 90 sec of immobility (FIGURE 1, C and D). At the end of each trial the mice were placed in a waiting box for a 30 sec intertrial interval.

The first series of experiments further investigated the involvement of endorphins in the development of pinch-induced catalepsy. In previous studies it was shown that blockade of endorphin receptors by a large dose of agloxone (i.e. 10 mg/kg) significantly attenuated the development of pinch-induced catalepsy.[7] A similar dose of naloxone had no effect on catalepsy once the response had been established (i.e., after eight acquisition trials). Thus, naloxone prevented the development of pinch-induced catalepsy but could not reverse it. In the present investigation mice were injected subcutaneously (s.c.) with different doses of naloxone (0.1–10 mg/kg) or morphine (0.1–10 mg/kg) 10 min before the first acquisition trial. Control mice were injected s.c. with saline (0.2 ml). As shown in FIGURE 2, naloxone pretreatment dose-dependently attenuated the development of pinch-induced catalepsy. In contrast, morphine pretreatment enhanced the development of catalepsy (FIGURE 3). In unpinched mice morphine stimulated motor activity at all doses tested.

Because treatment with naloxone produces a physiologic effect consistent with blockade of endorphin receptors and morphine can stimulate these receptors, these results strongly support a role for endorphin systems in the development of pinch-induced catalepsy. Previous studies have shown that the pituitary gland secretes increasing amounts of endorphins into the blood circulation in response to stress[6,17] and that endorphins in the circulation can gain access to the central nervous system (CNS).[18] That the pituitary gland might be the source of endorphins involved in the development of pinch-induced catalepsy was suggested by the following preliminary observations: (1) systemic administration of the glucocorticosteroid dexamethasone (400 and 200 µg/kg given 24 and 4 hr prior to testing, respectively), which abolishes stress-induced release of pituitary endorphins[19] and attenuated the development of pinch-induced catalepsy. (2) Bilateral adrenalectomy, which increases pituitary and plasma beta-endorphin,[20] markedly enhanced the development of catalepsy. The fact that adrenalectomy enhanced pinch-induced catalepsy also suggested that adrenal endorphins may not be significantly involved in pinch-induced catalepsy.

Blockade of dopamine receptors by haloperidol is known to produce profound catalepsy in rats.[21] This effect of haloperidol is not affected by naloxone[22] but it can be reversed by treatment with the dopamine receptor agonist, apomorphine.[23,24] In addition, apomorphine has been shown to antagonize the catalepsy induced by central injection of beta-endorphin.[23,24] Furthermore, it has been demonstrated that endorphins in the CNS interact with central dopaminergic mechanisms. There is a dense distribution of opiate receptors on central dopaminergic cell bodies and terminals[25,26] and opiates, including opioid peptides, have been shown to exert neurochemical effects consistent with blockade of dopaminergic transmission via these receptors.[27,28] To study the involvement of dopaminergic mechanisms in the development of pinch-induced catalepsy, mice were treated s.c. with various doses of apomorphine (0.1–10 mg/kg) or haloperidol (0.01–1 mg/kg) prior to the start of experimentation. As shown

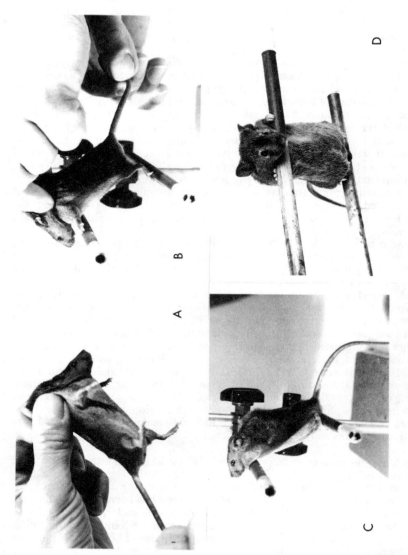

FIGURE 1. Pinch-induced catalepsy in mice. For description of method see text.

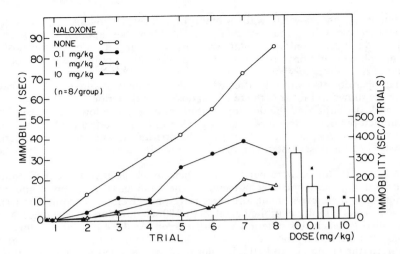

FIGURE 2. The effect of naloxone pretreatment on development of pinch-induced catalepsy. The points indicate means of catalepsy duration of saline or naloxone (0.1, 1, or 10 mg/kg)-treated mice at each testing trial. The bars and vertical lines on the right indicate means ±S.E.M. of total catalepsy time exhibited over eight trials. The asterisks indicate significant difference from saline-pretreated controls ($p < 0.05$, student's t tests).

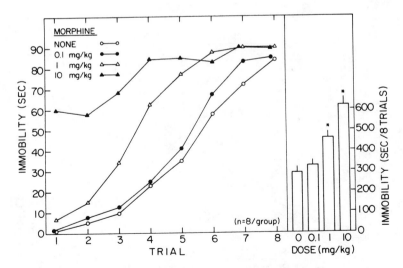

FIGURE 3. The effect of morphine pretreatment on development of pinch-induced catalepsy. For more details see legend to FIGURE 2.

in FIGURE 4, pretreatment with apomorphine 1 or 10 mg/kg, prevented the development of pinch-induced catalepsy. At 0.1 mg/kg, apomorphine slightly enhanced the development of catalepsy. This enhancing effect of the low dose of apomorphine could have been due to the presynaptic suppressive action of low doses of this compound.[29]

Haloperidol also variably affected the development of pinch-induced catalepsy. As shown in FIGURE 5, the two high doses of haloperidol (i.e., 0.1 and 1 mg/kg) markedly enhanced the development of catalepsy. The low dose (0.1 mg/kg) attenuated the development of catalepsy. This inhibitory effect could have been due to the presynaptic effect of low dose haloperidol to enhance dopaminergic activity.[30] At the doses tested haloperidol did not induce catalepsy in unpinched mice.

Additional studies were performed to determine the involvement of endorphin and dopaminergic mechanisms in the maintenance of pinch-induced catalepsy. In these experiments drug-free mice were given eight acquisition trials. In these series all mice exhibited catalepsy of 90 sec duration at least twice. Mice that failed to reach this criterion were discarded. At the end of the acquisition session the mice were injected s.c. with saline (controls), naloxone (1 mg/kg), or apomorphine (1 mg/kg) and 10 min later they were retested for eight additional trials. As shown in FIGURE 6, most saline-injected control mice displayed catalepsy of 90 sec duration in each of the eight testing trials. Similarly, naloxone-treated pinched mice displayed catalepsy of 90 sec duration in each of the eight testing trials. In contrast, apomorphine greatly shortened the duration of catalepsy; none of the apomorphine-treated mice remained cataleptic for 90 sec at any of the eight trials.

The finding with naloxone replicates the previous observation of a lack of

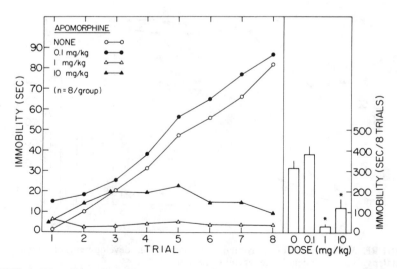

FIGURE 4. The effect of apomorphine pretreatment on development of pinch-induced catalepsy. For more details see legend to FIGURE 2.

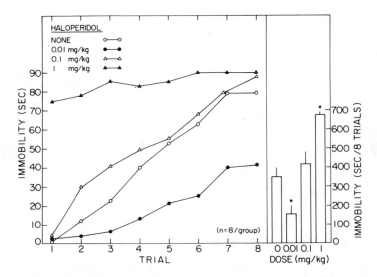

FIGURE 5. The effect of haloperidol pretreatment on development of pinch-induced catalepsy. For more details see legend to FIGURE 2.

effect of this opiate antagonist on maintenance of pinch-induced catalepsy.[7] According to these results, endorphin mechanisms may not be critically involved once the cataleptic response has been established. This is in contrast to endorphin's involvement in the development of pinch-induced catalepsy, as judged by naloxone's ability to prevent it. Apomorphine reversed ongoing pinch-induced catalepsy. This suggests that the maintenance of catalepsy involves functional blockade of central dopaminergic systems. Based on these findings and previous observations on the inhibitory relationship of central opiate and dopaminergic systems[27,28] it might be speculated that pinching to the scruff of the neck briefly activates central opiate mechanisms, which in turn cause activity within dopaminergic pathways involved in movement control to diminish. Inhibition within these dopamine pathways and the resultant catalepsy then perseverate independently of continued endorphin release. It remains to be determined if other endogenous factors might be involved in the process of dopaminergic blockade subserving the maintenance of pinch-induced catalepsy.

PINCH-INDUCED ANALGESIA

Pinch-induced catalepsy is accompanied by profound analgesia that is sensitive to naloxone. Thus, like many other stressful stimuli,[4-6] pinching to the scruff of the neck activates pain inhibitory systems mediated by endorphins.

In earlier studies of pinch-induced catalepsy it was observed that pinched mice failed to respond to needle pricking applied to different parts of the body. In

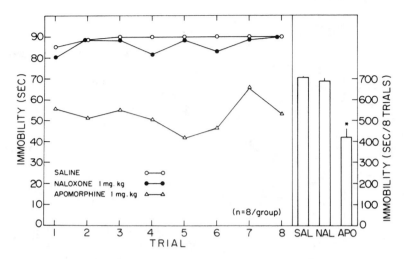

FIGURE 6. The effect of naloxone (1 mg/kg) and apomorphine (1 mg/kg) on the maintenance of pinch-induced catalepsy. Drugs or saline were administered immediately at the end of the eighth acquisition trial. Animals were retested for catalepsy 10 min later as described in the text. Details of the figure are the same as in FIGURE 2.

these experiments nociception was evaluated at the end of the acquisition session.[7] During retesting, naloxone-treated animals maintained cataleptic behaviors (as is shown in the present investigation) but analgesia was diminished and the mice responded vigorously to the needle pricking that was applied at the end of each testing trial. In a subsequent unpublished study, analgesia was assessed more systematically by heating the upper bar serving to support the mouse during catalepsy to 50°C and measuring the latency to withdrawal of the front paws. After eight acquisition trials animals were injected with saline or naloxone (1 mg/kg) and 10 min later subjected to the catalepsy/analgesia testing. Saline-treated pinched mice responded with catalepsy of over 50 sec duration on each of the five testing trials despite the heat stimulus that was applied to their front paws. In contrast, naloxone-treated pinched mice, which were previously shown to maintain catalepsy under normal testing conditions (bar at room temperature), failed to maintain catalepsy when the bar supporting their front paws was heated to 50°C. In these animals, catalepsy never lasted over 10 sec. These results support the proposition that pinching to the scruff of the neck activates endorphin-mediated pain inhibitory systems in addition to producing catalepsy. Moreover, the result suggests that the cataleptic and analgesic responses might be mechanistically interdependent—once the analgesia is disrupted by naloxone treatment and the animal is exposed to pain, catalepsy can no longer be maintained.

A subsequent study further investigated this possibility. This was warranted in view of the fact that the particular method used to assess the two pinch-induced responses did not allow independent evaluation of catalepsy and analgesia within the same animal—reversal of the analgesia by naloxone forced animals to remove their front paws from the catalepsy bar (that serve to apply the painful stimulus) and thus catalepsy was disrupted. In the present investigation, the painful heat stimulus was applied to the tail of cataleptic mice. Analgesia was tested by placing the tail in the light beam of a tail-flick apparatus that was situated below the parallel bars (FIGURE 7). The heat intensity of the light beam was calibrated, using naive unpinched mice, to elicit a tail flick response within 2 sec. The tail-flick apparatus was activated 5 sec after the start of a testing trial and the tail-flick latency was measured. The heat source was turned off when mice withdrew their tail or else after 8 sec. Catalepsy time was assessed simultaneously. Mice were given five analgesia-catalepsy testing trials starting 10 min after the last

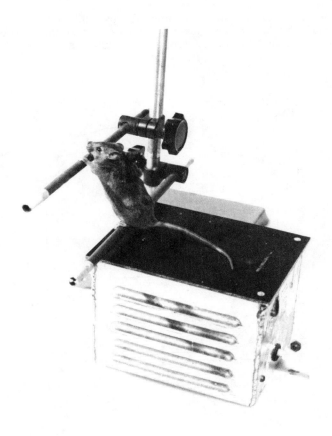

FIGURE 7. Simultaneous evaluation of catalepsy and analgesia (tail-flick test) in the same animal. Testing took place 10 min after the eighth acquisition trial as described in the text.

acquisition trial. Drugs were administered immediately after the last acquisition trial.

As shown in FIGURE 8, saline-treated pinched mice exhibited potent analgesia as well as catalepsy. The tail-flick latency in these mice ranged from 5 to 7 sec across the five trials compared to tail-flick latencies of 2.5 sec or less in unpinched controls. Catalepsy was not disrupted during analgesia testing in saline-treated pinched mice. Few animals did not reach the 90 sec cut-off time during the first few trials, but on subsequent trials 90 sec catalepsy occurred. Naloxone (1 mg/kg) abolished analgesia during pinch-induced catalepsy (FIGURE 8). The tail-flick latencies of these animals were as those of saline-treated unpinched control mice. However, naloxone had no effect on catalepsy. Apomorphine pretreatment (1 mg/kg) had no effect on pinch-induced analgesia (FIGURE 9) but it shortened catalepsy substantially.

Thus, while the mechanisms mediating catalepsy and analgesia are activated simultaneously by the pinching treatment and are parts of the same behavioral syndrome, they seem to be under the control of distinct neurochemical processes.

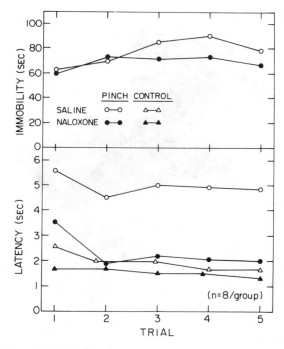

FIGURE 8. The effect of naloxone (1 mg/kg) on the maintenance of pinch-induced catalepsy (top) and analgesia (bottom). The drug was administered immediately after the eighth acquisition trial; animals were retested for five additional trials for both catalepsy and analgesia 10 min later. The points indicate means of catalepsy duration (top) or tail-flick latency (bottom). The saline- and naloxone-treated controls were unpinched animals used to evaluate baseline analgesia levels. For more details see text.

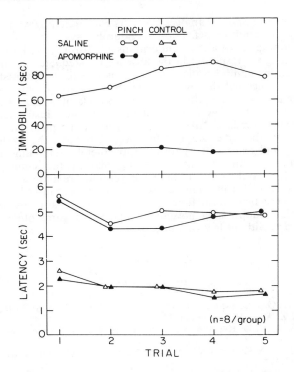

FIGURE 9. The effect of apomorphine (1 mg/kg) on the maintenance of pinch-induced catalepsy (top) and analgesia (bottom). For more details see legend to FIGURE 8.

Pinch-induced catalepsy is triggered by action of endorphins that presumably inhibit dopaminergic transmission. This inhibition, however, is subsequently maintained independently of further endorphin release. This is demonstrated by the ability of naloxone treatment to block but not to reverse catalepsy. In contrast, the analgesic response depends, entirely, on the functional integrity of endorphin mechanisms. It is selectively reversed by naloxone and it is unaffected by treatments that selectively disrupt catalepsy, e.g. apomorphine administration.

CONCLUSIONS

The studies described here show that a mild stressor, pinching to the scruff of the neck, elicits in mice two behavioral responses, catalepsy and analgesia, that are functionally interdependent, yet are mediated by two distinct neurochemical mechanisms. The first response, catalepsy, is triggered by action of endorphins (possibly of pituitary origin) to alter activity in dopamine-mediated systems involved in motor control. Once catalepsy is induced by action of endorphins to suppress dopaminergic activity, it perseveres independent of further endorphin action. The second response, analgesia, occurs concomitantly with catalepsy and like catalepsy it depends on activation of endorphin systems for its development. However, in contrast to catalepsy, endorphins are also required for the maintenance of the analgesic response; in the absence of adequate endorphin tone, as following naloxone administration, analgesia is selectively diminished.

It has been suggested that pinching to the scruff of the neck in mice may produce a sensation resembling the biting attack of a cat.[8] Pinch-induced catalepsy thus may be viewed as a defensive response instrumental for self-preservation, since predators likely ignore an immobile prey. The concomitant analgesia also might serve adaptive function; it reduces the likelihood that a cataleptic prey will react to the pain of injury thereby retracting the predator's attention. Catalepsy and analgesia are triggered by the same physiological stimulus, pinching to the scruff of the neck, yet they are maintained by separate neurochemical mechanisms. This allows a coordinated onset but independent control over these behavioral functions. Thus, injured animals can survive a predator attack by suppressing movement and remaining immobile and also may be able to escape without loss of analgesia.

REFERENCES

1. HAYES, R. L., G. J. BENNETT, P. NEWLON & D. J. MAYER. 1976. Brain Res. 155:69–90.
2. AMIR, S. & Z. AMIT. 1978. Life Sci. 23:1143–1152.
3. BODNAR, R. J., D. D. KELLY & M. GLUSMAN. 1978. Bull. Psychonomic Soc. 11:333–336.
4. TERMAN, G. W., Y SHAVIT, J. W. LEWIS, T. CANNON & J. C. LIEBESKIND. 1984. Science 226:1270–1277.
5. WATKINS, L. R. & D. J. MAYER. 1982. Science 216:1185–1192.
6. AMIR, S., Z. W. BROWN & Z. AMIT. 1980. Neurosci. Biobehav. Rev. 4:77–86.
7. AMIR, S., Z. W. BROWN, Z. AMIT & K. ORNSTEIN. 1981. Life Sci. 28:1189–1194.
8. ORNSTEIN, K. & S. AMIR. 1981. J. Comp. Physiol. Psychol. 95:827–835.
9. AMIR, S. & K. ORNSTEIN. 1981. Soc. Neurosci. Abstr. 7:49.
10. KLEMM, W. R. 1983. Experimentia 39:228–230.
11. KLEMM, W. R. 1983. Psychopharmacology 81:24–27.
12. CARLI, G., F. FARABOLLINI & G. FONTANI. 1981. Behav. Brain Res. 2:373–385.
13. CARLI, G. 1977. Psychol. Rec. 27 Suppl:123–143.
14. DE RYCK, M. & P. TEITELBAUM. 1984. Behav. Neurosci. 98:243–261.
15. ARIYANAYAGAM, A. D. & S. L. HANDLEY. 1975. Psychopharmacologia 41:165–167.
16. KATZ, R. J. 1980. Prog. Neuro-Psychopharmacol. 4:309–312.
17. GUILLEMIN, R., T. M. VARGO, J. ROSSIER, S. MINICK, N. LING, C. RIVIER, W. VALE & F. BLOOM. 1977. Science 197:1367–1369.
18. RAPOPORT, S. I., W. A. KLEE, K. D. PETTIGREW & K. OHNO. 1980. Science 207:84–86.
19. FRENCH, E. D., F. E. BLOOM, C. RIVIERE, R. GUILLEMIN & J. ROSSINER. 1978. Soc. Neurosci. Abstr. 4:408.
20. ROSSIER, J., E. FRENCH, C. GROS, S. MINICK, R. GUILLEMIN & F. E. BLOOM. 1979. Life Sci. 25:2105–2112.
21. DE RYCK, M., T. SCHALLERT & P. TEITELBAUM. 1980. Brain Res. 201:143–172.
22. SEGAL, D. S., R. G. BROWN, F. BLOOM, N. LING & R. GUILLEMIN. 1977. Science 198:411–414.
23. IZUMI, K., T. MOTOMATSU, M. CHRETIEN, R. F. BUTTERWORTH, M. LIS, N. SIDAH & A. BARBEAU. 1977. Life Sci. 20:1149–1156.
24. VAN LOON, G. R. & C. KIM. 1978. Res. Commun. Chem. Pathol. Pharmacol. 21:37–44.

25. GARDNER, E. L., R. S. ZUKIN & M. H. MAKMAN. 1980. Brain Res. **194**:232–239.
26. POLLARD, H., C. LLORENS-CORTES & J. C. SCHWARTZ. 1977. Nature **268**:745–747.
27. VAN LOON, G. R. & C. KIM. 1978. Life Sci. **23**:961–970.
28. VERSTEEG, D. H. G. 1980. Pharmac. Ther. **11**:535–557.
29. WALTERS, J. R., B. S. BUNNEY & R. H. ROTH. 1974. Neurology **9**:136–139.
30. PUECH, A. J., P. SIMON & J. R. BOISSIER. 1978. Eur. J. Pharmac. **50**:291–300.

Stress-Induced Analgesia: Its Effects on Performance in Learning Paradigms[a]

ZVI-HARRY GALINA AND ZALMAN AMIT

Center for Studies in Behavioral Neurobiology
Department of Psychology
Concordia University
Montreal, Quebec H3G 1M8

The organization of a behavioral response is governed by many interrelated factors. The most important are interactions between the internal state of the organism and the environmental circumstances at the time the behavior is expressed. Given the constant change in the state of both the internal and external environments of the organism, this interaction must be viewed as an ever-changing dynamic process. It follows logically that the behavior emitted by the organism at any time throughout its life is a product of this interaction. In recent years, we have been interested in determining how the pattern and organization of species-specific defensive behaviors are modulated by events in the immediate environment. We have chosen to examine simple conditioned and unconditioned responses and the manner in which they change as a consequence of varying physiological and environmental conditions.

Unconditioned noxious stimuli will elicit responses that may be construed as automatic. However, if the species-specific behavior results in a response that terminates or at least attenuates the intensity of the aversive stimuli, the probability of a recurrence of this response is increased. Thus the relationships between stimuli in both the external and internal environment and the behavior of the organism can be defined by well established laws of learning. Nevertheless, during certain environmental conditions, particularly those of acute stress, the usual organization and pattern of particular behaviors may not follow the prescriptions of the previously mentioned "lawful" relationship but instead appear to be compromised by an ensuing disorganization of the behavior.

Disorganization, however, is not always the immediate consequence of stressful events. Moderate levels of acute stress may in fact facilitate or activate physiological and behavioral coping mechanisms and strategies and result in an improved response pattern. Continued stress may lead to a breakdown in normal coping mechanisms and result in disruption of the species-specific response patterns. Even acute stressful stimuli can have diverse effects on the organism. Some researchers have postulated that acute stress can have both positive and negative consequences. Under certain conditions stress may disrupt behavior,

[a]Z.H.G. is the recipient of an NSERC scholarship award. Z. A. is a National Health Research Scholar (Canada).

while under different circumstances it can have an integrating effect on performance and behavioral response patterns.[1-3]

STRESS AS A CONTINUOUS INTERVENING VARIABLE

At this point in our discussion, it becomes important to define the term stress. Many words have been used synonymously with this term, yet all have clearly different connotations (e.g. activation and arousal). Perhaps a more useful way of distinguishing between stress and its synonyms is to regard those synonyms as representations of different locations along a single hypothetical continuum.

According to Selye[3] the term stress should be reserved for noxious stimuli that induce the same physiological syndrome. On the other hand, the term arousal, which was often used in the same context, was in fact describing concurrently stimulus dimensions such as intensity, duration, and frequency as well as psychological variables such as fear, reaction to novelty, and conflict. However, in general, stress was traditionally used to describe the nature of the stimulus while arousal was used to describe the status of the organism itself. Furthermore arousal was traditionally viewed as an adaptive process, while stress has traditionally been viewed as a maladaptive, even pathological process. However, it is more likely that stress and arousal, in this traditional frame of reference, simply describe different positions on the same continuum. In this case they merely constitute terms used to describe the response of an organism to different degrees, levels, or intensities of the same set of environmental stimuli impinging on the organism. Furthermore, arousal may describe the portion of the continuum where the response of the organism to the impinging stimuli is improved in its integrity and efficiency while stress describes a segment of the continuum where the response is disrupted and disintegrated. Therefore, our working hypothesis is that stress may be viewed as a position on an arousal continuum (i.e. too little or too much arousal) or that arousal constitutes a position on the stress continuum (i.e. a reaction to different intensities of a noxious stimulus). Clearly, the choice would depend on whether one focuses on the stimulus continuum or the continuum representing the status of the organism (for further discussion see Hennessy and Levine[4]).

An interesting and fruitful view of the stress/arousal continuum was put forward by Malmo.[2] As with other researchers, Malmo preferred his own terminology because he felt that it would better represent his own conceptualizations. In the context of the present discussion, it is interesting to note that Malmo speculated that an appropriate level of environmental stimulation ("activation") would sensitize the organism. Such activation at any given point on the continuum would be a consequence of an interaction between environmental and hormonal conditions. The hormonal conditions would not necessarily provide the directional impetus for a particular behavior (steering function) but would set up conditions to facilitate appropriate responding. In fact, Malmo delineated a specific experimental paradigm that included three levels of activation: low, moderate, and high. He went on to suggest that the expected corresponding performance levels of the organism under these three levels of activation would be low, optimal, and low, i.e. an inverted U-shaped curve. Stress, activation, and arousal in his schema have meaning only as relative terms determined by their position on the inverted U-shaped curve. It is imperative to note that the characterization of a behavioral response as high or low in this context is only meaningful in relation to their position on the curve. What follows from this line of reasoning is that experiments that employ only one level of stimulus intensity cannot yield meaningful data. We feel that this framework has particular merit and have therefore attempted whenever feasible to use this conceptual approach.

By adopting these notions into our conceptual scheme it becomes possible to better measure defensive reactions in terms of an integrated response to a stimulus configuration. This response, however, is necessarily constrained by the parameters of the experiment. The performance in the absence of stress becomes the baseline against which the behavioral response in all phases of the experiment is assessed. In this context all change in performance may be defined as the product of stress. For example, one of the adaptive responses of rodents to escapable footshock is avoidance. If the stimulus configuration impinging on the organism alters this adaptive response then this interaction is considered stressful. One must therefore conclude that despite the prevailing confusion in terminology, stress and arousal are by definition the intervening variables between environmental stimuli and the response. FIGURE 1 is a simplified graphic description of these concepts.

STRESS ANALGESIA IS ADAPTIVE

As stated above stress can be considered both as a disruptive or adaptive phenomenon. One of the observable results of stress is a diminished reaction to painful stimuli. This decreased sensitivity was termed stress-induced analgesia.[5,6] Appropriate and adaptive responses during the presence of noxious stimuli (i.e. avoidance, escape, freezing) may be disrupted or blocked due to accompanying pain. Within obvious limits, a diminished perception of pain would allow the organism to better focus its attention on a suitable response.[5] Therefore, SIA can and should be considered as an adaptive process.

A large body of literature has been gathered documenting the physiological and anatomical correlates of stress-induced analgesia. In addition, many of the variables that may be subsumed under the term stress have also been studied in terms of their capacity to modulate the perception of pain. It is now recognized that such factors as stimulus intensity and duration, as well as fear responses can determine not only the presence or absence of analgesia but also the type of analgesia that is manifested in response to stress.[7-9] Though the behavioral response patterns to different stressors may, in many cases, be the same, the underlying physiological substrate mediating the response may be different. For example, analgesia induced by the non-opiate–mediated cold water swim or the opiate-mediated prolonged intermittent footshock can both be measured by the tail-flick method. No apparent difference is seen in the behavior induced by the two stressors as measured by the tail-flick test yet the physiological substrate mediating this response seems quite different.[7-9]

Given the large data base that is available on stress-induced analgesia it seemed to us that we might be able to integrate the conceptual notions described above in the framework of more recent experimental data. To this end we have focused our attention on the analysis of the acquisition and extinction of avoidance behavior under conditions that also induce stress-induced analgesia.[10]

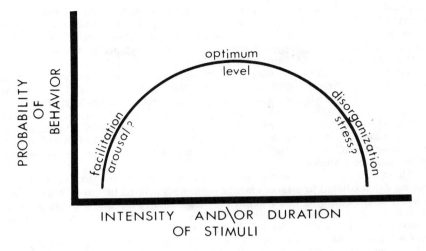

FIGURE 1. A graphic representation of our conceptual hypothesis concerning the term stress as a continuous variable. The probability of behavior is a function of the intensity or duration of stimuli. The stimulus variables will either facilitate, disrupt, or provide an optimum level of behavioral performance.

We were interested in determining at what point stress disrupts behavior or integrates it and what function does analgesia serve in these situations.

UNCONDITIONED RESPONSES

In our initial studies we chose a stimulus that was easily varied along the dimension of intensity. It consisted of short exposures (30 sec) to hot plates pre-heated to different temperatures. Some temperatures were only mildly aversive, while others were obviously highly aversive.

Initially we measured the effects of different intensities of heat on natural locomotor/exploratory behavior of rats exposed to novel environments. Four temperatures were used: 21, 47, 52, and 57°C. We found that the midrange levels of heat stress (47 or 52°C) increased while the higher level[57] depressed exploratory behavior relative to control groups.[21] In fact, the data could be expressed as an inverted U-shaped curve, representing a functional relationship between the intensity of stimuli and locomotion. A statistically significant quadratic trend was evident. This trend, in our conceptualization, may be a manifestation of the previously mentioned stress continuum as 47 and 52°C led to increased exploration, while 57°C led to depression of locomotor activity to a level below the control group.[11]

Using the same stimuli, we then determined the degree to which the pituitary adrenal axis was activated by the different levels of heat. Changes in the activity of this axis have long been associated with events that are considered stressful. In addition, this axis was of particular interest since some of the neuropeptides secreted by this axis have been considered to improve responding to motivationally relevant variables by enhancing environmental cues[12] or altering attentional variables.[13] This mechanism may then be responsible for the changes in the response at the different points on our continuum.

We observed that there was a relationship between the intensity of the heat and levels of plasma corticosterone.[11] The higher heat level induced the greatest release of corticosterone. By adrenalectomizing our rats we found that involvement of the adrenals was not necessary for the expression of the heat-stress generated locomotion. Hypophysectomy, however, significantly attenuated the behavior and this attenuation could be reversed by the pre-administration of a high dose of ACTH or mimicked by some doses of naloxone in non-hypophysectomized animals.[14]

These findings suggested that the reduced locomotor/exploratory effects of the stimuli are mediated to a large extent by pituitary-related factors. We were then interested in examining other behavioral responses, particularly stress-induced analgesia. As in the previous studies the rats were exposed to 30 sec of various levels of heat stress (hot plate). Following exposure to the hot plate they were immediately tested for analgesic responses. Five cm of the tail was submerged in 45°C water and the latency to withdraw the tail was recorded. Short exposures to the high intensity stressor induced an analgesia that lasted approximately 15 min as measured by tail-flick inhibition. This analgesia was not naltrexone reversible.[10] This latter finding suggested that a non-opiate analgesia was induced as a consequence of exposure to the higher intensity heat stimulus.

CONDITIONED RESPONSES

The one-way shuttle avoidance paradigm is a common procedure used in learning experiments with rats. Avoidance responding can be viewed as an integrated defensive reaction that would be functionally useful in natural settings. Rats will usually acquire this response within 20 trials. Since each trial in our paradigm lasts less than 1 min, the time needed to acquire the avoidance response is therefore well within the time frame of the analgesia induced by heat stress. Therefore, if the rat is exposed to the heat stimulus immediately before training we could then assess the affects of having a raised pain threshold on avoidance acquisition. This same paradigm can also be used to measure retention of the learned behavior. During the extinction phase of avoidance experiments subjects must in fact learn a new contingency; that the aversive stimulus is no longer present. The subject is not initially aware of this new situation and may continue to respond to the conditioned stimuli. This continued responding (avoidance) during extinction may be taken as a measure of retention.[15,16]

In our experiments utilizing the one-way avoidance paradigm, we included groups that were exposed to various intensities of heat as well as a control group that was not exposed to heat stimuli. In this way, we were able to assess the effects of pre-exposure to heat stimuli on avoidance learning. As Spear[16] has suggested, the physiological changes brought about by stimuli that precede avoidance testing become part of the stimulus complex. It follows that in the present experiment stress-induced analgesia was part of the stimulus complex for some of the groups.

Several groups of rats were exposed to the different levels of heat stress immediately before acquisition of avoidance. The groups were exposed to 21, 47, or 57°C heat for 30 sec before acquisition phase. An additional group received no hot-plate exposure (NHP) before training. The acquisition phase consisted of placing animals in one side of the shuttlebox, which triggered a relay that began a timed sequence of events. Ten seconds after being placed in the box, a door separating the two compartments was opened and a tone was sounded for 5 sec. Immediately following termination of the tone, an electric shock (0.5 mA, 1 sec, scrambled) was presented through a grid floor. The rat could avoid the shock presentation by shuttling to the other side during the tone or escape shock by shuttling to the other side during shock administration. Once the rat shuttled to the other side of the chamber, the door between compartments was shut and 10 sec elapsed before the animal was placed back in the original side for the next trial. The criterion for acquisition of avoidance responding in response to the tone was five consecutive avoidances. The animal was then returned to its home cage. Twenty-four hr later each animal was re-exposed to the shuttlebox procedure. The experimental conditions were identical except that no shock was presented to the animals and no heat stimulus was applied. Extinction criteria in this case were five consecutive non-avoidances. A successful non-avoidance consisted of not moving to the other side in response to the tone. After ten seconds the door separating the compartment was shut and the sequence was repeated.

Acquisition performance was unaffected by any of the stimuli. There was no difference in the number of trials necessary to acquire the avoidance response among the groups. A raised pain threshold therefore does not appear to affect acquisition of avoidance performance in this paradigm. However, it is possible to interpret the lack of significant differences between the 57°C group and the other groups as indicative of the presence of an adaptive mechanism. The reduction in pain allowed this group to function in a manner indistinguishable from controls thus allowing escape from a noxious stimuli. In other words, this should be compared to the animals' response pattern under the same pain-inducing stimuli but without pain reduction.

While we could not find differences in avoidance acquisition, when we exposed the groups to extinction trials 24 hr later we observed significant differences in the number of trials required to extinguish the avoidance response. There was a significant relationship between the intensity of the stimuli and rate of extinction (FIGURE 2). The results illustrated in FIGURE 2 suggest that higher stress levels prior to avoidance training were associated with faster extinction.

While it is possible that the results may simply reflect differences in the ability of the rats to perform the avoidance response, this is unlikely, since no differences were found in trials to acquisition. In addition, the differences in extinction reflect differences of non-avoidance (i.e. no movement).

It would appear then that the memory for the acquired behavior was differentially affected by exposure to different intensities of heat stimulus. These data, however, do not provide adequate evidence for an effect on memory processes per se. For example, the results of extinction training may be a reflection of alterations in sensory systems and not a direct effect on the memory trace.[17]

When the animals are undergoing extinction trials, re-exposure to the shuttle box is a necessary part of the stimulus complex. However, we did not re-administer the heat stimuli before the extinction phase, therefore only part of the stimulus complex was present. Nevertheless, this may have been enough to trigger the physiological changes associated with the previous days' experience. In other words, the animal that was exposed to 57°C heat stress before the acquisition

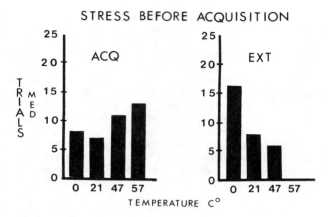

FIGURE 2. Acquisition and extinction of one-way avoidance. Heat stress was applied immediately before acquisition training. There was no difference in acquisition. A significant difference was found in extinction between groups (Kruskall-Wallis, $p < .05$). Group 57°C was significantly different from all other groups (Mann-Whitney U test $p < .05$).

phase may have undergone the acquisition in a different state than the animals in the other groups. It is probable that the total sensory experience of the shuttlebox was different for these animals. Upon re-exposure to the apparatus this altered sensory experience may have accounted for the faster extinction rates observed.

To further address the question of altered motoric or sensory effects we changed the experimental paradigm so that the same heat stressors were now applied immediately after acquisition criteria had been reached (five consecutive avoidances). Under these conditions, changes in performance 24 hr later could be interpreted as attributable to an effect of the stressor on memory. Since the heat stimulus comes after the acquisition it could not be expected to effect the original learning. Similar to the previous study, we found that different intensity levels of heat led to differences in extinction. This time these differences were not linear but curved. An inverted U-shaped curve depicting the relationship between stimulus intensity and extinction can be seen in FIGURE 3. Groups that were exposed to 21 or 47°C exhibited enhanced retention compared to the NHP group. More trials were needed in these groups to reach extinction. The group exposed to 57°C was indistinguishable from the NHP group.

Half the animals in each group of the previous avoidance experiments were further tested 24 hr after extinction. These animals were now once again exposed to the shock stimuli that were present during acquisition, but no heat stress was applied. Since the avoidance response was extinguished the rats had to, at least partially, re-acquire this response. Re-acquisition criteria of five consecutive avoidances was achieved by all groups regardless of previous heat stress experience within the first eight trials. This suggests that the differential effects seen in extinction are not present 24 hr later during re-acquisition of avoidance.

The inverted U-shaped curve depicting our extinction data (FIGURE 3) was

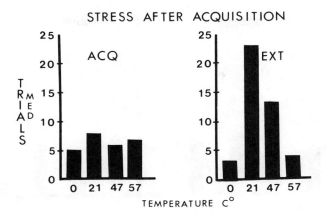

FIGURE 3. Acquisition and extinction of one-way avoidance. Heat stress was applied immediately after acquisition. There was no difference in acquisition. Significant differences were found in extinction (Kruskall-Wallis, $p < .05$). Groups 21 and 47°C were significantly different from 0 and 57°C (Mann-Whitney U test, $p < .05$).

reminiscent of data generated by other investigators through post-trial administration of ACTH in studies of retention of inhibitory avoidance.[18] Since we found that some locomotor/exploratory behavior was modulated by ACTH, we decided to further examine possible pituitary involvement in mediating this response.

Dexamethasone (DEX) is a synthetic steroid that inhibits the release of pituitary hormones including ACTH. Reversal or attenuation of behavior by DEX implies pituitary involvement in the observed behavior. DEX (0.5 or 1 mg/kg) was applied 2 hr before repeating the previous experiments. When the stress was applied before acquisition, DEX had no effect on acquisition of avoidance responding. However, DEX did affect extinction of the avoidance response when tested 24 hr following acquisition. In this latter case DEX reversed the effects of the high intensity heat stimulus when the heat stimuli was applied before avoidance acquisition (FIGURE 4). In the context of the present experiment, DEX seemed to induce a resistance to extinction at the highest intensity (57°C). However, when the heat stress was applied after acquisition DEX caused a resistance to extinction across all stress intensities (FIGURE 5). This suggests that DEX differentially affected extinction results depending on when the stress was applied.

At this stage of our research we have not yet established whether the effects of DEX were due to inhibition of ACTH (or other peptides) release or a direct effect of DEX on steroid receptors. Given the data that we collected earlier and the results of studies reported by others[17] we hypothesized that the effects we have observed are due to modulation of ACTH. This may occur in a number of ways. For example, the facilitation of retention, as demonstrated by resistance to extinction (FIGURE 2, extinction data), or the facilitated extinction by the same stimuli at different intensity levels may have been due to a direct effect of ACTH on central processes.[12] As stated earlier ACTH has been shown to affect learning in a biphasic manner.[17] It is also likely that as we continue to experiment other

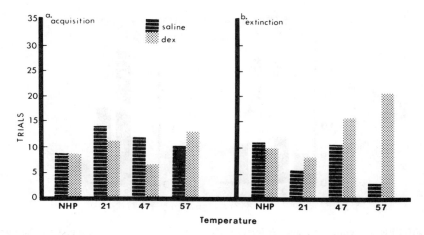

FIGURE 4. Acquisition and extinction of one-way avoidance. Heat stress was applied immediately before acquisition. Dexamethasone was injected 2 hr before acquisition.

peptides will be found to affect the induction of behaviors that we have observed in these experiments.

SUMMARY AND CONCLUSIONS

The results of the studies reported here indicate that the groups receiving the 57°C heat stimulus exhibited three different responses. These seemed to be dependent on the testing conditions employed. These testing conditions can be viewed as

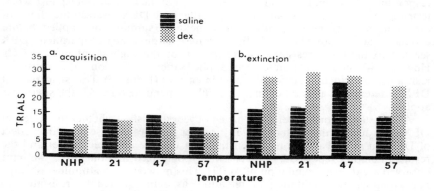

FIGURE 5. Acquisition and extinction of one-way avoidance. Heat-stress was applied immediately after acquisition. Dexamethasone was injected 2 hr before acquisition.

reflective of varying environmental circumstances. When the animal was placed in a novel environment and movement was not a critical adaptive component of the situation, the unconditioned response was one of reduced locomotion compared to controls. Concomitantly, these rats exhibited longer latencies to tail withdrawal in a tail-flick test indicating the presence of analgesia. Yet, when placed in a position where movement was the adaptive response (shuttle) the animals revealed that they can learn and perform the response as well as controls. Of particular interest, was the finding that although acquisition was not disrupted by exposure to the stimuli, the memory of the appropriate response was altered (as measured by latency to extinction). This would not seem to be an adaptive response. If the animal encounters the same stimuli again it would seem that remembering the previous encounter should facilitate current avoidance. However, a better explanation may be that since there is in fact no shock stimuli during extinction sessions, the recognition of this fact as reflected by the rapid extinction is adaptive. When the shock stimulus is present as was the case during re-acquisition sessions 24 hr later, the animals have shown that all groups re-acquire the avoidance response in the same amount of trials.

Attempts to incorporate these results into our concept of stress as discussed above reveal the existence of the following pattern. The animals' normal pattern of responding in our avoidance paradigm during extinction is to continue avoidance, as if the shock was still present. The animals that did not receive stress before acquisition have been conditioned to avoid at the sound of danger. The animals receiving the heat stimuli show progressively faster extinction as the heat intensity was increased. This indicates that even though these animals were also conditioned to avoid, they were not able to retain or retrieve this information 24 hr later. As explained earlier this pattern of differential rate of extinction was a function of the intensity of the stimuli.

Locomotor/exploratory behavior, performance of an acquired response 24 hr later, and pituitary adrenal response are all affected by the intensity of the stimuli. This pattern in many cases can be depicted by either an upright or inverted U-shaped curve. The behaviors become manifest as a result of factors in the environment and the internal conditions that prevail at the time of testing. We were able to change the background hormonal (and other) conditions by manipulating the intensity of stimuli. Given these results it may be appropriate to consider stress as the product of intensity and duration of stimuli. Changing the level of stimulation will determine at what point on the stress continuum the particular behavior is being measured. When experiments are designed to include more than one dimension of an agent the bell or Gaussian curve emerges.

At the outset of this paper we suggested that stress should be viewed on a continuum that would be best represented as an inverted U-shaped curve. At some locations on the curve stress could prove to be adaptive. Such was the case in the active avoidance paradigm where the rate of acquisition by the group receiving the higher intensity stimuli before avoidance training was not different than controls. We would suggest that this is possible because of the parallel activation of pain suppressive systems. The pain suppressive system acts in this situation as the agent that corrects or helps maintain adaptive responding. The findings presented here suggest that stress-induced analgesia can function as an adaptive mechanism that may facilitate responding in avoidance learning paradigms and by implication improve the nature of the animals' defensive response in noxious or dangerous situations.

ACKNOWLEDGMENTS

We would like to thank Yves Beauleau, Chris France, Stephen Nicoletti, Cathy Sutherland, James Sutherland, and Franc Rogan for their technical assistance. We would also like to thank Dr. B. R. Smith for helpful discussion during early drafts of the manuscript.

REFERENCES

1. HEBB, D. O. 1955. Psych. Rev. **62**:243–254.
2. MALMO, R. B. 1959. Psych. Rev. **66**:367–386.
3. SELYE, H. 1974. Stress Without Distress. Signet. New American Library. Scarborough, Ont.
4. HENNESSY, J. W. & S. LEVINE. 1979. *In* Progress in Psychobiology and Physiology Psychology. L. M. Sprague & A. N. Epstein, Eds. Academic Press. New York.
5. AMIR, S., Z. W. BROWN & Z. AMIT. 1980. Neurosci. Biobehav. Rev. **4**:77–86.
6. BODNAR, R. J., D. D. KELLY, M. BRUTUS & M. GLUSMAN. 1980. Neurosci. Biobehav. Rev. **4**:87–100.
7. BODNAR, R. J. & V. SIKORSKY. 1983. Learn Motiv. **14**:223–237.
8. CHANCE, W. T. 1980. Neurosci. Biobehav. Rev. **4**:55–67.
9. TERMAN, G. W., Y. SHAVIT, J. W. LEWIS, J. T. CANNON & J. C. LIEBESKIND. 1984. Science **226**:1270–1277.
10. GALINA, Z. H., F. ROGAN & Z. AMIT. 1983. Neurosci. Abstr. **13**:276.
11. GALINA, Z. H., C. J. SUTHERLAND & Z. AMIT. 1983. Pharmacol. Biochem. Behav. **19**:251–256.
12. DE WIED, D. *In* Neuropeptides and Neural Transmission. C. Ajmone Marsan & W. Z. Traczyk, Eds.: 217–226. Raven Press. New York.
13. SANDMAN, C. A. & A. J. KASTIN. 1981. Pharmac. Therap. **13**:39–60.
14. GALINA, Z. H., Z. AMIT & J. A. VAN REE. 1985. Peptides. (In press.)
15. RICCIO, D. C. & J. T. CONCANNON. 1981. *In* Endogenous Peptides in Learning and Memory Processes. pp. 117–142. Academic Press. New York.
16. SPEAR, N. E. 1973. Psychol. Rev. **80**:163–194.
17. GOLD, P. E. & S. F. ZORNETZER. 1983. Behav. Neural Biol. **38**:151–189.
18. GOLD, P. E. & R. B. VAN BUSKIRK. 1976. Behav. Biol. **16**:387–400.

Electroconvulsive Shock Activates Endogenous Opioid Systems: Behavioral and Biochemical Correlates

JOHN W. HOLADAY, FRANK C. TORTELLA,
JAMES L. MEYERHOFF, GREGORY LUCAS BELENKY,[a]
AND ROBERT J. HITZEMANN[b]

Department of Medical Neurosciences
[a]Department of Behavioral Biology
Division of Neuropsychiatry
Walter Reed Army Institute of Research
Washington, DC 20307-5100

[b]Department of Psychiatry
University of Cincinnati School of Medicine
Cincinnati, Ohio 45267

INTRODUCTION

Since the discovery of endogenous opioid peptides a decade ago, many hypotheses have evolved in an attempt to define the potential role of endogenous opioids in mental disorders.[1,2] The use of morphine to treat depression at the turn of the century was successful but short-lived due to the development of tolerance. Nonetheless, these clinical observations suggest that endogenous opioids and their receptors may be involved in affective disorders. We theorized that these endogenously activated opioid systems may play a therapeutic role in the antidepressant effects known to result from electroconvulsive therapy (ECT). In an initial test of this hypothesis, we subjected rats to electroconvulsive shock (ECS) and observed a spectrum of postictal responses with prominent opioid-like characteristics.[3-8] Most of these opioid-like behavioral and physiological effects of ECS were antagonized by the universal opioid antagonist, naloxone.[9]

The following review will briefly describe the effects of a single ECS as well as repeated daily ECS, emphasizing the use of this procedure as a model of stress-induced analgesia (SIA). Importantly, additional data demonstrating electroencephalographic (EEG), cataleptic, autonomic, anticonvulsant, and altered receptor binding characteristics produced by ECS are presented. These endpoints serve as important corollaries of the analgesic effects of ECS which may pertain to other models of SIA as well.

BEHAVIORAL, EEG, AND AUTONOMIC EFFECTS OF SINGLE ECS

Cataleptic and Analgesic Effects

ECS, produced in rats by transauricular electroshock (150 V, 60 Hz, 2 sec duration), resulted in an initial tonic-clonic seizure of approximately 40–50 sec duration. During the subsequent postictal interval, rats demonstrated an opioid-like catalepsy, characterized by rigidity with loss of righting reflexes and an inability to cling to an inclined wire screen.[3,6] Although the righting reflexes returned within 10 min, the stuporous cataleptic behavior (postictal depression) persisted for an hour or more in undisturbed rats.[6,7] Frenk and colleagues[10] have also observed a similar naloxone-sensitive postictal depression following kindled seizures in rats.

Tail-flick and hot-plate latencies measured during the postictal interval were also significantly elevated in ECS-treated rats.[3,6,8] The elevation of tail-flick latencies was short-lived (approximately 15 min) and naloxone pretreatment did not consistently block this antinociceptive response to ECS. By contrast, the increase in hot-plate escape latencies following ECS persisted for 90 min or longer and was reliably antagonized by naloxone pretreatment [3.0 or 10.0 mg/kg intraperitoneally (i.p.)]. Thus, this form of SIA appears to preferentially affect the centrally integrated hot-plate response more than the predominantly reflexive tail-flick response.

Selective opioid antagonists were used to determine the opioid receptor subtype involved in ECS-induced analgesia.[11] Pretreatment with the long-last μ antagonist, β-funaltrexamine [(β-FNA), 20 nmoles intracerebroventricularly (i.c.v.)] did not alter the usual pattern of hot-plate analgesia following ECS. However, the δ-antagonist ICI 154,129 (200 nmoles i.c.v.) significantly antagonized the analgesic effects of ECS. To confirm the receptor selectivity of these antagonist ligands, at these same doses and routes of administration, only the μ antagonist β-FNA (and not ICI 154,129) blocked the analgesic response to the classic μ agonist, morphine.[12,13] These results indicate that opioid peptides, activated by ECS, act upon central δ receptors to exert their analgesic actions.

Electroencephalographic and Anticonvulsant Effects

Tortella and colleagues[14,15] have characterized the pattern of cortical EEG response evoked by numerous opioid peptides. After the initial, transient polyspike epileptiform discharge (not accompanied by behavioral convulsions), a pattern of slow-wave, high voltage EEG was observed. The duration of this slow-wave EEG response correlated well with the duration of opioid-induced stuporous behavior (catalepsy). Naloxone pretreatment abolished these EEG and behavioral responses.

In more recent studies, it was shown that the postictal cortical EEG response following ECS was remarkably similar to the EEG pattern described for opioid peptides.[7] Furthermore, the duration of the EEG slow-wave, high voltage response evoked by ECS was highly correlated with the duration of postictal depression as measured by electromyography.[16] Both of these opioid-like responses were also blocked by naloxone.[7,16] These results have provided important correlations between the pharmacological actions of exogenous opioids and endogenous opioids activated by ECS.

Both alkaloid and peptide opioids are known to have anticonvulsant properties.[17-19] Although naloxone failed to alter the intensity or duration of seizures evoked by acute ECS in rats,[6,7] this is not surprising since endogenous opioid systems require a stressful stimulus for their activation. Once activated by ECS, the anticonvulsant effects of endogenously released opioids can be demonstrated. It was shown that a single ECS, like injected opioid peptides, elevates seizure thresholds when rats are subsequently challenged with exposure to the volatile convulsant, flurothyl.[18] Likewise, ECS delivered intermittently at 10 min intervals resulted in a progressive decrease in the severity and duration of seizures, and this effect was cross-tolerant in rats chronically exposed to morphine.[19] Both of these anticonvulsant effects of ECS were antagonized by naloxone, indicating another correlation between the pharmacological responses to injected opioids and the opioid-like responses produced by ECS. Of greater importance, these and other studies provide evidence that the endogenous opioid systems may participate in the limitation of seizures in various seizure disorders.[20]

Autonomic Effects

Like the classic opioid analgesics that depress respiration, respiratory depression is also a prominent characteristic of the postictal interval following seizures. Indeed, respiratory rates are profoundly reduced following ECS seizures, and naloxone pretreatment significantly antagonized this effect.[4,5,8] These results not only demonstrate a physiological role of endogenous opioid systems in respiratory function, but also confirmed their role in the etiology of respiratory depression produced by seizures.

As another autonomic corollary between opioids and the postictal responses to acute ECS, we evaluated the effects of naloxone pretreatment on the pattern of cardiovascular changes evoked by ECS.[5,8,21] As with ECT in humans, ECS in rats resulted in an initial surge of arterial pressure, followed by a return to normal values as the seizure intensity diminished (20 sec following ECS). Heart rate was erratic due to arrythmias during the seizure, however bradycardia was observed until 35 sec following ECS when heart rate returned to normal values. Pretreatment with naloxone (1.0 or 10.0 mg/kg i.p.) resulted in a significant overshoot of both arterial pressure and heart rate below normal values during the immediate postictal interval. Since opioids are known to blunt baroreceptor reflexes in animals and man,[21] these experiments provided evidence that the activation of baroreceptor reflexes by ECS also activates endogenous opioid systems that may serve to accelerate the return of normal cardiovascular function following seizures. Blockade of this system by naloxone prevented the usual inhibition of baroreceptor function by endogenous opioids and delayed the restoration of arterial pressure and heart rate to normal values. From these data and those of Zamir and Siegel,[22] increases in arterial pressure may be correlated with the subsequent analgesic effects of SIA stressors.

BEHAVIORAL, EEG, AND AUTONOMIC RESPONSES FOLLOWING REPEATED DAILY ECS TREATMENT

Behavioral, EEG, and Autonomic Effects

In humans, the therapeutic effects of ECT require repeated daily electroshock treatment for five to ten days in order to obtain maximum benefit.[23] Hong and colleagues[24] investigated the effects of repeated ECS on endogenous opioid concentrations in various tissues and found selective increases in enkephalin concentrations in specific brain regions (see below). Since single ECS appears to evoke the activation of endogenous opioid systems, we investigated the effects of repeated daily ECS on behavioral, EEG, and autonomic endpoints.[7,25]

Repeated daily ECS (once daily for nine days) resulted in rats that became progressively more cataleptic (longer intervals of postictal depression) and analgesic after ECS challenge when compared to single-ECS controls.[7,25] Additionally, the duration of the opioid-like EEG response and respiratory depression was also increased by repeated daily ECS.[25] This sensitization to the behavioral and EEG responses produced by daily ECS was also accompanied by a decreased efficacy of naloxone in reversing these opioid-like effects. These responses are opposite to those produced by chronic morphine treatment, which is known to result in a progressive tolerance to the effects of opioid challenge and enhanced sensitivity to naloxone.[26]

Further evidence dissociating the effects of repeated ECS and chronic morphine was obtained in cross-challenge experiments.[25] Instead of the expected decreased response to morphine in rats whose opioid systems were repeatedly activated by daily ECS (nine days) and pharmacologically challenged on day 10, rats were sensitized to the effects of 4 or 16 mg/kg morphine sulfate. Likewise, rats rendered tolerant to morphine (three pellets for three days) were also sensitized to the opioid-like effects of single ECS challenge. Thus, cross-sensitization instead of cross-tolerance was observed. Although Urca and colleagues[27] failed to replicate all aspects of these studies, these investigators also reported that repeated daily ECS enhanced responses to subsequent morphine challenge.

Repeated ECS and Opioid Receptors

In order to evaluate the potential mechanism(s) responsible for the cross-sensitization reviewed above, we investigated the effects of repeated daily ECS and chronic morphine treatment on opioid receptor binding variables. In initial studies using [^{3}H]D-Ala^2-D-Leu^5-enkephalin (^{3}H-DADL),[28] we found that repeated daily ECS (but not single ECS) resulted in an apparent increase in the number of opioid binding sites (B_{max}) without affecting the apparent receptor affinities (K_D). Likewise, chronic morphine exposure had the same effect (increased B_{max}) when compared to binding variables in control rats chronically treated with placebo pellets.

More recently, these results were confirmed and extended in further studies evaluating the effects of repeated daily ECS or chronic morphine on binding variables using the universal opioid ligand [^{3}H]diprenorphine, the δ ligand ^{3}H-DADL or the μ-ligand [^{3}H]morphine.[9,29] Although the number of binding sites for all three ligands increased in both repeated ECS rats and rats fed morphine pellet, by far the biggest effect on B_{max} was observed in the membranes treated with [^{3}H]diprenorphine (approximately 80%). Furthermore, brain membranes from repeated ECS rats demonstrated a proportionally greater increase in δ binding sites, whereas chronic morphine treatment resulted in a greater increase in μ binding.

This apparent up-regulation of opioid receptors produced by repeated ECS or chronic morphine treatment was only observed if binding assays were conducted in the absence of 100 mM NaCl. In the presence of NaCl, all groups of rats (repeated sham ECS, repeated ECS, single ECS, chronic morphine, or chronic placebo) demonstrated an equivalent B_{max} value.[9,29] Thus, one explanation for these findings is that repeated daily ECS or chronic morphine locks the receptor in the sodium-preferring (antagonist)[30] conformation. Nonetheless, although this may explain why morphine tolerance and concomitant increased naloxone efficacy occurs, repeated daily ECS has the converse effect, e.g. sensitization and decreased naloxone efficacy (see above). Further studies are underway to resolve these apparent discrepancies and to address the possibility that selective changes in opioid receptor subtypes may be involved.

Recently, Hitzemann et al.[31] have shown that the apparent increase in the number of opioid binding sites following repeated daily ECS is region specific within the brain (TABLE 1). Although both procedures increase the B_{max} values, they appear to produce different responses in different brain regions. Furthermore, there is a striking similarity between the areas of the brain that demonstrate increased binding sites and the regional increases in enkephalin concentrations reported by Hong et al.[24] (TABLE 1).

SUMMARY AND CONCLUSIONS

From the evidence reviewed above, there is little doubt that ECS activates endogenous opioids and modifies their receptors. Thus, this form of SIA is accompanied by many other corollaries of opioid-like actions, including catalepsy, similar EEG patterns, common autonomic effects, and increases in opioid receptor binding sites. Investigations have further indicated that the amnestic effects of ECS can also be attenuated by naloxone,[32] and that pituitary-

TABLE 1. Effects of Repeated Daily ECS

Brain Region	Increase in B_{max}[a]	Increase in Enkephalin[b]
Frontal cortex	0	0
Pyriform cortex	+	
Remaining cortex	0	0
Olfactory bulb	++	
N. accumbens	++	+
Striatum (N. caudatus)	++	+
Amygdala	+	+
Septum	+	++
Hippocampus	+	+
Hypothalamus	+	++
Midbrain	+	
Brainstem	0	0

Note: Effects of repeated daily ECS for nine days on opioid receptor numbers (B_{max}) and brain enkephalin concentrations as measured in brains removed one day following the last ECS seizure. B_{max} values were obtained using [^{3}H]diprenorphine as a ligand in the absence of NaCl, and enkephalin concentrations were determined by radioimmunoassay. "0" indicates no significant change from controls, + indicates 0–50% increase above controls, and ++ indicates >50% increase above controls. Open spaces indicate lack of available data.
[a]Data from Hitzemann et al.[31]
[b]Data from Hong et al.[24,36]

derived opioids may play an important role as a predominant source of opioids that contribute to these opioid-like effects following ECS.[33-35]

It is hoped that these many attempts to correlate SIA with other behavioral and physiological endpoints following ECS will provide a more global perspective on the role of endogenous opioid systems in ECS. From these results, it is suggested that other forms of SIA may also share many of these properties in common with ECS-induced SIA. Nonetheless, ECS and other forms of SIA, such as cold water exposure and restraint, share with ECS a common history of clinical use in the treatment of human depression.[6] It is possible that the common thread linking these experimental observations to endogenous opioid systems may provide new insights into the cause and treatment of mental disorders as well as the perception of pain.

ACKNOWLEDGMENT

We thank L. Robles and J. Kenner for their expert assistance in many of the studies reviewed in this manuscript.

REFERENCES

1. HOLADAY, J. W. & H. H. LOH. 1981. *In* Hormonal Proteins and Peptides: β-Endorphin. C. H. Li, Ed.:202–291. Academic Press. New York.
2. EMRICH, H. M., V. HOLLT, H. LASPE, M. FISCHLER, H. HEINEMANN, W. KISSLING, D. ZERSSEN & A. HERZ. 1979. *In* Neuro-psychopharmacology. Saletu, Berner & Hollister, Eds.:527–534. Pergamon Press. Oxford.
3. HOLADAY, J. W., G. L. BELENKY, H. H. LOH & J. L. MEYERHOFF. 1979. Soc. Neurosci. Abstr. **4**:409.
4. BELENKY, G. L. & J. W. HOLADAY. 1979. *In* Endogenous and Exogenous Opiate Agonists and Antagonists. E. L. Way, Ed. Pergamon Press. New York.
5. BELENKY, G. L. & J. W. HOLADAY. 1979. Brain Res. **177**:414–417.
6. HOLADAY, J. W. & G. L. BELENKY. 1980. Life Sci. **27**:1929–1938.
7. TORTELLA, F. C. A. COWAN, G. L. BELENKY & J. W. HOLADAY. 1981. Eur. J. Pharmacol. **76**:121–128.
8. HOLADAY, J. W., F. C. TORTELLA & G. L. BELENKY. 1981. *In* The Role of Endorphins in Neuropsychiatry. H. Emrich, Ed.:142–157. Karger. Basel.
9. HOLADAY, J. W., F. C. TORTELLA, J. B. LONG, G. L. BELENKY & R. J. HITZEMANN. 1986. Ann. N. Y. Acad. Sci. (This volume.)
10. FRENK, H., J. ENGEL, R. F. ACKERMANN, Y. SHAVIT & J. C. LIEBESKIND. 1979. Brain Res. **167**:435–440.
11. BELENKY, G. L., D. GELINAS-SORELL, J. R. KENNER & J. W. HOLADAY. 1983. Life Sci. **33**:585–586.
12. WARD, S. J. & J. W. HOLADAY. 1982 Soc. Neurosci. Abstr. **8**:388.
13. HOLADAY, J. W. & F. C. TORTELLA. 1984. *In* Central and Peripheral Endorphins: Basic and Clinical Aspects. E. E. Miller & A. R. Genazzani, Eds.:237–250. Raven Press. New York.
14. TORTELLA, F. C., J. E. MORETON & N. KHAZAN. 1978. J. Pharmacol. Exp. Ther. **206**:636–642.
15. ADLER, M. W. & F. C. TORTELLA. 1983. Pharmacologist **25**:152.
16. TORTELLA, F. C. & A. COWAN. 1982. Life Sci. **31**:881–888.
17. TORTELLA, F. C., A. COWAN & M. W. ADLER. 1981. Life Sci. **29**:1039–1045.
18. TORTELLA, F. C. & A. COWAN. 1982. Life Sci. **31**:2225–2228.

19. TORTELLA, F. C., J. B. LONG & J. W. HOLADAY. 1985. Brain Res. **332**:174–178.
20. TORTELLA, F. C. & J. B. LONG. 1985. Science **228**:1106–1108.
21. HOLADAY, J. W. 1983. Ann. Rev. Pharmacol. Toxicol. **23**:541–594.
22. ZAMIR, N. & M. SEGAL. 1979. Brain Res. **160**:170–173.
23. FINK, M. & J. O. OTTOSON. 1980. Psych. Res. **2**:49–61.
24. HONG, J. S., J. C. GILLIN, H.-Y. T. YANG & E. COSTA. 1979. Brain Res. **177**:273.
25. BELENKY, G. L. & J. W. HOLADAY. 1981. Life Sci. **29**:553–563.
26. WAY, E. L., H. H. LOH & F. H. SHEN. 1969. J. Pharmacol. Exp. Therap. **167**:1–8.
27. URCA, G., A. NOF, B. A. WEISSMAN & Y. SARNE. 1983. Brain Res. **260**:271–277.
28. HOLADAY, J. W., R. J. HITZEMANN, J. CURELL, F. C. TORTELLA & G. L. BELENKY. 1982. Life Sci. **31**:2209–2212.
29. HITZEMANN, R. J., B. HITZEMANN, S. BLATT, F. C. TORTELLA, J. R. KENNER, G. L. BELENKY & J. W. HOLADAY. 1985. (Submitted for publication.)
30. PERT, C. B. & S. H. SNYDER. 1974. Mol. Pharmacol. **10**:868–879.
31. HITZEMANN, R. J. *et al.* (In preparation.)
32. MESSING, R. B., R. A. JENSEN, J. L. MARTINEZ, J. R., V. R. SPIELER, B. J. VASQUEZ, B. SOUMIREU-MOURAT, K. C. LIANG & J. L MCGAUGH. 1979. Behav. Neural Biol. **27**:266–275.
33. LEWIS, J. W., J. T. CANNON, E. H. CHUDLER & J. C. LIEBESKIND. 1981. Brain Res. **208**:230–233.
34. TORTELLA, F. C., A. COWAN & J. W. HOLADAY. 1984. Peptides **5**:115–118.
35. LONG, J. B., J. W. HOLADAY & F. C. TORTELLA. 1984. IUPHAR 9th International Congress of Pharmacology Abstracts. 1460.
36. KANAMATSU, T., J. F. MCGINTY & J. S. HONG. 1984. Soc. Neurosci. Abstr. **10**:1110.

Somatovegetative Changes in Stress-Induced Analgesia in Man: An Electrophysiological and Pharmacological Study

JEAN CLAUDE WILLER AND MONIQUE ERNST

Laboratoire de Neurophysiologie Clinique
Faculte de Medecine Saint Antoine
75571 Paris Cedex 12
France

INTRODUCTION

While it appears obvious that the perception of pain in normal subjects depends on the physical characteristics of the noxious stimulus and on its site of application, it is also clear that the subjective pain response is dependent on psychological and social factors (see references in Beecher[1]). For instance, it has been shown that for a given intensity, an electrical stimulation was better tolerated by relaxed subjects than by anxious subjects.[2,3] In another experimental paradigm, when anticipating a liminal painful stimulus, naive subjects showed both increase and decrease in the pain threshold while trained subjects showed no change in the pain threshold.[4] However the changes in pain threshold observed in naive subjects habituated progressively within 30–40 minutes of the experimental session. This observation showed that naive subjects progressively became trained ones.[4] This is discussed in terms of the activation of various central nervous system structures and shows that naive subjects were more sensitive than trained ones to a specific anxiogenic situation induced by the anticipation of a very mild pain. This report raises several questions: (1) Can the anticipation of a painful stimulus produce a state of anxiety or of stress that would modify the pain sensation in trained subjects? (2) What level of intensity would be required for this conditioning painful stimulus? (3) Would these trained subjects exhibit any sign of habituation towards an intense pain?

Furthermore, since it has been shown in numerous animal studies that intermittent and inescapable foot-shock was able to induce, in certain conditions, a state of opiate-like naloxone-reversible analgesia,[5,6] one can wonder whether similar observations can be obtained from human studies, for which there is a clear lack of data.

The first part of this study was performed on trained volunteers. A repetitive signal announcing the occurrence or non-occurrence of an intense and inescapable noxious footshock induced a state of cumulative anxiety and of stress that resulted in a progressive analgesia associated with a decrease of nociceptive reflexes. This response was accompanied by a progressive somatovegetative response, i.e. polypnea, tachycardia, and by the facilitation of monosynaptic reflexes. These effects were found to be significantly modified by a double-blind injection of naloxone.

Since benzodiazepines are among the most widely used drugs, at least in the West, especially for their anti-stress and anxiolytic action, one could wonder if such drugs modify the subjective response as well as the somatovegetative reaction to the experimental stress observed in this study. Contradictory results appear in the literature. Some authors observed that diazepam reduced the catecholamine and corticosterone responses to stress.[7-9] Others reported that diazepam potentiated the analgesia induced by cold swim stress in rats.[10] The second part of this study demonstrated that a cross-over and double-blind diazepam treatment decreased the responses to the stress described in the first section.

METHODS

The experiment was performed on eight trained volunteers (four men and four women, 25–36 years old). Each subject had already participated in experiments involving the electrophysiological study of pain and was consequently familiar with the experimental procedure and atmosphere and with the electrical pain-inducing stimuli. All subjects were paid for their participation in the experiment. They had been fully informed of the aim and procedure of the study before signing a consent form in accordance with the principles of the Helsinki convention. During the session they were comfortably seated in an armchair in order to obtain muscular relaxation.

The threshold of the nociceptive reflex (RIII reflex) of the knee flexor muscle was studied because it has been previously found to be close to the threshold of pain.[11] Methodological details for stimulating the sural nerve and recording the reflex activity from the biceps femoris muscle have been extensively described elsewhere.[11,12] In brief, the sural nerve was stimulated at a 0.25 Hz rate through a pair of electrodes placed retromalleolary 2 cm apart on the degreased skin. The electrical stimulus consisted of a train of eight rectangular pulses (1 msec duration each) delivered over 20 msec by a constant-current stimulator. The intensity of stimulation varied randomly within a range of 0 to 30 mA. Electromyographic reflex responses were recorded from the ipsilateral biceps femoris muscle (Bi), using a pair of surface electrodes placed on the degreased skin overlying the muscle. These reflex responses (RIII,Bi) were full-wave rectified (time window of 100 msec, 80 msec after the stimulus onset). A stimulus intensity eliciting a liminal reflex response with a probability of 80–90% was defined as the reflex threshold.

The subjective quality and intensity of the sensation elicited by the sural nerve stimuli were evaluated by the subjects on a 10 point visual analogue scale (VAS), with "point 3" corresponding to the pain threshold as described in a previous report.[13]

In order to study the monosynaptic spinal excitability, the H reflex from the soleus muscle was elicited and recorded according to a well-known procedure:[14] The posterior tibial nerve was stimulated monopolarly at the popliteal fossa, and the ipsilateral soleus muscle (Sol) response was recorded via surface electrodes placed on the skin. The stimulus intensity was chosen so as to elicit a reflex response corresponding to 50% of the maximal H,Sol reflex amplitude.

The reflex responses (H,Sol and RIII,Bi) were elicited from alternate leg at a rate of 0.2 cm/sec. This procedure was considered reliable since we had previously verified the absence of any kind of interaction between these two reflex responses.[15]

Heart and respiratory rates were also studied since it has been shown that they are sensitive parameters of the vegetative response to attention, emotion, or stress.[16,17] The heart rate was measured via EKG using the V1 international derivation. The respiratory rate was recorded by means of a pneumograph, which is sensitive to respiratory movements, placed around the thorax.

All these parameters were displayed in parallel on a tape recorder (for further computed analysis), on a polygraph, and on a storage oscilloscope allowing permanent monitoring and control of the experiment.

The stress stimulation was produced according to a method described previously.[18,19] Briefly, during a 3–6 min conditioning period, three intense and inescapable highly noxious footshocks (70–80 mA; 7–8 times the pain threshold) and two very mild tactile ones (3–4 mA) were delivered to the sural nerve. The subjects were then asked to remember the noxious stimulus as the reference for intolerable pain. After this conditioning period, the subjects received a two-minute warning signal announcing the occurrence of the noxious stimulus or the tactile stimulus. The noxious stimulus and the tactile stimulus were given in randomized series during the session. This period, called stress period (S), was preceded by a rest period (R) also lasting 2 min, during which the subjects were asked to relax as much as possible. The R and S periods were repeated in this order 16–18 times during the session (FIGURE 1). Forty-five minutes after the beginning of the session, the subjects received (i.v.) either hydrochloride naloxone (0.08 mg/kg; 10 ml) or the equivalent volume of the naloxone vehicle, using a double-blind and cross-over procedure. Injections were performed through the cannula of an infusion of isotonic glucose placed into a vein of the forearm at the beginning of the session. This method had the advantage of facilitating drug injection and of preventing uncontrollable side-effects (anxiety, attention, emotion) resulting from a direct intravenous injection during the session.

For four days prior to the session, subjects received either a diazepam treatment at the standard dosage used for anxiety treatment (three capsules of 2 mg per day), or identical capsules of placebo, using a randomized cross-over and double-blind procedure. Each subject participated in four sessions at 10-day intervals, two diazepam sessions, and two placebo sessions, during which he(she) received naloxone and vehicle (i.v.) in both conditions. FIGURE 1 summarizes the experimental design.

The cumulative effects of repeated stress periods (S) were measured during the rest periods (R). Each parameter was recorded every 30 sec of rest period and was studied by means of individual and global means and variances. A two-way analysis of variance (ANOVA) was used for the analysis of the results.[20] The significance of the parameter variations as a function of the repetition of the stress in time was calculated by means of a paired t test and a linear regression analysis.

RESULTS

The cumulative effects of repetitive stress were studied on the threshold of both nociceptive reflex and pain sensation and on somatovegetative parameters, in subjects treated with diazepam or placebo, using a cross-over and double-blind procedure. In both conditions the effects of naloxone were studied in order to assess the involvement of endogenous opiates in the observed effects. We will consider the characteristics of the responses obtained during the placebo

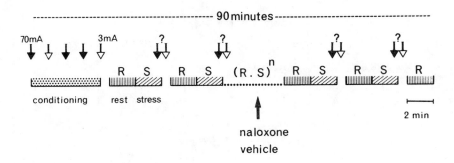

FIGURE 1. Diagram showing the whole experimental and pharmacological procedures of this study. DZP, diazepam and PBO, placebo.

treatment (as control values) and their modifications during the diazepam impregnation.

Characteristics of Control Responses (Placebo Treatment)

Before the conditioning period, all subjects showed homogeneous values of the nociceptive reflex threshold (10.2 ± 1 mA). The corresponding sural nerve stimulation elicited also homogeneous liminal pain sensation described as a pinprick sensation and rated at 3.3 ± 0.9 arbitrary units (a.u.) on the VAS. The heart rates was 37 ± 2 pulses/30 seconds and the respiratory rate was 7.3 ± 1.2. The homogeneity of the baseline values between subjects allowed further comparisons in experimental conditions such as repeated stress and after naloxone or vehicle injection.

In all subjects, the repetition of the stressor resulted in a progressive decrease in pain sensation and in the nociceptive reflex associated with a somatovegetative arousal. As shown in FIGURE 2 (lower graph), a stimulus intensity of 10.2 mA, eliciting a liminal pain sensation (3.3 a.u.), was progressively and significantly ($p < 0.01$) perceived as less and less painful, and finally as tactile (1.4 ± 0.6 a.u.) after 45 minutes of repeated stress. The depression of the nociceptive reflex ran parallel with these subjective changes since its threshold showed a significant 45% increase ($p < .05$) after 45 minutes of repetitive stress (FIGURE 3, lower graph). At the same time, the monosynaptic H reflex was significantly increased (+52%, $p < .05$) as well as the heart rate (21%) and the respiratory rate (66%). These electrophysiological characteristics are illustrated on the left part of each graph in FIGURE 4.

By the 45th minute of the session, the administration of naloxone produced a rapid (2–5 min) modification in all the changes observed above. As shown in FIGURE 2 (lower graph), naloxone significantly reversed the stress-induced analgesia ($p < .05$): the initial 10.2 mA stimulation was felt as very painful (rating

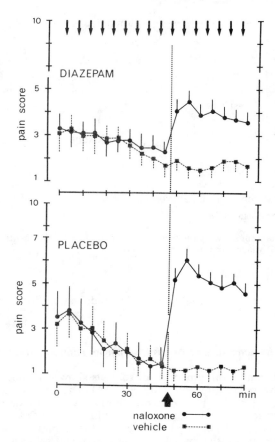

FIGURE 2. This figure shows the naloxone-reversible analgesic response induced by the repetitive stress (↓↓↓) during diazepam (upper) and placebo (lower). Dotted line and lower arrow indicate drug (naloxone and vehicle) injection. Each point represents the mean value of the pain rating score with its standard error mean (SEM).

score: 5–6 a.u. on the VAS) and the nociceptive reflex threshold exhibited a 50% decrease ($p < .01$) after naloxone injection (FIGURE 3, lower graph). In contrast, naloxone enhanced the facilitation of the H reflex (+50%) as well as the tachycardia (+16%) and the polypnea (+43%) observed during the 45 minutes of the session. These naloxone effects lasted between 20 and 30 minutes according to the parameter under consideration (lower graphs of FIGURES 2 and 3, FIGURE 4). The double-blind administration of the naloxone vehicle did not produce any significant modification in the parameters, when compared just before and 5 minutes after injection. However it is interesting to note that, in this case, the variations in the parameters reached a maximum by the 45–55th minute and

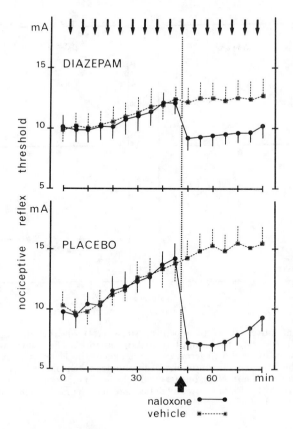

FIGURE 3. This figure shows the naloxone-reversible depression of nociceptive reflexes as expressed by the progressive increase in the threshold as a function of repetition of stress (↓↓↓) during diazepam (upper) and placebo (lower). Same legends as in FIGURE 2.

remained at this level until the end of the session. The linear regression analysis performed for the data obtained between 50 and 80 minutes did not show any significance in the variations as a function of time. These results are illustrated in FIGURES 2 and 3 (lower graphs) and 4.

Modifications of the Response to the Stress During Diazepam Treatment

As mentioned in the methods, a four-day treatment of diazepam (three tablets of 2 mg diazepam per day) was given to the subject prior to the session. This dosage was chosen since it is clinically known to produce only anxiolytic effects without hypnotic nor myorelaxant actions.

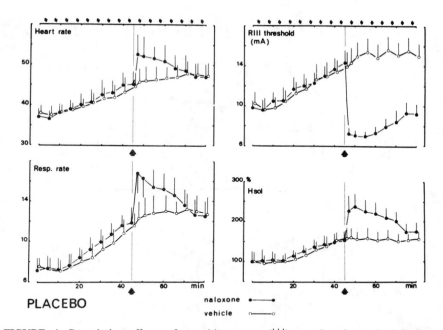

FIGURE 4. Cumulative effects of repetitive stress (↓↓↓) on the electrophysiological parameters studied during the control (placebo) situation. The values of heart and respiratory rates are expressed in terms of 30 sec epoch; the H reflex is expressed as a percentage of the baseline (unconditioned) amplitude, taken as 100%, while the RIII threshold is expressed in mA. Naloxone (●) and vehicle (○) injections (cross-over, double-blind) are indicated by the lower arrow and dotted line in each graph. Each point represents the mean value with 1 SEM.

The first modification induced by the diazepam treatment concerned the baseline values of the vegetative parameters: Both heart and respiratory rates showed a significant 10% decrease ($p < .05$) when compared with the baseline values of the control (placebo) condition. In contrast, diazepam did not affect the baseline value of the nociceptive reflex threshold (10.1 ± 0.9 mA) nor the corresponding liminal pain sensation (FIGURES 2 and 3). Moreover, diazepam did not modify significantly the baseline characteristics of the H reflex since the thresholds of the H and M responses and the $H_{maximum}/M_{maximum}$ ratio of the control condition (placebo) were similar to those of the diazepam condition.

During the R and S periods, diazepam induced a general slight moderating effect on the magnitude of the changes produced by the repetitive stress when compared with the control placebo condition.

As shown in FIGURE 2 (upper graph), a stimulus intensity of 10.1 mA, eliciting a liminal pain sensation of 3.2 ± 0.7 a.u. on the VAS, was progressively perceived as less painful (2 ± 0.5 a.u.) after 45 minutes of repeated stress. Similarly, the threshold of the nociceptive reflex showed a 20% increase during the same period (FIGURE 3, upper graph). The H reflex and the heart and respiratory rates increased respectively 17%, 15%, and 35% during the first 45 min of the session. These electrophysiological results are illustrated in FIGURE 5, on the left part of each graph.

The effects of naloxone, as described in control sessions, were still obtained, but, as above, were less marked than those from the placebo condition. The slight analgesia was reversed into a slight hyperalgesia, since the initial 10.1 mA stimulus was felt as just above pain threshold (rated at 4 a.u. on the VAS) (FIGURE 2, upper graph). Similarly, naloxone reversed the stress-induced depression of the nociceptive reflex by producing a 25% decrease in its threshold (FIGURE 3, upper graph). As with the control condition, but to a lesser extent, naloxone enhanced the facilitation of the H reflex (+32%), as well as the tachycardia (+10%) and the polypnea (14%) observed at the 45th minute of the repetitive stress during diazepam condition (FIGURE 5). These naloxone effects lasted between 15 and 30 min according to the parameter under consideration.

In contrast, the double-blind administration of naloxone vehicle did not produce any significant modification in the parameters values when compared just before and 5 min after injection. However, it is interesting to mention that here again, no significant change in the parameter values was observed between the 45th minute and the end (80th minute) of the session. It is also of interest to note that subjects did not report any clear hypnotic effect during the period of diazepam treatment. However they all reported to feel more relaxed in the daytime and during the session. This subjective observation was reported in two

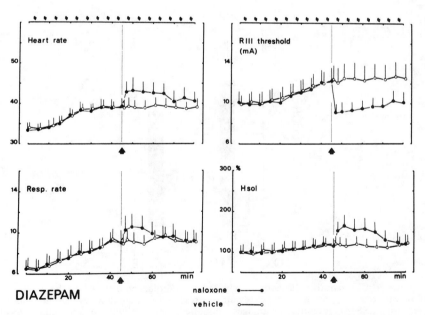

FIGURE 5. Cumulative effects of repetitive stress on the electrophysiological parameters during the diazepam situation. Same legends as FIGURE 4.

cases (1 man and 1 woman) during the placebo treatment. No sex difference nor habituating effect from one session to the other was noted in this randomized cross-over and double-blind study.

The last points to be considered concern (1) the quantitative aspects of the moderating diazepam action on the responses obtained during the repeated stress when compared to those obtained in the same stress condition during the control (placebo) condition and (2) the relationships between diazepam and the minor naloxone action compared to those obtained during placebo condition. In this purpose, the numerical data of each parameter obtained in each condition at the 45th minute of the session, i.e. just before naloxone or vehicle injection, were compared with those obtained at the maximum naloxone effect (5–10 min after injection) via a two-way analysis of variance. The results of these comparisons are illustrated in the histograms presented for each parameter in FIGURES 6 to 10. The maximum analgesia induced by the stressor during diazepam was 38% weaker than that obtained during the control condition ($p < .05$), and the subsequent naloxone-induced hyperalgesia was 21% less marked during diazepam (FIGURE 6). The maximum increase of the nociceptive reflex threshold was, during diazepam treatment, about 13% less important than that obtained during the placebo treatment and the naloxone reversal was 26% weaker during treatment with

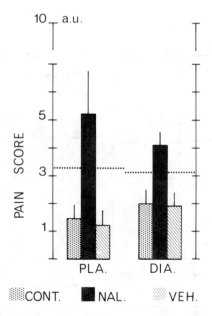

FIGURE 6. Comparative effects of placebo (PLA) and diazepam (DIA) on the maximum analgesic response produced by the repetitive stress and its naloxone reversibility. Dotted area (with 1 SEM) represents the analgesia obtained after 45 minutes of stressing (CONT). Black area (with 1 SEM) shows the effect of naloxone (NAL) while hatched area (with 1 SEM) shows the effect of double-blind administration of the naloxone vehicle (VEH). Dotted lines indicate the baseline level of the unconditioned pain score.

diazepam than with the placebo (FIGURE 7). For these two parameters, the statistical analysis clearly indicated that the weaker effects of naloxone during diazepam treatment were independent from the moderating action of this drug upon the depression of nociceptive reflexes induced by the stress. This will be discussed in terms of possible interactions between opiate and benzodiazepine receptors.

In contrast, for the three other parameters (H reflex, heart rate, and respiratory rate), the statistical analysis indicated that the moderating diazepam action upon the changes observed during stress was significantly related to the weaker effects of subsequent naloxone administration. As shown in FIGURE 8, during diazepam treatment the facilitation of the H reflex was attenuated 24% and 33% before and after naloxone, respectively, when compared to the control values. The vegetative parameters followed the same pattern of change. The polypnea observed during diazepam treatment was attenuated 24% and 40% before and after naloxone, respectively (FIGURE 9), and the tachycardia attenuated 13% and 18%, respectively (FIGURE 10).

DISCUSSION

The present study demonstrates that a repetitive stress induced by the anticipation of intense pain in trained volunteers can result in a distinct naloxone-

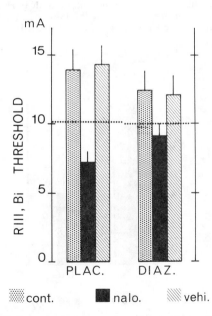

FIGURE 7. Comparative effect of the naloxone-reversible maximal increase of the threshold of the biceps femoris nociceptive reflex (RIII,Bi Threshold) during placebo (PLAC) and diazepam (DIAZ). Same legends as in FIGURE 6.

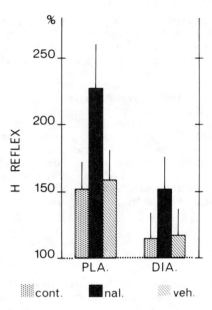

FIGURE 8. Comparative effect of placebo (PLA) and diazepam (DIA) on the naloxone-enhanced maximum facilitation of the monosynaptic reflex (H reflex) induced by the repetitive stress. Results are expressed in % of the baseline amplitude (as 100%) of the unconditioned H response Same legends as in FIGURES 6 and 7.

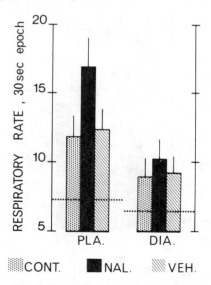

FIGURE 9. Comparative effect of placebo (PLA) and diazepam (DIA) on the naloxone-enhanced maximum polypnea induced by the repetitive stress. Same legends as in FIGURES 6 to 8.

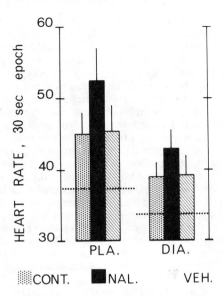

FIGURE 10. Comparative effect of placebo (PLA) and diazepam (DIA) on the naloxone-enhanced maximum tachycardia induced by the repetitive stress. Same legends as in FIGURES 6 to 9.

reversible analgesia and a depression of nociceptive spinal reflexes, associated with a facilitation of monosynaptic reflexes and an increase in both heart rate and respiratory rate. These latter changes were found to be enhanced after naloxone administration. This study also shows that a diazepam treatment can reduce by 50% all the changes described above.

These results will be discussed from several points of view. In the first section, we will consider the homogeneous pattern of variations in trained subjects when they anticipate an intense and inescapable pain during a control condition (placebo). In the second section, we will discuss the modifications induced by naloxone in terms of the involvement of the endogenous opioid pain suppressive system in the mechanism of the observed stress-induced analgesia. Finally, we will consider the moderating effects of diazepam treatment on the changes observed during stress, particularly as regards a possible relationship between opiate and benzodiazepine receptors.

A repetitive stress during a relatively short period (45–80 min) was able to produce homogeneous and stereotyped variations of pain sensation and of somatovegetative responses in normal trained volunteers. This pattern of responses, obtained with a painful conditioning stimulus applied to the sural nerve, has also been observed when the conditioning stimulation was applied elsewhere on the body skin.[18] Therefore it cannot be interpreted as a local hypothesis, i.e., localized control of spinal reflexes, but as a general behavior involving the whole body. The increase in heart and respiratory rates has been previously described in man as a sign of increased attention and/or emotion.[16,17] Similarly, the facilitation of monosynaptic reflexes associated with the depression of the nociceptive component of the exteroceptive reflexes and the pain threshold increase has also been observed in humans during increased attention or during non-specific arousal.[21] These variations are consistent with the results obtained from animal experiments that have shown that electrical stimulation of the mesencephalic reticular formation resulted in a stereotyped arousal including increase in respiratory and heart rates, facilitation of monosynaptic reflexes, and depression of nociceptive reflexes.[22,23] It is therefore tempting to suggest that in our study the cumulative effects of stress resulted in a progressive increase in the mesencephalic reticular activity. According to Routtenberg's hypothesis,[24] this would correspond to the activation of the arousal system I, which would be predominantly involved in the drive and organization of a general response to a stress stimulus induced by anticipation of a severe pain. However, when looking at the variation curves as a function of the repetition of the stress, it seems unlikely that two to three warnings would be necessary to initiate the above-described cumulative effects, especially those observed in respiration and spinal reflexes. One could suggest that this phenomenon corresponds to a general protective reaction from the stress. Similarly, the relative plateau observed in the variation of each parameter observed between the 45th and 80th minute of the session (during vehicle injection) can also be interpreted as another rate-limiting protective reaction against a too strong effect that could result from the cumulative effects of repetitive stress.

However, the observed progressive analgesia associated with the depression of nociceptive reflexes is in agreement with the animal studies,[6] which have shown the increase in the tail-flick latency associated with the increase in cerebral endogenous opiates in stressed rats. These observations clearly suggest the participation of the endogenous morphine-like system, which will be discussed in the following section.

The second kind of data obtained in this study shows that the specific opiate antagonist naloxone reversed the analgesia into hyperalgesia and induced the facilitation of nociceptive reflexes. These effects were associated with the exacerbation of both tachycardia and polypnea as well as the facilitation of monosynaptic reflexes. It is well known that morphine and endogenous opiates exert a depressive action not only on the nociceptive transmission (nociceptive reflexes here) but also on monosynaptic reflexes and vegetative parameters such as heart rate, blood pressure, and ventilation.[25-27] In normal and relaxed subjects there was no evidence of a tonic opiatergic regulation of these parameters, since we had previously observed that naloxone did not affect any of the above parameters in double-blind and cross-over studies.[28,29] Therefore, in the present study, our data strongly suggest that the cumulative effects of repetitive stress resulted in a progressive activation of some endogenous opiate system, since the double-blind administration of naloxone reversed the stress-induced analgesia, lowered the threshold of the nociceptive reflexes, and enhanced the variations of other parameters. These results show that endogenous opioids can exert a complex and multimodal influence, not only on the pain suppressive structures, but also on other central nervous regions involved in heart and respiratory regulation. As mentioned in a previous report,[30] it is tempting to suggest that three different mechanisms are involved in the bodily changes during the stress-induced analgesia. The first one, as mentioned in the first section, is a reticular activation (arousal system I) that would induce an increase in heart and respiratory rates, a facilitation of monosynaptic reflexes, and an inhibition of nociceptive ones, associated with analgesia. The second mechanism would involve a simultaneous and progressive activation of some endogenous opiatergic structure that would both modulate and reinforce the analgesia and the depression of nociceptive reflexes. This hypothesis is consistent with the effects of naloxone that we observed, i.e. a double action: exacerbation in the changes of some parameters (heart, respiration, H reflex) and reversal of the analgesia and of the depression of nociceptive reflexes into an hyperalgesia and facilitation of nociceptive reflexes. These latter data clearly show that endogenous opiates also exert a depressive effect on the central nervous structures, which would be responsible for the hyperalgesia and for the facilitation of nociceptive reflexes as evidenced by the effects of naloxone administration. Therefore it is possible to suggest that the activation of these structures represents a third mechanism, which would be implicated in the general reaction to stress. According to Routtenberg,[24] this mechanism, resulting from the activation of the arousal system II, involves some regions of the hypothalamus and part of the limbic system. This hypothesis is reinforced by other data that have shown that the activation of these latter structures produced hyperalgesic effects as well as facilitation of nociceptive reflexes and aggressive behavior.[23,31-35] Thus the cumulative effects of a repetitive stress would result in three concomitant and somewhat antagonistic mechanisms: predominant activation of reticular structures masking the effects of limbic and hypothalamic systems, all of them being modulated by the activation of endogenous opiatergic structures. In 1947 it was shown that adrenalectomized rates showed less analgesia to morphine than normal rats did.[36] Since then numerous multidisciplinary data clearly indicate that the pituitary-adrenal axis could be involved in the opioid part of the stress-induced analgesia.[6] It is tempting to suggest that in our study, such a system could be responsible for the morphine-like modulation of the changes observed during the cumulative effects of stress.

The third point discussed here concerns the effects of chronic administration of a weak dose of diazepam, using a cross-over and double-blind design. As described in the results section, diazepam alone was not analgesic, since, at the dosage used, the baseline values of both pain and nociceptive reflex threshold did not differ significantly from those obtained during the control (placebo) condition. These data are consistent with the results of others who have shown that low doses of diazepam had no effect on rat nociceptive thresholds.[10,37] Furthermore, as mentioned in the results, the diazepam treatment at a low dosage had no central or peripheral motor effect, since it did not affect the threshold of the M and H responses nor the $H_{maximum}/M_{maximum}$ ratio of the monosynaptic reflex. In contrast, we found that under diazepam, the baseline values of respiratory and heart rates were significantly reduced, showing that this drug exerted a toxic moderating action upon the vegetative activity. These latter data are clinically well-known and provide a satisfactory explanation for the anxiolytic action of diazepam administration. This effect was followed by an anti-stressing action, since all the responses obtained during the repetitive stress were clearly attenuated 50% when compared with the control (placebo) condition. During the diazepam treatment, the stress-induced analgesia and the associated depression of the nociceptive reflex were weaker than those obtained during the control condition. These data are in agreement with the predictive findings of other studies that have shown that diazepam and other related drugs were able to reduce both the corticosterone and catecholamine response to stress.[7-9] Furthermore, since we found a parallel modulation of pain sensation and of nociceptive reflexes by diazepam, one can assume that these diazepam effects can be explained by a decrease in the activation of some suprasegmental structures that are known to exert a descending inhibitory effect on the nociceptive transmission at the spinal level.[6] In contrast to these data, another group reported that diazepam potentiated the analgesia induced by cold-swim stress in rats.[10] This discrepancy in the results can be explained by the quite different procedure used by the latter authors working with rats while we worked with humans. Since diazepam is also known to be an hypothermisant drug, it is possible that this diazepam hypothermia may have potentiated or interacted with the hypothermia produced by exposing the animals to a cold-swim stress. This could possibly have resulted in a greater drop in the central body temperature, thus possibly potentiating the final analgesic response.

Finally, the last point worthy of discussion from this study concerns the possible relations between the effects of diazepam and the subsequent reduction of the naloxone action. As shown in the results, the slight hyperalgesia and the weak facilitation of the nociceptive reflex produced by naloxone administration during the diazepam treatment was not a direct consequence of the reduced stress response, i.e. a weaker analgesia and a smaller depression of the nociceptive reflex when compared with the control condition (placebo). In contrast, the weaker naloxone effect upon the other parameters (H reflex, heart and pulmonary rates) was found to be in direct relationship with the weaker response to stress during diazepam. These data clearly indicate that several different and complex mechanisms are involved in this neuropharmacological response. Some of them seem to be only related to the action of diazepam. Others, particularly those involved with the modulation of pain and of nociceptive reflexes, seem to be related to a possible interaction between diazepam and naloxone. In other words, diazepam would attenuate the reversal effect of naloxone. It is thus tempting to propose that some benzodiazepine brain type receptors exert a regulatory function upon the opiate receptors involved in pain control and in the depression of the nociceptive transmission at the spinal level. Unfortunately, there are no available data to our knowledge concerning these possible interactions. Further studies in this direction would be of great interest, particularly in a clinical setting, to better understand the interactions between pain and the neurovegetative (anxiolysis) therapies.

REFERENCES

1. BEECHER, H. K. 1957. The measurement of pain. Pharmacol. Rev. 9:59–209.
2. HILL, H. E., C. H. KORNETSKY, H. G. FLANARY & A. WIKLER. 1952. Studies on anxiety associated with anticipation of pain. I. Effects of morphine. Arch. Neurol. Psychiat. (Chic.). 67:612–619.
3. HALL, K. R. L. & E. STRIDE. 1954. The varying response to pain in psychiatric disorders. A study in abnormal psychology. Brit. J. Med. Psychol. 27:48–60.
4. WILLER, J. C. 1975. Influence de l'anticipation de la douleur sur les fréquences cardiaque et respiratoire et sur le réflexe nociceptif chez l'homme. Physiol. Behav. 15:411–415.
5. MADDEN, J., H. AKIL, R. L. PATRICK & J. D. BARACHAS. 1977. Stress-induced parallel changes in central opioid level and pain responsiveness in the rat. Nature (Lond.) 265:358–360.
6. TERMAN, G. W., Y. SHAVIT, J. W. LEWIS, J. T. CANNON & J. C. LIEBESKIND. 1984. Intrinsic mechanisms of pain inhibition: activation by stress. Science 226:1270–1277.
7. CORRODI, H., K. FUXE, P. LINDBRINK & L. OLSON. 1971. Minor tranquilizers, stress and central catecholamine neurons. Brain Res. 29:1–16.

8.   KEIM, K. L. & E. B. SIGG. 1977. Plasma corticosterone and brain catecholamines in stress: effect of psychotropic drugs. Pharmacol. Biochem. Behav. 6:79–85.

9.   TAYLOR, K. M. & R. LAVERTY. 1969. The effect of chlordiazepoxide, diazepam, and nitrazepam on catecholamine metabolism in regions of the rat brain. Eur. J. Pharmacol. 8:296–301.

10. LEITNER, D. S. & D. D. KELLY. 1984. Potentiation of cold swim stress analgesia in rats by diazepam. Pharmacol. Biochem. Behav. 21:813–816.

11. WILLER, J. C. 1977. Comparative study of perceived pain and nociceptive flexion reflex in man. Pain 3:69–80.

12. WILLER, J. C., F. BOUREAU & D. ALBE FESSARD. 1978. Role of large diameter cutaneous afferents in transmission of nociceptive messages: electrophysiological study in man. Brain Res. 152:358–364.

13. WILLER, J. C., A. ROBY & D. LE BARS. 1984. Psychophysical and electrophysiological approaches to the pain-relieving effects of heterotopic nociceptive stimuli. Brain 107:1095–1112.

14. HUGON, M. 1973. Methodology of the Hoffmann reflex in man. In New Developments in Electromyography and Clinical Neurophysiology. J. E. Desmedt, Ed. 3:277–293. Kager. Basel.

15. WILLER, J. C. & B. BUSSEL. 1980. Evidence for a direct spinal mechanism in morphine-induced inhibition of nociceptive reflexes in humans. Brain. Res. 187:212–215.

16. GAUTIER, H. 1972. Respiratory and heart rate responses to auditory stimulations. Physiol. Behav. 8:327–332.

17. PORGES, S. W. & D. C. RASKIN. 1969. Respiratory and heart rate components of attention. J. Exp. Psychol. 81:497–503.

18. WILLER, J. C. 1980. Anticipation of pain-produced stress: electrophysiological study in man. Physiol. Behav. 25:49–51.

19. WILLER, J. C., H. DEHEN & J. CAMBIER. 1981. Stress-induced analgesia in humans: endogenous opioids and naloxone-reversible depression of pain reflexes. Science 212:689–691.

20. SNEDECOR, G. W. & W. G. COCHRAN. 1957. Statistical Methods. 6th edit. The Iowa State University Press. Ames, Iowa.

21. WILLER, J. C., F. BOUREAU & D. ALBE FESSARD. 1979. Supraspinal influences on nociceptive flexion reflex and pain sensation in man. Brain Res. 179:61–68.

22. HUGELIN, A. & M. BONVALLET. 1957. Etude expérimentale des inter-relations reticulo-corticales. Proposition d'une théorie de l'asservissement réticulaire à un système diffus cortical. J. Physiol. (Paris) 49:1201–1223.

23. HUGELIN, A. 1972. Bodily changes during arousal, attention and emotion. In Limbic System. Mechanisms and Autonomic Function. C. H. Hockman, Ed.:P 202–218. C. C. Thomas. Springfield, IL.

24. ROUTTENBERG, A. 1968. The two-arousal hypothesis: reticular formation and limbic system. Psychol. Rev. 75:51–79.

25. ALDERMAN, E. L., W. H. BARRY, A. F. GRAHAM & D. C. HARRISSON. 1972. Hemodynamic effects of morphine and pentazocine differ in cardiac patients. New Engl. J. Med. 287:623–627.

26. FLOREZ, J., L. E. McCARTHY & H. L. BORISON. 1968. A comparative study in the cat of the respiratory effects of morphine injected intravenously and into the cerebrospinal fluids. J. Pharmacol. Exp. Ther. 163:448–455.

27. WIKLER, A. & K. FRANK. 1944. Hindlimb reflexes of chronic spinal dogs during cycles of addiction to morphine and methadone. J. Pharmacol. Exp. Ther. 80:176–187.

28. BOUREAU, F., J. C. WILLER & C. DAUTHIER. 1978. Study of naloxone in normal awake man: effects on spinal reflexes. Neuropharmacology 17:565–568.

29. WILLER, J. C., F. BOUREAU, C. DAUTHIER & M. BONORA. 1979. Study of naloxone in normal awake man: effects on heart rate and respiration. Neuropharmacology 18:469–472.

30. WILLER, J. C. & D. ALBE FESSARD. 1980. Electrophysiological evidence for a release of endogenous opiates in stress-induced "analgesia" in man. Brain Res. 198:419–426.

31. BONVALLET, M. & E. GARY-BOBO. 1973. La réaction de défense amygdalienne. Donnée historiques, histologiques et neurophysiologiques. Arch. ital. Biol. 3:642–656.
32. HUNSPERGER, R. W. & V. M. BUCHER. 1967. Affective behaviour produced by electrical stimulation in the forebrain and brainstem of the cat. In Structure and Function of the Limbic System. W. R. Adey & T. Tokizane, Eds. 27:103–127. Elsevier. Amsterdam.
33. KAADA, B. R. 1951. Somato-motor, autonomic and electrocorticographic responses to electrical stimulations of "rhinencephalic" and other structures in primates, cats and dogs. Acta Physiol. Scand. 24 (Suppl. 83):1–285.
34. KARLI, P. 1968. Système limbique et processus de motivation. J. Physiol. (Paris) 60:3–148.
35. KOIKEGAMI, H. 1964. Amygdala and other related limbic structures: experimental studies on the anatomy and function. II. Functional experiments. Acta Med. Biol. Niigata 12:73–266.
36. HARRIS, S. C. & F. J. FRIEND. 1947. Contribution of adrenals to morphine analgesia. Fed. Proc. 6:124.
37. KELLY, D. D., R. J. BODNAR, M. BRUTUS, C. F. WOODS & M. GLUSMAN. 1978. Differential effects upon liminal-escape pain thresholds of neuroleptic, antidepressant and anxiolytic agents. Fed. Proc. 37:470.

Multiple Endogenous Opiate and Non-Opiate Analgesia Systems: Evidence of Their Existence and Clinical Implications[a]

LINDA R. WATKINS

Department of Animal Physiology
Agriculture Experimental Station
University of California
Davis, California 95616

and

DAVID J. MAYER

Department of Physiology and Biophysics
Medical College of Virginia
Virginia Commonwealth University
Richmond, Virginia 23298

The observation that various environmental stimuli can profoundly modulate the response of animals to noxious stimuli[1] has stimulated widespread interest in this topic. This work is intimately related to the discovery of endogenous opiates;[2] and that discovery, in turn, stimulated further examination of analgesia systems. This chapter briefly reviews the development of these concepts, summarizes evidence that such systems can be activated by environmental stimuli, and reviews recent evidence for the existence of non-opiate analgesia systems.

A simple invariant relationship between stimulus intensity and the magnitude of pain perception is often not present. Earlier theories of pain perception recognized this fact, despite the lack of direct evidence to support it.[3,4] Interest in the detailed study of pain modulatory circuitry was spurred by the observation that electrical stimulation of specific brain areas could powerfully suppress the perception of pain.[5] Further investigation of stimulation-produced analgesia provided considerable detail about the neural circuitry involved.[6,7] Importantly, several similarities were recognized between these observations and information emerging from a concomitant resurgence of interest in the mechanisms of opiate analgesia.[6] The most important parallel facts revealed by these studies were (1) effective loci for both opiate analgesia[8,9] and stimulation-produced analgesia[6] lie within the periaqueductal and periventricular gray matter of the brain stem; (2) opiate analgesia[10,11] and stimulation-produced analgesia[12] are both mediated, at

[a]Supported in part by Public Health Service Grant DA 00576 to D. J. M.

273

least in part, by the activation of a centrifugal control system that exits from the brain via the dorsolateral funiculus of the spinal cord; and (3) the ultimate inhibition of the transmission of nociceptive information occurs in the spinal cord dorsal horn and homologous trigeminal nucleus caudalis by selective inhibition of neurons that respond to painful stimuli.[13]

In addition to these observations, studies of brain stimulation-produced analgesia provided direct evidence indicating that there are mechanisms within the central nervous system that depend upon endogenous opiates; that is (1) subanalgesic doses of morphine synergize with subanalgesic levels of brain stimulation to produce analgesia;[14] (2) tolerance, a phenomenon invariantly associated with repeated administration of opiates, is observed to the analgesic effects of brain stimulation;[15] (3) cross-tolerance between the analgesic effects of brain stimulation and opiates was demonstrated;[15] and (4) stimulation-produced analgesia could be at least partially antagonized by naloxone, a specific narcotic antagonist.[16,17] This last observation, in particular, could be most easily explained if electrical stimulation results in the release of an endogenous opiate-like factor.[18] Indeed, naloxone antagonism of stimulation-produced analgesia was a critical impetus leading to the eventual discovery of such a factor.[19]

Coincidental with this work, another discovery of critical importance for our current concepts of endogenous analgesia systems was made. Several laboratories, almost simultaneously, reported the existence of stereospecific binding sites for opiates in the central nervous system.[20-22] These receptor sites were subsequently shown to be localized to neuronal synaptic regions and to overlap anatomically with loci involved in the neural processing of pain.[23] The existence of an opiate receptor again suggested the likelihood of an endogenous compound with opiate properties to occupy it. Hughes and Kosterlitz reported the isolation from neural tissue of a factor (enkephalin) with such properties.[19] An immense amount of subsequent work has characterized this and other neural and extraneural compounds with opiate properties.[24,25] Importantly, as with the opiate receptor, the anatomical distribution of endogenous opiate ligands shows overlap with sites involved in pain processing.[26]

The demonstration of a well-defined neural system capable of potently blocking pain transmission suggests, but by no means proves, that the function of this system is to modulate the perceived intensity of noxious stimuli. If, in fact, this system has such a physiological role, then one might expect that the level of activity within the system would be influenced by impinging environmental stimuli. If environmental situations could be identified that produce analgesia, it would give credibility to the idea that invasive procedures, such as brain stimulation or narcotic drugs, inhibit pain by mimicking the natural activity within these pathways.

The first evidence for the environmental activation of an endogenous opiate analgesia system was provided by Mayer et al.[27,28] They showed that acupuncture analgesia in humans can be reversed by the narcotic antagonist naloxone. They suggested that such a result could be explained if acupuncture produced analgesia by the release of endogenous opiates.

A systematic search for environmental stimuli that activate pain inhibitory systems in animals was begun by Hayes et al.[1] They discovered that potent analgesia could be produced by such diverse stimuli as brief footshock, centrifugal rotation, and injection of intraperitoneal saline. These effects appeared to be specific to pain perception insofar as normal motor behavior, righting and corneal reflexes, vocalization, startle responses, and response to touch remain unimpaired. Two important additional concepts emerged from this work. First was the conclusion that exposure to stress was not sufficient to produce analgesia. Although all environmental stimuli that produce analgesia are stressors, the failure of classical stressors, such as ether vapors and horizontal oscillation, to produce pain inhibition indicated that stress was not the critical variable responsible. Second was the rather unexpected finding that the opiate antagonist, naloxone, did not block environmentally induced analgesias. Therefore, it appeared that non-opiate systems must exist, in addition to the opiate system described earlier.

Although the stimuli studied by Hayes *et al.* did not appear to activate an opiate system, subsequent investigations found clues that brain endorphins might be involved in at least some types of environmentally induced analgesias. Akil and co-workers[29] studied the analgesic effects of prolonged footshock. In contrast to the results of Hayes *et al.*[1] naloxone did partially antagonize the analgesia. This initial indication of opiate involvement led Akil and co-workers to look for biochemical evidence that footshock caused brain opiates to be released. They found that changes in brain opiate levels did indeed parallel the development of footshock-induced analgesia. When tolerance developed to the analgesic effects of footshock, brain opiate levels returned to control values. In agreement with these results, leu-enkephalin binding has been reported to decrease as analgesia increases.[30]

The controversy over the involvement of opiates in footshock-induced analgesia was resolved, in part, by Lewis *et al.*[31] They noted that the duration of footshock used by Hayes *et al.*[1] and Akil *et al.*[29] differed greatly and wondered whether this variable might explain the difference in their results. By comparing the effects of naloxone on analgesia produced by brief versus prolonged footshock, Lewis *et al.* showed that only the latter could be blocked by naloxone. This suggested that different analgesia systems become active as the duration of footshock increases.

Concurrent with this work of Lewis *et al.*, we made the observation that brief shock restricted to the front paws produced a naloxone-reversible analgesia as measured by the tail-flick assay.[32,33] We thought that this was rather puzzling since Hayes *et al.* and Lewis *et al.* found that brief shock produced non-opiate analgesia. This led us to test whether naloxone had different effects on analgesia produced by front paw versus hind paw shock. We found that naloxone does indeed have markedly different effects depending upon the body region shocked. An opiate system appears to be activated by front paw shock since low doses of naloxone antagonize this analgesia. In contrast, even high doses of naloxone failed to reduce hind paw shock–induced analgesia (FIGURE 1). Therefore, a non-opiate system seems to be involved in this response.

Definitive conclusions about opiate involvement in neural systems are tenuous when based exclusively on the effects of narcotic antagonists. Narcotic antagonists are known to have effects on non-opiate systems as well. Thus, additional lines of evidence are required to infer opiate involvement. To meet this criterion, we reasoned that if opiates are involved in front paw footshock–induced analgesia, then front paw footshock–induced analgesia should also be reduced in rats which have been made tolerant to opiates. When the rats were tested for front paw footshock–induced analgesia, analgesia was greatly reduced in morphine-tolerant rats.[34] Since front paw footshock–induced analgesia shows cross-tolerance with morphine and is antagonized by naloxone, the involvement of an endogenous opiate system in this type of analgesia stands on firm ground.

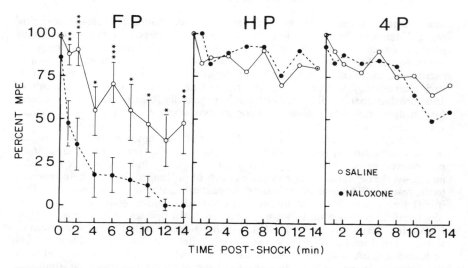

FIGURE 1. The effect of naloxone (two i.p. injections of 10 mg/kg) on analgesia induced by shock delivered to the front paws (FP), hind paws (HP), or to all four paws (4P). As measured by the tail-flick test, naloxone significantly antagonized front-paw FSIA (left) but had no effect on either hind-paw FSIA (center) or four-paw FSIA (right). (*$p < 0.05$; **$p < 0.01$; ***$p < 0.005$.) (From Watkins et al.[34] With permission from *Brain Research*.)

Using this same procedure, rats were tested to see whether cross-tolerance could be observed between morphine analgesia and hind paw footshock–induced analgesia. No cross-tolerance occurred.[34] The fact that hind paw footshock-induced analgesia is not affected by either high doses of naloxone or morphine tolerance demonstrates that this manipulation activates an independent non-opiate analgesia system and that factors other than exposure to stress determine whether non-opiate or opiate systems are activated.

We have studied front paw and hind paw footshock–induced analgesia in order to define how these opiate and non-opiate environmental analgesias are produced. In the following sections, the results of this work will be presented. The opiate analgesia produced by front paw shock will be discussed first. As will be seen, several similarities exist between the opiate analgesias produced by front paw shock and morphine.

The fact that endogenous opiates are involved in front paw footshock-induced analgesia (FSIA) does not prove that this effect is mediated by the same circuitry as morphine analgesia. A critical question was whether this could be accounted for by release of opiates from the pituitary or sympathetic-adrenal medullary axis since footshock has been shown to cause opiate release from these sites. Since hypophysectomy, adrenalectomy, and sympathetic blockade did not antagonize front paw footshock analgesia[35] our results also clearly show that this is not produced by opiates from the sympathetic nervous system. These data strongly suggest that front paw footshock analgesia, like morphine analgesia, is effected via opiate pathways within the central nervous system.

Based on these results, we began to search for the neural pathways involved in

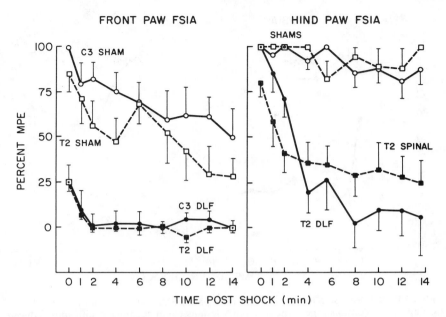

FIGURE 2. Effect of bilateral dorsolateral funiculus (DLF) lesions and spinal transection on front-paw FSIA and hind-paw FSIA. (Left) Bilateral DLF lesions at either the second thoracic (T2) or third cervical (C3) vertebral levels virtually abolish front-paw FSIA. Since DLF lesions at C3 leave intact all potential intraspinal connections between the level of stimulus input (front paws) and the lumbosacral cord (controlling the tail-flick response), direct intraspinal pathways cannot be involved in this analgesic response; pain inhibition must be mediated by supraspinal sites that inhibit pain via descending pathways within the DLF. (Right) Bilateral DLF lesions at T2 greatly attenuate but do not abolish hind-paw FSIA. Immediately after shock termination (0 min), profound analgesia is observed, which then slowly dissipates. No further significant reduction in analgesia is observed following T2 spinalization; spinalized rats remained analgesic through 12 min after hind-paw shock. These results imply that descending pathways involved in hind-paw FSIA exist only within the DLF and that intraspinal pathways account for the remaining potent analgesia. (From Watkins and Mayer.[33] With permission from *Science*.)

front paw footshock–induced analgesia. We found that front paw footshock analgesia is abolished by lesions of the dorsolateral funiculus of the spinal cord[36] (FIGURE 2). Furthermore, we have shown with brain lesion studies that, for front paw footshock analgesia as well as morphine analgesia, the descending pathway within the dorsolateral funiculus arises from a ventral medullary structure known as the nucleus raphe alatus (FIGURE 3).[37] In addition, we have shown that all of the critical circuitry for this analgesia effect exists below the level of the mesencephalon, since midcollicular decerebration has no effect on the analgesia.[38]

At this point, then, front paw footshock analgesia has been characterized as being a neural, opiate-mediated phenomenon. Analgesia is produced by activating brain sites that inhibit pain by way of descending pathways within the spinal cord dorsolateral funiculus. Yet none of this information pinpoints where the

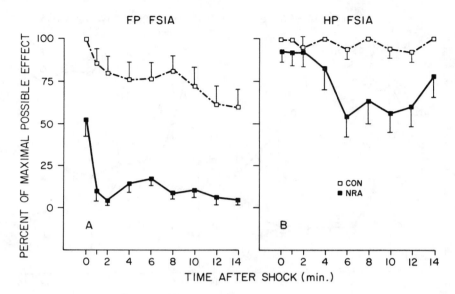

FIGURE 3. Effect of NRA lesions on front-paw FSIA (A) and hind-paw FSIA (B). Compared to controls (open squares), NRA lesions (solid squares) significantly reduced both front-paw FSIA and hind-paw FSIA. Since this lesions reduced front-paw FSIA (A) to a comparable degree as bilateral DLF lesions (FIGURE 2), it appears that the NRA is the origin of this descending pain-inhibitory pathway. In contrast, NRA lesions attenuated but did not abolish hind-paw FSIA (B). (From Watkins *et al.*[37] With permission from *Brain Research.*)

opiate synapse is located. Since we have found that spinal naloxone significantly antagonized front paw footshock analgesia, this demonstrates that an opiate synapse critical to the production of front paw footshock-induced analgesia exists within the spinal cord (FIGURE 4).[39]

One intriguing aspect of this naloxone effect is that naloxone can prevent but cannot reverse front-paw footshock–induced analgesia.[39] If this opiate antagonist is injected into the spinal cord immediately after a brief (90 sec) shock, analgesia is not reduced. Naloxone is effective only if it is delivered before the induction of analgesia (FIGURE 5). This implies that brief activation of this system produces a perseverative activity within the spinal cord that is no longer dependent upon continued opiate release. These results led us to speculate that these endogenous spinal opiates may act as neuromodulators of postsynaptic activity rather than as classical neurotransmitters.

A parallel series of experiments examined the non-opiate analgesia produced by hind paw shock. This work indicated that this effect is also neurally, rather than hormonally, mediated since analgesia was not reduced by removal of the pituitary or the adrenal glands.[35] Spinal lesion studies showed that this effect, like front paw footshock analgesia, is mediated via descending pathways within the spinal cord dorsolateral funiculus.[36] However since lesions of the ventral medulla only partially abolished hind paw footshock analgesia,[37] the neural substrate of

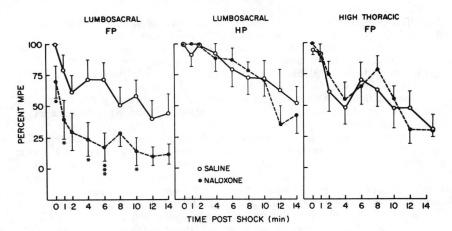

FIGURE 4. The effect of intrathecal injection of naloxone on front-paw and hind-paw FSIA. As measured by the tail-flick test, 1 μg of naloxone delivered to the lumbosacral cord significantly antagonized analgesia induced by front-paw shock (left). In contrast, this same dose of naloxine failed to attenuate hind-paw FSIA (center). The observed antagonism of front-paw FSIA by intrathecal injection of naloxone demonstrates that a critical opioid site exists within the spinal cord. This result cannot be explained by spread of the antagonist to supraspinal sites, since naloxone delivered to high thoracic cord (right) fails to attenuate front-paw FSIA. (From Watkins and Mayer.[33] With permission from *Science*.)

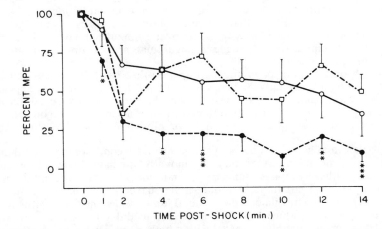

FIGURE 5. The differential effect of naloxone delivered before versus after induction of analgesia. In agreement with the results of experiment 1, 1 μg of naloxone delivered to the lumbosacral cord immediately prior to front-paw shock significantly attenuated the subsequent analgesia compared to saline controls. In contrast, this same dose delivered less than 1 min after front paw shock failed to attenuate the analgesia. The failure of post-shock naloxone to be effective at any time during the 14-min test is in no way accounted for by the temporal delay of naloxone injection, since, at maximum, there was only a 4-min difference in the time that these two groups received the drug. O, control; ●, naloxone pre-shock; □, naloxone post-shock. (*$p < 0.05$; **$p < 0.01$; ***$p < 0.005$.)

this effect is distinct from front paw footshock-induced analgesia at the level of the medulla. A further difference between the analgesias produced by front and hind paw shock is that hind paw footshock-induced analgesia is only reduced, not abolished, by either dorsolateral funiculus lesions or by transection of the spinal cord[36] indicating that an intraspinal as well as a descending pathway account for the potent analgesia induced by hind paw shock. As with front paw footshock analgesia, the supraspinal component of hind paw footshock-induced analgesia is mediated below the level of the mesencephalon, since it is unaffected by decerebration.[38]

An intriguing aspect of footshock-induced analgesia is that plasticity exists in the neural circuitry. Using a Pavlovian classical conditioning paradigm, Hayes *et al.*[1] found that rats readily associated environmental cues with the delivery of shock, such that they learned to activate their endogenous pain inhibitory systems when these cues were presented. In this study, the non-electrified shock chamber served as the conditioned stimulus, grid shock delivered to all four paws served as the unconditioned stimulus, and tail-flick inhibition served as the unconditioned response. Following pairings of shock with exposure to the grid, exposure to the non-electrified grid reliably induced analgesia in the total absence of shock.

Since we have now demonstrated that front paw footshock-induced analgesia is mediated via a well defined centrifugal opiate pathway, we used a classical conditioning paradigm to determine whether plasticity exists in opiate systems. The following section summarizes the evidence that animals can learn to activate their endogenous opiate systems to inhibit pain.[40]

Exposure to the nonelectrified grid became capable of producing potent analgesia after this stimulus was paired with front paw shock. That this effect is true classical conditioning is demonstrated by the observations that it shows extinction but cannot be produced by sensitization, backward conditioning, or pseudoconditioning. The fact that we have observed classically conditioned analgesia to be antagonized by systemic naloxone, spinal naloxone (FIGURE 6), and morphine tolerance strongly suggests that animals are learning to activate an endogenous opiate system.

Although opiate (front paw) and non-opiate (hind paw) footshock-induced analgesia can be differentially elicited, classically conditioned analgesia appears to always involve opiate pathways regardless of the body region shocked during conditioning trials. Classically conditioned analgesia can be antagonized by naloxone regardless of whether front paw or hind paw shock is used as the UCS.

The opiate analgesia produced by these classical conditioning paradigms appears to be neurally, rather than hormonally mediated, since it is not attenuated by either hypophysectomy or adrenalectomy.[35] Classical conditioning involves supraspinal circuitry since our studies have shown that conditioned analgesia is abolished by bilateral dorsolateral funiculus lesions.[40] Again, as with front paw footshock-induced analgesia, ventral medulla lesions abolish the effect.[37] However, as might be expected with a higher order behavior, decerebration abolishes the effect as well.[41] Finally, the role of the periaqueductal gray matter in the neural circuitry of endogenous analgesia systems is beginning to emerge since lesions of this structure reduce the conditioned effect but not the acute effects of footshock.[38]

In another series of experiments we have begun to examine the neurochemical bases of pain modulation. One approach was motivated both by the observation that cholecystokinin (CCK) has effects opposite those of opiates on a number of behaviors as well as by the finding that there is a striking overlap in the

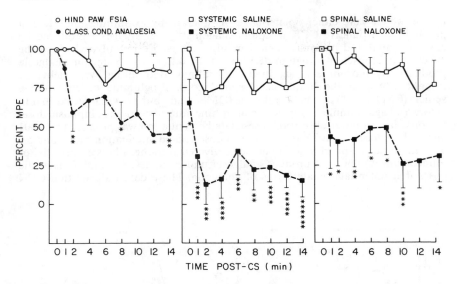

FIGURE 6. Naloxone reversibility of analgesia classically conditioned to hind paw shock. Hind paw shock (day 1) produced profound analgesia, as measured by the tail-flick test (left, open circles). This single exposure to shock was sufficient to classically condition analgesia, since placement of the rats on the nonelectrified grid on day 2 was sufficient to invoke significant analgesia (left, solid circles). Although hind paw FSIA has previously been demonstrated to be mediated by non-opiate systems, analgesia classically conditioned to hind paw shock does indeed appear to involve endogenous opioids. Compared to saline test days (center and right, open squares), both 10 mg/kg systemic (center, solid squares) and 1 µg lumbosacral (right, solid squares) naloxone significantly antagonized analgesia classically conditioned to hind paw shock. (*p 0.05; **$p < 0.01$; ***$p < 0.005$; ****$p < 0.0001$; *****$p < 0.0005$; ******$p < 0.0001$.) (From Watkins *et al.*[40] With permission from *Brain Research.*)

localization of CCK and opiates within the CNS.[42] We have made a number of intriguing observations about CCK and analgesia:[43] (1) cholecystokinin greatly reduces analgesia produced by systemic morphine, (2) it reduces environmentally produced opiate analgesias but not non-opiate analgesias, and (3) intrathecal cholecystokinin reduces front paw footshock analgesia, classically conditioned analgesia, and analgesia produced by intrathecal morphine. The effects produced by 3.6 ng intrathecal CCK are specific to CCK receptors since equimolar doses of unsulfated CCK (test for gastrin-like effects) do not antagonize the environmentally induced analgesias. Preliminary data suggest that gastrin-like neuropeptides may be involved as well, since 360 ng (100-fold increase in dose) unsulfated CCK does attenuate front-paw FSIA and classically conditioned analgesia. Thus, in every way we have examined so far, cholecystokinin is comparable to naloxone in its effects on analgesia systems.

These observations led us to hypothesize that endogenous CCK may function physiologically to oppose the analgesic effects of opiates. These data also suggest that tolerance resulting from repetitive opiate administration may be due to a compensatory increase in the activity of CCK systems. We tested these hypotheses in rats which were either opiate-naive or -tolerant by examining the effect of proglumide, a putative CCK receptor antagonist[44,45] on analgesia produced by environmental and pharmacological manipulations. We initially examined the effect of five doses of proglumide (0.001, 0.01, 0.1, 1, and 5 µg) on analgesia produced by morphine (1 µg in 0.5 µl saline). Both drugs were delivered intrathecally onto the lumbosacral spinal cord. Proglumide or equivolume vehicle (0.5 µl of 0.4% dimethyl sulfoxide (DMSO) and buffer) was injected 10 min before and again immediately before morphine administration. A biphasic dose-response function was observed; dose-related potentiation was produced by 0.001 and 0.01 µg doses, no effect by 0.1 µg, and dose-related attenuation by 1.0 and 5.0 µg.[46] Importantly, proglumide (whether delivered intrathecally, systemically, or intracerebrally) does not produce analgesia under our testing conditions at the doses that potentiate opiate forms of analgesia. These data indicate that CCK

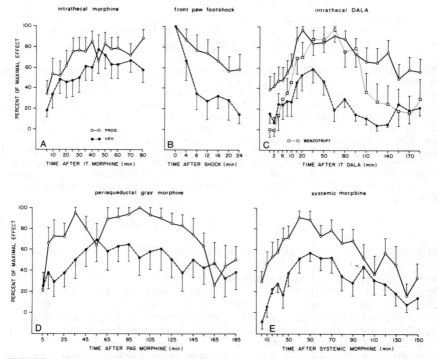

FIGURE 7. Potentiation (mean ± standard error) of opiate analgesia by proglumide (two injections of 0.01 µg, the optimum potentiating dose). (A) Enhancement of intrathecal morphine analgesia by intrathecal proglumide. (B) Enhancement of front paw footshock-induced analgesia by intrathecal proglumide. (C) Enhancement of intrathecal DALA analgesia by intrathecal proglumide. (D) Enhancement of PAG morphine analgesia by PAG proglumide. (E) Enhancement of systemic morphine analgesia by systemic proglumide. Data were evaluated by analyses of variance; for each comparison, $p < 0.0001$. (From Watkins et al.[48] With permission from *Brain Research*.)

systems are not tonically active but rather are activated in response to the activation of opiate systems.

Since these results suggest that endogenous CCK was able to oppose the antinociceptive actions of intrathecal morphine, we tested whether endogenous CCK might also attenuate analgesia induced by endogenous opiates. We examined the effect of 0.01 μg proglumide (the optimal potentiating dose for intrathecal morphine analgesia; the proglumide dose was delivered as two injections, 10 min apart) on analgesia produced by front paw footshock-induced release of endogenous opiates and on analgesia produced by intrathecal administration of the stable enkephalin analog D-ala-methionine enkephalinamide (DALA; 3 μg in 0.5 μl saline). In both cases, proglumide markedly potentiated these forms of opiate analgesia (FIGURE 7, B and C). Since another CCK receptor antagonist, benzotript,[47] was also observed to potentiate opiate analgesia induced by DALA,[48] potentiation of opiate analgesia does not appear to be a characteristic specific to proglumide but may reflect the effect of CCK receptor antagonists in general.

Extensions of these initial studies strongly suggest that proglumide potentiates analgesia by selectively interacting with opiate systems and that CCK-opiate interactions may be a widespread phenomenon in the CNS.

(1) Proglumide (0.01 μg) potentiates analgesia induced by morphine microinjected into the periaqueductal gray (3 μg morphine in 0.5 μl 0.4% DMSO-saline) (FIGURE 7, D). These data demonstrate that the ability of this CCK receptor blocker to interact with opiate systems is not unique to spinal circuitry. Combining these data with the striking degree of overlap of CCK and opiate systems within the CNS suggests that functional interactions between CCK and opiate systems may occur throughout the neuraxis.

(2) Naltrexone (10 mg/kg, i.p.) can both prevent and reverse potentiation by intrathecal proglumide (0.01 μg) of intrathecal DALA (3 μg) analgesia.[48] These data indicate that the enhancement of opiate analgesia produced by proglumide is due to selective enhancement of opiate pathways rather than actions through non-opiate systems.

(3) Proglumide differentially effects opiate and non-opiate forms of analgesia; Proglumide doses that potentiate opiate forms of analgesia tend to inhibit non-opiate forms of analgesia.[48] To date, we have examined three models of non-opiate analgesia: (1) norepinephrine (NE; 10 μg NE bitartrate in 5 μl saline) administered i.t. onto the lumbosacral cord (FIGURE 8, A), (2) brief hind paw shock delivered to spinally transected animals, and (3) brief hind paw shock delivered to neurally intact animals (FIGURE 8, B). These paradigms were chosen for study since the non-opiate analgesias induced by i.t. NE and hind paw shock are mediated by different neural mechanisms, as evidenced by the fact that hind paw FSIA is not attenuated by spinal depletion of NE.[49] The effects of hind paw shock were examined in both spinally transected and intact animals in order to compare the effects of proglumide on non-opiate analgesia mediated by intraspinal circuitry in the absence or presence, respectively, of concomitant activation of the centrifugal dorsolateral funiculus component of hind paw FSIA (FIGURE 2). Whereas 0.01 μl i.t. proglumide has been found to potentiate all forms of opiate analgesia examined, this same dose reliably attenuated each of the three models of nonopiate analgesia. The observation that proglumide can exert opposite effects on opiate and non-opiate analgesia is suggestive of the recent proposal that collateral inhibitory pathways modulate the activity of opiate versus non-opiate systems.[50]

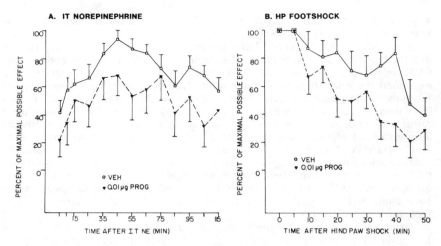

FIGURE 8. Effect of proglumide on two forms of non-opiate analgesia, (A) analgesia from i.t. application of norepinephrine and (B) analgesia from hind paw footshock. VEH = Vehicle and PROG = Proglumide.

Summarizing the data presented to this point, all evidence to date indicates that proglumide selectively hastens the onset, increases the peak level, and prolongs the duration of opiate analgesia. These observations raise the possibility that administration of CCK antagonists could decrease the dose of narcotics necessary to relieve pain and could enhance the effects of procedures such as acupuncture, which are mediated by environmentally induced release of endogenous opiates.[28] Because our control studies showed that proglumide does not affect basal pain sensitivity when delivered in the absence of opiates,[46] it appears that CCK systems are not tonically active but rather become active in response to the administration or release of opiates. CCK would thus appear to exert a negative feedback effect on opiate systems with the end result being a return of the organism toward basal pain responsivity. By such a mechanism, the balance of activity in CCK and opiate systems may determine the level of pain sensitivity experienced by the organism. Given the extensive neuroanatomical overlap of opiate and CCK systems, CCK/opiate interactions may be predicted to occur throughout the neuraxis leading to CCK modulation of diverse opiate actions.

If CCK antagonists are to be of clinical value for the management of pain, they should be effective after systemic administration. We therefore examined the effect of systemic proglumide (0.002 and 0.2 mg/kg, i.p.) delivered 10 min and again just before a 3 mg/kg i.p. injection of morphine. At a dose of 0.02 mg/kg, proglumide significantly potentiated morphine analgesia (FIGURE 7, E); 0.002 mg/kg produced a brief period of potentiation, and 0.2 mg/kg had no effect. Taken together with the recent observation that, in human volunteers, i.v. proglumide (50 µg) significantly potentiated the analgesic effects of i.v. morphine (4.2 mg/70 kg) without producing analgesia in the absence of opiates,[51] these data from rat and human studies strongly suggest that blockade of CCK systems could be a powerful tool for the management of clinical pain.

Another area of clinical importance that appears to be influenced by CCK systems is the development of opiate tolerance. Since the phenomenon of opiate tolerance is observed at the behavioral level as a decrease in the efficacy of opiates to produce analgesia and endogenous CCK is able to effect such a decrease, CCK may play an important role in tolerance. Long-term opiate administration may induce a compensatory increase in CCK synthesis or release, which in turn could result in a progressive antagonism of opiate analgesia. Based on this rationale, we examined whether systemic proglumide could attenuate tolerance to the analgesic effects of morphine. Low and high tolerance levels were produced by administering twice daily increasing doses of morphine (i.p.) over either 6 or 10 days, respectively. Upon completion of these regimens, rats were injected intraperitoneally either with one of a wide range of proglumide doses or with equivolume vehicle at 10 min and again immediately before an i.p. injection of morphine (4 mg/kg, a dose that produces potent analgesia in naive animals). This series of experiments (as well as a parallel series of experiments that examined the effect of i.t. proglumide on i.t. morphine tolerance) revealed that proglumide does indeed appear to be able to reverse morphine tolerance (FIGURE 9). Intriguingly, as the animals became more tolerant to the analgesic effects of morphine (either systemic or intrathecal), the dose of proglumide required to "re-instate" morphine analgesia also increased. These observations suggest that tolerance may develop, at least in part, from a progressive compensatory increase in the activity of CCK systems in response to prolonged opiate administration. If so, these results suggest that blockade of the CCK systems involved in pain modulation by drugs such as proglumide could potentially reverse or prevent development of narcotic tolerance in patients with chronic pain.

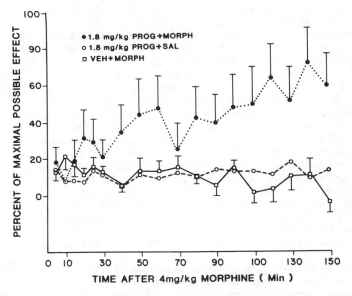

FIGURE 9. Effect of proglumide on morphine (4 mg/kg) analgesia in morphine-tolerant rats. Proglumide plus morphine results in significant analgesia while the same dose of morphine with saline produces no analgesia.

In another series of neurochemical studies we have begun to study the role of monoamines in various analgesias. A significant problem with studies examining the role of monoamines in the production of pain inhibition has been that many experiments have indiscriminately manipulated both spinal and supraspinal monoamines. Since these "transmitters" are present at more than one level of the neuraxis and, thus, may be having effects at more than one site, a more reasonable strategy, although not foolproof, seems to be to limit the anatomical locus of monoaminergic manipulations. In this series of studies, we have examined the effects of selective spinal cord monoaminergic manipulations on stimulation-produced analgesia, opiate analgesia, and environmental analgesias.

In one series of experiments,[52] the effects of spinal cord serotonin depletion or combined serotonin/norepinephrine depletion on analgesia elicited by electrical stimulation of, or morphine microinjection into, the periaqueductal gray were tested. Spinal cord serotonin was depleted by intrathecal injection of 5,7-dihydroxytryptamine (5,7-DHT) preceded by systemic desipramine, while 5,7-DHT alone was used to deplete both norepinephrine (NE) and serotonin. Selective serotonin depletion had no effect on analgesia induced by either method. Depletion of both monoamines had no effect on stimulation-produced analgesia. In contrast, depletion of both monoamines drastically attenuated morphine analgesia. Thus, although total CNS depletion of serotonin can reduce both stimulation-produced analgesia and morphine analgesia, medullospinal serotonin systems do not appear to be involved.

Although this lack of involvement of medullospinal serotonin systems may at first glance appear perplexing, a series of anatomical studies we have done makes this result more coherent. A critical fact concerning the organization of supraspinal neural systems that control pain is that the output pathway from the brain appears to descend to the spinal cord by way of the dorsolateral funiculus (DLF). DLF lesions greatly reduce or abolish analgesia produced by brain stimulation,[13] systemic morphine,[11] and morphine microinjection.[53] Thus, we felt it was of particular importance to describe carefully the origins of this pathway before undertaking behavioral and neurophysiological studies of brain centers involved in analgesia. Several studies utilizing a new horseradish peroxidase (HRP) gel technique developed in our laboratory[54] have examined the problem. We have shown that the population of neurons in the medullary raphe region contributing to the DLF consists of cells in the nucleus raphe magnus (NRM) and reticularis magnocellularis (Rmc), and roughly corresponds to the serotonergic cell group B3. We have named this region the nucleus raphe alatus (NRA), and this work has redefined the anatomical organization of the medullary raphe nuclei that contribute to the DLF.[55] The medullary nucleus raphe alatus (n. raphe magnus and n. reticularis paragigantocellularis), which gives rise to fibers that descend in the DLF, is a sensitive site for the production of analgesia by electrical[56] and pharmacological methods.[57] Indirect evidence suggests that descending serotonergic fibers from area B3 may play a role in descending inhibition. The cells of B3 show a similar distribution to those of NRA; however, there is no direct evidence that serotonergic fibers from B3 descend in the DLF.

In order to examine this question, we performed a study[58] in which the cell bodies of NRA were retrogradely labeled with HRP by implanting a small piece of HRP gel unilaterally into cervical DLF. Two days later, the method of Bowker et al.[59] was used to visualize simultaneously both retrogradely labeled cells and cells exhibiting serotonin-like immunoreactivity (SLI). Extremely few double-labeled cells were seen.[58] Retrogradely labeled cells of NRA exhibited a different distribution from SLI cells. The SLI cells of B3 lie ventral to NRA. Some intermingling of retrogradely labeled cells and SLI cells was seen, especially near the midline. At the level of the facial nucleus, 25 retrogradely labeled cells and 55 SLI cells were seen in a typical hemisection, while no more than two double-labeled cells could be identified. These results suggest that serotonin is not a major component of the DLF projection that originates in the NRA. This is consistent with evidence indicating that a descending serotonergic projection is unnecessary to elicit some types of analgesia.

A study examining the effects of these same monoamine manipulations on footshock-induced analgesia has been conducted.[60] Interestingly, while hind paw analgesia and classically conditioned analgesia were not attenuated by either of these neurochemical manipulations, front paw FSIA was significantly reduced by both serotonin depletion and combined serotonin/NE depletion (FIGURE 10). To assess the relative importance of spinal serotonin and NE in front paw FSIA, NE and serotonin antagonists were injected intraperitoneally prior to shock exposure. Attenuation of front paw FSIA by equimolar doses of the monoamine blockers was much greater following injection of the serotonin blocker than after the NE blocker (FIGURE 11).[60] These data indicate that spinal cord serotonin and, apparently to a lesser extent, spinal cord NE mediate front paw (opiate) FSIA whereas neither serotonin nor NE appears to mediate hind-paw (non-opiate) or

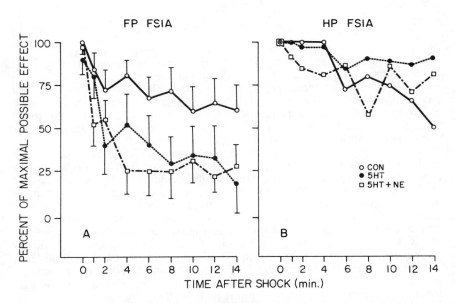

FIGURE 10. Effect of spinal cord serotonin depletion (5-HT) or combined serotonin and norepinephrine depletion (5-HT and NE) on front paw FSIA. Compared to controls (open circles), both 5-HT (solid circles) and 5-HT and NE (open squares) depletion reliably reduced analgesia induced by brief front paw shock.

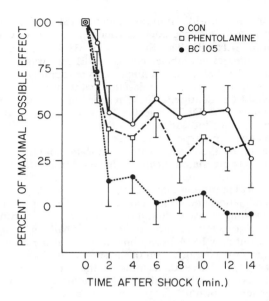

FIGURE 11. Intrathecal BC 105 (5-HT antagonist) and intrathecal phentolamine (NE antagonist) reduce front-paw FSIA. NE and 5-HT appear to be involved in the production of this analgesia at the level of the spinal cord.

classically conditioned analgesia. This study has complex but important implications. Since (1) the dorsolateral funiculus is necessary for front paw footshock-induced analgesia, (2) the nucleus raphe alatus is necessary for front paw footshock-induced analgesia, and (3) serotonergic output from nucleus raphe alatus does not descend via the dorsolateral funiculus, these results indicate that a synergism of serotonergic and non-serotonergic descending pathways may sometimes be necessary to produce analgesia.

We have also examined the potential involvement of nicotinic and muscarinic cholinergic systems in front paw FSIA, hind paw FSIA, and classically conditioned analgesia.[61] These experiments demonstrated that muscarinic cholinergic sites within the central nervous system are critically involved in the mediation of both hind paw (non-opiate) FSIA (FIGURE 12) and classically conditioned (opiate) analgesia (FIGURE 13) since scopolamine, but not mecamylamine, significantly attenuated analgesia. Equimolar methylscopolamine was also without effect indicating a CNS site of action. Furthermore, the primary muscarinic site(s) appears to exist at a supraspinal, rather than a spinal level, since intrathecal scopolamine was ineffective (FIGURE 14). Nicotinic systems do not appear to be importantly involved in any of these forms of environmentally induced analgesias since mecamylamine had no effect. These data and a review of the literature suggest that the critical cholinergic sites involved in hind paw FSIA exist within the caudal brainstem (probably in the vicinity of the parabrachial nucleus[62]) whereas cholinergic sites at more rostral brain levels probably mediate classically conditioned analgesia. These results again confirm

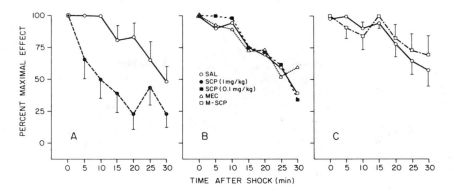

FIGURE 12. Effect of systemic scopolamine, mecamylamine, and methylscopolamine on hind paw (non-opiate) FSIA. (A) Comparison of the effect of 1 mg/kg scopolamine (filled circles) and equivolume saline (open circles) demonstrates that systemic administration of this muscarinic cholinergic antagonist markedly attenuates hind paw FSIA. (B) This antagonism appears to be dose-related since 0.1 mg/kg scopolamine (filled squares) does not antagonize hind paw FSIA compared to saline controls (open circles). Additionally, cholinergic mediation appears to be selective for muscarinic systems, since the nicotinic antagonist mecamylamine (1 mg/kg, open triangles) does not attenuate this form of non-opiate analgesia compared to saline controls (open circles). (C) Central muscarinic cholinergic sites are implicated in the effects produced by systemic scopolamine since the peripherally acting muscarinic antagonist methylscopolamine (open squares) does not attenuate hind paw FSIA compared to saline controls (open circles).

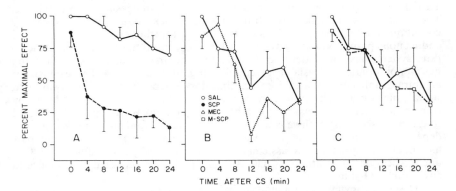

FIGURE 13. Effects of scopolamine, mecamylamine, and methylscopolamine on classically conditioned (opiate) analgesia. Muscarinic cholinergic systems within the central nervous system appear to be involved in classically conditioned analgesia since 1 mg/kg systemic scopolamine (filled circles, A) markedly attenuated, whereas 1.04 mg/kg of the peripherally acting methylscopolamine (open squares, C) does not attenuate, this form of opiate analgesia compared to saline controls (open circles). This effect appears to be relatively specific to muscarinic systems, since the nicotinic antagonist mecamylamine (1 mg/kg) has but a marginal effect on classically conditioned analgesia (open triangles, B).

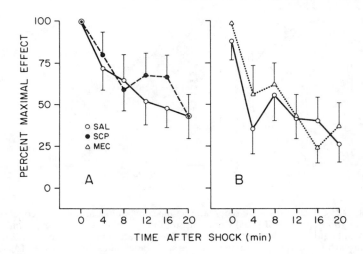

FIGURE 14. Effect of scopolamine and mecamylamine on front paw FSIA. Cholinergic systems do not appear to be involved in the opiate analgesia induced by front paw shock since neither 1 mg/kg scopolamine (A, filled circles) nor 1 mg/kg mecamylamine (B, open triangles) attenuated front paw FSIA compared to saline controls (open circles).

the existence of multiple systems for the modulation of nociceptive information on neurochemical grounds.

Before we proceed to clinical correlates of pain inhibitory systems, let us make a final summary of what environmentally induced analgesias have taught us. These studies of front paw and hind paw footshock analgesia and classically conditioned analgesia provide strong support for the existence of multiple endogenous pain modulatory systems within the central nervous system. At least three systems have been identified (FIGURE 15). The first two pathways mediate the neural non-opiate analgesia observed following hind paw shock. These consist of an intraspinal pathway and a descending dorsolateral funiculus pathway with supraspinal origin. The third is a neural opiate analgesia that is produced by front paw shock or by classical conditioning. This opiate analgesia is effected solely via descending pathways within the dorsolateral funiculus and is critically dependent upon an opiate synapse within the spinal cord. Thus, front paw footshock analgesia and classically conditioned analgesia provide the first unequivocal demonstrations of neural opiate pathways activated in response to environmental stimuli.

However, a review of the literature indicates that even these three systems do not account for all of the pain inhibitory responses that have been reported. Depending upon the analgesia-producing manipulation chosen, all combinations of opiate, non-opiate, neural, and endocrine-mediated pain inhibitory systems may be activated (TABLE 1). Although the details of this classification scheme can not be discussed here, it is important to point out that the scheme provides a framework for organizing analgesia systems.

At this point, we would like to make some parallels between our work and

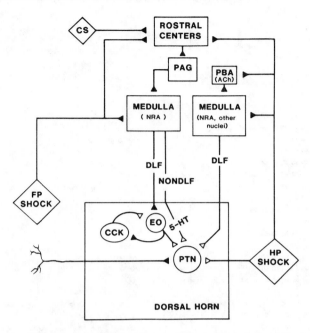

FIGURE 15. Neural circuitry of opiate and non-opiate analgesia induced by front paw and hind paw shock. Front paw shock activates the nucleus raphe alatus (NRA) within the ventral medulla. This nucleus sends a descending projection through the DLF to the dorsal horn of the spinal cord. A serotonergic pathway lying outside of the DLF (non-DLF) is recruited as well. In turn, endogenous opiates are released, inhibiting pain transmission neurons (PTN). Activation of endogenous opiates stimulates a negative feedback loop that utilizes CCK to reduce activity of endogenous opiate systems. Hind paw shock inhibits PTN via two non-opiate pathways: an intraspinal pathway and a descending DLF pathway. The latter originates from the nucleus raphe alatus and from some other yet unidentified medullary area(s). Classically conditioned (opiate) analgesia seems to result from activation of the same DLF output pathway as front paw (opiate) FSIA. After conditioning trials in which the conditioned stimulus is paired with either front paw or hind paw shock (the unconditioned stimulus), the conditioned stimulus becomes capable of activating rostral centers in the brain, which, in turn, activate the periaqueductal gray (PAG) and subsequently the nucleus raphe alatus. This results, via a descending DLF pathway, in the release of endogenous opiates within the dorsal horn, producing analgesia.

experimental and clinical studies in humans. This will be done in order to highlight the potential relevance of this work to the very difficult problem of treating pain syndromes in man. Throughout this discussion, it will be important to bear in mind that a number of distinct modulatory systems have been identified under controlled laboratory conditions. In the more naturalistic circumstances of clinical research, it is likely that more than one of these systems may be active at any given time, which may account for the variability and controversy in the clinical literature.

TABLE 1. Summary of Currently Available Data on Endogenous Analgesia Systems

	OPIATE	HORMONE	CIRCUITRY	NEUROCHEMISTRY

NEURAL/OPIATE
  BRIEF FPFS
  CCA
  SYSTEMIC MORPH
  IC MORPH (PAG)
  IT MORPH
  ECS
  CONDITIONED FEAR
  DEFEAT
NEURAL/NON-OPIATE
  BRIEF HPFS
  <OR=3 MIN 4-PFS
  2DG
HORM/OPIATE
  ACUPUNC (LO FREQ)
  30 MIN 4-PFS
  IMMOBILIZATION
  15 MIN COLD (4 C)
  EXERCISE
  PREGNANCY
  COND HELPLESS
  CCA
  FOOD DEP
  PROLONG TAILSHOCK
HORM/NON-OPIATE
  COLD WATER SWIMS
  BRIEF TAIL SHOCK
UNKNOWN/OPIATE
  SPA (PAG)
  SPA (VMM)

KINDLED SEIZURE	✓			
TNS-LO/FREQ-HI/IN	✓	✓		
VAGINAL PROBING	✓			
DNIC & PAIN (xFS)	✓			
CENTRIF ROTATION	✓			
PLACEBO	✓			
ANXIETY (HUMAN)	✓			
SEX (MALE)		>		
SPON HYPERTENSION	✓			
INT COLD WATER	✓			
20 C SWIM (MICE)	✓			
COLD WATER	✓			
WARM WATER (MICE)	✓	^		
HEAT (40 C)	✓			
RADIATION	✓			
NOVELTY (RAT)	✓			
UNKNOWN/NON-OPIATE				
SPA (PAG)	o	x	o	x
SPA (PB)	o	x	x	x
TNS (HI/F-LO/I)	o	x	x	x
ACUPUNC (HI FREQ)	o	x	x	x
HYPNOSIS	o	x	x	x
VAGINAL PROBING	o	x	x	x
CENTRIF ROTATION	o	x	x	x
30 C SWIM	o	x	x	x
FIREWALKING	o	x	x	x
VIBRATION	o	x	x	x
NOVELTY (CAT)	o	x	x	x
FEEDING (CAT)	o	x	x	x
IMMOBILIZATION	o	x	x	x
HORMONAL/UNKNOWN				
INSULIN				

A review of the literature reveals that four classes of analgesic manipulations can be identified: neural/opiate, hormonal/opiate, neural/non-opiate, and hormonal/non-opiate. The criteria used to classify analgesia as opiate include naloxone reversibility and cross-tolerance with morphine. Hormonal analgesia is characterized as being attenuated either by adrenalectomy, adrenal demedullation, or hypophysectomy. These latter criteria were chosen since all environmental stimuli that produce analgesia activate the pituitary-adrenal cortical and sympathetic-adrenal medullary axes. Regarding the neural substrates of these various analgesic responses, the most comprehensive data are available on the effect of dorsolateral funiculus (DLF) lesions, nucleus raphe alatus (NRA) lesions, and periaqueductal gray (PAG) lesions. As can be seen, DLF lesions attenuate all analgesic manipulations that have been tested, suggesting that the DLF may form a final common pathway for endogenous pain inhibitory systems. > = potentiation, < = attenuation, o = no effect, ? = conflicting data exist indicating either no effect or attenuation, blank = no data are available, x = inappropriate category.

There are at least two situations available for study of possible endogenous pain modulatory systems active in man. The first involves the basal, tonic activity within these systems and allows the experimenter to assess whether pain inhibition occurs continuously, at least to some degree. The second involves clinical manipulations that attempt to activate pain inhibitory systems.

Attempts have been made to determine whether pain modulatory systems are tonically active. The assumption made by these studies has been that administration of opiate antagonists should alter the perception of pain if opiate systems are tonically active. This change in pain perception would be recorded either as a decreased pain threshold or an increased level of ongoing pain. In general, however, naloxone has failed to affect pain thresholds of normal human volunteers. In contrast to these negative results, Buchsbaum et al.[63] found that naloxone lowered the thresholds of subjects with naturally high pain thresholds, yet had no effect in subjects with low pain thresholds.

Naloxone appears to be more consistently effective when delivered to experimental subjects who are experiencing some level of clinical pain.[64,65] Therefore, circumstances have been observed in which spontaneous activity of an endogenous opiate analgesia system occurs. Importantly, ongoing pain is one factor that appears to activate this system. In this regard, these results are consistent with the animal studies described above in which pain was observed to be a powerful activator of endogenous analgesia systems.

A number of manipulations are known to have some degree of clinical efficacy for the reduction of pain. Most of these procedures were developed before the recent explosion of information about endogenous pain control systems. Indeed, many of them evolved from theoretical approaches that are now outdated or incorrect. Nevertheless, the procedures are efficacious. It may be informative to re-examine them in the light of current knowledge.

The belief that an acute painful stimulus can be used to alleviate ongoing pain has been held since antiquity and is known as counter-irritation.[66] This procedure has a great deal in common with acupuncture and TNS. All use the application of somatic stimuli, either noxious or innocuous, to obtain relief from pain. Importantly, pain relief persists beyond the period of treatment in all cases. The site of treatment in relation to the painful area is highly variable, ranging from the painful dermatome, itself, to a theoretically unpredictable constellation of points in classical Chinese acupuncture. Lastly, the duration of treatment varies from less than a minute to hours. All of these factors, as we have seen, are important determinants of the effects produced by footshock in animals. Thus, the highly variable effects observed in the clinic would be predicted from animal research. Nevertheless, human data suggest the involvement of the same systems described above.

The involvement of an opiate system in these types of analgesia was first suggested by Mayer et al.[28] who showed that the increased pain thresholds produced by traditional acupuncture in man could be completely reversed by naloxone. Other investigators found that naloxone only partially reduced electroacupuncture analgesia. The differences in the magnitude of the effects seen in these studies are particularly enlightening considering the animal studies described above. Mayer et al. used the ho-ku points in the hands to induce analgesia in the teeth, an acupuncture point far removed from the painful region. In contrast, Chapman and Benedetti[67] stimulated the face to produce analgesia in the teeth and saw only a very small effect of naloxone. Thus, it seems likely that, as in animal experiments, stimulation of regions adjacent to the painful area

activate non-opiate analgesia systems, whereas stimulation of distant derma-
tomes activates opiate systems.

Other parameters of stimulation also appear to be critical in determining
whether opiate or non-opiate systems are involved. Sjolund and Eriksson[68] have
recently shown that high frequency/low intensity and low frequency/high
intensity nerve stimulation can both alleviate clinical pain. However, only the
analgesia produced by low frequency/high intensity stimulation could be
reversed by naloxone. From this work, it appears that noxious stimulation is
required for the activation of opiate inhibitory systems. In fact, that acupuncture
and transcutaneous nerve stimulation should be painful to produce maximal
effects has been pointed out by several workers.[66] This observation may explain
the failure of Chapman et al.[69] to replicate the results of Mayer et al.[28] since
Chapman et al. made an effort to minimize the discomfort produced by
acupuncture stimulation.

In conclusion, acupuncture and transcutaneous nerve stimulation appear to
be forms of counter-irritation that activate both opiate and non-opiate systems.
The variable clinical outcomes observed following these treatments probably
result from differential recruitment of segmental, extrasegmental, opiate, and
non-opiate pain inhibitory systems, all of which are now known to be activated by
these types of stimulation in animals.

Naloxone has also been used to examine whether endogenous opiates are
involved in placebo analgesia. Levine and co-workers[70] reported that naloxone
antagonized placebo effects. Although this conclusion has been questioned on
technical grounds,[71] no conflicting data have been published, and the possibility
that opiates are involved in some aspects of placebo analgesia appears particularly reasonable considering the fact that footshock analgesia can be classically
conditioned in rats. Placebo analgesia can easily be conceived of as a classical
conditioning paradigm wherein the placebo manipulation (i.e., injections and
pills) serves as the conditioned stimulus and prior medication or treatment serves
as the unconditioned stimulus.

Although explanations of this sort are clearly speculative, they are indicative
of the wealth of concepts from experimental pain research now available for
clinical evaluation. Our increasing knowledge of pain modulatory systems has
the potential not only of providing explanations of current therapies but of
suggesting new approaches for the control of pain. The preponderance of current
pain therapies involve either the surgical destruction of neural tissue or the use of
addictive drugs. Such procedures offer great difficulties for the prolonged
treatment of chronic pain. If multiple pain inhibitory systems could be activated
pharmacologically or otherwise in an alternating sequence, the problems of tissue
destruction and addiction could be circumvented.

ACKNOWLEDGMENT

We would like to thank Endo Labs for providing us with naloxone and A. H.
Robins for providing proglumide and funding for studies with proglumide.

REFERENCES

1. HAYES, R. L., G. J. BENNETT, P. NEWLON & D. J. MAYER. 1976. Analgesic effects of
certain noxious and stressful manipulations in the rat. Soc. Neurosci. Abs. 2:939.

2. HUGHES, J., T. W. SMITH, H. W. KOSTERLITZ, L. A. FOTHERGILL, B. A. MORGAN & H. R. MORRIS. 1975. Identification of two related pentapeptides from the brain with potent opiate agonist activity. Nature **258**:577–579.
3. MELZACK, R. & P. D. WALL. 1965. Pain mechanisms: A new theory. Science **150**:971–979.
4. NOORDENBOS, W. 1959. Pain. Elsevier-North Holland. Amsterdam.
5. MAYER, D. J., T. L. WOLFLE, H. AKIL, B. CARDER & J. C. LIEBESKIND. 1971. Analgesia from electrical stimulation in the brainstem of the rat. Science **174**:1351–1354.
6. MAYER, D. J. & J. C. LIEBESKIND. 1974. Pain reduction by focal electrical stimulation of the brain: An anatomical and behavioral analysis. Brain Res. **68**:73–93.
7. MAYER, D. J. & D. D. PRICE. 1976. Central nervous system mechanisms of analgesia. Pain **2**:379–404.
8. JACQUET, Y. F. & A. LAJTHA. 1973. Morphine action at central nervous system sites in rat: Analgesia or hyperalgesia depending on site and dose. Science **182**:490–491.
9. VIGOURET, J., H. J. TESCHEMACHER, K. ALBUS & A. HERZ. 1973. Differentiation between spinal and supraspinal sites of action of morphine when inhibiting the hindleg flexor reflex in rabbits. Neuropharmacology **12**:111–121.
10. HAYES, R. L., D. D. PRICE, G. J. BENNETT, G. L. WILCOX & D. J. MAYER. 1978. Differential effects of spinal cord lesions on narcotic and non-narcotic suppression of nociceptive reflexes: further evidence for the physiologic multiplicity of pain modulation. Brain Res. **155**:91–101.
11. WATKINS, L. R., D. A. OBELLI, P. FARIS, M. D. ACETO & D. J. MAYER. 1982. Opiate vs. non-opiate footshock-induced analgesia: The body region shocked is a critical factor. Brain Res. **242**:299–308.
12. BASBAUM, A. I., N. MARLEY & J. O'KEEFE. 1975. Effects of spinal cord lesions on the analgesic properties of electrical brain stimulation. In Advances in Pain Research and Therapy: Proceedings of the First World Congress on Pain. J. J. Bonica & D. G. Albe-Fessard, Eds. **1**:268. Raven Press. New York.
13. BENNETT, G. J. & D. J. MAYER. 1979. Inhibition of spinal cord interneurons by narcotic microinjection and focal electrical stimulation in the periaqueductal central gray matter. Brain Res. **172**:243–257.
14. SAMANIN, R. & L. VALZELLI. 1971. Increase of morphine-induced analgesia by stimulation of the nucleus raphe dorsalis. Eur. J. Pharmacol. **16**:298–302.
15. MAYER, D. J. & R. HAYES. 1975. Stimulation-produced analgesia: development of tolerance and cross tolerance to morphine. Science **188**:941–943.
16. AKIL, H., D. MAYER & J. LIEBESKIND. 1972. Comparaison chez le rat entre l'analgesie induite par stimulation de la substance grise periaqueducale et l'analgesia morphinique. C. R. Acad. Sci. **274**:3603–3605.
17. AKIL, H., D. J. MAYER & J. C. LIEBESKIND. 1976. Antagonism of stimulation-produced analgesia by the narcotic antagonist, naloxone. Science **191**:961–962.
18. MAYER, D. J. 1975. Pain inhibition by electrical brain stimulation: comparison to morphine. Neurosci. Res. Prog. Bull. **13**:94–99.
19. HUGHES, J. 1975. Search for the endogenous ligand of the opiate receptor. Neurosci. Res. Program Bull **13**:55–58.
20. HILLER, J. M., J. PEARSON & E. J. SIMON. 1973. Distribution of stereospecific binding of the potent narcotic analgesic etorphine in the human brain: predominance in the limbic system. Res. Commun. Chem. Pathol. Pharm. **6**:1052–1062.
21. PERT, C. B. & S. H. SNYDER. 1973. Opiate receptor: Demonstration in nervous tissue. Science **179**:1011–1013.
22. TERENIUS, L. 1973. Stereospecific interaction between narcotic analgesics and a synaptic plasma membrane fraction of rat cerebral cortex. Acta Pharmacol. Toxicol. **32**:317–320.
23. PERT, C. B., A. M. SNOWMAN & S. H. SNYDER. 1974. Localization of opiate receptor binding in synaptic membranes of rat brain. Brain Res. **70**:184–188.
24. AKIL, H., S. J. WATSON, E. YOUNG, M. E. LEWIS, H. KHACHATURIAN & J. M. WALKER. 1984. Endogenous opioids: Biology and function. Annu. Rev. Neurosci. **7**:223–256.
25. TAKATSUKI, K., Y. KAWAI, M. SAKANAKA, S. SHIOSAKA, E. SENBA & M. TOHYAMA. 1983.

Experimental and immunohistochemical studies concerning the major origins of the Substance-P-containing fibers in the lateral lemniscus and lateral parabrachial area of the rat, including the fiber pathways. Neurosci. **10**:57-72.

26. HUGHES, J. 1975. Isolation of an endogenous compound from the brain with pharmacological properties similar to morphine. Brain Res. **88**:295-308.

27. MAYER, D. J. 1975. Pain inhibition by electrical brain stimulation: comparison to morphine. Neurosci. Res. Prog. Bull. **13**:94-99.

28. MAYER, D. J., D. D. PRICE & A. RAFII. 1977. Antagonism of acupuncture analgesia in man by the narcotic antagonist naloxone. Brain Res. **121**:368-372.

29. AKIL, H., J. MADDEN, R. L. PATRICK & J. D. BARCHAS. 1976. Stress-induced increase in endogenous opiate peptides: Concurrent analgesia and its partial reversal by naloxone. *In* Opiates and Endogenous Opioid Peptides. H. W. Kosterlitz, Ed.: 63-70. Elsevier. North Holland.

30. DEVRIES, G. H., W. T. CHANCE, W. R. PAYNE & J. A. ROSECRANS. 1979. Effect of autoanalgesia on CNS enkephalin receptors. Pharmacol. Biochem. Behav. **11**:741-744.

31. LEWIS, J. W., J. T. CANNON & J. C. LIEBESKIND. 1980. Opioid and nonopioid mechanisms of stress analgesia. Science **208**:623-625.

32. COBELLI, D. A., L. R. WATKINS & D. J. MAYER. 1980. Dissociation of opiate and non-opiate footshock produced analgesia. Soc. Neurosci. Abs. **6**:247.

33. WATKINS, L. R. & D. J. MAYER. 1982. Organization of endogenous opiate and nonopiate pain control systems. Science **216**:1185-1192.

34. WATKINS, L. R., D. A. COBELLI, P. FARIS, M. D. ACETO & D. J. MAYER. 1982. Opiate vs. non-opiate footshock-induced analgesia: The body region shocked is a critical factor. Brain Res. **242**:299-308.

35. WATKINS, L. R., D. A. COBELLI, H. H. NEWSOME & D. J. MAYER. 1982. Footshock induced analgesia is dependent neither on pituitary nor sympathetic activation. Brain Res. **245**:81-96.

36. WATKINS, L. R., D. A. COBELLI & D. J. MAYER. 1982. Opiate vs non-opiate footshock induced analgesia (FSIA): Descending and intraspinal components. Brain Res. **245**:97-106.

37. WATKINS, L. R., E. G. YOUNG, I. B. KINSCHECK & D. J. MAYER. 1983. The neural basis of footshock analgesia: The role of specific ventral medullary nuclei. Brain Res. **276**:305-315.

38. WATKINS, L. R., I. B. KINSCHECK & D. J. MAYER. 1983. The neural basis of footshock analgesia: The effect of periaqueductal gray lesions and decerebration. Brain Res. **276**:317-324.

39. WATKINS, L. R. & D. J. MAYER. 1982. Involvement of spinal opioid systems in footshock-induced analgesia: antagonism by naloxone is possible only before induction of analgesia. Brain Res. **242**:309-316.

40. WATKINS, L. R., D. A. COBELLI & D. J. MAYER. 1982. Classical conditioning of front paw and hind paw footshock induced analgesia (FSIA): Naloxone reversibility and descending pathways. Brain Res. **243**:119-132.

41. KINSCHECK, I. B., L. R. WATKINS & D. J. MAYER. 1984. Fear is not critical to classically conditioned analgesia: The effects of periaqueductal gray lesions and administration of chlordiazepoxide. Brain Res. **298**:33-44.

42. STENGAARD-PEDERSEN, K. & L. I. LARSSON. 1981. Localization and opiate receptor binding of enkephalin, CCK and ACTH/Beta-endorphin in the rat central nervous system. Peptides **2**:3-19.

43. FARIS, P., B. KOMISURAK, L. WATKINS & D. J. MAYER. 1983. Evidence for the neuropeptide cholecystokinin as an antagonist of opiate analgesia. Science **219**:310-312.

44. HENRY, J. L. 1976. Effects of substance P on functionally identified units in cat spinal cord. Brain Res. **114**:439-452.

45. CHIODO, L. A. & B. S. BUNNEY. 1983. Proglumide: Selective antagonism of excitatory effects of cholecystokinin in central nervous system. Science **219**:1449-1451.

46. WATKINS, L. R., I. B. KINSCHECK & D. J. MAYER. 1985. Potentiation of morphine

analgesia by the cholecystokinin antagonist proglumide. Brain Res. **327**:169–180.

47. HAHNE, W. F., R. T. JENSEN, G. F. LEMP & J. D. GARDNER. 1981. Proglumide and benzotript: Members of a different class of cholecystokinin receptor antagonists. Proc. Natl. Acad. Sci. USA **78**:6304–6308.

48. WATKINS, L. R., I. B. KINSCHECK, E. F. S. KAUFMAN, J. MILLER, H. FRENK & D. J. MAYER. 1985. Cholecystokinin antagonists selectively potentiate analgesia induced by endogenous opiates. Brain Res. **327**:181–190.

49. WATKINS, L. R., J. N. JOHANNESSEN, I. B. KINSCHECK & D. J. MAYER. 1984. The neurochemical basis of footshock analgesia: The role of spinal cord serotonin and norepinephrine. Brain Res. **290**:107–117.

50. KIRCHGESSNER, A. L., R. J. BODNAR & G. W. PASTERNAK. 1982. Naloxazone and pain-inhibitory systems: Evidence for a collateral inhibition model. Pharmacol. Biochem. Behav. **17**:1175–1179.

51. PRICE, D. D. 1984. Antagonizing the endogenous opiate antagonists: a novel approach to pain control. Pain (Suppl.) **2**:S289.

52. JOHANNESSEN, J. N., L. R. WATKINS, S. M. CARLTON & D. J. MAYER. 1982. Failure of spinal cord serotonin depletion to alter analgesia elicited from the periaqueductal gray. Brain Res. **237**:373–386.

53. MURFIN, R., G. J. BENNETT & D. J. MAYER. 1976. The effects of dorsolateral spinal cord (DLF) lesions on analgesia from morphine microinjected into the periaqueductal gray matter (PAG) of the rat. Soc. Neurosci. Abstr. **2**:946.

54. GRIFFIN, G., L. R. WATKINS & D. J. MAYER. 1979. HRP pellets and slow release gels: Two new techniques for greater localization and sensitivity. Brain Res. **168**:595–601.

55. WATKINS, L. R., G. GRIFFIN, G. R. LEICHNETZ & D. J. MAYER. 1980. The somatotopic organization of the nucleus raphe magnus and surrounding brainstem structures as revealed by HRP slow-release gels. Brain Res. **181**:1–15.

56. ZORMAN, G., G. BELCHER, J. E. ADAMS & H. L. FIELDS. 1982. Lumbar intrathecal naloxone blocks analgesia produced by microstimulation of the ventromedial medulla in the rat. Brain Res. **236**:77–89.

57. TAKAGI, H. 1982. Critical review of pain relieving procedures including acupuncture. *In* Advances in Pharmacology and Therapeutics II. H. Yoshida, Y. Hagihara & S. Ebashi, Eds. **1**:79–92. Pergamon Press. New York.

58. JOHANNESSEN, J. N., L. R. WATKINS & D. J. MAYER. 1984. Non-serotonergic origins of the dorsolateral funiculus in the rat ventral medulla. J. Neurosci. **4**:757–766.

59. BOWKER, R. M., H. W. N. STEINBUSCH & J. D. COULTER. 1981. Serotonergic and peptidergic projections to the spinal cord demonstrated by a combined retrograde HRP histochemical and immunocytochemical staining method. Brain Res. **211**:412–417.

60. WATKINS, L. R., J. N. JOHANNESSEN, I. B. KINSCHECK & D. J. MAYER. 1984. The neurochemical basis of footshock analgesia: The role of spinal cord serotonin and norepinephrine. Brain Res. **290**:107–117.

61. WATKINS, L. R., Y. KATAYAMA, I. B. KINSCHECK, D. J. MAYER & R. L. HAYES. 1984. Muscarinic cholinergic mediation of opiate and nonopiate environmentally induced analgesias. Brain Res. **300**:231–242.

62. KATAYAMA, Y., D. S. DEWITT, D. P. BECKER & R. L. HAYES. 1984. Behavioral evidence for a cholinoceptive pontine inhibitory area: Descending control of spinal motor output and sensory input. Brain Res. **296**:241–262.

63. BUCHSBAUM, M. S., G. C. DAVIS & W. E. BUNNEY, JR. 1977. Naloxone alters pain perception and somatosensory evoked potentials in normal subjects. Nature **270**:620–621.

64. LASAGNA, L. 1965. Drug interaction in the field of analgesic drugs. Proc. R. Soc. Med. **58**:978–983.

65. LEVINE, J. D., N. C. GORDON & H. L. FIELDS. 1979. Naloxone dose dependently produces analgesia and hyperalgesia in postoperative pain. Nature **278**:740.

66. MELZACK, R. 1975. Prolonged relief of pain by brief, intense transcutaneous somatic stimulation. Pain 1:357–373.
67. CHAPMAN, C. R. & C. BENEDETTI. 1977. Analgesia following transcutaneous electrical stimulation and its partial reversal by a narcotic antagonist. Life Sci. 21:1645–648.
68. SJOLUND, B. H. & M. B. E. ERIKSSON. 1979. The influence of naloxone on analgesia produced by peripheral conditioning stimulation. Brain Res. 173:295–302.
69. CHAPMAN, C. R., C. BENEDETTI, Y. H. COLPITTS & R. GERLACH. 1983. Naloxone fails to reverse pain thresholds elevated by acupuncture: acupuncture analgesia reconsidered. Pain 16:13–32.
70. LEVINE, J. D., N. C. GORDON & H. L. FIELDS. 1978. The mechanism of placebo analgesia. Lancet 2:654–657.
71. KARCZYN, A. D. 1978. Mechanism of placebo analgesia. Lancet 2:1304–1305.

Relation of Stress-Induced Analgesia to Stimulation-Produced Analgesia[a]

GREGORY W. TERMAN AND JOHN C. LIEBESKIND

Department of Psychology
University of California
Los Angeles, California 90024

It has been twenty years since the gate control theory of Melzack and Wall[1] was published and began to focus so much attention on the field of pain research. In those years, major developments have occurred transforming this once sleepy field into one of the liveliest areas of behavioral, neuroscientific, and biomedical research. One exciting development portended by their theory has been the discovery of a central nervous system substrate whose normal function appears to be pain modulation. This substrate includes cells of the medial brain stem and fibers descending from them to the spinal cord dorsal horn. In the cord, the transmission of nociceptive inputs from peripheral fibers to ascending systems and reflex paths is modulated by these descending controls. Opioid peptides play a significant role in such processes of pain inhibition. We now know, however, that nonopioid mechanisms also exist, offering hope for the development of analgesic therapies lacking the unwanted properties of opiate drugs. Application of this new knowledge about intrinsic pain control systems has already been made by neurosurgeons adapting the techniques of direct medial brain stem stimulation from the original animal studies reporting dramatic stimulation-produced analgesia[2,3] to the alleviation of chronic pain symptoms in man.[4] The success of such clinical trials constitutes one of the clearest examples of the benefits of behavioral and neuroscientific research on laboratory animals, as recently cited by Miller.[5]

Until recently, most of the evidence suggesting the existence of an endgenous pain-suppressive system has come from studies of stimulation-produced analgesia. Electrically stimulating the midbrain periaqueductal gray matter and portions of the medial brain stem rostral and caudal to it causes profound analgesia in awake rats without reliably causing other sensory, motor, or motivational deficits. These findings suggested a natural pain-inhibitory role for these brain regions.[3] Before one could accept the existence of such a system, however, or credit it with more than epiphenomenal status, it would be essential to know under what circumstances it normally is used. In our earliest considera-tion of this matter,[6] we suggested that an endogenous analgesia substrate ought not be readily accessed or trivially employed; noxious stimuli generally hurt, and the warning signals they provide lead to important adaptive behavior. On the other hand, we reasoned, perhaps under certain conditions of dire emergency, when the perception of pain might disrupt effective defensive behavior or retreat, then pain suppression would have greater survival value than pain perception itself. The recent literature on stress-induced analgesia lends credence to this

[a]Supported by National Institutes of Health grant NS 07628.

view, suggesting that stress is one natural trigger for intrinsic pain-suppressive mechanisms.

Numerous reviews have appeared summarizing the extensive literatures on stimulation-produced and stress-induced analgesia.[7-10] Here, we shall attempt to touch upon only a few highlights in each field separately, then end by presenting some as yet unpublished evidence attesting to a common substrate these two analgesias share.

STIMULATION-PRODUCED ANALGESIA

The first solid evidence for the existence of endogenous pain-inhibitory systems came from early reports that electrical stimulation of the medial brain stem caused potent analgesia in rats.[2,3] This finding has since been replicated and extended numerous times in the rat, cat, monkey, and man.[4,11-13] Stimulation-produced analgesia has, for example, been found capable of completely inhibiting behavioral responses to various noxious somatic and visceral stimuli, including electric shocks applied to the tooth pulp[14] and limbs,[3] heating of the skin,[13] subcutaneous injections of formalin,[15] and intraperitoneal injections of hypertonic saline.[16] This reduction in pain responsiveness was found not to be regularly associated with either motor dysfunction or diminished sensory capacity in other than the nociceptive modality.[3] In a particularly clear demonstration of this point, Oliveras *et al.*[14] showed that whereas the jaw opening reflex to noxious tooth pulp stimulation was suppressed by stimulation-produced analgesia (SPA), a similar jaw opening response to innocuous tooth tap was not affected. The specificity of SPA in blocking responses to noxious stimuli has also been observed electrophysiologically in recordings from brain and spinal neurons.[17-19]

This analgetic specificity was reminiscent of the relatively specific pain suppressing effects of opiate drugs and suggested to us[3] that SPA might share sites and mechanisms of action with opiate analgesia. This hypothesis was supported by reports that the same periaqueductal region yielding profound SPA, is also exquisitely sensitive to morphine.[20,21] Mapping studies have since shown that many brain sites support both SPA and morphine analgesia.[22,23] In addition to sharing common sites of action, stimulation-produced and opiate analgesia have been associated in a number of other ways. For example, it has been shown that repeated brain stem stimulation manifests analgetic tolerance.[24] Also, animals made tolerant to morphine show reduced SPA, or cross-tolerance, again suggesting SPA and opiate analgesia are mediated by a common receptor.[24] Lesions of the dorsolateral funiculus of the spinal cord block both SPA and morphine analgesia, attesting to the critical importance of this descending path connecting the medial brain stem to the dorsal horn.[25] Opioid peptides and their receptors are well situated in the nervous system to function in a natural pain-inhibitory system.[8] They are found, among other places, in those brain regions where SPA and opiate microinjections appear to work best. Injections of small amounts of opioid peptides into many of these areas cause significant increases in pain thresholds.[26,27]

Perhaps the most salient finding associating the mechanisms of stimulation-produced and opiate analgesic action was the demonstration that the opiate antagonist drug, naloxone, significantly reduced SPA in the rat.[28,29] This observation suggested that SPA and opiate drugs share a common receptor site, presumably the opiate receptor.[29] Although some authors were unable to replicate this finding,[30,31] others were successful.[32,33] Recent work from our laboratory seems to resolve these discrepancies. We find that whereas SPA can be elicited equally well from dorsal and ventral portions of the rat's periaqueductal gray matter, only SPA from ventral stimulation sites in the dorsal raphe and subjacent tegmentum is antagonized by naloxone.[34] Moreover, even very low doses of the drug (5 μg via the intraperitoneal route) significantly reduce SPA from these naloxone-sensitive placements, suggesting antagonism occurs at a high affinity receptor site.[34] The localization of adjacent naloxone-sensitive and naloxone-insensitive SPA regions in the rat midbrain may explain both the failure of some investigators to obtain naloxone-sensitive SPA and the curious observation[29,34] that even when SPA is reduced by naloxone it is only partially reduced by the drug. That anatomically distinct opioid and nonopioid mechanisms of SPA exist was further supported by our findings[35] that bulbar raphe lesions disrupt only the naloxone-sensitive SPA from more ventral periaqueductal regions.[36] It seems that not one but multiple intrinsic analgesia systems exist, some opioid-mediated, some not. As will be seen below, this same conclusion is reached from the literature on stress-induced analgesia.

STRESS-INDUCED ANALGESIA

The earliest studies of stress-induced analgesia (SIA),[37–42] while agreeing that numerous stressors had potent analgesic effects, differed as to whether or not such effects were blocked by naloxone or showed tolerance or cross-tolerance with morphine. Our first work in this area,[43] using a single stressor, inescapable footshock of constant intensity, showed that varying the temporal parameters of the footshock (brief, continuous versus longer duration, and intermittent) caused comparable analgesia; however, only that from the intermittent shock was blocked by naloxone. We went on to confirm the existence of opioid-mediated and nonopioid-mediated stress analgesia systems by applying criteria other than naloxone antagonism. Thus, repeated exposure to these footshocks resulted in the development of analgesic tolerance only to the naloxone-sensitive form; and only this form showed cross-tolerance in morphine-tolerant animals.[44]

The pituitary/adrenal axis has long been recognized for the role it plays in the adaptive response to stress. As described above, pain suppression may be thought of as an adaptive response to stress under certain circumstances; hence, participation of the pituitary/adrenal system in stress analgesia seemed likely. We showed[45] that hypophysectomy attenuates only the opioid form of stress analgesia. But hypophysectomy comprises function of the adrenal medulla as well as the adrenal cortex,[46] and the adrenal medulla contains enkephalin-like peptides and secretes them in response to sympathetic activation.[47] The effects of hypophysectomy on opioid stress analgesia, therefore, might be attributable to a reduction in adrenal as well as hypophyseal opioids. Indeed, we found[48] that adrenalectomy, adrenal demedullation, and adrenal medulla denervation all cause profound and selective blockade of opioid SIA. This form of stress analgesia seems dependent on adrenal medullary enkephalin-like peptides.[48]

We have recently found that even SIA from continuous footshock is not a unitary phenomenon.[10] By varying the severity of continuous footshock, reliable opioid and nonopioid SIA can be seen. The parameters of continuous footshock used in our earlier work (3 min; 2.5 mA) appear now to be intermediate between those producing clearer opioid and nonopioid SIA. Thus, opioid SIA results from lowering the severity of this footshock (e.g., 2.5 mA for 1 min or 2.0 mA for 3 min) and nonopioid SIA from raising the severity (e.g., 2.5 mA for 4 min or 3.5 mA for 3 min).[49] Very low doses of opiate antagonists (as little as 0.05 mg/kg of naltrexone) block this opioid SIA as they do that from intermittent footshock.[50] Opioid SIA from less severe continuous footshock and opioid SIA from intermittent footshock share several other defining characteristics of opioid involvement. Both manifest tolerance after 14 daily stress exposures, and both manifest cross-tolerance in morphine-tolerant rats.[10] The nonopioid SIA from more severe continuous footshock (e.g., 2.5 mA for 4 min) does not diminish with repetition and is unchanged in morphine-tolerant animals. In fact, the two opioid forms of SIA show mutual cross-tolerance with each other.[10] As expected, repeated exposure to nonopioid SIA does not affect either opioid form, nor does nonopioid SIA change in animals made tolerant to either form of opioid SIA.[10]

From these data[10] it is apparent that when the temporal pattern of footshock is held constant (continuous footshock), the severity of the shock, defined in terms either of its duration or intensity, determines whether or not the analgesia is opioid mediated. On the other hand, when the exact same total amount of footshock causing nonopioid SIA (4 min; 2.5mA) is applied intermittently (on for 1 of every 5 sec) rather than continuously, it causes opioid analgesia. Thus, by holding constant shock intensity and shock "on" time, variations in the temporal pattern of the shock can be made the critical factor in determining the opioid or nonopioid basis of SIA.

Important differences have also been seen between the two opioid forms of SIA.[10] As before,[45,48] opioid SIA from intermittent footshock is blocked by adrenalectomy and hypophysectomy; but opioid SIA from continuous footshock (and, for that matter, nonopioid SIA) is unaffected by these procedures.[10] Opioid and nonopioid SIA from continuous footshock are also unaffected by deep pentobarbital anesthesia (55 mg/kg), whereas opioid SIA from intermittent shock completely disappears in anesthetized rats. Spinal transections and lesions of the spinal dorsolateral funiculus reduce all forms of SIA[7,10,51,52] as they do SPA,[25] indicating the critical importance of centrifugal or descending controls in mediating these types of analgesia. However, decerebration blocks SIA from intermittent footshock without altering opioid or nonopioid continuous foot-shock SIA.[10] Supporting the conclusion that only the opioid SIA from long duration intermittent footshock relies on higher brain function, we have seen in a collaborative study with Maier[53] that only this type of footshock is perceived by rats as inescapable, as evidenced by the development of "learned helplessness." This learning that the footshock is inescapable appears to rely on prolonged shock exposure[53] and may be critical for the production of such forms of opioid SIA.[10,53-55] In this regard, the muscarinic cholinergic drug, scopolamine, known to interfere with various paradigms of learning, including learned helplessness,[56] has a selective inhibitory effect on opioid SIA from the intermittent shock.[57,58]

Providing generality to the concept of three independent forms of SIA, we have recently shown that they can be faithfully reproduced in another species, the mouse, using footshock parameters similar to those used in rats.[59] Comparing two strains of mice, one known to be deficient in central opioid binding sites (CXBK) and one normal in this regard (C57), we found that although the C57 strain showed robust opioid and nonopioid SIA, the CXBK strain showed normal nonopioid SIA but reduced SIA of both opioid types.

A final note of interest concerning opioid and nonopioid mechanisms of SIA: We have been able to show that intermittent footshock yielding opioid SIA, but not continuous footshock yielding nonopioid SIA, suppresses an important index of immune system function (natural killer cell cytotoxicity)[60] and enhances the development of an experimental tumor.[61] These effects are blocked by naltrexone.[60,61] By bringing under control the parameters of footshock stress activating opioid and nonopioid mechanisms of analgesia, we have begun not only to explain some of the apparent discrepancies in the stress analgesia literature but also to account for some of the variance previously obscuring the relationship between stress and immune function and tumor growth.

A summary of the major findings described in this section is provided in TABLE 1.

EVIDENCE THAT SPA AND SIA SHARE A COMMON SUBSTRATE

A study recently conducted in our laboratory[62] seems to provide direct evidence that at least opioid-mediating forms of SPA and SIA share a common substrate. This study sought to determine the commonality between opioid substrates of SPA and SIA by assessing the development of cross-tolerance between them.

All rats were implanted with SPA electrodes in dorsal and ventral regions of the periaqueductal gray matter (PAG) shown by Cannon et al.[34] to yield naloxone-insensitive and naloxone-sensitive analgesia, respectively. Baseline SPA thresholds were assessed one week after surgery. The next day, animals were assigned

TABLE 1. Characteristics of Three Forms of Stress-Induced Analgesia

	Opioid-mediated
	  reduced by low doses of opiate antagonists
	  demonstrates tolerance and cross-tolerance with morphine, opioid-mediated SPA, and other forms of opioid stress analgesia

Long Duration Intermittent
(20 min, 2.5 mA)
(1 sec on every 5 sec)
	absent in mice deficient in μ_1 opiate receptors
	Dependent on adrenal medullary enkephalins
	Supraspinally mediated (blocked by spinal transection and DLF lesions)
	Dependent on learning that shock is inescapable
	  reduced by decerebration, anesthesia, and scopolamine
	  associated with learned helplessness and immunosuppression

Low Severity Continuous (e.g., 1 min, 2.5 mA)	Opioid-mediated Unaffected by hypophysectomy or adrenalectomy Supraspinally mediated Unaffected by decerebration or deep pentobarbital anesthesia
High Severity Continuous (e.g., 4 min, 2.5 mA)	Nonopioid-mediated Unaffected by hypophysectomy or adrenalectomy Supraspinally mediated Unaffected by decerebration or deep pentobarbital anesthesia

to one of four groups, and footshock stress was begun. Three groups received 14 daily sessions of one or another of the three types of footshock paradigms described above. The fourth group served as unshocked controls. One day after the last stress treatment, dorsal and ventral PAG SPA thresholds were determined for each rat, as before. Results derived from 69 electrode placements, of which 33 lay in the region of the dorsal raphe nucleus and comprised the ventral group and 36 were found more dorsally within the PAG and comprised the dorsal group. Assignment of electrode sites to dorsal and ventral groups was performed blind to the behavioral results.

Fourteen daily exposures to either the continuous or the intermittent form of opioid SIA significantly increased SPA thresholds at ventral but not dorsal placements compared to unshocked controls. Repeated exposure to the non-opioid form of SIA caused no significant change in either dorsal or ventral SPA thresholds. Thus, SPA only from the more ventral PAG sites found by Cannon et al.[34] to be naloxone-sensitive, demonstrates cross-tolerance to opioid forms of SIA.

Studies of stress-induced analgesia derive conceptually from earlier work on stimulation-produced analgesia. They have as one major goal the identification of environmental stimuli normally activating endogenous pain-inhibitory systems. The critical properties of such stimuli are gradually being elucidated by experiments such as ours and those of many others described in these *Annals*. In this context, it is noteworthy that SIA studies are now beginning to interdigitate closely with the parent series of SPA experiments. The finding that cross-tolerance occurs between opioid forms of SPA and SIA, by providing evidence for a common substrate these two analgesias share, strengthens the assertion that SPA studies relate to natural systems of pain modulation.

ACKNOWLEDGMENT

We thank Edna Shavit for assisting in the preparation of this manuscript.

REFERENCES

1. MELZACK, R. & P. D. WALL. 1965. Pain mechanisms: A new theory. Science **150**:971–979.
2. REYNOLDS, D. V. 1969. Surgery in the rat during electrical analgesia induced by focal brain stimulation. Science **164**:444–445.
3. MAYER, D. J., T. L. WOLFLE, H. AKIL, B. CARDER & J. C. LIEBESKIND. 1971. Analgesia from electrical stimulation in the brainstem of the rat. Science **174**:1351–1354.
4. YOUNG, R. F., R. A. FELDMAN, R. KROENING, W. FULTON & J. MORRIS. 1984. Electrical stimulation of the brain in the treatment of chronic pain in man. *In* Advances in Pain Research and Therapy. L. Kruger & J. C. Liebeskind, Eds. **6**:289–303. Raven Press. New York.
5. MILLER, N. E. 1985. The value of behavioral research on animals. Am. Psychologist **40**:423–440.
6. LIEBESKIND, J. C., G. J. GIESLER, JR. & G. URCA. 1976. Evidence pertaining to an endogenous mechanism of pain inhibition in the central nervous system. *In* Sensory Functions of the Skin in Primates. Y. Zotterman, Ed. **1**:561–573. Pergamon Press. Oxford.
7. WATKINS, L. R. & D. J. MAYER. 1982. The organization of endogenous opiate and nonopiate pain control systems. Science **216**:1185–1192.

8. AKIL, H., S. J. WATSON, E. YOUNG, M. E. LEWIS, H. KHACHATURIAN & J. M. WALKER. 1984. Endogenous opioids: Biology and function. Ann. Rev. Neurosci. 7:223–255.
9. BASBAUM, A. I. & H. L. FIELDS. 1984. Endogenous pain control systems: Brainstem spinal pathways and endorphin circuitry. Ann. Rev. Neurosci. 7:309–338.
10. TERMAN, G. W., Y. SHAVIT, J. W. LEWIS, J. T. CANNON & J. C. LIEBESKIND. 1984. Intrinsic mechanisms of pain inhibition: Activation by stress. Science 226:1270–1277.
11. GOODMAN, S. J. & V. HOLCOMBE. 1976. Selective and prolonged analgesia in monkey resulting from brain stimulation. In Advances in Pain Research and Therapy. J. J. Bonica & D. Albe-Fessard, Eds. 1:495–502. Raven Press. New York.
12. LIEBESKIND, J. C., G. GUILBAUD, J. M. BESSON & J. L. OLIVERAS. 1973. Analgesia from electrical stimulation of the periaqueductal gray matter in the cat: behavioral observations and inhibitory effects on spinal cord interneurons. Brain Res. 50:441–446.
13. MAYER, D. J. & J. C. LIEBESKIND. 1974. Pain reduction by focal electrical stimulation of the brain: an anatomical and behavioral analysis. Brain Res. 68:73–93.
14. OLIVERAS, J. L., A. WODA, G. GUILBAUD & J. M. BESSON. 1974. Inhibition of the jaw opening reflex by electrical stimulation of the periaqueductal gray matter in the awake, unrestrained cat. Brain Res. 72:328–331.
15. MELZACK, R. & D. F. MELINKOFF. 1974. Analgesia produced by brain stimulation: evidence of a prolonged onset period. Exp. Neurol. 43:369–374.
16. GIESLER, G. J. JR & J. C. LIEBESKIND. 1976. Inhibition of visceral pain by electrical stimulation of the periaqueductal gray matter. Pain 2:43–48.
17. MORROW, T. J. & K. L. CASEY. 1976. Analgesia produced by mesencephalic stimulation: effect on bulboreticular neurons. In Advances in Pain Research and Therapy. J. J. Bonica & D. Albe-Fessard, Eds. 1:503–510. Raven Press. New York.
18. OLESON, T. D., D. A. TWOMBLY & J. C. LIEBESKIND. 1978. Effects of pain-attenuating brain stimulation and morphine on electrical activity in the raphe nuclei of the awake rat. Pain 4:211–230.
19. DUGGAN, A. W. & C. R. MORTON. 1983. Periaqueductal gray stimulation: An association between selective inhibition of dorsal horn neurones and changes in peripheral circulation. Pain 15:237–248.
20. JACQUET, Y. F. & A. LAJTHA. 1974. Paradoxical effects after microinjection of morphine in the periaqueductal grey matter in the rat. Science 185:1055–1057.
21. SHARPE, L. G., J. E. GARNETT & T. J. CICERO. 1974. Analgesia and hyperreactivity produced by intracranial microinjections of morphine into the periaqueductal gray matter of the rat. Behav. Biol. 11:303–313.
22. MAYER, D. J. & D. D. PRICE. 1976. Central nervous system mechanisms of analgesia. Pain 2:379–404.
23. YAKSH, T. L. & T. A. RUDY. 1978. Narcotic analgetics: CNS sites and mechanisms of action as revealed by intracerebral injection techniques. Pain 4:299–359.
24. MAYER, D. J. & R. L. HAYES. 1975. Stimulation-produced analgesia: development of tolerance and cross-tolerance to morphine. Science 188:941–943.
25. BASBAUM, A. I., N. J MARLEY, J. O'KEEFE & C. H. CLANTON. 1977. Reversal of morphine and stimulus produced analgesia by subtotal spinal cord lesions. Pain 3:43–56.
26. BELLUZZI, J. D., N. GRANT, V. GARSKY, D. SARANTAKIS, C. D. WISE & L. STEIN. 1976. Analgesia induced in vivo by central administration of enkephalin in rat. Nature 260:625–626.
27. URCA, G., H. FRENK, J. C. LIEBESKIND & A. N. TAYLOR. 1977. Morphine and enkephalin: analgesic and epileptic properties. Science 197:83–86.
28. AKIL, H., D. J. MAYER & J. C. LIEBESKIND. 1972. Comparaison chez le rat entre l'analgésie induite par stimulation de la substance grise peri-aqueducale et l'analgésie morphinique. C. R. Acad. Sci. (Paris) 274:3603–3605.
29. AKIL, H., D. J. MAYER & J. C. LIEBESKIND. 1976. Antagonism of stimulation-produced analgesia by naloxone, a narcotic antagonist. Science 191:961–962.
30. PERT, A. & M. WALTER. 1976. Comparison between naloxone reversal of morphine and electrical stimulation induced analgesia in the rat mesencephalon. Life Sci. 19:1023–1032.

31. YAKSH, T. L., J. C. YEUNG & T. A. RUDY. 1976. An inability to antagonize with naloxone the elevated thresholds resulting from electrical stimulation of the mesencephalic central gray. Life Sci. **18**:1193–1198.

32. HOSOBUCHI, Y., J. E. ADAMS & R. LINCHITZ. 1977. Pain relief by electrical stimulation of the central gray matter in humans and its reversal by naloxone. Science **197**:183–186.

33. OLIVERAS, J. L., Y. HOSOBUCHI, F. REDJEMI, G. GUILBAUD & J. M. BESSON. 1977. Opiate antagonist, naloxone, strongly reduces analgesia induced by stimulation of a raphe nucleus (centralis inferior). Brain Res. **120**:221–229.

34. CANNON, J. T., G. J. PRIETO, A. LEE & J. C. LIEBESKIND. 1982. Evidence for opioid and nonopioid forms of stimulation-produced analgesia in the rat. Brain Res. **243**:315–321.

35. PRIETO, G. J., J. T. CANNON & J. C. LIEBESKIND. 1983. N. raphe magnus lesions disrupt stimulation-produced analgesia from ventral but not dorsal midbrain areas in the rat. Brain Res. **261**:53–57.

36. LOVICK, T. A. 1985. Ventrolateral medullary lesions block the antinociceptive and cardiovascular responses elicited by stimulating the dorsal periaqueductal grey matter in rats. Pain **21**:241–252.

37. AKIL, H., J. MADDEN, R. L. PATRICK & J. D. BARCHAS. 1976. Stress-induced increase in endogenous opiate peptides; concurrent analgesia and its partial reversal by naloxone. *In* Opiates and Endogenous Opioid Peptides. H. W. Kosterlitz, Ed. **1**:63–70. Elsevier. Amsterdam.

38. CHESHER, G. B. & B. CHAN. 1977. Footshock induced analgesia in mice: its reversal by naloxone and cross-tolerance with morphine. Life Sci. **21**:1569–1574.

39. HAYES, R. L., G. J. BENNETT, P. G. NEWLON & D. J. MAYER. 1978. Behavioral and physiological studies of non-narcotic analgesia in the rat elicited by certain environmental stimuli. Brain Res. **155**:69–90.

40. AMIR, S. & Z. AMIT. 1978. Endogenous opioid ligands may mediate stress-induced changes in the affective properties of pain related behavior in rats. Life Sci. **23**:1143–1152.

41. BODNAR, R. J., D. D. KELLY, A. SPIAGGIA, C. EHRENBERG & M. GLUSMAN. 1978. Dose-dependent reductions by naloxone of analgesia induced by cold-water stress. Pharmacol. Biochem. Behav. **8**:667–672.

42. BODNAR, R. J., D. D. KELLY, A. SPIAGGIA & M. GLUSMAN. 1978. Biphasic alterations of nociceptive thresholds induced by food deprivation. Physiol. Psych. **6**:391–395.

43. LEWIS, J. W., J. T. CANNON & J. C. LIEBESKIND. 1980. Opioid and nonopioid mechanisms of stress analgesia. Science **208**:623–625.

44. LEWIS, J. W., J. E. SHERMAN, & J. C. LIEBESKIND. 1981. Opioid and nonopioid stress analgesia: assessment of tolerance and cross-tolerance with morphine. J. Neurosci. **1**:358–363.

45. LEWIS, J. W., E. H. CHUDLER, J. T. CANNON & J. C. LIEBESKIND. 1981. Hypophysectomy differentially affects morphine and stress analgesia. Proc. West. Pharmacol. Soc. **24**:323–326.

46. POHORECKY, L. A. & R. J. WURTMAN. 1971. Adrenocortical control of epinephrine synthesis. Pharmacological Rev. **23**:1–35.

47. VIVEROS, O. H., E. J. DILIBERTO JR., E. HAZUM & K. J. CHANG. 1980. Enkephalins as possible adrenomedullary hormones: storage, secretion, and regulation of synthesis. *In* Neural Peptides and Neuronal Communications, Advances in Biochemical Psychopharmacology. E. Costa & M. Trabucchi, Eds. **22**:191–204. Raven Press. New York.

48. LEWIS, J. W., M. G. TORDOFF, J. E. SHERMAN & J. C. LIEBESKIND. 1982. Adrenal medullary enkephalin-like peptides may mediate opioid stress analgesia. Science **217**:557–559.

49. FANSELOW, M. 1984. Shock-induced analgesia on the formalin test: effects of shock severity, naloxone, hypophysectomy, and associative variables. Behav. Neurosci. **98**:79–95.

50. TERMAN, G. W., J. W. LEWIS & J. C. LIEBESKIND. 1983. The sensitivity of opioid-

mediated stress analgesia to narcotic antagonists. Proc. West. Pharmacol. Soc. 26:49–53.

51. LEWIS, J. W., G. W. TERMAN, L. R. WATKINS, D. J. MAYER & J. C. LIEBESKIND. 1983. Opioid and nonopioid mechanisms of footshock-induced analgesia: role of the spinal dorsolateral funiculus. Brain Res. 267:139–144.

52. WATKINS, L. R., R. C. DRUGAN, R. L. HYSON, T. B. MOYE, S. M. RYAN, D. J. MAYER & S. F. MAIER. 1984. Opiate and non-opiate analgesia induced by inescapable tail-shock: Effects of dorsolateral funiculus lesions and decerebration. Brain Res. 291:325–336.

53. MAIER, S. F., J. E. SHERMAN, J. W. LEWIS, G. W. TERMAN & J. C. LIEBESKIND. 1983. The opioid/nonopioid nature of stress-induced analgesia and learned helplessness. J. Exp. Psych.: Animal Behav. Proc. 9:80–90.

54. GRAU, J. W., R. L. HYSON, S. F. MAIER, J. MADDEN IV & J. D. BARCHAS. 1981. Long-term stress-induced analgesia and activation of the opiate system. Science 213:1409–1410.

55. MAIER, S. F., R. C. DRUGAN & J. W. GRAU. 1980. Controllability, coping behavior and stress-induced analgesia. Pain 12:47–56.

56. ANISMAN, H., G. REMINGTON & L. S. SKLAR. 1979. Effect of inescapable shock on subsequent escape performance: Catecholaminergic and cholinergic mediation of response initiation and maintenance. Psychopharmacology 61:107–124.

57. LEWIS, J. W., J. T. CANNON & J. C. LIEBESKIND. 1983. Involvement of central muscarinic cholinergic mechanisms in opioid stress analgesia. Brain Res. 270:289–293.

58. TERMAN, G. W. & J. C. LIEBESKIND. 1985. Differential effects of scopolamine on three forms of stress analgesia. Brain Res. 361:405–407.

59. MOSKOWITZ, A. S., G. W. TERMAN & J. C. LIEBESKIND. 1985. Stress-induced analgesia in the mouse: strain comparisons. Pain 23:67–72.

60. SHAVIT, Y., J. W. LEWIS, G. W. TERMAN, R. P. GALE & J. C. LIEBESKIND. 1984. Opioid peptides mediate the suppressive effect of stress on natural killer cell cytotoxicity. Science 223:188–191.

61. LEWIS, J. W., Y. SHAVIT, G. W. TERMAN, L. R. NELSON, R. P. GALE & J. C. LIEBESKIND. 1983. Apparent involvement of opioid peptides in stress-induced enhancement of tumor growth. Peptides 4:635–638.

62. TERMAN, G. W., E. R. PENNER & J. C. LIEBESKIND. 1985. Stimulation-produced and stress-induced analgesia: Cross-tolerance between opioid forms. Brain Res. 360:374–378.

The Role of Brain and Spinal Cord Norepinephrine in Autoanalgesia

WILLIAM T. CHANCE

Department of Surgery
University of Cincinnati Medical Center
Cincinnati, Ohio 45267-0558

The existence of endogenous mechanisms of pain control has been suggested by ancedotal accounts of pain inhibition during periods of extreme arousal or anxiety.[1,2] Thus in life and death situations it is advantageous and probably necessary for survival to prevent conscious recognition of even normally disabling pain for a period of time. However, the counterproductivity of long-term activation of such a system is also obvious, since the organism does need to seek repair after an injury. Therefore, important characteristics of such endogenous nociceptive control must be very rapid activation and reasonably short duration.

Based on neurophysiological observation, the theoretical framework of such an endogenous analgesic system was outlined by Melzack and Wall in the gate control theory of pain.[3] These scientists suggested a gating mechanism at the spinal cord that would reduce the conscious appreciation of pain when additional somatosensory input was applied. Perhaps more important for endogenous control of pain was the second postulate of the gate control theory, suggesting the existence of descending central nervous system (CNS) control of pain perception in accord with past experience and current CNS activity.[4]

Working under the second postulate of the gate control theory of pain, we in 1976[5] demonstrated that the extreme hyperemotionality of septal-lesioned rats (increased CNS activity) and the fear classically conditioned to the environmental stimuli associated with the analgesia test (past experience) induced significant analgesia as assessed by standard tail-flick tests.[6] Subsequent experimentation indicated that the analgesia exhibited by these lesioned rats was indeed secondary to their hyperemotionality, since both the antinociception and emotionality were reduced by the minor tranquilizer, diazepam.[7] We also demonstrated that the analgesia of fear-conditioned rats was specific to the environmental stimuli associated with the fear, since removal of these stimulus cues significantly reduced the analgesia.[8] Rather than referring specifically to each of these paradigms as hyperemotionality-induced analgesia, acute footshock-induced analgesia, or classically conditioned fear-induced analgesia, we chose instead to refer collectively to all of these paradigms of behaviorally induced antinociception as autoanalgesic phenomena.[9] This term seemed applicable since the analgesia is self-generated under appropriate behavioral conditions and therefore must result from the neuronal activity of endogenously synthesized effectors.

The first experiments investigating the neurochemical basis of analgesia following long periods (30–60 min) of intense footshock (3 mA) reported increased brain endorphin activity (as suggested by reduced binding of [³H]naloxone) that paralleled the analgesia.[10,11] Early experiments by us demonstrated decreases in CNS binding of [³H]N-leucine enkephalin[12] and [³H]-etorphine[9] that were proportional to the increase in tail-flick latency in the classical conditioning paradigm. Thus, merely placing the rats in the specific fear-producing environment elicited analgesia and increased brain opioid peptide activity. However, our subsequent experiments de-emphasized the role of endogenous opioid peptides as primary mediators of autoanalgesic phenomena. Thus, opiate antagonists did not reduce autoanalgesia[13] and rats made tolerant to morphine still exhibited the analgesic effects of acute footshock and conditioned fear.[14] In addition, removal of pituitary endorphins by hypophysectomy had no effect on autoanalgesia.[15] Although other investigators have reported significant antagonism of footshock-induced analgesia by opiate antagonist drugs, these reductions in antinociception were observed only when multiple tail-flick tests were conducted at one minute intervals.[16,17] Thus in these paradigms opiate antagonism of the analgesia is usually observed only on the second or third tail-flick test. These tests at one minute intervals are a marked departure from the traditional use of tail-flick procedures in pharmacological studies of analgesia. As such, these tests may be in danger of generating data that are confounded by local tail damage and increased temporal summation at the spinal cord. However, if these data do reflect nonconfounded results, they indicate opiate and nonopiate involvement in endogenous analgesic mechanisms. Lewis et al.[16] have suggested that acute footshock activates nonopioid analgesia, while more chronic footshock-induced analgesia is mediated by endogenous opiates. The generally observed absence of naloxone antagonism of analgesia immediately after footshock suggest that nonopioid mechanisms may be involved in the activation of the analgesia, while opioids may have a role in maintaining it.

In 1979, we reported that the alpha-2 adrenergic antagonist, yohimbine, completely abolished autoanalgesia elicited either by acute footshock[18] or classically conditioned fear.[19] This antagonism was observed on the tail-flick test immediately following presentation of the analgesia-producing stimulus in each paradigm. Therefore, this reduction in autoanalgesia represents pharmacological antagonism of the activation of endogenous antinociceptive mechanisms. Since yohimbine has been reported to have serotonergic antagonist properties[20] as well as alpha-2 adrenergic blocking ability,[21] the remainder of this manuscript will be devoted to investigating the role of norepinephrine (NE) and serotonin (5-HT) in mediating autoanalgesia.

THE AUTOANALGESIA PARADIGM

Since emotionality can affect tail-flick latencies, all rats were handled daily for at least one week to gentle them. Antinociception was assessed using a modification of a radiant heat tail-flick apparatus[6] consisting of a 100 W lamp mounted in a concave reflector and focused on a photocell. The lamp and photocell were connected to a timer so that activation of the photocell, by the rat flicking its tail, interrupted the circuit to give a reaction time to the nearest hundredth of a second. The intensity of the lamp was controlled by a rheostat and was set to elicit tail-flick latencies of approximately 3 sec in control rats. A latency cut-off criterion of 8 sec was also maintained in most experiments to minimize tail damage. Shock was delivered by a Lafayette A 615C shocker (Lafayette Instruments, Lafayette, IN) to a 21 × 21 cm grid platform. The grids were 3 mm in diameter and were spaced 15 mm apart. The grid platform was elevated by 8 cm and was used to support the rats during the tail-flick tests.

Within the autoanalgesia paradigm, analgesia elicited acutely by footshock as well as by classically conditioned fear was assessed. Individual rats in the experimental group were removed from the home cage by a gloved hand. Each rat was placed on the shock grid, the tail was placed over the photocell and a baseline tail-flick latency was obtained. Ten seconds later continuous footshock (1 mA) was administered for 15 sec while the rate was held in place on the grid. Ten seconds after the termination of the footshock, the tail-flick latency was determined again, which was the acute analgesic response to footshock. The rat was then returned to its home cage. On the following day, which was day 1 of classically conditioned analgesia, the rat was removed from its cage with a gloved hand, placed on the grid, and the tail-flick latency was assessed. Ten seconds later, footshock (1 mA, 15 sec) was administered, after which the rat was returned to its home cage. This procedure was continued until the rat exhibited asymptotic tail-flick latencies, which usually occurred in four to six days. Control rats were handled in the same manner, except that footshock was not administered. FIGURE 1 presents data obtained from seven experimental and seven control rats. Although both groups exhibited similar baseline tail-flick latencies, the response 10 sec after footshock (solid triangle) was increased significantly. Acquisition of conditioned fear-induced autoanalgesia is illustrated on days 1–4, with the rats in the shocked group exhibiting increased tail-flick latencies prior to the administration of footshock across these four days. Thus, presentation of the environmental stimuli associated with footshock, such as the glove and grid, was sufficient stimuli to elicit the analgesia.

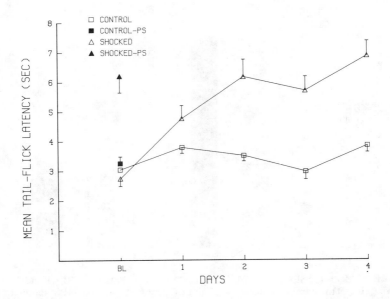

FIGURE 1. Mean (± SEM) tail-flick latencies of rats 10 sec prior to or 10 sec following (BL, solid triangle) the administration of footshock. For each group, $N = 7$.

EFFECTS OF NORADRENERGIC AND SEROTONERGIC ANTAGONISTS

In these experiments the effects of the alpha-2 adrenergic antagonist, yohimbine; the alpha-1 adrenergic antagonist, phentolamine; and the serotonergic blocker, methysergide, on autoanalgesia were investigated.

In the first experiment basal tail-flick latencies (BL-1, FIGURE 2) were determined on 16 adult, male Sprague-Dawley (SD) rats (Charles River Laboratories, Wilmington, MA). Yohimbine (10 mg/kg, free base; Sigma Chemical Co., St. Louis, MO) was administered i.p. to eight of these rats, while the remaining animals were treated with normal saline. Thirty minutes later, tail-flick latencies were again determined (BL-2, FIGURE 2), after which footshock (1 mA, 15 sec) was administered. As indicated in FIGURE 2, yohimbine dramatically reduced the postshock (PS) analgesia that was observed in the saline group. In a subsequent experiment the effects of yohimbine on autoanalgesia elicited by conditioned fear were investigated. Fear was conditioned to the tail-flick procedure as previously described in 18 adult, male Sprague-Dawley rats. An additional 16 rats served as nonconditioned controls. As illustrated in FIGURE 3, these fear-conditioned rats exhibited rapid acquisition of autoanalgesia. On day 6, each group of rats was randomly divided into two equal groups for the administration of saline or yohimbine (5 mg/kg, i.p.) 30 min prior to the determination of the tail-flick latencies. It is obvious from FIGURE 3 that the yohimbine treatment reduced ($p < 0.01$) the tail-flick latency of the fear-conditioned rats to control levels and

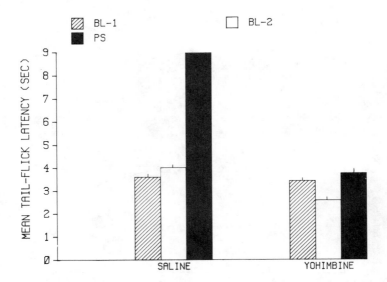

FIGURE 2. Mean ($\pm$ SEM) tail-flick latencies 24 hr after footshock (BL-1) and 30 min following (BL-2) the administration of yohimbine (10 mg/kg). Solid bars (PS) represent the analgesic effects of footshock in control and yohimbine-treated rats. For each group, $N = 8$.

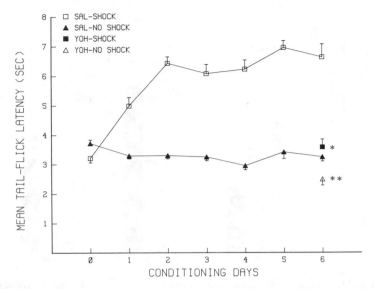

FIGURE 3. Mean (± SEM) tail-flick latencies 24 hr after footshock (open symbols, N = 18) or control manipulations (solid triangles, N = 16). On day 6 each group was halved and yohimbine (5 mg/kg) or saline was administered 30 min prior to the tail-flick test. *p < 0.01, **p < 0.05 versus the respective saline-treated group.

also lowered (p < 0.05) the basal responses of the control group. The reductions in autoanalgesia and the hyperalgesic effects of yohimbine suggest that this drug may be removing descending inhibitory influences to the spinal cord. Since alpha-2 adrenergic receptors are inhibitory to the release of NE,[22] the reversal of autoanalgesia by yohimbine may be linked to increased release and neuronal activity of NE in the CNS. In support of this interpretation, Westerink[23] has reported that 5 mg/kg of yohimbine increases NE turnover in several brain areas.

In order to determine whether yohimbine would reduce autoanalgesia when injected directly into the brain, stainless steel cannulae (24 gauge) were implanted into the lateral ventricle of 22 rats at the following stereotaxic coordinates[24] taken from bregma: A. − 0.5 mm, L. ± 1.5 mm, V. − 4.5 mm. After a recovery period of two weeks the rats were tested for autoanalgesia following footshock that was administered 10 min after the intracranial injection (5 μl) of yohimbine (10 μg) or saline. As illustrated in FIGURE 4, this dose of yohimbine did reduce (p < 0.01) the analgesia following the footshock. However, the analgesic response was not normalized, as it was following the systemic administration of the drug, and no hyperalgesia was observed in the BL-2 measures. In the second phase of this experiment, autoanalgesia was conditioned for eight days and intraventricular (ivt.) yohimbine (10 μg in 5 μl) was administered 10 min prior to the tail-flick test. From FIGURE 5 it may be observed that yohimbine did reduce (p < 0.05) the conditioned analgesia but did not restore the tail-flick latencies to baseline (p < 0.01 versus control group). Therefore it is apparent that yohimbine was not as effective when administered via the ivt. route as when injected systemically.

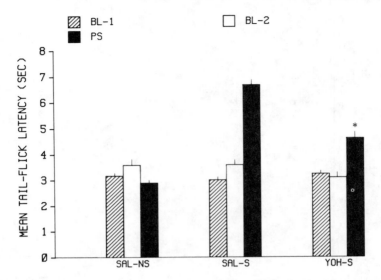

FIGURE 4. Mean (± SEM) tail-flick latencies prior to (BL-1) and 10 min after (BL-2) the intraventricular administration of yohimbine (10 μg, YOH) or 5 μl of saline (SAL). Solid bars (PS) represent the acute effects of footshock (S) or control handling (NS) in these groups. For SAL-S and YOH-S groups $N = 7$, while $N = 8$ in the SAL-NS group. *$p < 0.01$ versus SAL-S (PS) or SAL-NS (PS) groups.

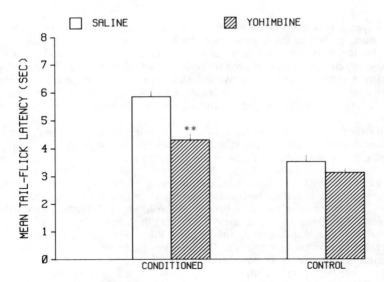

FIGURE 5. Mean (± SEM) tail-flick latencies of rats classically conditioned to exhibit autoanalgesia or control rats following (10 min) the intraventricular injection of yohimbine (10 μg) or saline (5 μl) on the previous day. For each group, $N = 7$. **$p < 0.05$ versus saline-conditioned group and $p < 0.01$ versus yohimbine-control group.

One reason for this difference may be that the ivt. dose was too small. However, 10 µg is a large dose for direct intracranial injection. In addition, yohimbine has been reported to be more potent in eliciting hyperalgesia at lower doses.[25] Another possibility for these differences in antagonsim of autoanalgesia may be that the alpha-2 receptors of the spinal cord must also be blocked to completely antagonize the analgesia. Resolution of these different possibilities will require dose-response analyses of intraventricularly and intrathecally administered yohimbine.

The next experiment investigated whether antagonism of alpha-adrenergic receptors with phentolamine or serotonergic receptors with methysergide would reduce autoanalgesia. The intrathecal administration of each of these drugs has been reported to reduce the analgesic effect of injecting morphine into the periaqueductal gray area of the brainstem.[26] In this experiment basal tail-flick latencies were determined for 29 adult male Sprague-Dawley rats. Phentolamine (10 mg/kg, i.p.; CIBA Pharmaceuticals, Summit, NJ), methysergide (10 mg/kg, i.p.; Sandoz Pharmaceuticals, E. Hanover, NJ), or saline was administered to separate groups ($N = 7$) of rats and tail-flick latencies were again determined 30 min later. Footshock (1 mA, 15 sec) was next given to the drug-treated and half of the saline-injected rats, with tail-flick latencies again being determined 10 sec later. As shown in FIGURE 6, significant analgesia was observed in all of the footshock groups. Thus neither of the drug treatments reduced the antinociception following footshock to a significant degree. This experiment was continued for four days to allow classical conditioning of the analgesia. On day 4, phentolamine (10 mg/kg, i.p.), methysergide (10 mg/kg, i.p.), or saline was again administered 30

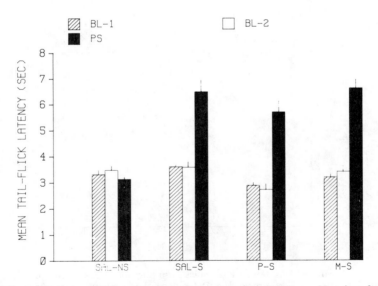

FIGURE 6. Mean (± SEM) tail-flick latencies prior to (BL-1) or 30 min after the administration of saline (SAL), phentolamine (P; 10 mg/kg), or methysergide (M; 10 mg/kg). Solid bars represent the tail-flick response 10 sec after footshock (S) or control handling (NS). For each group, $N = 7$.

min prior to the determination of antinociception. FɪɢᴜʀᴇF 7 illustrates that these rats exhibited significant acquisition of analgesia across these conditioning days. Although phentolamine had no significant effect on tail-flick latencies, conditioned analgesia was reduced by methysergide ($p < 0.05$) treatment. Thus, alpha-1 adrenergic blockade was ineffective in antagonizing autoanalgesia elicited by acute footshock or conditioned fear. However, even though methysergide had no significant effect on analgesia acutely elicited by footshock, it did reduce the conditioned analgesia assessed 24 hr after the last footshock. The data of these experiments employing neurotransmitter receptor blockers emphasize the significance of alpha-2 adrenergic receptors in mediating autoanalgesia and suggest a serotonergic input in the activation of endogenous antinociceptive mechanisms in the absence of footshock. These data are similar to a previous report of the lack of effect of phenoxybenzamine (alpha-1 antagonist) and effectiveness of BC-105 (serotonergic antagonist) in blocking analgesia elicited acutely by footshock.[27] Although we did not observe methysergide antagonism of analgesia immediately following the footshock, BC-105 may block acute stress-induced analgesia because of potency or receptor affinity differences. However, in other experiments, we have tested the efficacy of BC-105 (10 mg/kg, i.p., Sandoz) on the conditioned analgesia paradigm and have not observed any antagonism of the antinociception (BC-105: TF = 6.86 ± 0.14 sec; saline: TF = 7.51 ± 0.32; controls: TF = 2.52 ± 0.16 sec). At present we have no explanation for differences in effectiveness of these antagonists.

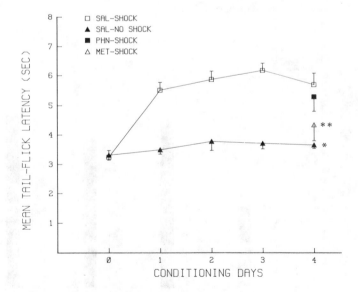

FIGURE 7. Mean ($\pm$ SEM) tail-flick latencies 24 hr after footshock (open squares, $N = 21$) or control handling (solid triangles, $N = 7$). On day 4 the footshock group was divided into three groups of seven rats each for the administration of saline, phentolamine (10 mg/kg), or methysergide (10 mg/kg) 30 min prior to the tail-flick test. *$p < 0.01$; **$p < 0.05$ versus SAL-Shock group.

EFFECTS OF SEROTONIN DEPLETION

In order to more fully investigate the role of endogenous serotonin (5-HT) neurons in autoanalgesic phenomena, CNS 5-HT stores were depleted in 21 adult, male, Sprague-Dawley rats by the injection (10 mg/kg, i.p.) of *para*-chloroamphetamine (PCA, Sigma Chemical Co.). We[28] and other[29] investigators have observed long-term reduction in brain levels of 5-HT and the metabolite, 5-hydroxyindoleacetic acid (5-HIAA), following a single systemic injection of PCA. In this experiment an additional 18 rats received control injections of normal saline. Baseline tail-flick latencies were determined on all rats 16 days after these injections. Following the baseline tests, footshock (1 mA, 15 sec) was administered to 12 PCA-treated and 10 saline-treated rats, with tail-flick latencies being determined again 10 sec afterward. As illustrated in FIGURE 8, both shocked groups exhibited significant analgesia following the footshock. This experiment was continued as the acquisition of conditioned analgesia was investigated across the next four days. FIGURE 9 shows that there was rapid acquisition of autoanalgesia by both PCA-treated and saline-treated groups. Therefore, the PCA treatment had no effect on either paradigm of autoanalgesia. To determine the degree and specificity of neurochemical changes following PCA treatment, each rat in this experiment was decapitated immediately following the tail-flick test of day 5. The brains were removed rapidly and dissected into forebrain and

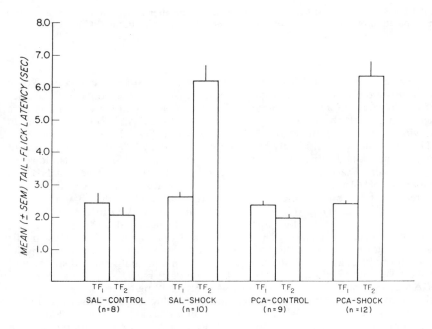

FIGURE 8. Mean ($\pm$ SEM) tail-flick responses prior to (TF_1) and following (TF_2) footshock or control handling of rats treated previously (16 days) with saline (SAL) or *para*-chloroamphetamine (PCA, 10 mg/kg).

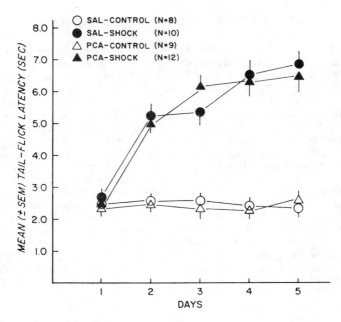

FIGURE 9. Mean (± SEM) tail-flick latencies 24 hr after a daily footshock or control manipulation of saline (SAL)-injected and *para*-chloroamphetamine (PCA)-treated rats.

brainstem areas by a vertical cut just anterior to the superior colliculus. These sections were frozen in liquid nitrogen. Following homogenization in 10 volumes of 1 N formic acid/acetone (15/85), amine neurotransmitter concentrations were determined by high performance liquid chromatography (HPLC) according to previously published procedures.[30,31] As indicated in TABLE 1, concentrations of 5-HT were reduced significantly by 66% and 5-HIAA by 72% in the forebrains of PCA-treated rats. Brainstem levels of both 5-HT and 5-HIAA were also lowered by 51% each. TABLE 2 suggests that forebrain and brainstem levels of NE and dopamine (DA) were not affected by the PCA treatment. However, there were increases in forebrain concentrations of the DA metabolites, 3,4-dihydroxy-phenylacetic acid (DOPAC), and homovanillic acid (HVA) in the PCA-shock group, perhaps due to the removal of 5-HT–mediated inhibition of DA neurotransmission.[32] Although we did not measure spinal cord amines in this experiment, we recently replicated this experiment to obtain those values. In the replication, PCA treatment again had no effect on autoanalgesia and spinal cord 5-HT levels were reduced by 49% (634 ± 23 ng/g versus 326 ± 54 ng/g) and 5-HIAA concentrations were lowered by 44% (352 ± 19 ng/g versus 197 ± 24 ng/g). Therefore these experiments demonstrate that reduction of CNS 5-HT and 5-HIAA by at least 72% to 44% had no effect on autoanalgesic phenomena. Thus these data do not support 5-HT as having a major role as a primary mediator of autoanalgesia. A similar absence of effect of 5-HT depletion on analgesia elicited by electric stimulation of the dorsal raphe nucleus has been reported.[33] In

TABLE 1. Tryptophan, Serotonin, and 5-Hydroxyindoleacetic Acid

Brain Area	Group	N	TRP (µg/g)	5-HT (ng/g)	5-HIAA (ng/g)
Forebrain	SAL-Control	8	3.3 ± 0.1	713 ± 38	361 ± 10
	SAL-Shock	10	3.2 ± 0.1	685 ± 29	375 ± 15
	PCA-Control	9	3.3 ± 0.1	235 ± 21[a]	103 ± 13[a]
	PCA-Shock	12	3.6 ± 0.1	247 ± 19[b]	103 ± 5[b]
Brainstem	SAL-Control	8	3.3 ± 0.1	1056 ± 47	667 ± 29
	SAL-Shock	10	3.3 ± 0.1	1067 ± 24	703 ± 22
	PCA-Control	9	3.1 ± 0.1	537 ± 27[a]	331 ± 13[a]
	PCA-Shock	12	3.2 ± 0.1	509 ± 13[b]	338 ± 8[b]

Mean (± SEM) forebrain and brainstem levels of tryptophan (TRP), serotonin (5-HT), and 5-hydroxyindoleacetic acid (5-HIAA) in adult male rats sacrificed three weeks after treatment with *para*-chloroamphetamine (PCA, 10 mg/kg, i.p.) or saline (SAL) and 24 hours after the last of four daily footshocks (1 mA, 15 sec).
[a] $p < 0.01$ versus SAL-Control and [b] $p < 0.01$ versus SAL-Shock.

addition, analgesia elicited by acute stress and assessed by the hot plate technique was potentiated when spinal cord 5-HT concentrations were depleted.[34] Differences in these results undoubtedly reflect differences in stressors and methods of of assessing analgesia.

EFFECTS OF CLONIDINE TOLERANCE

The alpha-2 agonist drug, clonidine, has been reported to elicit potent analgesia in rats.[35] Yohimbine has also been reported to effectively antagonize clonidine-induced analgesia, while the alpha-1 adrenergic antagonist, phenoxybenzamine, was without effect.[35,36] Thus clonidine analgesia has pharmacologic similarities with autoanalgesia. Therefore, in this experiment, we examined whether rats would exhibit analgesic tolerance to clonidine and the degree of cross-tolerance of these rats to autoanalgesia.

The duration of clonidine analgesia was assessed following the injection (i.p.) of 0.5 mg/kg ($N = 8$) or 1.0 mg/kg ($N = 8$) of the drug (gift from Boehinger Ingelheim, Ridgefield, CT) or normal saline ($N = 7$) into adult male Sprague-Dawley rats. Results from this test indicated that peak analgesia for both doses of the drug occurred 30 min after the injections. Analgesic tolerance to clonidine was induced in the next phase of the experiment by the continued administration of these doses of clonidine or saline to the respective groups across the next seven days. On each of these days tail-flick latencies were determined 30 min after the injections to indicate the development of tolerance. As indicated in FIGURE 10, significant analgesic tolerance did develop to clonidine. Although there was no difference between the different doses of the drug, the tail-flick latencies for both clonidine-treated groups decreased significantly ($p < 0.01$) across the eight test days. On day 9 a more stringent test of tolerance was employed by assessing the analgesic effects of 2 mg/kg of the drug in all treatment groups. Again, analgesic tolerance to clonidine is indicated in FIGURE 10 by the differential effects of this larger dose. Thus, the analgesic response of the saline group to 2 mg/kg of

TABLE 2. Effects of PCA Treatment

Group	N	TYR (μg/g)	DA (ng/g)	3-MT (ng/g)	DOPAC (ng/g)	HVA (ng/g)	NE (ng/g)
Forebrain							
SAL-Control	8	10.6 ± 0.6	1503 ± 44	15 ± 1	111 ± 3	103 ± 4	619 ± 22
SAL-Shock	10	10.1 ± 0.4	1470 ± 44	14 ± 1	111 ± 5	111 ± 4	652 ± 15
PCA-Control	9	11.2 ± 0.6	1504 ± 56	17 ± 1	133 ± 12	138 ± 19	627 ± 29
PCA-Shock	12	11.6 ± 0.5	1528 ± 39	18 ± 1	147 ± 5[a]	152 ± 5[a]	614 ± 19
Brainstem							
SAL-Control	8	11.8 ± 0.7	119 ± 9	11 ± 1	34 ± 2	47 ± 4	693 ± 53
SAL-Shock	10	11.5 ± 0.3	116 ± 4	10 ± 1	40 ± 2	48 ± 5	744 ± 35
PCA-Control	9	11.1 ± 0.2	117 ± 5	10 ± 2	36 ± 2	47 ± 6	708 ± 41
PCA-Shock	12	11.6 ± 0.4	103 ± 3	11 ± 2	33 ± 2	52 ± 6	712 ± 20

Mean (± SEM) forebrain and brainstem levels of tyrosine (TYR), dopamine (DA), 3-methoxytyramine (3-MT), 3,4-dihydroxyphenylacetic acid (DOPAC), homovanillic acid (HVA), and norepinephrine (NE) in adult male rats sacrificed 3 weeks after treatment with *para*-chloroamphetamine (PCA, 10 mg/kg, i.p.) or saline (SAL) and 24 hours after the last of four daily footshocks (1 mA, 15 sec).

[a] $p < 0.01$ versus SAL-Shock.

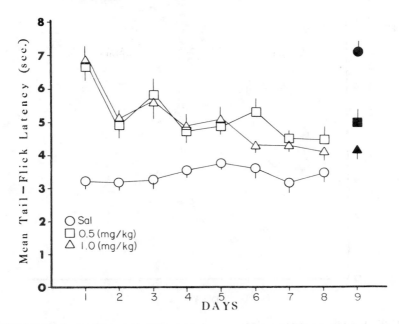

FIGURE 10. Mean (± SEM) tail-flick latencies of rats 30 min following the daily administration of saline, 0.5 mg/kg or 1.0 mg/kg of clonidine. On day 9, all rats were injected with 2 mg/kg of clonidine to assess analgesic tolerance. (From W.T. Chance. Life Sci. 1983. **33**:2241–2246. With permission from *Life Sciences*.)

clonidine was greater ($p < 0.01$) than that of either drug group. In addition, the differential development of tolerance was suggested by the greater analgesic response of the 0.5 mg/kg, as compared to the 1.0 mg/kg group ($p < 0.05$), to this larger dose of the drug. On the following day, cross-tolerance of clonidine analgesia to autoanalgesia was investigated. The effects of acute footshock and classically conditioned fear in inducing autoanalgesia were assessed in these animals according to methods described previously. Clonidine tolerance was maintained throughout the duration of these analgesic tests by the continued administration of 0.5 mg/kg or 1.0 mg/kg of the drug to the respective treatment groups. Since analgesia induced by classical conditioning procedures is very resistant to extinction,[8] it was possible to test all animals for autoanalgesia again eight days after the conclusion of the cross-tolerance tests. To reduce clonidine tolerance, no drug was administered during this time and no additional footshocks were given. The results of this cross-tolerance study are illustrated in FIGURE 11. Differential cross-tolerance to autoanalgesia elicited acutely by footshock is suggested by the tail-flick latencies following the footshock (day 1, filled symbols). Although the saline and 0.5 mg/kg clonidine groups did not differ, the analgesic response of the 1.0 mg/kg clonidine group was reduced significantly ($p < 0.01$) as compared to either of the other groups. A similar pattern of reduced autoanalgesia was observed in the conditioning phase of the

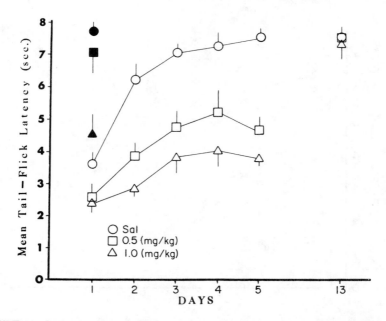

FIGURE 11. Cross-tolerance of clonidine antinociception to autoanalgesia. Open symbols on day 1 are mean (± SEM)basal tail-flick latencies of all groups. Solid symbols on day 1 illustrate the differential analgesic response of all groups to acute footshock. Tail-flick latencies on days 2–5 are the analgesic responses prior to footshock of tolerant and nontolerant groups. The responses on day 13 demonstrate autoanalgesia of the groups after a week of no drug or shock treatments. (From W.T. Chance. Life Sci. 1983. **33**:2241–2246. With permission from *Life Sciences*.)

experiment, with both clonidine-tolerant groups exhibiting significantly ($p <$ 0.01) less analgesia than did the saline group. Furthermore a repeated measures analysis of variance showed the 1.0 mg/kg group to have significantly ($p < 0.01$) shorter tail-flick response latencies than observed in the 0.5 mg/kg group, suggesting a greater degree of cross-tolerance. In addition, after eight days of no drug treatments (day 13) all groups responded to presentation of the conditioned stimuli with near maximal analgesia. Thus, after the clonidine tolerance had dissipated, autoanalgesic responses returned to values observed in nontreated subjects. Although little is known concerning the neurochemical basis of analgesic tolerance to clonidine, these results suggest that similar mechanisms subserve both clonidine analgesia and autoanalgesia.

In an attempt to generate data that might suggest neurochemical changes associated with clonidine tolerance, clonidine (1 mg/kg) was administered daily to 15 rats for 10 days. Tail-flick latencies were determined 30 min after each of these injections. On day 10 these clonidine-tolerant rats were divided into two groups and saline or clonidine (1 mg/kg) was administered, with the rats being sacrificed 30 min later. An additional 10 rats were sacrificed 30 min after their first injection of clonidine (1 mg/kg) and 18 rats were decapitated 30 min after an injection of normal saline. The results of this experiment are summarized in TABLE 3. As in the preceding study, analgesic tolerance was observed following the repeated administration of clonidine. The major neurochemical changes observed were increased ($p < 0.01$) brain levels of NE 30 min after the injection of clonidine and elevated concentrations of 5-HT ($p < 0.01$) in the clonidine-tolerant groups. Two-way analyses of variance indicated that statistically significant ($p < 0.01$) increases in both NE and 5-HT were associated with analgesic tolerance to clonidine. The changes in 5-HT levels may be due to decreased release and metabolism of this amine, since concentrations of 5-HIAA did not show parallel increases. Although the same interpretation may be true for the increase in NE associated with clonidine tolerance, the absence of metabolite data does not allow a specific explanation. Westerink[23] has reported decreased turnover of NE in several brain areas following the injection of clonidine, which would lead to increased levels of NE in the brain samples. Therefore it appears that clonidine tolerance may be associated with decreased CNS activity of both NE and 5-HT neuronal systems.

EFFECTS OF NOREPINEPHRINE DEPLETION

The effectiveness of yohimbine in atgaonizing autoanalgesia and the cross-tolerance of clonidine analgesia to autoanalgesia suggest a role of NE in mediating endogenous antinociception. To permit direct investigation of this hypothesis, acquisition of autoanalgesia was studied in rats in which endogenous stores of NE had been depleted by the intracranial injection of the neurotoxin, 6-hydroxydopamine (6-OHDA, Sigma Chem. Co.). In one group of adult, male Sprague-Dawley rats ($N = 7$), 6-OHDA (30 µg in 3 µl, free base) was injected bilaterally into the locus coeruleus (LC) through a 30 gauge needle at the following stereotaxic coordinates taken from the interaural line: A. − 1.6 mm, L. ± 1.1 mm and V. − 3.0 mm.[24] In another group of rats ($N = 8$), 6-OHDA was injected (200 µg in 20 µl) into the cisterna magna (CM) through a 27 gauge needle. Control rats ($N = 14$) were subjected to all experimental treatments except that no injections were made into the LC. One week after these treatments basal tail-flick latencies were determined for all rats. Ten seconds later all of the 6-OHDA and half of the control rats were subjected to footshock (1 mA, 15 sec). Tail-flick latencies were assessed again 10 sec after the termination of the footshock to determine the acute autoanalgesic response. Across the next six days, tail-flick latencies were determined prior to the footshock to measure the acquisiton of conditioned autoanalgesia. Immediately following the tail-flick test of day 6, each rat was sacrificed and the brain was removed and dissected into forebrain and brainstem sections. The spinal columns were dissected free and the spinal cords were blown free of the columns with compressed air. All tissues were frozen immediately in liquid nitrogen prior to their assay for amine neurotransmitter content by HPLC.

As illustrated in FIGURE 12, the acute analgesic response to footshock was reduced significantly ($p < 0.05$) in both LC and CM treatment groups. However, these tail-flick latencies were not normalized, with both LC ($p < 0.01$) and CM ($p < 0.05$) groups exhibiting significant analgesia. Similar intermediate responses were observed in the conditioned autoanalgesia phase of the experiment (FIGURE 13). Thus, the LC and CM groups were significantly ($p < 0.01$) less analgesic than the nontreated conditioned group. However, they did exhibit longer tail-flick

TABLE 3. Effects of Clonidine and Clonidine Tolerance on Tailflick Latencies and Neurotransmitters

Group	N	TF	NE	DE	5-HT	5-HIAA
Saline	18	3.58 ± 0.16	447 ± 9	848 ± 23	786 ± 12	479 ± 14
Acute clonidine	10	6.77 ± 0.40	547 ± 14[a]	855 ± 29	831 ± 24	469 ± 17
Clonidine-tolerant saline	8	3.12 ± 0.20	510 ± 17	858 ± 18	862 ± 22[a]	500 ± 23
Clonidine-tolerant clonidine	7	4.72 ± 0.40	578 ± 17[a]	895 ± 29	929 ± 33[a,b]	483 ± 27

Mean (± SEM) effects of clonidine (1 mg/kg, ip) and clonidine tolerance, induced by 10 days of clonidine treatment (1.0 mg/kg/day), on tailflick latencies (sec) and whole brain concentrations (ng/g) of norepinephrine (NE), dopamine (DA), serotonin (5-HT), and 5-hydroxyindoleacetic acid (5-HIAA) of rats.

[a] $p < 0.01$ versus Saline group.
[b] $p < 0.01$ versus Acute clonidine group.

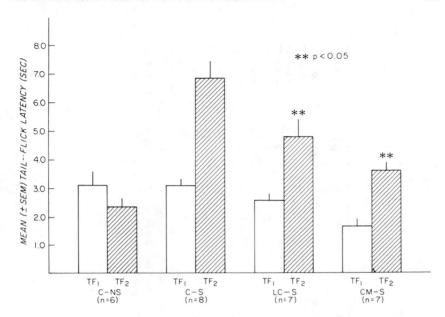

FIGURE 12. Mean (± SEM) tail-flick latencies prior to (TF$_1$) and following (TF$_2$) control handling (NS) or the administration of footshock (S) to rats injected previously (7 days) with 6-hydroxydopamine into the locus coeruleus (LC) or cisterna magna (CM). **$p < 0.05$ versus control shock group.

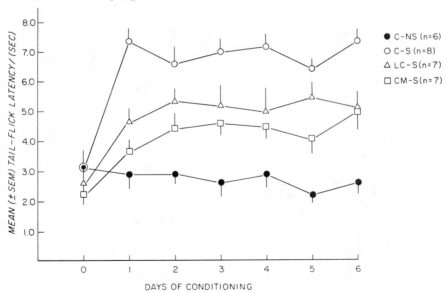

FIGURE 13. Mean (± SEM) tail-flick latencies 10 sec prior to the daily administration of footshock (open symbols) or control manipulations (filled symbols) in control (C) rats and 6-hydroxydopamine-treated (LC & CM) rats.

TABLE 4. Effects of 6-OHDA on Neurotransmitters

CNS Area	Group	N	NE	DA	DOPAC	5-HT	5-HIAA
Forebrain	C-NS	6	597 ± 16	1663 ± 60	149 ± 7	869 ± 30	399 ± 11
	C-S	8	632 ± 11	1707 ± 53	176 ± 11	957 ± 54	452 ± 28
	LC-S	7	235 ± 51[a]	1530 ± 101	138 ± 8	940 ± 62	437 ± 28
	CM-S	7	311 ± 54[a]	1181 ± 190	143 ± 10	939 ± 27	454 ± 22
Brainstem	C-NS	6	703 ± 17	163 ± 3	64 ± 5	1282 ± 27	620 ± 15
	C-S	8	705 ± 21	161 ± 3	55 ± 7	1242 ± 20	640 ± 16
	LC-S	7	336 ± 29[a]	158 ± 10	58 ± 3	1214 ± 57	634 ± 15
	CM-S	7	394 ± 32[a]	148 ± 8	68 ± 6	1284 ± 50	779 ± 53
Spinal cord	C-NS	6	418 ± 20	64 ± 2	24 ± 3	839 ± 30	300 ± 21
	C-S	8	474 ± 14	64 ± 3	21 ± 2	776 ± 14	288 ± 10
	LC-S	7	79 ± 18[a]	57 ± 3	23 ± 3	779 ± 31	283 ± 17
	CM-S	7	44 ± 18[a]	64 ± 2	26 ± 4	804 ± 28	292 ± 12

Mean (± SEM) concentrations (ng/g) of norepinephrine (NE), dopamine (DA), 3,4-dihydroxyphenylacetic acid (DOPAC), serotonin (5-HT), and 5-hydroxyindoleacetic acid (5-HIAA) in the forebrain, brainstem, and spinal cord of rats sacrificed 24 hours after footshock (S) or control manipulations (NS) and 14 days after the injection of saline (C) or 6-hydroxydopamine into the locus coeruleus (LC) or cisterna magna (CM).

[a] $p < 0.01$ versus C-S group.

latencies ($p < 0.01$) than did the nonconditioned control group. Examination of the neurochemical data (TABLE 4) indicates that the depletions of NE were specific to this neurotransmitter. The largest depletions of NE were observed in the spinal cord, with LC rats showing 82% reductions and CM rats exhibiting decreases of 90%. Forebrain and brainstem levels of NE were reduced to a lesser extent, with depletions ranging approximately 50% to 60%.

Although these results do not support NE as the sole mediator of auto-analgesia, they do suggest that normal levels of NE are necessary for the normal activation of autoanalgesic mechanisms. Watkins *et al.*[37] have investigated the role of spinal cord NE in stress-induced analgesia and report no effect of spinal NE depletion on acute footshock-induced analgesia or classically conditioned analgesia. These results may reflect major differences in the experimental paradigms. In the present experiment, levels of forebrain and brainstem NE were also reduced, which may increase the antagonism, while in the experiment reported in the Watkins *et al.* paper only spinal cord NE was depleted. Another major difference is that tail-flick latencies were detemined every min for over 10 min in the experiments reported by Watkins *et al.* Thus the possibility exists of tail damage confounding the results.

EFFECTS OF YOHIMBINE ON OPIATE-MEDIATED STRESS-INDUCED ANALGESIA

Terman *et al.*[38] recently reported that a variety of footshock magnitude-duration combinations could elicit opiate or nonopiate-mediated analgesia. Thus, continuous footshock at 2.5 mA for 1 to 2 min elicited analgesia that was blocked by naltrexone, while extending the duration to 4 to 5 min or increasing the intensity rendered naltrexone ineffective. In the present experiment, we replicated the opiate antagonism of continuous footshock-induced analgesia and investigated the effects of yohimbine in this same paradigm.

In this experiment, basal tail-flick latencies were determined on 18 rats. These rats were next treated with saline, naltrexone (5 mg/kg, i.p.; gift from Endo Laboratories, Garden City, NY), or yohimbine (10 mg/kg, i.p., Sigma Chemical Co.). Twenty to 30 min later tail-flick latencies were again determined, after which each rat was placed in a $30.5 \times 30.5 \times 30.5$ cm shock box and continuous footshock (2.5 mA) was administered for 90 sec. At the termination of the footshock each rat was removed from the box and tail-flick latencies were determined every min for the next 10 min, as described by Terman *et al.*[38] As can be observed in FIGURE 14, the footshock treatment elicited significant analgesia across the 10 min period. Although naltrexone did antagonize the analgesia a significant reduction in tail-flick latencies was not observed until the 4 min test. Yohimbine also antagonized the tail-flick response to footshock, with significant antagonism occurring at the 1 min tail-flick test. Thus, the alpha-2 adrenergic antagonist, yohimbine, was more effective in reducing this opiate-mediated analgesia than was the opiate antagonist, naltrexone. These data emphasize the problem with classifying a behavioral response as opioid solely on the basis of the effectiveness of opiate antagonist drugs. These results also continue to support the role of NE in at least mediating partially analgesia resulting from even severe stress. It should also be mentioned that the rats in the saline-shock group, and to a lesser extent in the naltrexone group, exhibited severe tail damage on the day following these tests. This observation again emphasizes, as have other investi-

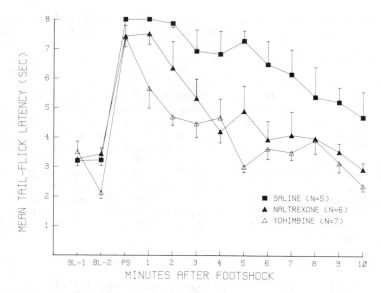

FIGURE 14. Mean (± SEM) tail-flick latencies prior to (BL-1) and following (BL-2) the injection of saline, naltrexone, or yohimbine. Footshock (2.5 mA, 90 sec) was administered to the rats after (20–30 min) drug treatments and tail-flick latencies were determined immediately (PS) and at 1 min intervals thereafter.

gators,[39] the possibility of confounding results due to heat or shock damage to the tail.

CONCLUSIONS

Much evidence is accumulating concerning the alpha-2 adrenergic receptor and descending inhibition of nociceptive reflexes. Yohimbine was reported to block tonic descending inhibition of spinal reflexes in the cat.[40] More recently the intrathecal administration of yohimbine antagonized antinociception elicited by electrical stimulation of the lateral reticular nucleus[41] or by the injection of carbachol into the nucleus raphe magnus.[42] In addition, injection of NE into the lateral reticular nucleus decreased tail-flick latencies,[43] suggesting that the ability of yohimbine to antagonize this reflex may be due to increased NE turnover. Conversely, the alpha-2 agonist, clonidine, reduces the release and turnover of NE and elicits analgesia. Therefore, activation of descending inhibition of nociception appears to be related, at least in part, to decreased turnover of NE.

In the experiments reported in this paper, yohimbine was the only treatment that consistently antagonized autoanalgesia. The reduction in this antagonism following the ivt. injection of yohimbine suggests that brainstem and spinal cord sites are perhaps more important than forebrain areas for this inhibition. The ineffectiveness of phentolamine indicates that antagonism of alpha-1 postsynaptic receptors does not yield similar blockade of autoanalgesia. Additional emphasis on the importance of alpha-2 receptors is also suggested by the cross-tolerance of clonidine analgesia to autoanalgesia. A role for NE in mediating autoanalgesia is also suggested by the partial antagonism of the analgesia by CNS NE depletion, which may have destroyed a portion of the neurons that subserve the behavior. Although methysergide reduced conditioned autoanalgesia, it was without effect immediately following footshock, suggesting subtle differences in these paradigms that may involve 5-HT. However, reduction of CNS 5-HT stores had no effect on autoanalgesic phenomena, indicating that it probably does not have a primary role in activating the analgesia. Considering that yohimbine has been reported to antagonize both 5-HT[20] and NE[21] neurons, it may present the ideal combination of receptor antagonism to completely block endogenous antinociceptive mechanisms. More research is required to separate putative NE and 5-HT mechanisms of autoanalgesia in the brain and spinal cord.

REFERENCES

1. BEECHER, H. K. 1959. Measurement of Subjective Responses. Oxford University Press. New York.
2. LIVINGSTON, W. K. 1953. Sci. Am. **88**:59–66.
3. MELZACK, R. & P. D. WALL. 1965. Science **150**:971–979.
4. MELZACK, R. & K. L. CASEY. 1968. Sensory motivational and central control determinants of pain. *In* The Skin Senses. D. Kenshalo, Ed.: 423–435. Thomas Press. Springfield, IL.
5. ROSECRANS, J. A. & W. T. CHANCE. 1976. Proc. Soc. Neurosci. **2**:919.
6. D'ARMOUR, F. E. & D. L. SMITH. 1941. J. Pharmac. Exp. Ther. **72**:74–79.
7. CHANCE, W. T., G. M. KRYNOCK & J. A. ROSECRANS. 1977. Fed. Proc. **36**:394.
8. CHANCE, W. T., G. M. KRYNOCK & J. A. ROSECRANS. 1978. Pain **4**:243–252.
9. CHANCE, W. T., A. C. WHITE, G. M. KRYNOCK & J. A. ROSECRANS. 1977. Eur. J. Pharmac. **44**:283–284.
10. AKIL, H., J. MADDEN IV, R. L. PATRICK & J. D. BARCHAS. 1976. Stress-induced increase in endogenous opiate peptides: concurrent reversal by naloxone. *In* Opiates and Endogenous Opioid Peptides. H. W. Hosterlitz, Ed.: 63–70. Elsevier/North Holland. Amsterdam.
11. MADDEN IV, J., H. AKIL, R. L. PATRICK & J. D. BARCHAS. 1977. Nature **265**:358–360.
12. CHANCE, W. T., A. C. WHITE, G. M. KRYNOCK & J. A. ROSECRANS. 1978. Brain Res. **141**:371–374.
13. CHANCE, W. T. & J. A. ROSECRANS. 1979. Pharmac. Biochem. Behav. **11**:643–646.
14. CHANCE, W. T. & J. A. ROSECRANS. 1979. Pharmac. Biochem. Behav. **11**:639–642.
15. CHANCE, W. T., G. M. KRYNOCK & J. A. ROSECRANS. 1979. Psychoneuroendocrinology **4**:199–205.
16. LEWIS, J. W., J. T. CANNON & J. C. LIEBSKIND. 1980. Science **208**:623–625.
17. WATKINS, L. R. & D. J. MAYER. 1982. Science **216**:1185–1192.
18. CHANCE, W. T. & M. D. SCHECHTER. 1979. Proc. Soc. Neurosci. **5**:607.
19. CHANCE, W. T. & M. D. SCHECHTER. 1979. Eur. J. Pharmac. **58**:89–90.
20. LAMBERT, G. A., W. J. LANG, E. FRIEDMAN, E. MELLER & S. GERSHON. 1978. Eur. J. Pharmac. **49**:39–48.
21. STARKE, K., E. BOROWSKI & T. ENDO. 1975. Eur. J. Pharmac. **34**:385–388.
22. ANDEN, N. E., M. GRABOWSKA & U. STROMBOM. 1976. Naunyn-Schmiedeberg's Arch. Pharmac. **292**:43–52.
23. WESTERINK, B. H. C. 1984. J. Neurochem. **42**:934–942.
24. PELLEGRINO, L. J. & A. J. CUSHMAN. 1967. A Stereotaxic Atlas of the Rat Brain. Appleton-Century-Crofts. New York.

25. PAALZOW, G. H. M. & L. K. PAALZOW. 1983. Naunyn-Schmiedeberg's Arch. Pharmac. **322**:193–197.
26. YAKSH, T. L. 1979. Brain Res. **160**:180–186.
27. SNOW, A. E., S. M. TUCKER & W. L. DEWEY. 1982. Pharmac. Biochem. Behav. **16**:47–50.
28. CHANCE, W. T., M. VON MEYENFELDT & J. E. FISCHER. 1983. Pharmac. Biochem. Behav. **18**:115–121.
29. SANDERS-BUSH, E., J. A. BUSHING & F. SULSER. 1975. J. Pharmac. Exp. Ther. **192**:33–41.
30. LOULLIS, C. C., D. L. FELTEN & P. A. SHEA. 1979. Pharmac. Biochem. Behav. **11**:89–93.
31. CHANCE, W. T., Y. BERLATZKY, K. MINNEMA, O. TROCKI, J. W. ALEXANDER & J. E. FISCHER. 1985. J. Trauma **25**:501–507.
32. DRAY, A., J. DAVIES, N. R. OAKLEY, P. TONGROACH & S. VELLUCI. 1978. Brain Res. **151**:431–442.
33. JOHANNESSEN, J. N., L. R. WATKINS, S. M. CARLTON & D. J. MAYER. 1982. Brain Res. **237**:373–386.
34. HUTSON, P. H., M. D. TRICKLEBANK & G. CURZON. 1982. Brain Res. **237**:367–372.
35. PAALZOW, G. & L. PAALZOW. 1976. Naunyn-Schmiedeberg's Arch. Pharmac. **292**:119–126.
36. FIELDING, S., J. WILKER, M. HYNES, M. SZEWCZAK, W. J. NOVICK & H. LAL. 1978. J. Pharmac. Exp. Ther. **207**:899–905.
37. WATKINS, L. R., J. N. JOHANNESSEN, I. B. KINSCHECK & D. J. MAYER. 1984. Brain Res. **290**:107–118.
38. TERMAN, G. W., Y. SHAVIT, J. W. LEWIS, J. T. CANNON & J. C. LIEBESKIND. 1984. Science **226**:1270–1277.
39. CHATTERJEE, T. K. & G. F. GEBHART. 1984. Brain Res. **323**:380–384.
40. KOSS, M. C. & P. J. BERNTHAL. 1979. Neuropharmac. **18**:295–299.
41. GEBHART, G. F. & M. H. OSSIPOV. 1984. Proc. Soc. Neurosci. **10**:98.
42. PROUDFIT, H. K. & M. S. BRODIE. 1984. Proc. Soc. Neurosci. **10**:99.
43. OSSIPOV, M. H. & G. F. GEBHART. 1984. Proc. Soc. Neurosci. **10**:98.

Opioid and Catecholaminergic Mechanisms of Different Types of Analgesia

E. O. BRAGIN

Laboratory of Neurochemistry and Histochemistry
Central Institute of Reflexotherapy
Moscow 103051, U.S.S.R.

The facts established by the experiments performed by several investigators are that different factors affecting human and animal organisms may frequently cause analgesia. A significant decrease in pain sensitivity occurs when a large spectrum of stress stimuli is in action (immobilization,[3] footshock, cold swimming stress,[4,7,8,10,39] insulin stress,[6,21] or 2-deoxy-D-glucose stress[5]). Besides these effects, significant analgesia was also observed under electrostimulation of different brain sites (periaqueductal grey, nuclei Raphe, reticular formation, thalamus, hypothalamus, etc.[1,22,44,45]), auricular and peripheral electroacupuncture,[9,10,14,24,31,32,37,41–43,50] vaginal probe,[15,25] sexual excitement, etc.[49]

In the investigations using a wide range of neurochemical agonists and antagonists, it was demonstrated that different neurochemical systems are participating in the mechanism of analgesia—opioid, catecholamine, and serotonin systems. However, there are a lot of conflicting points in the results of investigations aimed at studying the mechanisms of different types of analgesia. For instance, it is demonstrated that stress-induced analgesia is partly suppressed by naloxone,[28,29] but other investigators[19,40,52] do not report on naloxone effect in these cases. Conflicting results have been obtained in experiments studying the role of the opioid mechanisms in acupuncture analgesia,[11,31,32,41,42] as well as the analgesia elicited by periaqueductal grey (PAG) stimulation.[22,36] All these data indicate that analgesia caused by different stimuli might be mediated by different neurochemical mechanisms. The results of certain brilliant works[12,13,27–29,52,53,55–59] have shown that incorporation of different neurochemical systems into the mechanisms of analgesia depends on the type of stimulus: its intensity, localization, frequency, time of exposure, and biological significance. Because different types of stimuli may involve different volumes of cerebral neuroelements in the excitation process, one may think that in each case the morphological structure of the nociceptive and antinociceptive systems must be varied. The heterogeneous distribution of neurochemical elements implies that effects of different stimuli must also be followed by different degrees of activations of neurochemical mechanisms involved in the regulation of pain sensitivity.

Therefore, it becomes apparent that the analgesia, as well as pain excitation, occurring in each case might be mediated by a selective and specific morphoneurochemical mechanism.

The aim of this work was to study the selective and differential support of various types of analgesia and pain excitation by a complex of neurochemical mechanisms possessing specific neurochemical and morphological structures.

NALOXONE EFFECT ON THE ANALGESIA INDUCED BY SOME TYPES OF STIMULI

The present data concerning the role of the opioid systems in different types of analgesia mechanisms were obtained mainly from experiments using a systematically administered opiate antagonist. The results of these experiments have a lot of conflicting points. This fact first of all might be explained by different degrees of activations of opioid systems involved in different types of analgesia. Secondly, it is important that in a series of experiments different technical approaches were used for measurements of pain, and for this reason the interpretation of the obtained data was limited.

Therefore, in the first series of experiments to elucidate the functional significance of the opioidergic mechanisms, a comparative analysis of the naloxone effect on analgesia produced by auricular electroacupuncture (AEA), peripheral electroacupuncture (PEA), and footshock was performed.

Methods

The experiments were carried out on 40 rats (250–300 g weight). AEA (16 rats) was induced by electrostimulation of the *lung* point in the ear,[9,10,37] (current 0.8–1.0 mA, 1 msec, 15 min). PEA (10 rats) was carried out at the same current, but in *Zsu-san-li* point. Footshock was induced by direct current (2 mA, 8 impulses/min for 10 min). Pain sensitivity was evaluated by the latency period of the tail-flick reaction 10–12 min prior to the effect and after it at certain intervals. The animals were divided into two equal groups. The first received 10 mg/kg of naloxone-HCl intraperitoneally just after the tail-flick measurement. The second group received saline (control). All the results were estimated by Student's *t*-test for independent or paired samples.

Results and Discussion

The analgesia models of AEA, PEA, and footshock used in the experiments differed from each other by a number of parameters. In the first two cases the stimuli varied only by localization. In the last case the stimuli were of a higher intensity and frequency and also of different biological significance. This is supported by the fact that the animals' behavior under AEA and PEA stimulation roughly differs from the behavior during footshock. For instance, during AEA and PEA the rats are very calm, passive, sometimes sleepy. But the footshock was accompanied by vocalizations, high motor activity, and considerable aggression. However, FIGURE 1 shows that all the types of stimulation increase tail flick reaction as compared to the baseline in the saline-pretreated (dotted) and naloxone-pretreated rats (solid). The comparison of the results obtained in the control and experimental group after AEA or PEA shows that tail-flick latencies were significantly shorter in the naloxone-pretreated rats than in the saline-pretreated ones. In the rats subjected to footshock, naloxone significantly suppressed tail-flick latencies only at the fifth minute.

Therefore, the observed data suggest that the analgetic effects of AEA, PEA, and footshock are mediated by both opioid and non-opioid systems. FIGURE 1 shows that the degree of the antagonistic effect of naloxone depends on the type

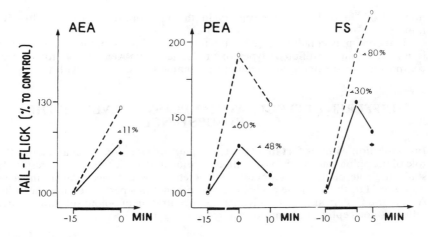

FIGURE 1. The influence of naloxone (10 mg/kg i.p.) and saline (i.p.) on the dynamics of the tail-flick reaction (compaired to control − Baseline) after auricular electroacupuncture (AEA), peripheral electroacupuncture (PEA), and footshock (FS). (♦), significant differences between naloxone and saline. (—), naloxone; (———), saline.

of analgesia; it has a slight effect on AEA analgesia and a more pronounced effect on PEA and footshock analgesia.

The degree to which opioid mechanisms are implicated in the analgesia can be explained by the fact that AEA and PEA stimulation differ only by the location of the electrode. The same results were obtained in the experiments[55,56] that demonstrated that shocking the rats' forepaws induced naloxone-reversible analgesia, but shocking the hindpaw or all four paws with the same current parameters induced the non-naloxone suppression of pain threshold.

FIGURE 1 indicates that at definite intervals of the recovery period, after the cessation of PEA and footshock, the antinociceptive effects are provided by mechanisms with different neurochemical elements. This is especially apparent in the footshock experiments. It is certainly demonstrated that naloxone prevents the analgesic effect beginning from the fifth minute, and does not influence analgesia at earlier periods.

The same results were obtained by the electrostimulation of PAG in the rat[36] and cold swimming stress.[4] In the experiments of the cold swimming stress at 8°C or 2°C, the analgesia wasn't prevented by naloxone for the first minutes of the recovery period, until after 30 min, when it reached its minimum values. In response to the extremely intensive stimulus, such as footshock or the PAG stimulation, the analgesic phenomenon is provided by a maximum number of a wide range of neurochemical systems. Thus, naloxone does not affect the duration of tail-flick latency at those periods of time. In the following intervals, the significance of non-opioid systems decreases and the role of opioid systems increases. This could explain the naloxone suppression of the analgesic effects of footshock at the fifth minute. These facts are in agreement with the data.[27,29,39] It has been demonstrated by Pert and Bowie[39] that cold swim stress increases the number of "loaded" opiate receptors in the rats' brain only at the 10–15th minute.

Thus, one may conclude that the functional significance of the opioid systems is not the same in different types of analgesia. Moreover, the neurochemical composition of the analgesic mechanisms changes dynamically with time.

DIFFERENT EFFECTS AT THE PLASMA LEVEL OF THE OPIOID SUBSTANCE

In connection with the fact that the experiments using naloxone characterize the role of the opioid mechanisms of pain formation and analgesia, it is interesting to study the role of those peripheral (extracerebral) opioid mechanisms in these processes. For this purpose a series of experiments was performed together with A. Pert and C. Pert, aimed at studying the concentration of opioid substances after different nociceptive and antinociceptive stimulations.

Methods

The experiments were performed on 48 rats divided into three groups. In the first group the rats were subjected to footshock (seven rats) and to sham footshock (seven rats).

In the second group, AEA (seven rats) and sham AEA (seven rats) was applied. The conditions were described in the previous chapter. In the third group, pain was induced by subcutaneous injection in the rear part of the hip of 1 ml 4% KCl solution (five rats), 12.5% formalin solution (five rats), 1% acetic acid (five rats), or saline (five rats).

Two minutes later the rats were decapitated and blood was gathered. Opioid peptides were extracted and their quantity measured by the radio-receptor method.[37]

Results and Discussion

The animals' behavior during AEA and FS is described in the previous chapter. After the subcutaneous injections of the irritative stimulus, squeaking, writhing, and licking of the injection site were noted, as compared to the control rats. Biochemical research (FIGURE 2) generalized data versus controls have shown that plasma Radioreceptor activity (RRA) content in the control rats was as follows: $2.49 \pm 1.17 \times 10^{-12}$ moles/ml for the first group and $2.47 \pm 0.44 \times 10^{-12}$ for the second group. In the experimental group the evident increase in the RRA material by 60% was noticed after footshock, but the changes were not significant after AEA or KCl or acetic acid injection. After prolonged footshock, plasma β-endorphin is also increased;[21,46] moreover, it is known that dexamethasone, which suppresses the peptide synthesis in the pituitary, prevents the effects of β-endorphin increases[47] and analgesia[10] during footshock. Thus, one may consider that the pituitary β-endorphin is involved in stress-induced analgesia. It has also been demonstrated by the experiments on the hypophysectomized animals. The suppression of the analgesic effect after the hypophysectomy was noticed in experiments using different stress models: footshock,[33] cold swim stress, and

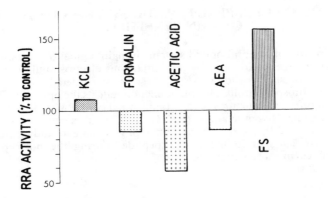

FIGURE 2. The level of the opioid material in plasma after nociceptive stimuli (subcutaneous administration of KCl, formalin, acetic acid, footshock) and auricular electroacupuncture. (♦), $p < 0.05$ for comparisons between footshock and sham footshock.

insulin shock.[5] However, hypophysectomy does not inhibit the development of analgesia in every case.[6] For instance, when morphine is used in the dosage of 1–2.5 mg/kg or in the shock induced by 2-dioxy-D-glucose at the dosage of 100–200 mg/kg, no differences between latency periods in the control and hypophysectomized rats were observed. Increasing the morphine dosage to 5–10 mg/kg or the 2-dioxy-D-glucose dosage to 400–600 mg/kg in the hypophysectomized rats enhanced the analgesia. Hypophysectomy does not affect the development of analgesia during the low intensity electrostimulation of the front paw of the rats.[59]

The same effect was displayed in the animals subjected to analgesia by conventional footshock.[59] In some cases the effects of footshock were different.[54]

The absence of changes in plasma opioid material after AEA indicates that the opioid mechanisms of the hypophysis are not involved in this kind of analgesia, and this correlates well with available data.[17] But is has been shown that in the case of stimulating *Zsu-san-li* points, hypophysectomy suppresses the analgesia.[43] Therefore, one may conclude that the pituitary opioid mechanisms are not always involved in the analgesia induced by different types of stress and acupuncture.

On the other hand, regarding footshock and AEA as nociceptive effects and comparing changes of plasma opioid levels caused by other effects (FIGURE 2), one may conclude that in the formation of pain excitation in each case a definite mechanism is involved. The findings suggest that different effects would have different impact on peripheral endorphin systems of the body. It is obviously connected with the fact that in response to different biologically significant stimuli the organism reacts by forming an antinociceptive system specific for this situation. Moreover, the morpho-functional and, consequently, the neurochemical structure of this system depend on the character of the triggering stimulus.

REACTION OF CEREBRAL PEPTIDE SYSTEMS TO THE DROP OF PAIN SENSITIVITY

The participation of cerebral opioid systems in pain regulation is testified to by the fact that analgesias induced by transcutaneous electrostimulation,[48,51] PAG stimulation,[23] footshock, and AEA[9,10,35,37] are accompanied by an increase of opioids in cerebrospinal fluid. This phenomenon reflects the opioid mechanisms' activation in different structures of the brain (spinal cord, PAG, medial thalamus (MT), basomedial hypothalamus (BMH), and letral septum (LS)). In the experiments with A. Pert and C. Pert an attempt was made to study the character of quantitative changes in the opioid peptides during the nociceptive and analgesic effects in those structures.

Methods

The experiments were performed on 57 rats (250–300 g). Footshock (six rats) and sham footshock (six rats), AEA (six rats), and sham (five rats) were effected through the methods described above. Moreover, the analgesia was induced in six rats by vaginal probe during 5 min[15,25] (constant pressure of 300–500 g for 5 min). The control group consisted of six rats. Electrostimulation (1.5–3 mA, 100 Hz, 50 msec, 5 min) of PAG of the midbrain by implanted electrodes (coordinates AP − 0.0 mm; L$^\pm$ 0.5; VD − 1.0 mm) was brought about in five experimental rats (control-sham stimulation in five rats). The experimental intensive pain was induced by thermal paw stimulation. The rats were put on a hot plate (60°C) for 3 min (six rats). The control group of six rats was exposed to the same conditions, but without thermal stimulation.

Pain sensitivity was measured by the latencies 10 minutes before and just after the procedure.

The cerebral substance extraction and the opioid substance quantitative measurement were performed by the method described by Pert et al.[37]

Results and Discussion

It was demonstrated that footshock, AEA, vaginal probe, and PAG stimulation induced an increase in the hot plate and tail flick reaction as compared to the control group of rats.

Biochemical analysis shows (FIGURE 3) that the drop of pain sensitivity is accompanied by a definite profile of correlation in the opioid concentrations in brain. For the PAG, MT, BMH, and LS structures, the respective values (expressed as the percentage of control values with ^{a} indicating a significant difference as compared to control) are: 70^a, 30^a, 40^a, and 130, after AEA stimulation; 102, 65^a, 100, and 81^a, after PAG stimulation; and 75^a, 114, 105, and 73^a, after vaginal probe. After nociceptive stimulation the values were 60^a, 48^a, 68^a, and 79 footshock and 117, 75^a, 80^a, and 108 for intensive thermal pain stimulation.

The sharp drop of the opioid level in SC was revealed only after the thermal pain effect.

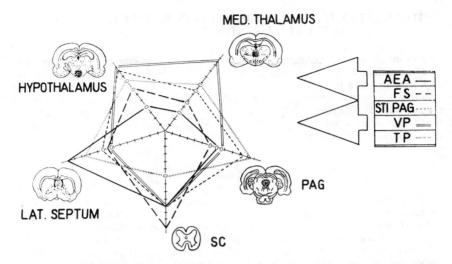

FIGURE 3. The morphological profile of the opioid systems after different stimuli. (AEA), auricular electroacupuncture, (FS), footshock, (STI PAG), electrostimulation of the midbrain PAG, (VP), vaginal probe, and (TP) thermic pain. (O), significant differences in the content of opioid material as compaired to appropriate control (sham stimuli).

A significant feature is that nonhomogeneous changes of the opioid substance concentration in different cerebral structures as a result of various stimuli are accompanied by analgesia.

The biochemical results show that the specific behavioral reactions of the animals, induced by certain external stimuli, are mediated by the antinociceptive mechanisms with a definite morphological structure in each case. As for the neurochemical mechanisms, particularly the opioid ones, the findings suggest that the character of the involvement and the specific contribution to the total systems' activity and to each structural unit have their own qualitative and quantitative specificity.

Hence, the character of the morphological profile of the opioid mechanisms' activity depends on and apparently is determined by the type of the effect and its specific parameters (location, intensity, frequency, biological significance, and the organism's functional condition). It is supported by our data obtained in the biochemical determination of β-endorphin in the pituitary and hypothalamus of the rat after low frequency (2 Hz) and high frequency (200 Hz) AEA. It has been shown that under AEA the content of β-endorphin in the pituitary had not changed as compared to control either at the high or at the low frequency stimulation. However, in the hypothalamus it was noticed that a low frequency AEA induces significant decrease of β-endorphin content to $128.5 \pm 17 \times 10^{-15}$ moles/mg as compared to the control ($213 \pm 35 \times 10^{-15}$ moles/mg). After the high frequency stimulation β-endorphin content was near the control level ($210 \pm 38 \times 10^{-15}$).

THE SYSTEMIC CATECHOLAMINERGIC MECHANISMS OF DIFFERENT KINDS OF ANALGESIA

The monoamine mechanisms as well as the opioid systems play an important role in different types of analgesia.[1,3,12,15,18,24,26,32,35] But the results of those experiments have the same number of conflicting points. The present series of experiments were carried out for studying the role of the monoaminergic regulation in different types of analgesia. The role of the catecholamine mechanisms in analgesia was studied using a systemic administration of catecholamine antagonists.

Methods

Four series of experiments in 84 rats were carried out. In the first series the antagonist of the β-adrenergic receptors, propranolol (5 mg/kg, i.p., five rats), or saline (five rats) was administered 15 min before AEA. In the second series the inhibitor of dopamine receptors, haloperidol (0.05 mg/kg i.p., 14 rats), or saline (14 rats) was injected 60 min before AEA or footshock. The footshock experiments were performed on seven rats treated with haloperidol and on seven rats treated with saline. AEA analgesia was induced in seven rats treated with haloperidol or in seven rats treated with saline.

In the third series of experiments 30 rats were divided into two equal groups and each group received AMPT (150 mg/kg) or saline 2.5 hr before the experiments. In the footshock experiments (carried out together with A. Pert) eight experimental and eight control rats were used. For studying AEA analgesia seven experimental and seven control rats were used. In the next series, eight rats received 6-OHDA (200 mg/kg i.p.) in order to inactivate the peripheral catecholamine systems. Another eight rats received saline. The experiments were carried out 1.5 week after the injections. The footshock and AEA parameters were described above. Pain sensitivity was estimated by hot plate and tail flick reactions.

Results and Discussion

TABLE 1 shows that the dosage of haloperidol that inhibits only the dopamine receptors also reduces the analgesic effect of AEA and footshock. This fact agrees with the results of the experiments on the rats subjected to the stimulation of PAG and peripheral electroacupuncture.[1,12] But there are experiments,[23] in which the analgesic effect was enhanced with the combination of acupuncture and haloperidol. The discrepancy between our results and the results of these experiments may be explained by different dosages of haloperidol and stimulation methods. The depression of the antinociceptive reactions was also discovered (TABLE 1) after the treatment of animals with propranolol. It is important to note that in the rats that received the inhibitors the suppression of the pain reactions after AEA and footshock was marked in later recovery intervals. Immediately after the cessation of AEA and footshock, the latency periods were higher than the baseline but did not differ from the control level. It suggests that in the first minutes of the recovery period the analgesia is provided by a complex of neurochemical mechanisms, but in later periods predominantly by the dopamine and β-adrenergic mechanisms.

TABLE 1. The Influence of Propranolol and Haloperidol on the Change in Pain Latency Periods Before and After Footshock and Auricular Electroacupuncture

	Baseline	Percent of Baseline (min)				
		0	5	10	20	30
Hot plate						
Saline + AEA	8.4 ± 1.1	253[a]	203[a]	232[a]	239[a]	171
P + AEA	8.9 ± 1.4	133[b]	100[b]	103[b]	100[b]	98
Only P	8.8 ± 1.4	133	106	120	120	108
Hot plate						
saline + FS	10.3 ± 1.4	540[a]	442[a]	–	520[a]	417[a]
H + FS	10.4 ± 0.9	521[a]	360[a,b]	–	257[a,b]	233[a,b]
Tail flick						
saline + AEA	5.2 ± 0.7	215[a]	–	180[a]	155[a]	142[a]
H + AEA	5.6 ± 0.7	200[a]	–	137[a]	120[a,b]	110[a,b]

[a] $p < 0.05$ for comparisons to baseline.
[b] $p < 0.05$ for comparisons of experiments rats to control (Student's t-test).
Propranolol (P), haloperidol (H), footshock (FS), and auricular electroacupuncture (AEA).

TABLE 2 shows that in the rats pretreated with AMPT, AEA and footshock do not cause reduction of analgesia. In other works, when catecholamine synthesis was depressed by AMPT or reserpine,[12] the depression of analgesia was noticed after high frequency stimulation of the acupuncture peripheral zones.

Since AMPT evokes the exhaustion of the catecholamine neurons both in the cerebral tissues and in the periphery, one may suppose that the absence of the inhibitory effect of AMPT on the development of analgesia is associated with the

TABLE 2. The Influence of AMPT on the Change of Pain Latency Periods before and after FS and AEA

	Baseline	Percent of Baseline (min)				
		0	5	10	20	30
Hot plate						
Saline + FS	11.2 ± 0.8	220[a]	193			
AMPT + FS	10.9 ± 0.8	252[a]	206			
Tail flick						
Saline + FS	3.5 ± 0.2	220[a]	160			
AMPT + FS	3.6 ± 0.4	214[a]	169			
Hot plate						
Saline + AEA	9.0 ± 0.9	145[a]	160[a]	126[a]	144[a]	141[a]
AMPT + AEA	10.3 ± 1.0	117	155[a]	138[a]	118	137[a]
Tail flick						
Saline + AEA	2.7 ± 0.2	148[a]	140[a]	133[a]	144[a]	133[a]
AMPT + AEA	3.1 ± 0.3	135[a]	132[a]	122[a]	112[a,b]	106[b]

[a] $p < 0.05$ for comparisons to baseline.
[b] $p < 0.05$ for comparisons of experiments rats to control (Student's t-test).

fact that the central and peripheral systems play different functional roles in this process. This assumption is confirmed by the experiments in animals subjected to chemical sympathectomy by intraperitoneal injection of 6-OHDA. It is shown (FIGURE 4) that in peripherally sympathectomized rats the analgesia after footshock is more marked than in controls. It agrees with the data[20] of experiments showing enhancement of the morphine and β-endorphin analgesia in adrenalectomized rats.

These results confirm the fact that under normal conditions the function of the peripheral catecholamine system is directed to the suppression of the antinociceptive reactions.

The findings indicate that under normal conditions the peripheral catecholamine system suppresses antinociceptive mechanisms.

But in the analysis of the dynamics of the footshock analgesia in sympathectomized rats, as well as in previous experiments, it was revealed that in the first moments after the end of footshock the tail flick reaction is significantly higher ($p < 0.001$) as compared to the initial period, and does not differ from the control. After 5 and 10 min latency periods were significantly higher ($p < 0.01$ and < 0.02) when comparing both to the initial period and the control. This also confirms that at different time intervals the antinociceptive mechanisms have different neurochemical structures, i.e. it changes dynamically in time.

THE ROLE OF THE CENTRAL NORADRENERGIC SYSTEMS IN ANTINOCICEPTIVE PROCESSES

The present study was undertaken to assess the role of central catecholaminergic mechanisms of analgesia induced by different types of stimulation. One of the structures responsible for catecholaminergic control of the antinociceptive processes is A-I nucleus of reticular formation, the catecholaminergic neurons of which project to the spinal cord.[16] Moreover, it has been shown[38] that lesions of

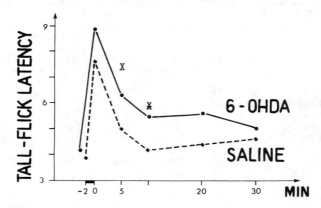

FIGURE 4. The role of the peripheral catecholaminergic system on the dynamics of tail-flick latency after footshock. (X), $p < 0.05$ and (X), $p < 0.01$ for comparisons between 6-OHDA (200 mg/kg i.p.) and saline.

catecholamine neurons of A-I lead to changes in the morphine-induced analgesia. The A-I lesion was considered to influence the analgesia induced by footshock, AEA, cold swim stress, and vaginal probe.

Methods

Fifty-five rats weighing 200–250 g, were used as subjects. Neurosurgical intervention was performed in anesthetized animals (8% solution of chloral-hydrate, 4.5 ml/kg; i.p.). Lesion of the lateral reticular nuclei (A-I) was carried out by injection of 6-hydroxydopamine (6-OHDA) (Sigma, 6 mg/2 ml), using the following stereotaxic coordinates: AP − 6.0; L$^{\pm}$ 2.0; VP − 3.2 mm.[34] The control group was injected with sterile saline (2 ml), at the same stereotaxic points of the brain.

The experiments were performed 12–15 days after surgery. Cold swim stress was induced by swimming in water (0°C) for a period of 3 min (12 rats: 6 sham and 6 lesion). The methods of AEA (5 sham and 5 lesion), footshock (9 sham and 9 lesion), and vaginal probe (8 sham and 7 lesion) were used as previously. Pain sensitivity was assessed by measuring the hot plate and tail flick latency. Norepinephrine concentrations in the brain and the spinal cord were determined in all the rats 24–36 hours after the experiments. The brains of five rats were histologically examined to locate the cannula.

Results and Discussion

Administration of the 6-OHDA in A-I led to a sharp decrease of nor-adrenaline only in the spinal cord. AEA or footshock (the footshock experiments were carried out in cooperation with A. Pert) did not cause any decrease in pain sensitivity as compared to the baseline (FIGURE 5). However, AEA and footshock result in a marked increase in hot plate and tail flick reactions in sham-operated rats compared to baseline and experimental rats (FIGURE 5). The results suggest that catecholamines of A-I and descending from them spinal systems play a leading role in the analgesia induced by AEA and footshock. A stronger stimulus, for instance cold swim stress, caused a significant increase in the latency period compared to the initial level immediately after the cessation of the stimulation (FIGURE 5). At the fifth minute after cold swim stress the latency period decreased and was significantly shorter than in sham-operated rats. This phenomenon suggests that the antinociceptive activation during cold swim stress and immedi-ately after its cessation are not mediated by catecholamine systems of A-I. At later intervals of the recovery period the significance of catecholamine A-I systems increases.

The vaginal probe (FIGURE 5) caused a significant increase in tail flick reaction in both groups of animals. However, a significant difference ($p = 0.05$) between lesioned and control rats was only estimated up to the end of the first minute. The lesioned rats showed a shorter tail flick reaction. During all the other intervals no differences were found between control and experimental rats. Thus, one may suppose that catecholamine systems of A-I, as well as of other neurochemical systems play an important role in the antinociceptive mechanisms activated by vaginal probe during the first minutes; but in later periods the analgesic effect is provided either by other chemical mechanisms of A-I or by other cerebral structures.

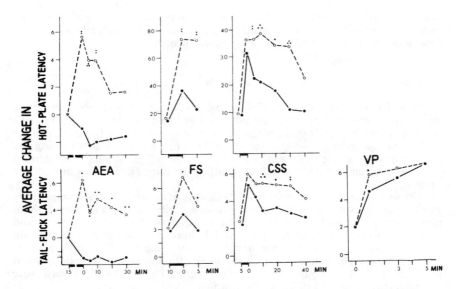

FIGURE 5. The effect of an A-I catecholaminergic lesion on the dynamics of pain reaction after auricular electroacupuncture (AEA), footshock (FS), cold swimming stress (CSS), and vaginal probe (VP). (———), lesioned rats and (– – – –), sham-lesioned rats. $^*p < 0.05$; $^{**}p < 0.02$; $^\ddagger p < 0.001$; $^{**}p < 0.002$ for comparisons between sham-lesioned and lesioned rats.

All these facts provide evidence for the existence of a dynamic process of formation of the antinociceptive mechanisms with selective involvement of neurochemical components that depend on the character of the stimuli.

The findings suggest that catecholamine systems of A-I and their projections to the spinal cord would be involved in the antinociception at AEA, footshock, cold swim stress, and vaginal probe. The functional significance of these systems in antinociception is not homogeneous in different types of stimulation. Alongside with catecholamines, other neurochemical systems are involved in antinociception formation. It is important that correlation between these systems and their specific roles in the final analgesic effect are different and depend on the type of the stimulus. Therefore one may suppose that the processes of involvement of the neurochemical systems in antinociceptive mechanisms depend on the specific thresholds of activation.

CONCLUSION

The neurochemical and neuropharmacological findings show that pain excitation and analgesia are mediated by the integral complex of mechanisms with a selective and dynamically changing neurochemical and neuromorphological structure that is determined by the type of the stimuli.

REFERENCES

1. AKIL, H. & J. LIEBESKIND. 1975. Brain. Res. **94**:279-296.
2. AKIL, H., J. MADDEN, R. L. PATRICK & J. D. BARCHAS. 1976. *In* Opiates and Endogenous Opioid Peptides. H. W. Kosterlitz, Ed.: 63-70. North Holland. Amsterdam.
3. BHATTACHARYA, S. K. 1978. Eur. J. Pharmacol. **50**(1):83-85.
4. BODNAR, R. & V. SIKORSZKY. 1983. Learn. Motiv. **14**(2):223-237.
5. BODNAR, R. J., D. D. KELLY, M. BRUTUS & M. GLUSMAN. 1978. Pharmacol. Biochem. Behav. **9**:763-768.
6. BODNAR, R. J., D. D. KELLY, A. MANSOUR & M. GLUSMAN. 1979. Pharmacol. Biochem. Behav. **11**:303-308.
7. BODNAR, R. J., M. GLUSMAN, M. BRUTUS, A. SPIGAGIA & D. D. KELLY. 1979. Physiol. Behav. **23**:53-62.
8. BODNAR, R. J., D. D. KELLY, A. SPIGAGIA, C. EHRENBERG & M. GLUSMAN. 1978. Pharmacol. Biochem. Behav. **8**:667-672.
9. BRAGIN, E. O. & R. A. DURINYAN. 1983. Pain **17**:225-234.
10. BRAGIN, E. O., G. F. VASILENKO & R. A. DURINYAN. 1983. Pain **16**:33-40.
11. CHAPMAN, C. R., C. BENEDETTI, Y. COLPITTS & R. GERLACH. 1983. Pain **16**:13-31.
12. CHENG, R. S. S. & B. POMERANZ. 1981. Brain Res. **215**:77-92.
13. CHENG, R. S. S., B. POMERANZ & G. YU. 1979. Life Sci. **24**:1481-1486.
14. CLEMENT-JONES, V., L. MCLAUGHLIN, P. J. LOWRY, G. M. BESSER, L. H. REESE & H. L. NEN. 1979. Lancet **8139**:380-382.
15. CROWLEY, W. H., R. JACOBS, J. VOLPE, J. F. RODRIGUEZ-SIERRA & B. R. KOMISSARUK. 1976. Physiol. Behav. **16**:483-488.
16. DAHLSTROM, A. & A. FUXE. 1965. Acta Physiol. Scand. **64**(247):5-36.
17. FU TSU-CHING, S. P. HALENDA & W. DEWEY. 1980. Brain Res. **202**(1):33-39.
18. GRIERSMITH, B. T., A. W. DUGGAN & R. A. NORTH. 1981. Brain Res. **204**:147-158.
19. HAYES, R. L., D. D. PRICE, G. J. BENNETT, G. L. WILCOX & D. J. MAYER. 1978. Brain Res. **155**:91-101.
20. HOLADAY, J. W., P.-Y. LAW, H. H. LOH & C. H. LI. 1979. J. Pharmacol. Exp. Ther. **208**:176-183.
21. HOLLT, V., P. PRZEWLOCKI & A. HERZ. 1978. Naunyn-Schmiedeberg's Arch. Pharmacol. **303**:171-174.
22. HOSOBUCHI, Y., J. ROSSIER, F. E. BLOOM & R. GUILLEMIN. 1978. Science **203**:279-281.
23. HOSOBUCHI, Y., J. ROSSIER, F. E. BLOOM & R. GUILLEMIN. 1979. Adv. Pain Res. Ther. **3**:515-523. Raven Press. New York.
24. JELLINGER, K. 1984. Deutsche Zeitschrift Akupunkt. **4**:77-93.
25. KOMISSARUK, B. R. & J. WALLMAN. 1977. Brain Res. **137**:85-107.
26. KULKARNI, S. K. 1980. Life Sci. **27**:185-188.
27. LEWIS, J. W., T. CANNON & J. C. LIEBESKIND. 1980. Science **208**:623-625.
28. LEWIS, J. W., J. E. SHERMAN & J. C. LIEBESKIND. 1981. J. Neurosci. **1**:358-363.
29. LEWIS, J. W., G. W. TERMAN, L. R. WATKINS, D. J. MAYER & J. C. LIEBESKIND. 1983. Brain Res. **267**:139-144.
30. MADDEN, J. H., H. AKIL, R. L. PATRICK & J. D. BARCHAS. 1977. Nature **265**:358-360.
31. MAYER, D. J., D. D. PRICE & A. RAFII. 1977. Brain Res. **121**:368-372.
32. MCLENNAN, H., K. GILFILLAN & Y. HEAP. 1977. Pain **3**:229-238.
33. MILLAN, M. J. 1981. *In* Modern Problems in Pharmacopsychiatry. H. M. Emrich, Ed. **17**:49-67. Basel.
34. PELLEGRINO, L. J., A. S. PELLEGRIN & A. J. CUSHMAN. 1979. A stereotaxic atlas of the rat brain. Plenum Press. New York.
35. PERT, A. 1982. Adv. Neurol. **33**:107-122.
36. PERT, A. & M. WELTER. 1976. Life Sci. **19**:1023-1032.
37. PERT, A., R. DIONNE, L. NG, E. BRAGIN, T. MOODY & C. PERT. 1981. Brain Res. **224**:83-93.
38. PERT, A., J. MASSARY, Y. TIZABI, T. L. O'DONOHUE & D. JACOBOWITZ. 1980. *In* Endogenous and Exogenous Opiate Agonists and Antagonists. E. L. Way, Ed.: 151-154. Pergamon Press. New York.

39. PERT, C. & D. L. BOWIE. 1979. *In* Endorphins and Mental Health Res. E. Usdin, Ed.: 145–161. McMillan Press. London.
40. PEZALLA, P. D. 1983. Brain Res. **278**:354–358.
41. POMERANZ, B. 1978. Adv. Biochem. Psychopharmacol. **18**:351–359.
42. POMERANZ, B. & D. CHIU. 1976. Life Sci. **19**:1757–1762.
43. POMERANZ, B., R. CHENG & P. LAW. 1977. Exp. Neurol. **54**:172–178.
44. REYNOLDS, D. V. 1969. Science **164**:444–445.
45. RICHARDSON, D. E. 1982. Appl. Neurophysiol. **45**:116–122.
46. ROSSIER, J., E. D. FRENCH, C. RIVIER, C. LING, R. GUILLEMIN & F. E. BLOOM. 1977. Nature **270**:618–620.
47. ROSSIER, J., E. FRENCH, C. RIVIER, T. SHIHASAKI, R. GUILLEMIN & F. E. BLOOM. 1980. Proc. Natl. Acad. Sci. USA **77**:666–669.
48. SJOLUND, B., L. TERENIUS & M. ERIKSSON. 1977. Acta Physiol. Scand. **100**:382–384.
49. SZECHTMAN, H., M. HERSHKOWITZ & R. SIMANTOV. 1981. Eur. J. Pharmacol. **70**:279–285.
50. TAKESHIGE, C., Y. KAMADA & T. HISAMITSU. 1981. Acupunct. Electro-Ther. Res. **6**(1):57–74.
51. TERENIUS, L. 1978. Ann. Rev. Pharmacol. Toxicol. **18**:189–194.
52. TRIKLEBANK, M. D., P. H. HUTSON & G. CURZON. 1982. Neuropharmacology **21**:51–56.
53. TRIKLEBANK, M. D., P. H. HUTSON & G. CURZON. 1984. Psychopharmacology **82**:185–188.
54. VIDAL, C., J.-M. GIRAULT & J. JACOB. 1982. Brain Res. **233**(1):53–64.
55. WATKINS, L. R., D. A. COBELLI & D. J. MAYER. 1982. Brain Res. **245**:97–106.
56. WATKINS, L. R., D. A. COBELLI, P. FARIS, M. D. ACETO & D. J. MAYER. 1982. Brain Res. **242**:299–308.
57. WATKINS, L. R., P. L. FARIS, B. R. KOMISSARUK & D. J. MAYER. 1984. Brain Res. **294**:59–65.
58. WATKINS, L. R., D. A. COBELLI, H. H. NEWSOME & D. J. MAYER. 1982. Brain Res. **245**:81–96.
59. WATKINS, L. R. & D. J. MAYER. 1982. Science **216**:1185–1192.

Neuropharmacological and Neuroendocrine Substrates of Stress-Induced Analgesia[a]

RICHARD J. BODNAR

Department of Psychology
Queens College
City University of New York
Flushing, New York 11367

The ability of a number of stressful and other environmental stimuli to elicit a transient analgesic response following acute exposure is well established[1] and serves as a useful, noninvasive means for activating intrinsic pain-inhibitory pathways. However, given the diversity in the profiles of the analgesic responses induced by such stimuli,[2-4] it appears that multiple pain-inhibitory systems exist. Two major dimensions by which analgesic stressors have been categorized are whether they are mediated by the endogenous opioids or by purely neural or neurohormonal mechanisms.[3] The physiological mechanisms subserving inescapable footshock analgesia are covered in other chapters of this volume; this chapter will focus on the physiological profiles of two other analgesic environmental stressors studied extensively by our laboratory: cold-water swims (CWS) and 2-deoxy-D-glucose (2DG) glucoprivation. Both stimuli produce increases in pituitary-adrenal stress responses, and also have the advantage of eliciting other measurable physiological responses in addition to analgesia. Therefore, by analyzing the analgesic and hypothermic responses following CWS, and the analgesic and hyperphagic responses following 2DG, one can determine whether a given manipulation is affecting analgesic pain-inhibitory systems selectively, or rather changing multiple responses to a stressor. The issues that will be reviewed are opiate involvement, neuroendocrine involvement, hypothalamic involvement, neuropharmacological profiles, and an interactive model of opiate and nonopiate pain-inhibitory systems.

OPIATE INVOLVEMENT IN CWS AND 2DG ANALGESIA

Since the initial interest in developing environmental models of analgesic systems was to identify the precise role of endogenous opioids in this response, we initially examined whether CWS and 2DG analgesia developed tolerance, developed cross-tolerance with morphine, and was reversed or attenuated by opiate antagonists. That CWS (2°C for 3.5 min) analgesia was the consequence of the stressful properties of the swim, and not an epiphenomenon of its hypo-

[a]Supported by National Institutes of Health grant AGO4425 and PSC/City University of New York grant 6-64187.

thermic or other nonspecific effects, was confirmed by the observation that the
analgesic, but not the hypothermic response adapted following chronic daily
exposure to the swims.[5] Although the time course of adaptation appeared to
mimic that of morphine tolerance, FIGURE 1 indicates the total lack of cross-
tolerance between continuous CWS analgesia and morphine analgesia.[6] Like the
effects observed for inescapable footshock analgesia,[3,4] this effect is dependent
upon the swim parameters employed: intermittent CWS elicits analgesia that
adapts with repeated exposures and is fully cross-tolerant with morphine.[7] The
nonopiate nature of continuous CWS analgesia was reinforced by our further
finding (FIGURE 2) that naloxone (1–20 mg/kg) failed to alter CWS analgesia.[8]
Again, subsequent studies showed that this effect was dependent upon the swim
parameters employed: exposure to intermittent swims produces a naloxone-

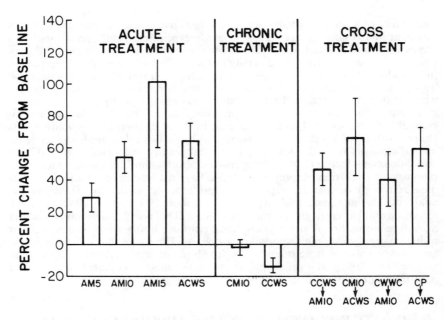

FIGURE 1. Lack of cross-tolerance between cold-water swim (CWS) analgesia and
morphine analgesia as measured by the jump test in rats. The ordinate displays the percent
change in jump thresholds from baseline with an increase over baseline indicating the size
of the analgesic effect. The left panel illustrates that the analgesic response following the
first day (acute) of exposure to CWS (ACWS) is equivalent in magnitude to that of acute
exposure to a 10 mg/kg dose of morphine (AM10). The CWS consisted of a 3.5 min swim in
a bath temperature of 2°C. The middle panel shows that chronic exposure to CWS (CCWS)
over 14 days results in adaptation in much the same way that chronic exposure to morphine
(CM10) over 14 days results in tolerance. The right panel shows that animals previously
exposed to CWS over 14 days (CCWS-AM10) display morphine analgesia that is
indistinguishable from analgesia elicited by acute morphine (AM10). Further, animals
previously exposed to morphine over 14 days (CM10-ACWS) display CWS analgesia that is
indistinguishable from analgesia elicited by acute CWS (ACWS). (From Bodnar et al.[6] With
permission from *Pharmacology, Biochemistry and Behavior.*)

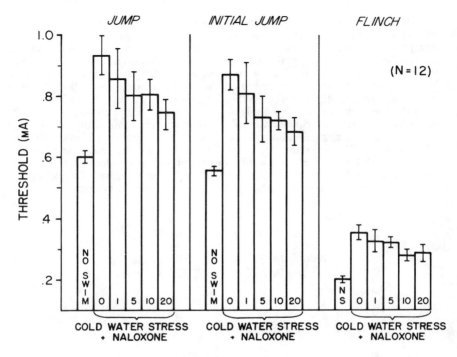

FIGURE 2. Inability of naloxone to significantly reduce the analgesia induced by cold-water swims (CWS) on the flinch-jump test. The ordinate displays jump thresholds of rats that were either exposed to a no-swim (baseline) condition, or were exposed to a CWS condition in conjunction with a vehicle or naloxone injection. Jump thresholds were assessed 30 min following the swim. The figure shows that while exposure to CWS without naloxone produced the greatest analgesic effect, no dose of naloxone (1, 5, 10, or 20 mg/kg) was capable of significantly reducing CWS analgesia. However, this effect may be subject to individual differences as described in the text. (From Bodnar et al.[8] With permission from *Pharmacology, Biochemistry and Behavior*.)

reversible analgesia.[9] Further, while continuous swims in a 2°C bath produced a nonopiate analgesia, continuous swims in a 15°C bath elicited analgesia that was reversed by naloxone.[10] Moreover, naloxone produced a partial antagonism of continuous CWS analgesia in some animals subjected to 2°C bath, but not in others. A significant positive correlation emerged between the magnitude of CWS analgesia and the ability of naloxone to partially antagonize this effect. This suggested that animals with small analgesic responses to CWS were activating nonopiate pain-inhibitory systems, while animals with large analgesic responses to CWS were activating both nonopiate and opiate systems with the latter affected by naloxone pretreatment.[10] The relative inability of naloxone to reverse CWS analgesia has also been replicated in mice.[11] The use of naloxone to discriminate definitively between opiate or nonopiate analgesic responses is problematic since it is short-acting and interacts with a number of opioid receptor subtypes. Hence, we then evaluated CWS analgesia following pretreatment with the irreversible and selective mu-1 receptor antagonist, naloxazone,[12] which eliminates supraspinal analgesia elicited by agonists of the mu, kappa, delta, and epsilon receptors.[12-14] FIGURE 3 shows that naloxazone pretreatment significantly reduced morphine analgesia, yet significantly potentiated CWS analgesia.[15] A reciprocal relationship emerged when rats were pretreated with a putative anti-enkephalinase, D-phenylalanine:[16] it potentiated the analgesic response following morphine, yet significantly reduced CWS analgesia.[17]

Like CWS analgesia, 2DG analgesia appeared to be the consequence of the stressful properties of glucoprivation and not an epiphenomenon of its other actions, since the analgesic, but not the hyperphagic response, adapted following chronic daily 2DG injections.[18] FIGURE 4 indicates that the analgesic responses following 2DG and CWS develop full and reciprocal cross-tolerance.[19] However, unlike CWS, 2DG appears to interact with opiate mechanisms in eliciting an analgesic response. FIGURE 4 shows that while morphine-tolerant rats fail to

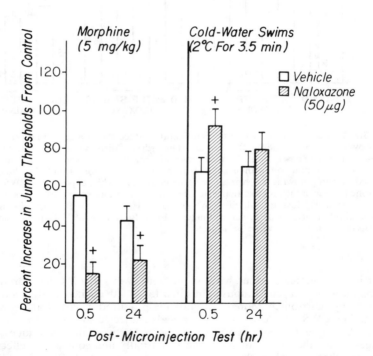

FIGURE 3. Naloxazone, an antagonist of the high-affinity binding site of the opiate receptor, produces differential effects upon opiate and nonopiate analgesia on the jump test in rats. The left panel indicates that the magnitude of morphine analgesia is reduced in rats pretreated with this opiate receptor antagonist. The right panel indicates that the magnitude of CWS analgesia is increased in rats pretreated with this opiate receptor antagonist. These data are discussed in support of a collateral inhibition model between different pain-inhibitory systems. (From Kirchgessner *et al.*[15] With permission from *Pharmacology, Biochemistry and Behavior.*)

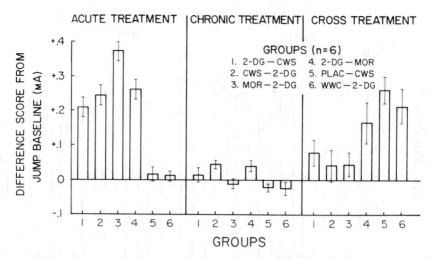

FIGURE 4. Reciprocal cross-tolerance occurs between 2-deoxy-D-glucose (2DG) and CWS analgesia and between 2DG and morphine analgesia on the jump test in rats. As in FIGURE 1, the left panel displays the increase in jump thresholds 30 min following acute exposure to either 2DG, CWS, or morphine. The middle panel indicates that chronic exposure to either 2DG, CWS, or morphine over 14 consecutive days (chronic) results in adaptation or tolerance to the analgesic responses. The right panel shows the following relationships. Rats exposed to 14 daily injections of 2DG fail to display CWS analgesia (Group 1). Rats exposed to 14 daily CWS fail to display 2DG analgesia (Group 2). Rats exposed to 14 daily injections of morphine fail to display 2DG analgesia (Group 3). Finally, rats exposed to 14 daily injections of 2DG display a significant attenuation in morphine analgesia. (From Spiaggia et al.[19] With permission from *Pharmacology, Biochemistry and Behavior.*)

display 2DG analgesia, 2DG-adapted rats exhibit a marked reduction in morphine analgesia. This is supported further by the analgesic synergy obtained by pairing subanalgesic doses of 2DG and morphine.[20] However, FIGURE 5 shows that 2DG analgesia does not appear to interact with the opiate system through the mu receptor since naloxone fails to alter this analgesic response.[20]

NEUROENDOCRINE INVOLVEMENT IN CWS AND 2DG ANALGESIA

The pituitary-adrenal axis is a critical locus for the mediation of many stress responses.[21] Given the nonopiate, yet stress-related actions of CWS analgesia, we initially examined whether CWS analgesia was present in hypophysectomized animals. FIGURE 6 illustrates that whereas intact and hypophysectomized animals display similar escape response patterns, acute exposure to CWS decreases escape responding in normal, but not hypophysectomized animals.[22] The reduction in CWS analgesia in hypophysectomized animals has been replicated over several nociceptive tests, but is not accompanied by concomitant changes in CWS

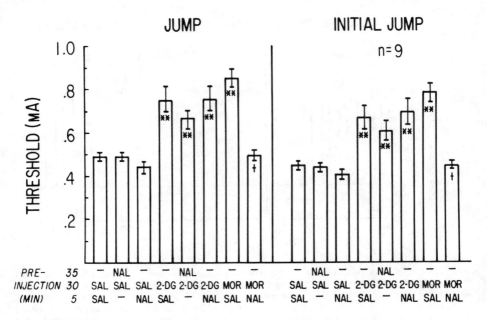

FIGURE 5. Inability of naloxone to significantly reduce the analgesia induced by 2DG on the jump test. The ordinate displays jump thresholds of rats that were either exposed to a 2DG (600 mg/kg, i.p.) or morphine (10 mg/kg, s.c.) in conjunction with a vehicle or naloxone (10 mg/kg, s.c.) injection. Jump thresholds were assessed 30 min following the injection. (From Bodnar et al.[20] With permission from *Pharmacology, Biochemistry and Behavior.*)

hypothermia. Since one of the major neuroendocrine responses to CWS is activation of the adrenocortical axis, further research examined whether this system was critical for the full expression of CWS analgesia. Several lines of evidence supported this notion. First, removal of the posterior and intermediate lobes of the pituitary gland failed to affect CWS analgesia.[23] Second, adrenalectomy potentiated CWS analgesia.[24,25] The reason why this latter finding is consistent with adrenocortical involvement in CWS analgesia is that glucocorticoid release produces negative feedback upon subsequent adrenocortical activity, particularly adrenocorticotrophic hormone (ACTH) release.[21] Third, adrenal demedullation and peripheral exposure to 6-hydroxydopamine, which produces peripheral catecholamine depletion, failed to alter CWS analgesia.[26] These treatments eliminate output from the sympathomedullary branch of the adrenal glands and suggest further that it is the adrenal cortex and not the adrenal medulla that is responsible for potentiated CWS analgesia following adrenalectomy. If the adrenocortical axis is important, then direct stimulation or interference with the negative feedback loop should also alter CWS analgesia. In this regard, CWS analgesia is reduced by administration of the synthetic glucocorticoid, dexamethasone, and is potentiated by corticosteroid synthesis inhibition.[25,27,28]

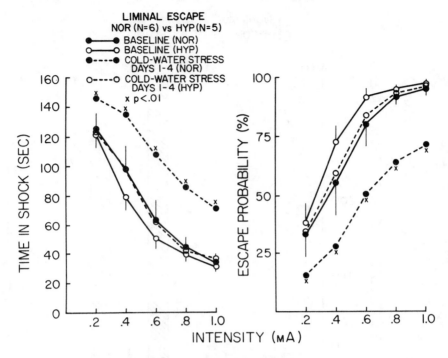

FIGURE 6. Total hypophysectomy attenuates the analgesic response to CWS on the liminal escape test in rats. To allow the hypophysectomized animals to survive in a normal laboratory environment, supplements of corticosterone, thyroxin, and electrolytes were administered. Such supplements were ineffective in altering CWS analgesia in normal rats. (From Bodnar *et al.*[22] With permission from *Physiology and Behavior.*)

    Although 2DG analgesia appears to be activated by the stressful consequences of glucoprivation, interruption of the pituitary-adrenal axis results in a different pattern of effects from that observed for CWS analgesia.[29] FIGURE 7 shows that hypophysectomized animals display marked potentiations in 2DG analgesia. Indeed, hypophysectomized animals also display the same potentiations following administration of morphine, indicating yet another similarity between 2DG analgesia and opiate analgesia. It should be noted that not all opiate-mediated analgesic stressors show the same pattern of neuroendocrine effects as morphine. For instance, while prolonged intermittent footshock analgesia is reversed by opiate antagonists and cross-tolerant with morphine,[30,31] it is reduced in hypophysectomized,[32,33] adrenalectomized, and adrenal demedullated rats.[34] Further, the opiate-mediated analgesia elicited by forepaw shock is not affected by neuroendocrine manipulations.[3] Thus, while opiate/ neural and opiate/neurohormonal classifications may serve to distinguish some forms of opiate-mediated stressors, there appear to be further dichotomies among them, including the relative contributions of the pituitary, the adrenal cortex, and adrenal medulla.

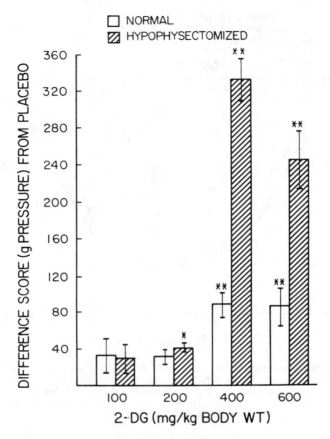

FIGURE 7. In contrast, total hypophysectomy potentiates 2DG analgesia on the foot pinch test across a range of doses. (From Bodnar et al.[29] With permission from *Pharmacology, Biochemistry and Behavior.*)

HYPOTHALAMIC INVOLVEMENT IN CWS AND 2DG ANALGESIA

The medial-basal hypothalamus regulates many homeostatic and autonomic anterior pituitary functions through the production and disposition of releasing factors delivered through the hypothalamohypophysial portal system.[35] Since the preceding data suggested a neuroendocrine, and particularly an adrenocortical modulation of CWS analgesia, one would expect that interruption of the functions of the medial-basal hypothalamus would produce similar effects to that observed following hypophysectomy. One noninvasive means of producing relatively selective destruction of the medial-basal hypothalamus is through the neurotoxic effects of neonatal administration of monosodium glutamate (MSG).[36] FIGURE 8 shows that neonatal MSG treatment reduces CWS analgesia in

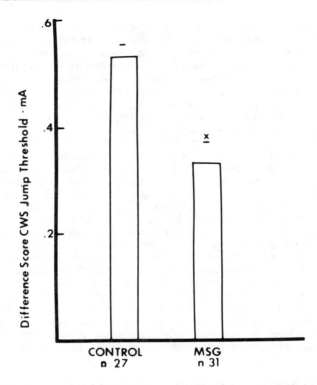

FIGURE 8. Neonatal administration of monosodium glutamate (MSG) to rats produces selective destruction of the circumventricular system, particularly the medial-basal hypothalamus. Such treatment profoundly decreases the analgesic response to CWS, indicating that this effect is dependent upon the integrity of the hypothalamohypophysial axis for its expression (From Badillo-Martinez et al.[38] With permission from *Neuroendocrinology.*)

adult rats in much the same way as hypophysectomy.[37,38] However, it should be noted that while hypophysectomy decreased CWS analgesia but not CWS hypothermia, neonatal MSG treatment produced similar shifts in both CWS analgesia and hypothermia. This suggests that MSG treatment produces more global changes in an animal's physiological responses to stress, rather than a selective effect upon a given endogenous pain-inhibitory system. Further work revealed that the physiological profiles underlying CWS analgesia and 2DG analgesia differed following manipulations of the hypothalamohypophyseal axis. Unlike the reductions in CWS analgesia, 2DG analgesia is potentiated in animals neonatally treated with MSG. Moreover, the analgesic potentiation is selective since it is accompanied by significant impairments in 2DG hyperphagia.[38] Given that neonatal MSG treatment resulted in both a potentiation in opiate-mediated 2DG analgesia and the elimination of both beta-endorphin and met-enkephalin perikarya in the medial-basal hypothalamus,[37,39] it would appear that different forms of opiate analgesia should be reduced by neonatal MSG pretreatment. However, effects of MSG treatment vary as a function of the opiate or opioid administered with decreases observed in analgesia on the jump test following morphine, no changes in analgesia following beta-endorphin, and potentiations in analgesia following D-ala-D-leu-enkephalin. The differential alterations of various forms of opiate-mediated analgesia by MSG appear to be due to changes in sensitivity among opiate receptor subtypes.[37,40,41] Again, the simple classification of opiate-mediated analgesia may not reflect the complexities in underlying mechanisms subserving stress-induced analgesia.

Several other questions emerge concerning the modulatory role that the hypothalamus-pituitary-adrenal axis plays in the mediation of some forms of stress-induced analgesia. For instance, it is not clear whether activation of this system by a given stressor initiates the analgesic response or maintains it after activation by central processes. In the latter case, the neural medial-basal hypothalamic mechanism could conceivably be the means by which short-duration neural signals of pain inhibition are translated into the longer-duration analgesic responses that are observed following some stressors. Indeed, the duration of some analgesic stressors sensitive to neurohormonal manipulations (CWS, 2DG) far outlast the transient effects of analgesic stressors sensitive to neural mechanisms (forepaw and hindpaw footshock). Other stimulation studies have also indicated the existence of a hypothalamic gating mechanism that controls noxious input in the brainstem.[42] Thus, when considering the role of different levels of the nervous system in some forms (particularly neuro-hormonally mediated forms) of stress-induced analgesia, the hypothalamic area must be considered in addition to the midbrain periaqueductal gray, the medullary nucleus raphe magnus, and the spinal cord dorsal horn.[43,44]

NEUROPHARMACOLOGICAL PROFILES OF CWS AND 2DG ANALGESIA

In addition to making a distinction between the opiate and nonopiate involvement in an analgesic response to a given stressor, three additional approaches have been employed: the neuroendocrine involvement that has just been reviewed, involvement of descending centrifugal mechanisms described previously for morphine and stimulation-produced analgesia,[45-47] and involvement of specific transmitter and peptide systems by the use of pharmacological interventions. Given the hormonal component of CWS and 2DG analgesia, research in our laboratory has centered upon the third approach rather than the second approach, which is reviewed elsewhere in this volume as well as in other reviews.[4,48]

A major emphasis in our recent research has centered upon the examination of the relationship between stress-induced analgesia, particularly CWS analgesia, and the vasopressin system. This interest was sparked by our initial work with Brattleboro rats, which are genetically deficient in vasopressin.[49] These animals were found to be hyperalgesic, and this effect could be corrected by peripheral treatment with a long-lasting vasopressin analogue. More importantly, FIGURE 9 shows that CWS analgesia is markedly reduced in the Battleboro rat,[50] yet morphine analgesia is unimpaired. Nonopiate CWS analgesia was linked further to a vasopressinergic mechanism by the discovery that vasopressin could elicit a nonopiate analgesic response.[51-55] While vasopressin analgesia is unaffected by

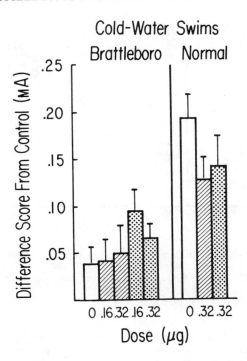

FIGURE 9. Failure of the Brattleboro rat, which is genetically deficient in vasopressin, to display CWS analgesia in the jump test in rats. (From Bodnar *et al*.[50] With permission from *Life Sciences*.)

either morphine tolerance or naloxone pretreatment, it is eliminated by pretreatment with a vasopressin antagonist.[52,53,55] Further, hyperalgesia can be induced in normal rats following pretreatment with an antiserum raised against vasopressin.[56]

The anatomical distribution of vasopressin makes it a viable candidate for the modulation of analgesic, and especially stress-related analgesic responses. Vasopressin-containing neurons from the hypothalamic paraventricular nucleus project to the posterior lobe of the pituitary gland, to the zona externa of the median eminence, and to extrahypothalamic structures, with the latter projection including pain control neurons in the midbrain, medulla, and the dorsal horn of the spinal cord.[57-59] Hypophysectomy fails to alter vasopressin analgesia.[51] This is not inconsistent with the observed reduction in CWS analgesia following hypophysectomy,[22] because vasopressin projects to the posterior lobe, which when excised results in a normal analgesic response to CWS.[23] The vasopressinergic projection to the zona externa of the median eminence appears to be indirectly involved in analgesic processes because MSG treatment eliminates this projection and potentiates vasopressin analgesia.[60] However, as illustrated in FIGURE 10, vasopressin analgesia is eliminated in animals with lesions placed in

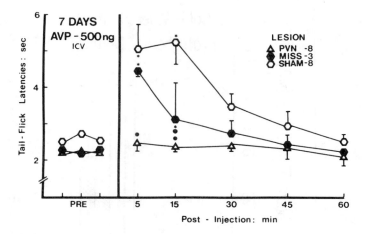

FIGURE 10. Failure of rats with lesions placed in the hypothalamic paraventricular nucleus to display vasopressin analgesia on the tail-flick test 7 days after the lesion. This effect was subsequently replicated in a second group of rats 35 days after the lesion.

the hypothalamic paraventricular nucleus.[61] Current work in our laboratory is determining whether similar effects are observed for CWS analgesia.

The role of catecholaminergic systems in CWS and 2DG analgesia has also been studied using neuropharmacological techniques. In this regard, it appears that norepinephrine and dopamine exert reciprocal actions upon the analgesic responses. If norepinephrine availability is increased by pretreatment with either clonidine, a noradrenergic receptor stimulant or desiprimine, a noradrenergic reuptake blocker, CWS analgesia is potentiated.[62,63] In contrast, lesions placed in the noradrenergic locus coeruleus decrease CWS analgesia.[64] Neuropharmacological manipulations with dopamine exert the opposite pattern of effects: dopamine receptor stimulation with apomorphine reduces both CWS and 2DG analgesia,[65] and dopamine receptor blockade potentiates both responses.[66] Interestingly, neither serotonin, which is intimately related to opiate analgesic mechanisms,[67] nor GABA alter CWS analgesia.[68,69] The effects of acetylcholine and thyrotropin-releasing hormone on both CWS and 2DG analgesia are reviewed elsewhere in this volume.

A COLLATERAL INHIBITION MODEL

In this review, many instances have been cited in which a given manipulation alters an opiate-mediated response and a nonopiate-mediated response in opposite ways. Given these dissociations, our laboratory[1,15] has proposed that a form of collateral inhibition exists between endogenous pain-inhibitory systems. Their very existence suggests that they respond differentially or specifically to incoming environmental stimuli, rather than the potentially maladaptive circumstance of immediate and equal activation in response to any nociceptive stimulus. A model of collateral inhibition would predict a parsimonious hierarchy of analgesic responses with less appropriate systems held in reserve. Thus, activation of one pain-inhibitory system (A) by endogenous or exogenous stimuli should inhibit the activity of another (B) with the magnitude of the effect dependent upon each system's tonic activational state and the magnitude of the activational stimuli. If the A system acts through the endogenous opioids, then it should be enhanced and reduced by respectively increasing and decreasing endogenous opioid levels. Concurrently, B analgesia would be modulated by endogenous opioid availability in an opposite manner. Thus, blockade of the mu-1 receptor with naloxazone reduces morphine analgesia and potentiates CWS analgesia. In contrast, increased availability of endogenous opioids following an antienkephalinase increases morphine analgesia and reduces CWS analgesia. Elimination of a crucial part of the B system should also disinhibit the A system. Thus, while hypophysectomy reduces CWS analgesia, it potentiates morphine analgesia. Similarly, a nonopiate form of footshock analgesia is potentiated by some manipulations that reduce an opiate form of footshock analgesia.[32,34,70] So, despite the existence of distinct heterogeneous pain-inhibitory systems, they appear to interact through an orderly process by which other pain-inhibitory systems are preserved for readiness in case an activated system fails.

ACKNOWLEDGMENTS

I would like to thank my students (J. Kordower, D. Simone, D. Badillo-Martinez, P. Butler, E. Sperber, E. Kramer, A. Kirchgessner, L. Truesdell, P. Mann, and M. Romero) for their unfailing support in this research.

REFERENCES

1. BODNAR, R. J. 1984. Types of stress that induce analgesia. *In* Stress-Induced Analgesia. M. Tricklebank & G. Curzon, Eds.: 19–33. J. Wiley. New York.
2. BODNAR, R. J., D. D. KELLY, M. BRUTUS & M. GLUSMAN. 1980. Stress-induced analgesia: neural and hormonal determinants. Neurosci. Biobehav. Rev. 4:87–100.
3. WATKINS, L. R. & D. J. MAYER. 1982. The neural organization of endogenous opiate and nonopiate pain control systems. Science 216:1185–1192.
4. TERMAN, G. W., Y. SHAVIT, J. W. LEWIS, J. T. CANNON & J. C. LIEBESKIND. 1984. Intrinsic mechanisms of pain inhibition and their activation by stress. Science 226:1270–1277.
5. BODNAR, R. J., D. D. KELLY, A. SPIAGGIA & M. GLUSMAN. 1978. Stress-induced analgesia: adaptation following chronic cold-water swims. Bull. Psychon. Soc. 11:337–340.
6. BODNAR, R. J., D. D. KELLY, S. S. STEINER & M. GLUSMAN. 1978. Stress-produced analgesia and morphine-produced analgesia: lack of cross-tolerance. Pharmacol. Biochem. Behav. 8:661–666.
7. GIRADOT, M. N. & F. A. HOLLOWAY. 1984. Intermittent cold-water stress analgesia in rats: cross-tolerance to morphine. Pharmacol. Biochem. Behav. 20:631–633.
8. BODNAR, R. J., D. D. KELLY, A. SPIAGGIA, C. EHRENBERG & M. GLUSMAN. 1978. Dose-dependent reductions by naloxone of analgesia induced by cold-water stress. Pharmacol. Biochem. Behav. 8:667–672.
9. GIRADOT, M. N. & F. A. HOLLOWAY. 1984. Cold water stress analgesia in rats: differential effects of naltrexone. Physiol. Behav. 32:547–555.
10. BODNAR, R. J. & V. SIKORSZKY. 1983. Naloxone and cold-water swim analgesia: parametric considerations and individual differences. Learning Motiv. 14:223–237.

11. O'CONNOR, P. & R. E. CHIPKIN. 1984. Comparisons between warm and cold water swim stress in mice. Life Sci. **35**:631–639.
12. PASTERNAK, G. W., S. R. CHILDERS & S. H. SNYDER. 1980. Opiate analgesia: evidence for mediation by a subpopulation of opiate receptors. Science **208**:514–516.
13. PASTERNAK, G. W. 1980. Multiple opiate receptors: (^{3}H)ethylketocyclazocine receptor binding and ketocyclazocine analgesia. Proc. Natl. Acad. Sci. USA **77**:3691–3694.
14. PASTERNAK, G. W. 1981. Opiate, enkephalin and endorphin analgesia: relations to a single subpopulation of opiate receptors. Neurology **31**:1311–1315.
15. KIRCHGESSNER, A. L., R. J. BODNAR & G. W. PASTERNAK. 1982. Naloxazone and pain-inhibitory systems: evidence for a collateral inhibition model. Pharmacol. Biochem. Behav. **17**:1175–1179.
16. EHRENPREIS, S., R. C. BALAGOT, J. E. COMATY & S. MYLES. 1979. Naloxone reversible analgesia in mice produced by D-phenylalanine and hydrocinnamic acid inhibitors of carboxypeptidase A. Adv. Pain Res. Ther. Vol. 3.
17. BODNAR, R. J., M. LATTNER & M. M. WALLACE. 1980. Antagonism of stress-induced analgesia by d-phenylalanine, an anti-enkephalinase. Pharmacol. Biochem. Behav. **13**:829–833.
18. BODNAR, R. J., D. D. KELLY, M. BRUTUS & M. GLUSMAN. 1978. Chronic 2-deoxy-D-glucose treatment: adaptation of its analgesic, but not hyperphagic properties. Pharmacol. Biochem. Behav. **9**:763–768.
19. SPIAGGIA, A., R. J. BODNAR, D. D. KELLY & M. GLUSMAN. 1979. Opiate and non-opiate mechanisms of stress-induced analgesia: cross-tolerance between stressors. Pharmacol. Biochem. Behav. **10**:761–765.
20. BODNAR, R. J., D. D. KELLY & M. GLUSMAN. 1979. 2-deoxy-D-glucose analgesia: influences of opiate and non-opiate factors. Pharmacol. Biochem. Behav. **11**:297–301.
21. AXELROD, J. & T. D. REISINE. 1984. Stress hormones: their interaction and regulation. Science **224**:452–459.
22. BODNAR, R. J., M. GLUSMAN, M. BRUTUS, A. SPIAGGIA & D. D. KELLY. 1979. Analgesia induced by cold-water stress: attenuation following hypophysectomy. Physiol. Behav. **23**:53–62.
23. GLUSMAN, M., R. J. BODNAR, D. D. KELLY, C. SIRIO, J. STERN & E. A. ZIMMERMAN. 1979. Attenuation of stress-induced analgesia by anterior hypophysectomy in the rat. Soc. Neurosci. Abstr. **5**:609.
24. GLUSMAN, M., R. J. BODNAR, A. MANSOUR & D. D. KELLY. 1980. Enhancement of stress-induced analgesia by adrenalectomy in the rat. Soc. Neurosci. Abstr. **6**:56.
25. MAREK, P., I. PONOCKA & G. HARTMANN. 1982. Enhancement of stress-induced analgesia in adrenalectomized mice: its reversal be dexamethasone. Pharmacol. Biochem. Behav. **16**:403–405.
26. BODNAR, R. J., N. S. SHARPLESS, J. H. KORDOWER, M. POTEGAL & G. A. BARR. 1982. Analgesic responses following adrenal demedullation and peripheral catecholamine depletion. Physiol. Behav. **29**:1105–1109.
27. MOUSA, S., C. H. MILLER & D. COURI. 1981. Corticosteroid modulation and stress-induced analgesia in rats. Neuroendocrinology **33**:317–319.
28. MOUSA, S., C. H. MILLER & D. COURI. 1983. Dexamethasone and stress-induced analgesia. Psychopharmacology **79**:199–202.
29. BODNAR, R. J., D. D. KELLY, A. MANSOUR & M. GLUSMAN. 1979. Differential effects of hypophysectomy upon analgesia induced by two glucoprivic stressors and morphine. Pharmacol. Biochem. Behav. **11**:303–307.
30. LEWIS, J. W., J. T. CANNON & J. C. LIEBESKIND. 1980. Opioid and nonopioid mechanisms of stress analgesia. Science **208**:623–625.
31. LEWIS, J. W., J. E. SHERMAN & J. C. LIEBESKIND. 1981. Opioid and non-opioid stress analgesia: assessment of tolerance and cross-tolerance with morphine. J. Neurosci. **1**:358–363.
32. LEWIS, J. W., E. H. CHUDLER, J. T. CANNON & J. C. LIEBESKIND. 1981. Hypophysectomy differentially affects morphine and stress analgesia. Proc. West. Pharmac. Soc. **24**:323–326.

33. MILLAN, M. J., R. PRZEWLOCKI & A. HERZ. 1980. A non beta-endorphinergic adenohypophysial mechanism is essential for an analgetic response to stress. Pain 8:343-353.
34. LEWIS, J. W., M. G. TORDOFF, J. E. SHERMAN & J. C. LIEBESKIND. 1982. Adrenal medullary enkephalin-like peptides may mediate opioid stress analgesia. Science 217:557-559.
35. KRIEGER, D. T. & A. S. LIOTTA. 1979. Pituitary hormones in brain: where, how and why. Science 205:366-372.
36. OLNEY, J. W. 1969. Brain lesion, obesity and other disturbances in mice treated with monosodium glutamate. Science 164:719-721.
37. BODNAR, R. J., G. W. ABRAMS, E. A. ZIMMERMAN, D. T. KRIEGER, G. NICHOLSON & J. S. KIZER. 1980. Neonatal monosodium glutamate: effects upon analgesic responsivity and immunocytochemical ACTH/B-lipotropin. Neuroendocrinology 30:280-284.
38. BADILLO-MARTINEZ, D., N. NICOTERA, P. D. BUTLER, A. L. KIRCHGESSNER & R. J. BODNAR. 1984. Impairments in analgesic, hypothermic and glucoprivic stress responses following neonatal monosodium glutamate. Neuroendocrinology 38:438-446.
39. ROMAGNANO, M. A., T. L. CHAFEL, W. H. PILCHER & S. A. JOSEPH. 1982. The distribution of enkephalin in the mediobasal hypothalamus of the mouse brain: effects of neonatal administration of MSG. Brain Res. 236:497-504.
40. BADILLO-MARTINEZ, D., A. L. KIRCHGESSNER, P. D. BUTLER & R. J. BODNAR. 1984. Monosodium glutamate and morphine analgesia: test-specific effects. Neuropharmacology 23:1141-1149.
41. BODNAR, R. J., T. PORTZLINE & G. NILAVER. 1985. Differential alterations in opioid analgesia following neonatal monosodium glutamate treatment. Brain Res. Bull. 15:299-305.
42. CARR, K. D. & E. E. COONS. 1982. Lateral hypothalamic stimulation gates nucleus gigantocellularis-induced aversion via a reward-independent process. Brain Res. 232:293-316.
43. FIELDS, H. L. & A. I. BASBAUM. 1978. Brainstem control of spinal pain-transmission neurons. Ann. Rev. Physiol. 40:217-248.
44. BASBAUM, A. I. & H. L. FIELDS. 1984. Endogenous pain control systems: brainstem spinal pathways and endorphin circuitry. Ann. Rev. Neurosci. 7:309-338.
45. MAYER, D. J. & D. D. PRICE. 1976. Central nervous system mechanisms of analgesia. Pain 2:379-404.
46. YAKSH, T. L. & T. A. RUDY. 1978. Narcotic analgesics: CNS sites and mechanisms of action as revealed by intrathecal injection. Pain 4:299-359.
47. GEBHART, G. F. 1982. Opiate and opiate peptide effects on brainstem neurons: relevance to nociception and antinociceptive mechanisms. Pain 12:93-140.
48. MAYER, D. J. & L. R. WATKINS. 1984. Multiple endogenous opiate and nonopiate analgesia systems. Adv. Pain Res. Ther. 6:253-276.
49. VALTIN, H. 1967. Hereditary diabetes insipidus in rats (Brattleboro strain): a useful animal model. Am. J. Med. 42:814-827.
50. BODNAR, R. J., E. A. ZIMMERMAN, G. NILAVER, A. MANSOUR, L. W. THOMAS, D. D. KELLY & M. GLUSMAN. 1980. Dissociation of cold-water swim and morphine analgesia in Brattleboro rats with diabetes insipidus. Life Sci. 26:1581-1590.
51. BERNTSON, G. G. & B. S. BERSON. 1980. Antinociceptive effects of intraventricular or systemic administration of vasopressin in the rat. Life Sci. 26:455-459.
52. BERKOWITZ, B. A. & S. SHERMAN. 1982. Characterization of vasopressin analgesia. J. Pharmacol. Exp. Ther. 220:329-334.
53. BERSON, B. S., G. G. BERNTSON, W. ZIPF, M. W. TORELLO & W. T. KIRK. 1983. Vasopressin-induced antinociception: an investigation into its physiological and hormonal basis. Endocrinology 113:337-343.
54. KORDOWER, J. H., V. SIKORSZKY & R. J. BODNAR. 1982. Central antinociceptive effects of lysine vasopressin and an analogue. Peptides 3:613-617.
55. KORDOWER, J. H. & R. J. BODNAR. 1984. Vasopressin analgesia: specificity of action and non-opioid effects. Peptides 5:747-756.

56. BODNAR, R. J., G. NILAVER, M. M. WALLACE, D. BADILLO-MARTINEZ & E. A. ZIMMERMAN. 1984. Pain threshold changes in rats following central injection of beta-endorphin, met-enkephalin, vasopressin or oxytocin antisera. Int. J. Neurosci. **24**:149–160.

57. NILAVER, G., E. A. ZIMMERMAN, J. WILKINS, J. MICHAELS, D. HOFFMAN & A. J. SILVERMAN. 1980. Magnocellular hypothalamic projections to the lower brain stem and spinal cord of the rat: immunocytochemical evidence for the predominance of the oxytocin-neurophysin system as compared to the vasopressin-neurophysin system. Neuroendocrinology **30**:150–158.

58. SWANSON, L. W. & H. G. J. M. KUYPERS. 1980. The paraventricular nucleus of the hypothalamus: cytoarchitectronic subdivisions and the organization of projections to the pituitary, dorsal vagal complex, and spinal cord as demonstrated by retrograde fluorescence double-labeling methods. J. Comp. Neurol. **194**:555–570.

59. SWANSON, L. W., P. E. SAWCHENKO, S. J. WIEGAND & J. L. PRICE. 1980. Separate neurons in the paraventricular nucleus project to the median eminence and to the medulla or spinal cord. Brain Res. **198**:190–195.

60. BODNAR, R. J., L. S. TRUESDELL, J. HALDAR, J. H. KORDOWER & G. NILAVER. 1984. Elimination of vasopressin analgesia following lesions placed in the rat hypothalamic paraventricular nucleus. Soc. Neurosci. Abstr. **10**:676.

61. BODNAR, R. J., L. S. TRUESDELL & G. NILAVER. 1985. Potentiation of vasopressin analgesia in rats treated neonatally with monosodium glutamate. Peptides **6**:621–626.

62. BODNAR, R. J., K. P. MERRIGAN & E. S. SPERBER. 1983. Potentiation of cold-water swim analgesia and hypothermia by clonidine. Pharmacol. Biochem. Behav. **19**:447–451.

63. BODNAR, R. J., P. E. MANN & E. A. STONE. 1985. Potentiation of cold-water swim analgesia by acute, but not chronic desipramine administration. Pharmacol. Biochem. Behav. **23**:749–752.

64. BODNAR, R. J., M. M. WALLACE, J. H. KORDOWER, A. KIRCHGESSNER, D. SIMONE, K. MERRIGAN, J. SCALISI & M. LATTNER. 1980. Analgesic responses to stress and opiates following selective destruction of either catecholaminergic, serotonergic or substance P pathways. Soc. Neurosci. Abstr. **6**:56.

65. BODNAR, R. J., D. D. KELLY, M. BRUTUS, C. B. GREENMAN & M. GLUSMAN. 1980. Reversal of stress-induced analgesia by apomorphine, but not by amphetamine. Pharmacol. Biochem. Behav. **13**:171–175.

66. BODNAR, R. J. & N. NICOTERA. 1982. Neuroleptic and analgesic interactions upon pain and activity measures. Pharmacol. Biochem. Behav. **16**:411–416.

67. MESSING, R. B. & L. D. LYTLE. 1977. Serotonin-containing neurons: their possible role in pain and analgesia. Pain **4**:1–21.

68. BODNAR, R. J., J. H. KORDOWER, M. M. WALLACE & H. TAMIR. 1981. Stress and morphine analgesia: alterations following parachlorophenylalanine. Pharmacol. Biochem. Behav. **14**:645–651.

69. BODNAR, R. J. & E. S. SPERBER. 1982. Cold-water swim analgesia following pharmacological manipulation of GABA. Behav. Neur. Biol. **36**:311–314.

70. KORDOWER, J. H., R. J. BODNAR, M. M. MANNING & W. H. SAWYER. 1983. Vasopressin analgesia: specificity of action and nonopioid effects. Soc. Neurosci. Abstr. **9**:202.

Involvement of Humoral Factors in the Mechanism of Stress-Induced Analgesia in Mice

PRZEMYSŁAW MAREK, IZABELLA PANOCKA, AND
BOGDAN SADOWSKI

Department of Behavioral Physiology
Institute of Genetics and Animal Breeding
Polish Academy of Sciences
Jastrzębiec, 05-551
Mroków, Poland

Since the demonstration that exposure to stressful stimuli decreases nociception in rodents, a great deal of effort has been expended to investigate the mechanism of this phenomenon. Most of this research focused on the involvement of newly discovered endogenous substances—opioid peptides—in mediating the analgesic effect of stress.[1,2] One of these substances (β-endorphin) was found to be released concomitantly with ACTH by the pituitary in response to experimental and traumatical stress.[3] The stress-evoked increase of β-endorphin blood level was prevented either by hypophysectomy or by pretreatment with synthetic gluco-corticoid, dexamethasone.[3,4] On the other hand, after adrenalectomy, increased levels of β-endorphin and ACTH were observed.[3] These results clearly demon-strated that the release of pituitary β-endorphin is regulated by a mechanism similar to that controlling the activation of the pituitary-adrenal axis in the stress reaction. Due to potent analgesic action,[5] β-endorphin became one of the putative mediators involved in stress-induced analgesia (SIA). Another indication of such a possibility was the finding that chronically repeated exposure to stress causes a gradual decrease of SIA similar to the tolerance produced by repeated opiate administration.[1] However, in the case of β-endorphin involvement in the mechanism of SIA, the antinociceptive effect of stress should have opiate-like character and so should be blocked by the specific opiate antagonist naloxone. The results of experiments investigating the influence of naloxone on SIA are conflicting. Naloxone pretreatment diminished analgesic effect of some stressors (immobilization and food deprivation), but not others (cold water swimming, 2-deoxy-D-glucose administration).[1,2] Additionally, as it was demonstrated by Lewis et al.,[6] even the single stressor, footshock, when delivered in different paradigms is able to induce either opiate or non-opiate analgesia. Prolonged (30 min) exposure to this stressor produced analgesia that was antagonized by naloxone and displayed tolerance and cross-tolerance with morphine analgesia, while the same criteria were not fulfilled with brief (3 min) footshock SIA.[7] The authors concluded that SIA is promoted by at least two separated mechanisms, one involving opioid peptides and the other not.

The existence of neurochemically separate pain inhibitory systems was also supported by a demonstration that analgesia induced by brief electrical stimulation restricted to the front paw is of opiate character, whereas the same type of shock on the hind paw evokes non-opiate analgesia. Such resolution was based on experiments applying naloxone and morphine cross-tolerance tests.[2]

The story of opioid involvement in SIA was further complicated by finding that both the number of shocks applied and the controllability of stress by the subject may determine the type of analgesia induced by electrical stimulation of the tail.[8]

Similar to the results of studies on opioid involvement, removal of the pituitary differentially affected analgesias induced by various forms of stress. The lack of effect of hypophysectomy eliminated the possibility of pituitary β-endorphin involvement in some forms of opiate SIA, including those evoked by front paw shock and conditioning to footshock.[2] Differential effects of the removal of the pituitary were also observed in non-opiate types of SIA. For example, this procedure attenuated cold water swimming SIA[9] and enhanced 3 min[10] but not affected 10 sec[11] footshock SIA.

All these data indicate that SIA is a complex rather than unique phenomenon and led Watkins and Mayer[2] to classify the forms of SIA into the four groups: neural opiate and non-opiate and humoral opiate and non-opiate. According to their criteria, in the rat pituitary β-endorphin may be involved in the mechanism of immobilization and prolonged footshock SIA only, both being opiate in nature and attenuated by hypophysectomy.

It must be noted that all the conclusions presented so far were based on experiments with rats, and care must be taken in extrapolating them to other species. A review of the literature reveals that the role of opioids in SIA mediation may differ even between closely related species such as rats and mice.

Generally, the SIA in the mouse shows greater susceptibility to the naloxone blockade independent of the kind of stressor used. It was demonstrated that in mice 1 mg/kg of naloxone completely blocks the analgesia induced by short (30 sec)[12] and long (10 min)[13] duration footshock. Additionally, 10 min footshock was incapable of producing analgesia in morphine-tolerant animals.[13] A still lower dose of naloxone (0.1 mg/kg) completely antagonized pain threshold elevation produced by 3 min room temperature water (20°C) swimming.[14] More recent studies have revealed that in mice warm water (32°C) swimming SIA is attenuated by naloxone and displays tolerance and cross-tolerance with morphine.[15] Briefly, up to the present naloxone was found to be effective in attenuating all the forms of SIA tested in mice including those evoked by social conflict,[16] food deprivation,[17] and immobilization.[18]

Results of several experiments implicated the role of the hypophysis in pain modulatory mechanisms in mice. Thus the integrity of the pituitary was shown to be crucial for the appearance of naloxone hyperalgesia.[19] Moreover, acupuncture analgesia was shown to be attenuated either after hypophysectomy[20] or dexamethasone pretreatment.[21]

Bearing these results in mind, we decided to test the influence of adrenalectomy and dexamethasone pretreatment on room temperature water swimming SIA in mice. We have chosen this form of SIA because of its opiate character by which it differed from cold water swimming SIA in rats (only partially blocked by 20 mg/kg of naloxone).[1]

Animals were randomly divided into two groups. In the first group (ADREX) a bilateral adrenalectomy was performed under ether anesthesia. Animals from the second group (SHAM) were assigned as controls and subjected to a sham operation that consisted of incising and suturing the skin without removing the glands.

A day before the operation all animals were exposed to a 3 min room temperature (21°C) water swimming stress. Prior to swimming and two minutes after its termination, pain threshold was estimated by means of the hot plate method. The temperature of the plate was kept at 56°C and the hind paw flick was regarded as a pain reaction. Animals not responding within 60 sec (cut-off time) were removed from the plate.

Both swimming and testing the pre- and poststress nociceptive threshold were repeated on the eighth and ninth postoperative days. On the eighth day, all animals were preinjected intraperitoneally with a 0.9% NaCl solution. On the ninth day, part of both groups received dexamethasone (Decadron Phosphate, Merck Sharp and Dohme) at a dose of 0.5 mg/kg, while others were preinjected again with saline. All injections were given 100 min before the estimation of the prestress pain threshold because of the finding that a similar dexamethasone protocol reversed opiate hypersensitivity in adrenalectomized mice.[22]

The results of the experiment are presented in FIGURE 1. Exposure to swimming caused significant (by about 255%) increase of hind paw flick latencies. This analgesic effect of swimming was even more potent than that originally observed by Willow et al.[14] who reported 79% of increase in hind paw flick latencies. Such comparison is admittable since both stress and hot plate parameters applied by these authors were almost identical with ours. We assume that such differences might result from using different strains of mice (QS by Willow et al.[14] and CFW by us).

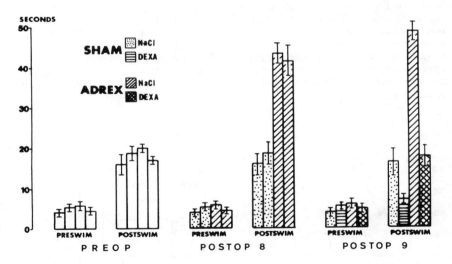

FIGURE 1. Hind paw flick latencies (±SEM) before and after 3 min room temperature water swimming: preop = before the surgery, postop 8 and postop 9 = on the eighth and the ninth day following the removal of adrenals (ADREX) or after sham adrenalectomy (SHAM). Each group was labeled according to the surgery and preinjection with dexamethasone (DEXA) or 0.9% NaCl (NaCl) on the ninth postoperative day. All animals were preinjected with saline on the eighth day. The statistical significance of both adrenalectomy and dexamethasone effects was confirmed by three-way analysis of variance (in all groups $p < 0.001$, details described elsewhere[30]).

On the eighth postoperative day the magnitude of postswim analgesia was similar to that observed during the preoperative test in sham-operated, but significantly increased in adrenalectomized animals. The adrenalectomy enhancement of analgesia was also observed on the ninth postoperative day in mice receiving saline injections, but was completely reversed in those receiving dexamethasone. An even more potent effect of this synthetic glucocorticoid was noted in sham-operated animals in which it completely blocked the swim-induced analgesia. Interestingly, neither adrenalectomy nor dexamethasone influenced the baseline pain reaction latencies, which remained at the same level in all groups throughout the course of the experiment.

The results of the first experiment indicated that the mechanism of swimming SIA in mice may depend on the activation of the pituitary-adrenal axis. However, the question has arisen as to whether such effects of adrenalectomy and dexamethasone are not specific for this form of stress. Therefore we undertook the next experiment to test the influence of adrenalectomy and dexamethasone on 10 min footshock SIA, determined by Chesher and Chan to be opiate.[13]

The surgery, pharmacological treatment, and analgesimetric test were the same as those used in the previous experiment, but the protocol was modified by using non-repeated measures and adding the group of non-operated animals.

Each mouse was exposed to 10 min footshock (0.5 mA rms) delivered in 10 sec on/10 sec off schedule. Pain threshold was assayed just before and immediately after the stress termination.

As shown in FIGURE 2, exposure to footshock caused significant increase in hind paw flick latencies in all animals' groups receiving saline injections. This analgesic action of footshock did not differ between sham and intact animals, but was significantly enhanced in mice with adrenal glands removed. Dexamethasone pretreatment significantly decreased the analgesic action of footshock in sham-operated and adrenalectomized animals and completely blocked the appearance of analgesia in intact animals. As in the first experiment, neither adrenalectomy nor dexamethasone pretreatment influenced the baseline pain sensitivity.

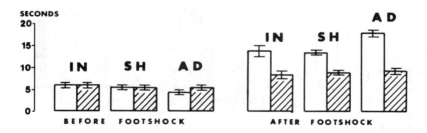

FIGURE 2. Hind paw flick latencies (±SEM) before and after 10 min footshock in intact (IN), adrenalectomized (AD), and sham-operated (SH) mice. White columns = animals pretreated with 0.9% NaCl and dashed columns = animals pretreated with dexamethasone. Three-way analysis of variance revealed that adrenalectomized animals displayed greater analgesia in comparison with intact and sham-operated ones ($p < 0.001$). The analgesic effect of footshock was significantly decreased after dexamethasone administration ($p < 0.05$, details described elsewhere[31]).

The results of both experiments suggest involvement of the pituitary-adrenal axis in the mechanism of SIA in mice. Such involvement is especially interesting since pain threshold elevation induced by both stressors was shown to be blocked completely by naloxone.[13,14] Since Chesher and Chan, who originally demonstrated opiate character of footshock analgesia in mice applied the abdominal constriction response as the only analgesimetric test,[13] we carried out an experiment in which we confirmed the opiate character of 10 min footshock SIA by blocking it with 1 mg/kg of naloxone (Naloxone hydrochloride, Endo Laboratories) in the hot plate test (FIGURE 3).

The observation of a parallel dexamethasone and naloxone attenuation of SIA forms an interesting comparison with the rat in which only severe footshock SIA was blocked by naloxone and dexamethasone.[6] In the rat brief (up to 3 min) footshock SIA is completely resistant to 10 mg[6] while cold water swimming SIA is only partially reversed by 20 mg/kg of naloxone.[1] The species specificity in the mechanism of SIA is also indicated by different stress susceptibility of rats and mice with regard to analgesic response. Thus, room temperature swimming procedure is unable to induce analgesia in the rat in which cold water (2, 8, or 15°C) is necessary.[9]

Although the dexamethasone and adrenalectomy effects observed in both experiments may suggest involvement of pituitary β-endorphin in SIA mechanism in mice, several data argue against such resolution. First adrenalectomy per se increases circulating β-endorphin concentration.[3] Thus, in the case of pituitary β-endorphin mediation in SIA we should also expect a baseline pain threshold increase. However, such effect was not observed either in the first or second experiment. The lack of change in the baseline pain sensitivity in adrenalectomized mice is in agreement with reports of Holaday et al. who suggested that it may result from the development of functional tolerance.[22] It must be noted that both experiments were carried out eight days after adrenalectomy.

Another argument against involvement of pituitary β-endorphin in SIA was based on the finding that the intravenous doses of this peptide necessary to produce analgesia are unphysiologically high.[23] An interesting resolution of this paradox was proposed by Lewis et al. who hypothesized that analgesic concentration of pituitary opioids may be reached in the brain areas responsible for pain inhibition via the hypophyseal portal system or cerebrospinal fluid (CSF).[6] This

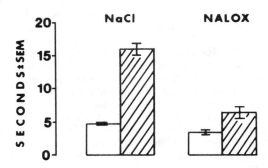

FIGURE 3. Hind paw flick latencies before (white columns) and after footshock (dashed columns) in mice pretreated with saline (NaCl) and naloxone (NALOX).

hypothesis is especially suggestive in the mouse in which such a humoral pathway was proposed by Fu and Dewey as crucial in morphine antinociception.[24] According to these authors antinociceptive effect of morphine in mice is not direct, but mediated by substance(s) released from supraspinal stuctures, transported down by CSF and acting at the spinal level. This conclusion was based on the finding that even total transection of the spinal cord does not influence the morphine antinociception in mice provided that free flow of the CSF to the lower parts of the spinal cord is maintained. It must be noted at this point that in the rat the spinal cord descending pathways play an important role in morphine and electrical stimulation of the brain produced analgesia.[25] Destruction of the descending pathway lying in the dorsolateral funiculus attenuated both opiate and non-opiate forms of four paw footshock SIA[26] and totally abolished front paw footshock SIA.[2]

Thus, the question has arisen whether the indirect action of morphine in mice is specific for this form of antinociception or whether it results from the organization of endogenous pain inhibitory system. To answer this question we undertook the next experiment to test whether the mechanism of stress-induced antinociception in mice may depend on the substances transported to the spinal cord by the CSF. The positive result would support the presumption that the organization of the pain inhibitory system may differ between rats and mice. It would also confirm the hypothesis of Lewis et al. that analgesic concentration of endogenous substances may reach pain inhibitory centers via the CSF.

Two groups of mice spinalized differentially according to the method published by Fu and Dewey[24] were used in the experiment. Some mice (LIGATED) were spinalized by ligating the spinal cord together with dura and others by squeezing the spinal cord but leaving the dura intact (DURA-INTACT). The first preparation was aimed to block, while the latter to leave intact the CSF flow to the caudal part of the spinal cord.

Since spinalized animals were to be used in the experiment we had to change both the form of stress and the nociception measurement test. As a stressor we chose the front paw shock, whose analgesic effect in the rat was found to be opiate in nature and completely dependent upon the integrity of the spinal cord pathways descending in the dorsolateral funiculus.[2] Antinociception was assayed with the tail-flick test.

Both groups of animals were exposed to the footshock (1 mA rms) restricted to the front paw only. Footshocking lasted 30 min and was delivered on a 10 sec on/10 sec off schedule. The nociceptive threshold testing was carried out immediately prior to footshock and during the first, fifth, 10th, 20th, and 30th min after its termination. The latency at each indicated time point was calculated as a mean of four measurements separated by 30 sec intervals. The light intensity was adjusted to keep the average baseline response at about 2 sec. A 5 sec cut-off time was applied to avoid tissue damage. Animals not responding within 4 sec during baseline testing were not used in the experiment. One hour prior to footshocking some of the animals from both groups received physiological saline, whereas others were preinjected intraperitoneally with naloxone (1 mg/kg).

As presented in FIGURE 4 front paw shock caused slight, but significant increase of nociceptive threshold in the DURA-INTACT group. This antinociceptive effect appearing 5–30 min after footshocking (but not immediately) was completely antagonized by naloxone pretreatment. The opposite effect of footshock, i.e. decrease in nociceptive threshold was observed in the LIGATED group (FIGURE 4, B). This effect, noted upon the first poststress measurement only, was also reversed by naloxone. These results demonstrate that front paw shock

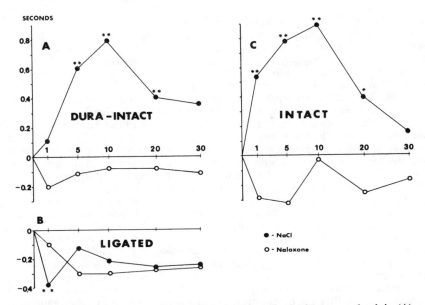

FIGURE 4. Mean changes in tail-flick latencies after 30 min front paw shock in (A) mice spinalized to allow free passage of the CSF to the lower parts of the spinal cord; (B) spinalized with blockage of CSF flow; and (C) intact animals. (NaCl, Naloxone) mice pretreated with 0.9% NaCl or naloxone, respectively. 1, 5, 10, 20, 30 = postfootshock minutes. *$p < 0.05$, **$p < 0.01$ (Newman-Keuls).

was capable of inducing antinociception only in DURA-INTACT mice. Although the degree of this antinociceptive effect was rather low, it did not differ from what we observed in an earlier experiment carried out on intact animals (FIGURE 4, C). It must be noted, however, that in DURA-INTACT mice the onset of antinociceptive effect was delayed in comparison with intact ones in which a significant (though not maximal) increase of nociceptive threshold was observed immediately after footshock termination.

The poststress increase of nociceptive threshold only in those animals prepared in the manner allowing free flow of CSF to the lower parts of the spinal cord suggests that the antinociceptive effect of front paw shock in mice is exerted at the spinal level by substances released from supraspinal structures and transported down in the CSF. The complete reversal of nociceptive threshold elevation by naloxone implicates opioid involvement in this form of antinociception. These results support the idea that the antinociceptive effect of stress may be mediated by substances released into the CSF. They also indicate that the antinociceptive effect of front paw shock in mice is mediated by a mechanism similar to that proposed by Fu and Dewey for morphine analgesia in this species.[24]

The scarce data available allow only speculation as to which substance(s) reaching the CSF may be involved in the proposed mechanism. The putative candidate seems to be β-endorphin whose release increases under condition of stress. Additionally, this peptide was found to be present in the CSF[27] and shows analgesic activity when delivered into the subarachnoid space.[28] But Fu and Dewey argue against involvement of pituitary opioids in the mechanism of morphine antinociception in mice because of the finding that the action of this narcotic is not altered in hypophysectomized animals.[24] Fu *et al.* also reported that removal of the pituitary does not change acupuncture analgesia in mice.[29] The authors suggest that β-endorphin originating from the hypothalamus rather than from the pituitary may be involved in this form of analgesia.

Unlike the animals from the DURA-INTACT group the mice spinalized with a block of CSF flow to the lower parts of the spinal cord displayed significant decrease of tail-flick latencies after exposure to front paw shock. This effect indicates that simultaneously with the antinociceptive mechanism stress may also activate a pronociceptive one. Such dual action of stress might explain the delay in the appearance of antinociception observed in the DURA-INTACT animals. It is possible that the lack of changes in the nociceptive threshold noted in this group immediately after the footshock termination resulted from the concomitant action of two antagonistic mechanisms. On the other hand, intact animals displayed significant antinociception already during the first poststress measurement. It must be noted, however, that the degree of this antinociception was also lower than in the 10th postfootshock minute when the maximal effect (similar to the DURA-INTACT group) was observed. We suppose that in the DURA-INTACT mice the effect of pronociceptive mechanism activation (observed as a lack of changes in tail-flick latencies during the first postfootshock minute) could have been enhanced in comparison with the intact animals by postsurgery changes in the velocity of the CSF flow.

The decrease of postfootshock latencies in the LIGATED mice in which the caudal portion of the spinal cord was devoid both neural and humoral (via the CSF) connections with supraspinal structures indicated that stress-induced facilitation of nociceptive reflex was exerted at the spinal level by factor(s) reaching the spinal sites through the bloodstream. It is likely that the hypernociception could be caused by substances released from structures of the pituitary-adrenal axis under the stress conditions. The next experiment was planned to examine the influence of synthetic glucocorticoid dexamethasone on nociception in spinal mice. Although in the two first experiments dexamethasone did not decrease the baseline pain sensitivity, such effect could result from a compensatory action of supraspinal structures. Thus, we supposed that the spinal cord ligation should unmask the supposed pronociceptive properties of dexamethasone, similarly as this preparation revealed the pronociceptive effect of front paw shock in the LIGATED mice.

Twenty mice spinalized by ligation (LIGATED) and 20 intact animals (INTACT) were used in the experiment. Both LIGATED and INTACT animals were randomly divided into two groups assigned to receive either physiological saline or dexamethasone (0.5 mg/kg, intraperitoneally). Injections were made immediately after the estimation of baseline tail-flick latencies by the same means described in the previous experiment. The nociceptive threshold was then estimated again 10, 20, 30, 40, and 50 min after injection.

As presented in FIGURE 5, saline administration influenced the nociception in neither the LIGATED nor the INTACT group. Dexamethasone injection had no effect on tail-flick latencies in INTACT, but decreased them in the LIGATED mice. Although this dexamethasone produced decrease was slight, the postinjection latencies were significantly shorter with respect to baseline.

LIGATED   **INTACT**

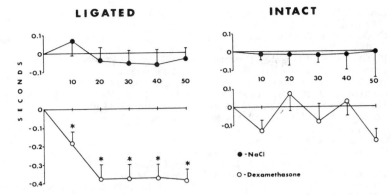

FIGURE 5. Mean changes in tail-flick latencies ±SEM in spinal (LIGATED) and intact (INTACT) mice pretreated either with 0.9% NaCl (NaCl) or dexamethasone. 10, 20, 30, 40, 50 = minutes after injection. *$p < 0.05$ (Newman-Keuls).

Such action of dexamethasone indicates that poststress hypernociception observed in the LIGATED mice in the previous experiment might be mediated by glucocorticoids released under the stress and acting on the spinal cord. However, the mechanism of such glucocorticoid action remains unclear and it should be determined whether the dexamethasone-produced decrease in tail-flick latencies results from the increased sensitivity to noxious stimuli or rather from glucocorticoid action on the spinal cord motor neurons.

ACKNOWLEDGMENTS

We gratefully acknowledge a gift of naloxone hydrochloride from Endo Laboratories.

REFERENCES

1. BODNAR, J. R., D. D. KELLY, M. BRUTUS & M. GLUSMAN. 1980. Neurosci. Biobehav. Rev. **4**:87–100.
2. WATKINS, L. R. & D. J. MAYER. 1982. Science **216**:1185–1192.
3. GUILLEMIN, R., T. VARGO, J. ROSSIER, S. MINICK, N. LING, C. RIVIER, W. VALE & F. E. BLOOM. Science **197**:1367–1369.
4. FRENCH, E. D., F. E. BLOOM, C. RIVIER, R. GUILLEMIN & J. ROSSIER. 1978. Neurosci. Abstr. **4**:408.
5. TSENG, L. F., H. H. LOH & C. H. LI. 1976. Nature **263**:239–240.
6. LEWIS, J. W., J. T. CANNON & J. C. LIEBESKIND. 1980. Science **208**:623–625.
7. TERMAN, G. W., J. W. LEWIS & J. C. LIEBESKIND. 1983. Brain Res. **260**:147–150.
8. HYSON, R. L., L. J. ASHCRAFT, R. C. DRUGAN, J. W. GRAU & S. F. MAIER. 1982. Pharmacol. Biochem. Behav. **17**:1019–1025.
9. BODNAR, R. J., M. GLUSMAN, M. BRUTUS, A. SPAGGIA & D. D. KELLY. 1979. Physiol. Behav. **23**:53–62.

10. LEWIS, J. W., E. H. CHUDLER, J. T. CANNON & J. C. LIEBESKIND. 1981. Proc. West. Pharmacol. Soc. **24**:323-326.
11. CHANCE, W. T., G. N. KRYNOCK & J. A. ROSECRANS. 1979. Psychoendocrinology **4**:199-205.
12. BUCKET, W. R. 1979. Eur. J. Pharmacol. **58**:169-178.
13. CHESHER, G. B. & B. CHAN. 1977. Life Sci. **21**:1569-1574.
14. WILLOW, M., J. CARMODY & P. CARROLL. 1980. Life Sci. **26**:219-224.
15. CHRISTIE, M. J., P. TRISDIKOON & G. B. CHESHER. 1982. Life Sci. **31**:839-845.
16. TESKEY, G. C., M. KAVALIERS & M. HIRST. 1984. Life Sci. **35**:303-315.
17. KONECKA, A. M., I. SROCZYŃSKA & R. PRZEWŁOCKI. 1985. Arch. Int. Physiol. Biochim. (In press.)
18. GREENBERG, R. & E. H. O'KEEFE. 1982. Life Sci. **31**:1185-1188.
19. GREVERT, P., E. R. BAIZMAN & A. GOLDSTEIN. 1978. Life Sci. **23**:723-728.
20. POMERANZ, B., R. CHENG & P. LAW. 1977. Expl. Neurol. **54**:172-178.
21. CHENG, R., B. POMERANZ & G. YU. 1979. Life Sci. **24**:1481.
22. HOLADAY, J. W., P-Y LAW, H. H. LOH & C. H. LI. 1979. J. Pharmacol. Exp. Ther. **208**:176-183.
23. ROSSIER, J., E. D. FRENCH, C. RIVIER, N. LING, R. GUILLEMIN & F. E. BLOOM. 1977. Nature **270**:618-620.
24. FU, T-C & W. L. DEWEY. 1979. Life Sci. **25**:53-60.
25. BASBAUM, A. I., N. J. E. MARLEY, E. H. O'KEEFE & C. H. CLANTON. 1977. Pain **3**:43-56.
26. LEWIS, J. W., G. W. TERMAN, L. R. WATKINS, D. J. MAYER & J. C. LIEBESKIND. 1983. Brain Res. **267**:139-144.
27. NAKAO, K., OKI, I. TANAKA, K. HORII, Y. NAKAI, T. FURVI, M. FUKUSHIMA, A. KUWAYAMA, N. KAGEYAMA & H. IMURA. 1980. J. Clin. Invest. **66**:1383-1390.
28. TSENG, L. F. 1981. Life Sci. **29**:1417-1424.
29. FU, T-C, S. P. HALENDA & W. L. DEWEY. 1980. Brain Res. **202**:33-39.
30. MAREK, P., I. PANOCKA & G. HARTMANN. 1982. Pharmacol. Biochem. Behav. **16**:403-405.
31. MAREK, P., I. PANOCKA & B. SADOWSKI. 1983. Pharmacol. Biochem. Behav. **18**:167-169.

The Relationship between Cardiovascular and Pain Regulatory Systems

NADAV ZAMIR

Hypertension–Endocrine Branch
National Heart, Lung, Blood Institute
National Institutes of Health
Bethesda, Maryland 20892

and

WILLIAM MAIXNER

National Institute of General Medical Science
and Neurobiology and Anesthesiology Branch
National Institute of Dental Research
Bethesda, Maryland 20892

INTRODUCTION

The body responds to increased physical and psychological demands by activating certain components of the peripheral and central nervous systems. In addition, hormones (e.g. ACTH, beta-endorphin, prolactin) are released from the anterior pituitary, glucocorticoids from the adrenal cortex, epinephrine from the adrenal medulla, and norepinephrine from the sympathetic nerves. These hormonal and neural responses serve to adapt the body to a variety of psychological and physical stressors, which range in affect and intensity. Reactions to stressors typically involve either short or long-term compensatory changes in the cardiovascular, energy-producing, endocrine, immune, and somatosensory systems, which tend to maintain adequate physiological function in the face of the imbalance created by the stressors. When the intensity or the duration of the requisite adjustment exceeds the limits of these adaptive mechanisms, pathological changes may occur. Selye called these changes "diseases of adaptation" and include diseases such as hypertension, gastric ulceration, and neurological disorders.[97,98] Little is known about the manner in which different systems coordinate their responses to a stressor and operate collectively in the intact organism. A greater understanding of the interactions between peripheral and central systems involved in cardiovascular regulation and pain perception would illuminate factors associated with the onset and maintenance of "diseases of adaptation."

GENERAL HISTORICAL ASPECTS OF BLOOD PRESSURE AND SOMATOSENSORY INTERACTIONS

Several recent observations have provided indirect evidence that supports the view that somatosensory and cardiovascular regulatory systems are functionally linked. Pharmacologically, drugs that affect blood pressure such as alpha-adrenergic agonists, also modify response to pain,[26,36,38,60,68,92] and analgesic drugs like morphine affect blood pressure.[32,37,62,63,66,71,112] In addition, many neuro-anatomical substrates that support opioid analgesia and stimulation-produced analgesia are also implicated in the central regulation of blood pressure.[2-4,14,19,21-23,27,29-32, 35,39,40,45,52,54,58,62,69,70,72,77,80,88-90,93,94,96,103,107,109,114,116]

More direct evidence for the proposed interaction comes from the findings that acute or chronic arterial hypertension is associated with a behavioral hypoalgesia. In rats, experimentally induced renal hypertension, deoxycorti-costerone acetate (DOCA) salt-induced hypertension, and social deprivation-induced hypertension are associated with a naloxone-reversible hypoalgesia.[83] The onset and magnitude of the hypoalgesia is time-linked to the increase in arterial pressure.[75,118,123] In addition, the response appears to be dependent upon elevated arterial pressure since lowering the arterial pressure by ganglionic blockade or removing the renal artery stenosis greatly attenuates or abolishes the hypoalgesic behavior.[75,89,118,122] Spontaneously hypertensive rats (SHR) and hypertension-prone SABRA rats also exhibit reduced pain sensitivity.[75,95,101,118,120,123] The onset of the hypoalgesia exhibited by SHRs is related to the onset of the arterial hypertension and can be reversed by ganglionic block-ade.[75,123]

Perhaps the most convincing evidence that hypertension is associated with a hypoalgesia, which is related to diminished pain perception, is the finding that pain threshold to noxious tooth pulp stimulation is elevated in unmedicated essential hypertensive humans.[119,123] Thus it appears that various forms of hypertension, which result from different etiologies, are all associated with an intrinsic hypoalgesia. It still remains an open issue as to how changes in blood pressure can influence nociception.

The underlying mechanisms responsible for the hypoalgesia have not been fully delineated. However, it is unlikely that the diminished responsiveness to noxious stimuli results from a pathological change in primary nociceptor afferent activity secondary to hypertension since a hypoalgesic response is also observed following acute elevations in blood pressure and is also present at the onset of the development of hypertension in SHR.[75] It is also apparent that the hypoalgesia exhibited by chronically hypertensive rats does not result from a general motor deficit since open field exploratory activity and general motor activity are either equal to or greater than normotensive controls.[123] In addition, SHR are hyperreactive to certain intensities of electrical stimuli.[20,89] The observation that systemically administered naloxone diminishes or abolishes the hypoalgesic behavior in SHR, hypertension-prone SABRA rats, and renal hypertensive rats suggests that endogenous opioid peptides may contribute to the hypoalgesia associated with chronic forms of hypertension. This endogenous opioid system does not appear to contribute to the maintenance of the hypertension since systemically administered naloxone (at doses that diminish the hypoalgesia) fails to change blood pressure.[118,120]

Further support for the view that chronic elevation of arterial blood pressure results in an opioid-mediated hypoalgesia is the finding that renal hypertensive rats exhibit significantly higher levels of opioid activity in their cervical spinal cord as compared to normotensive controls.[120] Similarly, hypertension-prone SABRA rats have a significantly higher level of endogenous opioids in their cervical spinal cord, hypothalamus, and pituitary gland compared to parental SABRA rats.[120] Interestingly, there is significantly lower [³H]naloxone binding in the dorsal horn of the cervical spinal cord of renal hypertensive and hypertension-prone SABRA rats as compared with normotensive controls.[121] Increased levels of opioid peptides and decreased opioid receptor-binding at the same site may be associated with the development of receptor desensitization, which resulted from a relative increase in opioid peptides available to the receptors. Further studies are needed to reveal the kinetics of these changes during the development of hypertension and their functional significance. These alterations in the spinal opioid system may contribute to the hypoalgesia observed in the hypertensive rats because it is known that opiates can act at the spinal level to produce analgesia.[116] In addition, the dorsal horn is a site involved in the modulation of nociceptive transmission and contains regions that are abundant in both opioid receptors and opioid peptides.[5,6,109,114,116]

Recent findings support the view that carotid sinus, cardiopulmonary, and possibly aortic baroreceptor pathways may play an important role in cardiovascular and somatosensory interactions.[36,74,75,89–91,123] Historically, the baroreceptor system has been viewed as a homeostatic regulator of cardiovascular function.[16,59] This system can be stimulated or engaged by elevating arterial (carotid sinus baroreceptors) pressure or venous (cardiopulmonary baroreceptors) pressure.[16,59,89] The behavioral effects of baroreceptor manipulations have not been popularized but appear relevant to the proposed influence of blood pressure on nociception. The activation of carotid sinus baroreceptors produces a generalized inhibitory effect characterized by diminished muscle tone and cortical activity.[15,25,111] Sham-rage is attenuated in decerebrate cats by carotid sinus baroreceptor stimulation and augmented by bilateral common carotid occlusion (a procedure that diminishes carotid sinus nerve activity).[7] Though not specifically related to nociception, it is evident that stimulation of carotid sinus baroreceptors results in a generalized inhibition.

A number of recent findings support the view that carotid sinus baroreceptor pathway stimulation modulates behavioral responses to noxious stimuli.[89] Acute elevation in arterial blood pressure produced by the alpha-adrenoreceptor agonist phenylephrine, decreases escape-avoidance responses to aversive electrical stimulation in the rat.[36] Similarly, phenylephrine-induced hypertension is associated with a reduced tail-flick reflex evoked by noxious radiant heat.[90] Both of these effects are attenuated by carotid sinus baroreceptor denervation.[36,90] A number of findings also suggest that cardiopulmonary baroreceptor pathways play a role in nociception. First, the hypoalgesia exhibited by SHR is markedly attenuated by resecting the right cervical vagus (a procedure that diminishes cardiopulmonary baroreceptor afferent input).[75] Second, the physiological activation of cardiopulmonary baroreceptor afferents produced by increasing central venous pressure elevates tail-flick latencies.[74] Recent electrophysiological studies also support this finding since the direct electrical stimulation of primate cardiac or cervical vagal afferents diminishes the response of dorsal horn spinothalamic neurons to noxious stimuli applied to their receptive fields.[89] Third, the pharmacological activation of cardiopulmonary baroreceptors by intravenous administration of [D-Ala²]-met-enkephalinamide produces an analgetic-like response in the rat that is abolished by bilateral cervical vagotomy.[91]

Finally, the integrity of cardiopulmonary baroreceptor pathways is required for the full expression of footshock-induced analgesia since resection of the right vagal nerve trunk attenuates the "analgesic" response to prolonged foot-shock.[74]

FUTURE DIRECTIONS AND SIGNIFICANCE

The above discussion serves to illustrate that cardiovascular and pain regulatory pathways are functionally linked and may play a role in the organism's adaptive response to stress. Currently, we know very little about the central network that is responsible for this interaction. FIGURE 1 represents a number of potential central and peripheral sites that may participate in this interaction. The putative role of many of these areas in cardiovascular and somatosensory regulation has been recently discussed.[89] Indeed, future studies are required to determine the extent to which somatosensory and cardiovascular regulatory systems interact at various levels of the neuroaxis. It is likely that the local neural circuitry of these regions is complex and provides a vast range of physiological responses to various environmental stressors. FIGURE 1 also points out that various emotional stressors may also interact with central components of the baroreceptor reflex by engaging the defense reaction (a discussion of this proposed interaction is presented by Randich and Maixner, this volume).

To what degree baroreceptors are activated in response to a stressor has not been systematically evaluated. However, many of the stressors used to produce conditioned analgesia in rats and man can increase sympathetic tone, heart rate, and arterial and central venous pressures.[17,49-51,56,61,85,104] In this regard, an increase in heart rate is observed in humans trained to anticipate the onset of painful, inescapable footshock.[115] The onset of the signal that announces the occurrence of noxious stimuli results in a progressive increase in heart rate, which is associated with suppression of the polysynaptic RIII nociceptive reflex.[115] Thus, it seems plausible that stressors that increase sympathetic tone and venous and/or arterial pressure impair pain perception by stimulating baroreceptor pathways.

Other forms of analgesia produced by peripheral stimulation may be partially mediated by arterial and/or venous pressor responses that stimulate baroreceptor pathways.[17,49-51,56,85,104] In a series of studies on freely moving spontaneously hypertensive rats (SHR) and Wistar-Kyoto (WKY) rats, it has been shown that low frequency sciatic nerve stimulation, at intensities that activate A-delta (Group III) afferent fibers, increases arterial blood pressure and heart rate.[117] Following stimulation, a transient decrease in pain sensitivity and a prolonged depressor response is observed in both SHR and WKY.[117] The systemic administration of naloxone (1.0 mg/kg) reverses the hypoalgesia but fails to alter the depressor response.[91] The authors suggest that the activation of high threshold afferent nerve fibers, which elicit the sensation of deep pain, is required to obtain an effective opioid-mediated hypoalgesia. Other forms of noxious peripheral stimulation that engage diffuse noxious inhibitory controls may also be partially mediated by stimulating baroreceptor pathways.[64,65] For some time it has been recognized that pain can inhibit pain. A painful stimulus applied to one body site activates intrinsic pain modulatory systems that attenuate the behavioral and electrophysiological responses to another painful stimulus applied to a remote body region.[64,65] It seems plausible that many forms of peripheral stimulation (i.e. acupuncture, transcutaneous nerve stimulation, and pain may activate peripheral and/or central components of the baroreceptor pathways that modulate noci-

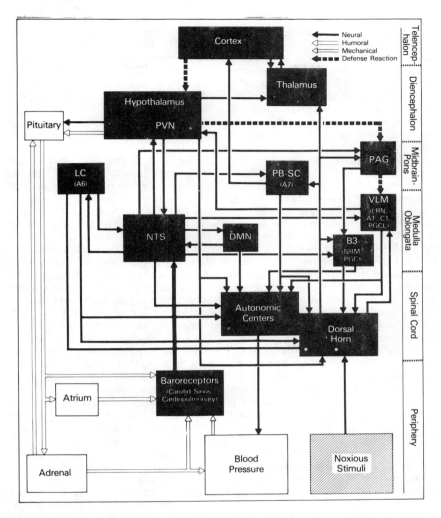

FIGURE 1. Some possible interactions between cardiovascular and pain regulatory systems. Autonomic Centers = Intermediolateral cell column, B3 = nucleus raphe magnus, (NRM), paragigantocellular nucleus (PGL), DMN = Dorsal motor nucleus of the vagus, NTS = nucleus of the solitary tract, VLM = Ventral lateral medulla (VLM), which includes the lateral reticular nucleus (LRN), catecholamine regions A1 and C1, lateral paraganto-cellular nucleus (PGCL), LC = locus coeruleus, PB-SC = Parabrachial-subcoeruleus region; A7 catecholamine region, PAG = Periaqueductal central gray, and PVN = Para-ventricular nucleus.

ceptive responses. In this regard, many types of noxious stimuli (i.e. electrical shock, radiant heat, and cold) increase both arterial and venous pressures, which can stimulate various baroreceptor pathways.[1,41,54,99] In addition, the full expression of footshock-induced analgesia produced by prolonged inescapable footshock is diminished by unilateral cervical vagotomy (a procedure that diminishes cardiopulmonary baroreceptor activity).[74] Though not conclusive, these findings support the view that baroreceptor systems may play a role in the antinociceptive behaviors elicited by different types of peripheral stimulation. Whether various types of noxious or "stressful" peripheral stimuli engage various aspects of the baroreceptor network that modulates nociceptive responses still remains an open issue.

Chronic and acute forms of hypertension in humans and animals are accompanied by altered activity of the hypothalamus-pituitary-adrenal axis.[18,41,42,44,57,78,100,124] However, the role of the pituitary gland in pain regulation is controversial.[113] Several studies suggest involvement of pituitary gland in hypoalgesia based upon the observations that total hypophysectomy may produce hyperalgesia in the rat as tested by responses to electric footshock[46] or to formalin injected to the paw,[4] and that analgesia induced by stress (immobilization, cold-water swim, footshock, and electroacupuncture) is reduced or abolished by total hypophysectomy.[4,14,79,87] On the other hand, other studies have shown involvement of the pituitary in hyperalgesic responses based upon the arguments that hypophysectomy may induce analgesia in humans suffering from cancer pain[81,82] and may increase baseline pain threshold (hot-plate test)[53] and that the hyperalgesic responses of naloxone were abolished by hypophysectomy in mice.[47] Finally, the lack of any effect of hypophysectomy on basal nociception has also been reported.[4,47,55,79]

Many putative mechanisms have been proposed to account for this phenomenon. The prevailing one is that there is a loss of some hypophyseal hormones with analgesic properties. Pituitary opioid peptides, such as β-endorphin, met-enkephalin, leu-enkephalin and dynorphin-related peptides,[125] may be suitable candidates. However, it should be understood that the concentration of plasma β-endorphin are not sufficient to alter pain perception, even after stress.[48] However, hypophyseal hormones may have more direct access to brain via release into the inverse portal system or into the cerebrospinal fluid.[8,84] Indeed, a naloxone-reversible analgesia has been observed in rats bearing hypersecretory hypophyseal tumors.[43] The loss of variable non-opioid pituitary peptides with antinociceptive properties, such as vasopressin,[9–11,13,28,33] neurotensin,[24] α-MSH,[108] bombesin,[86] or substance P[76,106] may also be involved in the hyperalgesic effects of hypophysectomy. In line with this idea, Brattleboro rats, which are genetically deficient in hypothalamo-neurohypophyseal vasopressin, have been reported to exhibit basal hypersensitivity to pain.[13]

Many studies that have demonstrated that hypophysectomy results in a hypoalgesia have used the argument that the hypoalgesia results from the loss of humoral substances with hyperalgesic properties such as ACTH.[12,46] Some variations in experimental designs, such as differences in species (mouse, rat, human) in pain tests (tail flick, hot-plate, flinch jump, formalin) and the type of stressor (inescapable footshock, immobilization, cold water swim, etc.) may influence the relative participation of such analgetic and hyperalgesic pituitary hormones and thus might account for the diverse effects of hypophysectomy on pain sensitivity. In addition, caution needs to be exercised in interpreting data from hypophysectomized animals because their poor physical state most likely influences their behavior.

The adrenal gland may also be relevant to pain perception. Adrenalectomy blocks the opioid form of stress analgesia but potentiates the analgesic response to morphine.[67] Unlike stress analgesia, morphine analgesia is unaffected by adrenal demedullation and denervation, showing that the adrenal cortex, but not the medulla, is involved.[67] Other findings support this view. For example, hypophysectomy potentiates morphine analgesia as does adrenalectomy[55] and normal morphine responsiveness is restored by hormonal replacement.[73] Also, the affinity of opiate receptors to etorphine or morphine is increased by both adrenalectomy and hypophysectomy.[67] Therefore adrenalectomy may potentiate opiate analgesia by increasing the affinity of receptors for opiate drugs in response to the loss of adrenocortical hormones, but decreases opioid stress analgesia by eliminating an important source of enkephalin-containing peptides, the adrenal medulla.[67]

Recently, the cardiac atrium has been shown to be an important endocrine organ, containing atrial natruiretic peptides.[102] Some of these peptides may activate vagal afferents and thus may alter pain perception.[110] Many of the above-mentioned hormones may exert their action on pain regulatory systems, peripherally through actions on the baroreceptor systems or centrally through the brain to modify activity of the baroreceptors.[34] Further studies are needed to untangle the intricate relationship between hormones and somatosensory systems.

To what degree stress alters normal homeostatic regulation to produce pathophysiological conditions has been an area of great interest. Many diseases such as hypertension, gastric ulceration, mental disorders, and recently immune disorders, are thought to ensue as the homeostatic responses to various stressors are exceeded. In the short term, however, the physiological responses produced by various stressors may be of value since they may provide the organism with a variety of means of dealing with life-threatening situations. In this regard, stress-induced elevations in arterial and/or venous pressure may engage intrinsic neural networks, such as baroreceptor pathways, that decrease the perceived magnitude or motivational-affective aspects of a stressor. It has been proposed that baroreceptor stimulation and hypertension may produce "rewarding" properties to an organism under stress and that repeated pairings of stress and acute pressor responses may lead to more enduring forms of hypertension, which diminish the psychophysiological aspects and aversity of environmental stressors.[36,75,89] In support of such a view is the tight covariance of hypertension and pain sensitivity.[75,118,124] In addition, it has recently been reported that rats exposed to short-term social deprivation (i.e. isolation) exhibit a profound arterial hypertension and a naloxone-reversible hypoalgesia.[83] Reintroduction to their normal living environment reduces both arterial blood pressure and the nociceptive threshold. However, future studies are required to delineate the putative reward or reinforcing properties of baroreceptor stimulation and/or hypertension. Studies of this type will provide additional evidence regarding the causal as opposed to the associative relationship between cardiovascular and pain regulatory networks.

The present discussion serves to illustrate the complexities of an organism's response to stress. The putative interaction between cardiovascular and somatosensory systems represents only a small fraction of the known responses to a stressor. Even with respect to the proposed cardiovascular somatosensory interactions, we do not yet know if baroreceptor activation specifically alters nociception or whether perception in other sensory modalities is also influenced. In addition, we do not yet know if alterations in arterial and venous pressure alter the sensory-discriminative and/or affective aspect of pain.

The proposed interaction between the cardiovascular and somatosensory systems represent our current synthesis of ideas given the available information. It is not our intention that these concepts and speculations be treated as dogmas but rather as testable hypotheses that can be modified as new information is gathered.

SUMMARY

An increasing amount of anatomical, physiological, and pharmacological evidence suggest that pain inhibitory circuitry is linked with cardiovascular regulatory systems in man and laboratory animals.

Induction of hypertension in rats by different methods (mineralocorticoid treatment, stenosis of renal artery, or social deprivation) is associated with reduced responsiveness to noxious thermal stimuli (hot-plate) or to noxious mechanical stimuli (paw pressure). Genetically hypertension-prone rats derived from the SABRA strain and spontaneously hypertensive rats derived from Wistar/Kyoto strain also display a similar hypoalgesia. Acute increases in blood pressure are associated with reduced sensitivity to painful stimuli. Additionally, the interaction between blood pressure and pain perception has also been supported by the demonstration that various experimental interventions that diminish the magnitude of hypertension also attenuate the hypoalgesia. Recent clinical findings are also in agreement with the laboratory animal findings since sensory and pain thresholds have been shown to be significantly higher in unmedicated essential hypertensive subjects compared to normotensive controls. Thus, the human data corroborate animal data and suggest that a relation between blood pressure and pain sensitivity is likely to be a general phenomenon. It is unlikely that damage to peripheral pain fibers caused by a change in blood pressure contributes to the observed hypoalgesia. Naloxone, which has no effect on blood pressure, returns the pain sensitivity to normal levels. Behavioral tests (open field and motor activity cage) of normotensive and of renal and genetically (SBH and SHR) hypertensive rats exclude the possibility of a general motor deficit in hypertensive rats.

Endogenous opioid peptides in central and peripheral nervous systems as well as in endocrine organs are implicated, although non-opioid mechanisms are also evident. Activation of baroreceptor afferents by acute or chronic increases in arterial or venous blood pressure may play an important role in the somatosensory responses associated with the increase in blood pressure. Coordinated cardiovascular-pain regulatory responses may be part of an adaptive mechanism that helps the body to face stressful events.

REFERENCES

1. ABRAM, S. E., D. R. KOSTREVA, F. A. HOPP & J. P. KAMPINE. 1983. Cardiovascular responses to noxious radiant heat in anesthetized rats. Am. J. Physiol. **245**:R576–R580.
2. AKIL, H. & J. C. LIEBESKIND. 1975. Monoaminergic mechanisms of stimulation-produced analgesia. Brain Res. **94**:279–296.
3. AMARAL, D. G. & H. M. SINNAMON. 1977. The locus coeruleus: Neurobiology of a central noradrenergic nucleus. Prog. Neurobiol. **9**:147–196.
4. AMIR, S. & Z. AMIT. 1978. The pituitary gland mediates acute and chronic pain responsiveness in stressed and non stressed rats. Life Sci. **24**:439–448.

5. ATWEH, S. F. & M. J. KUHAR. 1977. Autoradiographic localization of opiate receptors in rat brain. I. Spinal cord and lower medulla. Brain Res. 124:53-67.
6. ATWEH, S. F. & M. J. KUHAR. 1977. Autoradiographic localizations of opiate receptors in rat brain. II. The brain stem. Brain Res. 129:1-12.
7. BARTORELLI, C., E. BIZZI, A. LIBRETTI & A. ZANCHETTI. 1968. Inhibitory control of sinocarotid pressoceptive afferents on hypothalamic autonomic activity and sham rage behavior. Arch. Ital. Bio. 98:308-326.
8. BERGLAND, R. M. & R. B. PAGE. 1978. Can the pituitary secrete directly to the brain? (Affirmative anatomical evidence). Endocrinology 102:1325-1338.
9. BERKOWITZ, B. & S. SHERMAN. 1982. Characterization of vasopressin analgesia. J. Pharmacol. Exp. Ther. 220:329-334.
10. BERNTSON, G. G. & B. S. BERSON. 1980. Antinociceptive effects of intraventricular or systemic administration of vasopressin in the rat. Life Sci. 26:455-459.
11. BERSON, B. S., G. G. BERNSTON, W. ZIPF, M. W. TORELLO & W. T. KIRK. 1983. Vasopressin-induced antinociception: An investigation into its physiological and hormonal basis. Endocrinology 113:337-343.
12. BERTOLINI, A., R. POGGIOLI & W. FERRARI. 1980. Possible physiological role of ACTH-peptides in nociception. Adv. Biochem. Psychopharmacol. 22:109-119.
13. BODNAR, R. J., E. A. ZIMMERMAN, G. NILAVER, A. MANSOUR, L. W. THOMAS, D. D. KELLY & M. GLUSMAN. 1980. Dissociation of cold-water swim and morphine analgesia in Brattleboro rats with diabetes insipidus. Life Sci. 26:1581-1590.
14. BODNAR, R. J., D. D. KELLY, M. BRUTUS & M. GLUSMAN. 1980. Stress-induced analgesia: Neural and hormonal determinants. Neurosci. Biobehav. Rev. 4:87-100.
15. BONVALLET, M., P. DELL & G. HIEBEL. 1954. Tonus sympathique et activite electrique corticqle. Electroencephalogr. Clin. Neurophysiol. 6:119-144.
16. BROWN, A. M. 1980. Receptors under pressure: An update on baroreceptors. Circul. Res. 46:1-10.
17. BUCKLEY, J. P., E. E. VOGIN & W. J. KINNARD. 1966. Effects of pentobarbital acetylsalicylic acid and reserpine on blood pressure and survival of rats subjected to experimental stress. J. Pharm. Sci. 55:572-575.
18. BURSTYN, P. G. & D. F. HORROBIN. 1970. Possible mechanism of action for aldosterone-induced by hypertension. Lancet 973-976.
19. CABOT, J. B., J. M. WILD & D. H. COHEN. 1979. Raphe inhibition of sympathetic preganglionic neurons. Science 203:184-186.
20. CAMPBELL, R. J. & L. V. DiCARA. 1977. Running-wheel avoidance behavior in the Wistar/Kyoto spontaneously hypertensive rat. Physiol. Behav. 19:473-480.
21. CHAN, S. H. H. & J. S. KUO. 1980. Interaction of gigantocellular reticular nucleus with reflex bradycardia and tachycardia in the cat. Brain Res. 182:457-460.
22. CHAN, S. H. H., J. S. KUO, Y. H. CHEN & J. Y. HWA. 1980. Modulatory actions of the gigantocellular reticular nucleus on baroreceptor reflexes in the cat. Brain Res. 196:1-9.
23. CHEN, Y. H. & S. H. H. CHAN. 1980. The involvement of gigantocellular reticular nucleus in clonidine-promoted hypotension and bradycardia in experimentally-induced hypertensive cats. Neuropharmacology 19:939-945.
24. CLINESCHMIDT, B. & J. MCGUFFIN. 1977. Neurotensin administered intracisternally inhibits responsiveness of mice to noxious stimuli. Eur. J. Pharmacol. 46:395-396.
25. COLERIDGE, H. M., J. C. COLERIDGE & F. ROSENTHAL. 1976. Prolonged inactivation of cortical pyramidal tract neurons in cats by distension of the carotid sinus. J. Physiol. 256:635-649.
26. COLVILLE, K. T. & E. CHAPLIN. 1964. Sympathomimetics as analgesics: Effects of methoxamine, methamphetamine, metaraminol, and norepinephrine. Life Sci. 3:315-322.
27. COOTE, J. H., S. M. HILTON & W. ZBROZYNA. 1973. The pons-medullary area integrating the defense reaction in the cat and its influence on muscle blood flow. J. Physiol. 229:257-274.

28. CRINE, A. F. & P. G. CARLIER. 1984. Vasopressin as a putative mediator in SHR hypoalgesia. Med. Hypothesis 14:297-300.
29. DAHLSTROM, A. & K. FUXE. 1964. Evidence for the existence of monoamine-containing neurons in the central nervous system. I. Demonstrations of monoamines in the cell bodies of the brain stem neurons. Acta Physiol. Scand. 62 (Suppl. 232):1-55.
30. DAHLSTROM, A. & K. FUXE. 1965. Evidence for the existence of monoamine-containing neurons in the central nervous system. II. Experimentally induced changes in the intraneuronal amine levels of bulbospinal neuron system. Acta Physiol. Scand. 64 (Suppl. 247):5-36.
31. DEFEUDIS, F. V. 1982. The link between analgesia and cardiovascular function. Role of GABA and endogenous opioids. Prog. Neurobiol. 19:1-17.
32. DE JONG, W., M. PETTY & J. M. A. SITSEN. 1983. Role of opioid peptides in brain mechanisms regulating blood pressure. Chest 2:306-308.
33. DORIS, P. A. 1984. Vasopressin and central integrative processes. Neuroendocrinology 38:75-85.
34. DRURY, R. A. & R. M. GOLD. 1977. Differential effects of ovarian hormones on reactivity to foot-shock in rats. Physiol. Behav. 20:187-191.
35. DUGGAN, A. W. & C. R. MORTON. 1983. Periaqueductal grey stimulation: An association between selective inhibition of dorsal horn neurons and changes in peripheral circulation. Pain 15:237-248.
36. DWORKIN, B. R., R. J. FILEWICH, N. E. MILLER, N. CRAIGMYLE & T. G. PICKERING. 1979. Baroreceptor activation reduces reactivity to noxious stimulation: Implications for hypertension. Science 205:1299-1301.
37. FELDBERG, W. & E. WEI. 1978. Central sites at which morphine acts producing cardiovascular effects. J. Physiol. 275:57P.
38. FIELDING, S., J. WILKER, M. HYNES, M. SZEWCZAK, W. J. NOVICK & H. LAL. 1978. A comparison of clonidine with morphine for antinociceptive and antiwithdrawal action. J. Pharmacol. Exp. Ther. 207:899-905.
39. FIELDS, H. L. & A. I. BASBAUM. 1978. Brain stem control of spinal pain-transmission neurons. Ann. Rev. Physiol. 40:217-248.
40. FLOREZ, J. & A. MEDIAVILLA. 1977. Respiratory and cardiovascular effects of met-enkephalin applied to the ventral surface of the brain stem. Brain Res. 138:585-590.
41. FOLKOW, B. 1982. Physiological aspects of primary hypertension. Physiol. Rev. 62:347-504.
42. FRASER, R. et al. 1976. The adrenal cortex and hypertension: Some observations on a possible role for mineralocorticoids other than aldosterone. J. Steroid Biochem. 7:963-970.
43. GALEANO, C., M. BOURASSA, M. CHRETIEN & M. LIS. 1980. Analgesic action of chronic high levels of endogenous neuropeptides in rats bearing the MtT-F_4 tumor. Life Sci. 27:151-156.
44. GALOSY, R. A., L. K. CLARKE, M. R. VASKO & I. L. CRAWFORD. 1981. Neurophysiology and neuropharmacology of cardiovascular regulation and stress. Neurosci. Biobehav. Rev. 5:137-175.
45. GEBHART, G. F. 1982. Opiate and opioid peptide effects on brain stem neurons: Relevance to nociception and antinociceptive mechanisms. Pain 12:93-140.
46. GISPEN, W. H., J. B. VAN WIMERSMA-GREIDANUS & S. SPECTOR. 1970. Effects of hypophysectomy and $ACTH_{1-10}$ on responsiveness to electric shock in rats. Physiol. Behav. 5:143-146.
47. GREVERT, P., E. R. BAIZMAN & A. GOLDSTEIN. 1978. Naloxone effects on a nociceptive responds in hypophysectomized and adrenalectomized mice. Life Sci. 23:723-728.
48. GUILLEMIN, R., T. VARGO & J. ROSSIER. 1977. β-endorphin and adrenocorticotropin are secreted concomitantly by the pituitary gland. Science 197:1367-1369.
49. HALL, C. E. & O. HALL. 1959. Augmentation of hormone-induced hyperactive

cardiovascular disease by simultaneous exposure to stress. Acta Endocrinol. **30**:557-566.

50. HALL, C. E. & O. HALL. 1959. Enhancement of somatotrophic hormone-induced hypertensive cardiovascular disease by stress. Am. J. Physiol. **197**:702-704.

51. HALLBACK, M. & B. FOLKOW. 1974. Cardiovascular responses to acute mental "stress" in spontaneously hypertensive rats. Acta Scand. Physiol. **90**:684-698.

52. HAYES, R., G. BENNETT, P. NEWLON & D. MAYER. 1978. Behavioral and physiological studies of non-narcotic analgesia in the rat elicited by certain environmental stimuli. Brain Res. **155**:69-90.

53. HEYBACH, J. P. & J. VERNIKOS-DANELLIS. 1978. The effect of pituitary-adrenal function in the modulation of pain sensitivity in the rat. J. Physiol. **283**:331-340.

54. HILTON, S. M. 1975. Ways of veiwing the central nervous control of the circulation— old and new. Brain Res. **87**:213-219.

55. HOLADAY, J. W., P. Y. LAW, L. F. TSENG, H. H. LOH & C. H. LI. 1977. β-endorphin: Pituitary and adrenal glands modulate its action. Proc. Natl. Acad. Sci. USA **74**:4628-4632.

56. HUDAK, W. J. & J. P. BUCKLEY. 1961. Production of hypertensive rats by experimental stress. J. Pharm. Sci. **50**:263-264.

57. IAMS, S. G., J. P. MCMURTRY & B. WEXLER. 1979. Aldosterone, deoxycorticosterone, and prolactin changes during the lifespan of chronically and spontaneously hypertensive rats. Endocrinology **104**:1357-1363.

58. KHACHATURIAN, H., M. E. LEWIS, M. K.-H. SCHAFER & S. J. WATSON. 1985. Anatomy of the CNS opioid systems. Trends Neurosci. **8**(3):111-119.

59. KORNER, P. I. 1979. Central nervous control of autonomic cardiovascular function. *In* Handbook of Physiology: The Cardiovascular System. R. M. Berne, N. Sperelakis & S. R. Geiger, Eds.: 691-739. American Physiological Society. Baltimore, MD.

60. KOSTOWSKI, W. & M. JERLICZ. 1978. Effects of lesions of the locus coeruleus and the ventral noradrenergic bundle on the antinociceptive action of clonidine in rats. Pol. J. Pharmacol. Pharm. **30**:647-651.

61. LAMPRECHT, F., R. B. WILLIAMS & I. J. KOPIN. 1973. Serum dopamine-beta-hydroxylase during development of immobilization-induced hypertension. Endocrinology **92**:953-956.

62. LAUBIE, M. & H. SCHMITT. 1980. Action of the morphinometic agent, fentanyl, on the nucleus tractus solitarii and the nucleus ambiguous cardiovascular neurons. Eur. J. Pharmacol. **67**:403-412.

63. LAUBIE, M. & H. SCHMITT. 1981. Indication for central vagal endorphinergic control of heart rate in dogs. Eur. J. Pharmacol. **71**:401-409.

64. LE BARS, D., A. H. DICKENSON & J. M. BESSON. 1979. Diffuse noxious inhibitory controls (DNIC) II. Lack of effects on non-convergent neurones, supra spinal involvement and theoretical implications. Pain **6**:305-327.

65. LE BARS, D., A. H. DICKENSON & J. M. BESSON. 1979. Diffuse noxious inhibitory controls (DNIC) I. Effects on dorsal horn convergent neurons in the rat. Pain **6**:283-304.

66. LEMAIRE, I., R. TSENG & S. LEMAIRE. 1978. Systemic administration of β-endorphin: Potent hypotensive effect involving a serotonergic pathway. Proc. Natl. Acad. Sci. USA **75**:6240-6242.

67. LEWIS, J. W., M. G. TORDOFF, J. E. SHERMAN & J. C. LIEBESKIND. 1982. Adrenal medullary enkephalin-like peptides may mediate opioid stress analgesia. Science **217**:557-559.

68. LITTLE, H. J. & J. M. H. REES. 1978. Naloxone antagonism of sympathomimetic analgesia. *In* Characteristics and Functions of Opioids. J. M. Van Ree & L. Terenius, Eds.: 433-434. Elsevier/North Holland. Amsterdam.

69. LOEWY, A. D. & S. MCKELLAR. 1980. The neuroanatomical basis of central cardiovascular control. Fed. Proc. **39**:2495-2503.

70. LOEWY, A. D., J. H. WALLACH & S. MCKELLAR. 1981. Efferent connections of the ventral medulla oblongata in the rat. Brain Res. Rev. **3**:63-80.

71. LOH, H. H., L. F. TSENG, E. WEI & C. H. LI. 1976. β-endorphin is a potent analgesic agent. Proc. Natl. Acad. Sci. USA **73**:2895-2898.
72. LOVICK, T. A. 1985. Ventrolateral medullary lesions block the antinociceptive and cardiovascular responses elicited by stimulating the dorsal periaqueductal grey matter in rats. Pain **21**:241-252.
73. MACLENNAN, J. A., R. C. DRUGAN, R. L. HYSON, S. F. MAIER, J. MADDEN & J. BARCHAS. 1982. Corticosterone: A critical factor in an opioid form of stress-induced analgesia. Science **215**:1530-1532.
74. MAIXNER, W. & A. RANDICH. 1984. Role of the right vagal nerve trunk in antinociception. Brain Res. **298**:374-377.
75. MAIXNER, W., K. B. TOUW, M. J. BRODY, G. F. GEBHART & J. P. LONG. 1982. Factors influencing the altered pain perception in the spontaneously hypertensive rat. Brain Res. **237**:137-145.
76. MALICK, J. B. & J. M. GOLDSTEIN. 1978. Analgesic activity of substance P following intracerebral administration in rats. Life Sci. **23**:835-844.
77. MAYER, D. J. & D. D. PRICE. 1976. Central nervous system mechanisms of analgesia. Pain **2**:379-404.
78. MELBY, J. C. & S. L. DALE. 1979. Adrenocorticosteroids in experimental and human hypertension. J. Endocrinol. **81**:93P-106P.
79. MILLAN, M. J., R. PREZEWLOCKI & A. HERZ. 1980. A non-β endorphinergic adenohypophyseal mechanism is essential for an analgetic response to stress. Pain **8**:343-353.
80. MILLAN, M. J., C. GRAMSCH, R. PREZEWLOCKI, V. HOLLT & A. HERZ. 1980. Lesions of the hypothalamic arcuate nucleus produce a temporary hyperalgesia and attenuate stress-evoked analgesia. Life Sci. **27**:1513-1523.
81. MISFELDT, D. S. & A. GOLDSTEIN. 1977. Hypophysectomy relieves pain not via endorphins. N. Eng. J. Med. **297**:1236-1237.
82. MORICCA, G. 1974. Chemical hypophysectomy for cancer pain. Adv. Neurol. **4**:707-714.
83. NARANJO, J. R. & J. A. FUENTES. 1985. Association between hypoalgesia and hypertension in rats after short-term isolation. Neuropharmacology **24**:167-171.
84. OLIVER, C., R. S. MICAL & J. C. PORTER. 1977. Hypothalamic pituitary vasculature: Evidence for retrograde blood flow in the pituitary stalk. Endocrinology **101**:598-604.
85. PERHACH, J. L., H. C. FERGUSON & G. P. McKINNEY. 1975. Evolution of antihypertensive agents in the stress-induced hypertensive rat. Life Sci. **16**:1731-1736.
86. PERT, A., T. W. MOODY, C. B. PERT, L. A. DEWALD & J. RIVIER. 1980. Bombesin: Receptor distribution in brain and effects on nociception and locomotor activity. Brain Res. **193**:209-222.
87. POMERANZ, B., R. CHUNG & P. LAW. 1977. Acupuncture reduces electrophysiological and behavioral responses to noxious stimuli; pituitary is implicated. Exp. Neurol. **54**:172-178.
88. PRICE, M. T. C. & H. C. FIBIGER. 1975. Ascending catecholamine systems and morphine analgesia. Brain Res. **99**:189-193.
89. RANDICH, A. & W. MAIXNER. 1984. Interactions between cardiovascular and pain regulatory systems. Neurosci. Biobehav. Rev. **8**:343-367.
90. RANDICH, A. & C. HARTUNIAN. 1983. Activation of the sinoaortic baroreceptor reflex arc induces analgesia: Interactions between cardiovascular and endogenous pain inhibition systems. Physiol. Psychol. **11**:214-220.
91. RANDICH, A. & W. MAIXNER. 1984. [D-Ala^2]-Methionine enkephalinamide reflexively induces antinociception by activating vagal afferents. Pharmacol. Biochem. Behav. **21**:441-448.
92. REDDY, S. V. R., J. L. MAERDRUT & T. L. YAKSH. 1980. Spinal cord pharmacology of adrenergic agonist-mediated antinociception. J. Pharmacol. Exp. Ther. **213**:525-530.
93. RICARDO, J. A. & E. T. KOH. 1978. Anatomical evidence of direct projections from the

nucleus of the solitary tract to the hypothalamus, amygdala, and other forebrain structures in the rat. Brain Res. **153**:1–26.
94. ROSENFELD, J. P. & S. STOCCO. 1980. Differential effects of systemic versus intracranial injection of opiate on central, orofacial, and lower body nociception: Somatotypy in bulbar analgesia systems. Pain **9**:307–318.
95. SAAVEDRA, J. M. 1981. Naloxone reversible decrease in pain sensitivity in young and adult spontaneously hypertensive rats. Brain Res. **209**:245–249.
96. SASA, M., K. MUNEKIYO, Y. OSUMI & S. TAKAORI. 1977. Attenuation of morphine analgesia in rats with lesions of the locus coeruleus and dorsl raphe nucleus. Eur. J. Pharmacol. **42**:53–62.
97. SELYE, H. 1950. The Stress of Life. McGraw Hill Book Company. New York.
98. SELYE, H. 1976. The general adaptation syndrome and the diseases of adaptation. J. Clin. Endorcinol. **6**:117–130.
99. SHAPIRO, A. P. 1961. An experimental study of comparative responses of blood pressure to different noxious stimuli. J. Chronic Dis. **13**:293–311.
100. SHARE, L. & J. T. CROFTON. 1984. The role of vasopressin in hypertension. Fed. Proc. **43**:103–106.
101. SISTEN, J. M. & W. DE JONG. 1983. Hypoalgesia in genetically hypertensive rats (SHR) is absent in rats with experimental hypertension. Hypertension **5**:185–190.
102. SKOFITSCH, G., D. M. JACOBOWITZ, R. L. ESKAY & N. ZAMIR. 1985. Distribution of atrial natriuretic factor-like immunoreactive neurons in the rat brain. Neuroscience. **16**:917–948.
103. SMITH, O. A. & J. L. DEVITO. 1984. Central neural integration for the control of autonomic responses associated with emotions. Ann. Rev. Neurosci. **7**:43–65.
104. SMOOKLER, H. H., K. H. GOEBEL, M. T. SIEGEL & D. E. CLARKE. 1973. Hypertensive effects of prolonged auditory, visual and motion stimulation. Fed. Proc. **32**:2105–2110.
105. STEIN, L. 1978. Reward transmitters: Catecholamines and opioid peptides. *In* Psychopharmacology: A Generation of Progress. M. Wipton, A. Moscio & K. Killan, Eds.: 469–581. Raven Press. New York.
106. STEWART, J. M., C. J. GETTO, K. NELDNER, E. B. REEVE, W. A. KRIVOY & E. ZIMMERMAN. 1976. Substance P and analgesia. Nature **262**:784–785.
107. SWANSON, L. W. & P. E. SAWCHENKO. 1980. Paraventricular nucleus: A site for the integration of neuroendocrine and autonomic mechanisms. Neuroendocrinology **31**:410–417.
108. SZEKELY, J. I., E. MIGLECZ, Z. DUNAI-KOVACS, I. TARNAWA, A. Z. RONAI, L. GRAF & S. BAJUSZ. 1979. Attenuation of morphine tolerance and dependence by α-melanocyte stimulating hormone (α-MSH). Life Sci. **24**:1931–1938.
109. TERMAN, G. W., Y. SHAVIT, J. W. LEWIS, J. T. CANNON & J. C. LIEBESKIND. 1984. Intrinsic mechanisms of pain inhibition: Activation by stress. Science **226**:1270–1277.
110. THOREN, P., D. MORGAN, T. P. O'NEILL, P. NEEDLEMAN, A. MARK & M. J. BRODY. 1985. Atrial natriuretic factor activates vagal afferents in rats. Fed. Proc. Absts. 8616.
111. TOURANDE, A. & S. MALMEJAC. 1929. Diversite des actions reflexes que declenche l'excitation du nerf. C. R. Soc. Biol. **100**:708–711.
112. TSENG, L. F., H. H. LOH & C. H. LI. 1976. β-endorphin as a potent analgesic by intravenous injection. Nature **263**:239–240.
113. VIDAL, C., J.-M. GIRAULT & J. JACOB. 1982. The effect of pituitary removal on pain regulation in the rat. Brain Res. **233**:53–64.
114. WATKINS, L. R. & D. J. MAYER. 1982. Organization of endogenous opiate and non-opiate pain control systems. Science **216**:1185–1192.
115. WILLER, J. C. & D. ALBE-FESSARD. 1980. Electrophysiological evidence for a release of endogenous opiates in stress-induced analgesia in man. Brain Res. **198**:419–426.
116. YAKSH, T. L. 1981. Spinal opiate analgesia: Characteristics and principles of action. Pain **11**:293–346.
117. YAO, T., S. ANDERSSON & P. THOREN. 1982. Long-lasting cardiovascular depressor

response following sciatic stimulation in spontaneously hypertensive rats. Evidence for the involvement of central endorphin and serotonin systems. Brain Res. **244**:295–303.

118. ZAMIR, N. & M. SEGAL. 1979. Hypertension-induced analgesia: Changes in pain sensitivity in experimental hypertensive rats. Brain Res. **160**:170–173.

119. ZAMIR, N. & E. SHUBER. 1980. Altered pain perception in hypertensive humans. Brain Res. **201**:471–474.

120. ZAMIR, N., R. SIMANTOV & M. SEGAL. 1980. Pain sensitivity and opioid activity in genetically and experimentally hypertensive rats. Brain Res. **184**:299–310.

121. ZAMIR, N., M. SEGAL & R. SIMANTOV. 1981. Opiate receptor binding in the brain of the hypertensive rat. Brain Res. **213**:217–222.

122. ZAMIR, N., M. SEGAL, D. BEN-ISHAY & R. SIMANTOV. 1980. Pain sensitivity and endogenous opiates in hypertension. *In* Neurotransmitters and Their Receptors. U. Z. Littauer, Y. Dudai, I. Silman, V. I. Teichberg & Z. Vogel, Eds.: 485–491. John Wiley & Sons, Ltd. New York.

123. ZAMIR, N. 1981. Interactions between cardiovascular and pain regulatory systems in the rat. Ph.D. dissertation. Weizmann Institute of Science. Rehovot, Israel.

124. ZAMIR, N., D. BEN-ISHAY, J. WIEDENFELD & R. SIEGEL. 1983. Stress induced secretion of ACTH, corticosterone and prolactin in experimentally and genetically hypertensive rats. Endocrinology **112**:580–586.

125. ZAMIR, N., D. ZAMIR, L. E. EIDEN, M. PALKOVITS, M. J. BROWNSTEIN, R. L. ESKAY, E. WEBER, A. I. FADEN G. FUERSTEIN. 1985. Methionine- and leucine-enkephalin in rat neurohypophysis: Different responses to osmotic stimuli and T_2 toxin. Science **228**:606–608.

The Role of Sinoaortic and Cardiopulmonary Baroreceptor Reflex Arcs in Nociception and Stress-Induced Analgesia[a]

ALAN RANDICH

Department of Psychology
The University of Iowa
Iowa City, Iowa 52242

and

WILLIAM MAIXNER

Neurobiology and Anesthesiology Branch
The National Institute of Dental Research
National Institutes of Health
Bethesda, Maryland 20205

INTRODUCTION

Sinoaortic and cardiopulmonary baroreceptor reflex arcs represent the primary mechanisms for maintaining circulatory homeostasis. These arcs utilize both peripheral receptors and central nervous system (CNS) components to control the circulation through reflex adjustments of sympathetic and parasympathetic efferents to the heart and vasculature.[1,2] There is also evidence to indicate that peripheral activation of baroreceptor reflex arcs by cardiovascular stimuli concomitantly engages endogenous CNS systems that inhibit pain. It is possible, therefore, that some stress-induced analgesias (SIAs) may be mediated by either stress-induced cardiovascular responses or the stress-induced release of substances that activate these arcs. In our view, at least three different peripheral physiological events are known to occur following the application of experimental stressors that bear upon possible mediation of SIAs by the baroreceptor reflex arcs. These stress-induced events include the release of opioid-like substances into the peripheral circulation, the release of vasoconstrictors, such as norepinephrine, that result in elevations of arterial blood pressure, and changes in the distribution of blood towards the heart, such as during the cardiovascular defense reaction, resulting in increased central blood volume. In the discussion that follows, we will show that hypoalgesia, a diminished sensitivity to tissue-damaging stimuli,[3] results from experimental manipulations which can be thought of as modeling these physiological reactions to stress. These manipulations include i.v. administration of [D-Ala²]methionine enkephalinamide, i.v.

[a]Supported by a grant from the National Institutes of Health (NS 18341) and a research fellowship from the Alfred P. Sloan Foundation to A. Randich. A. Randich is an Alfred P. Sloan Research Fellow.

administration of the peripheral vasoconstrictor phenylephrine, and administration of the volume-expander Ficoll. We then provide some evidence to show the involvement of these arcs in SIA that results from prolonged exposure to electric footshock.

BACKGROUND

In the original formulation of interactions between cardiovascular and pain inhibitory systems,[4] we proposed a working hypothesis asserting that either peripheral or central activation of the sinoaortic baroreceptor reflex arc and/or the cardiopulmonary baroreceptor reflex arc results in both circulatory and antinociceptive reflex adjustments. The cardiovascular adjustments to peripheral baroreceptor activation have been well studied and primarily involve an increase in parasympathetic tone to the heart, resulting in a negative chronotropic and inotropic action, and a decrease in sympathetic tone to the various vascular beds resulting in vasodilatation. The antinociceptive actions of baroreceptor activation are just beginning to be systematically studied, but historically were anticipated by diverse findings ranging from baroreceptor-induced inhibition of sham rage in decerebrate cats[5] to induction of a sleep-like state in dogs.[6] It is likely that baroreceptor activation also inhibits cardiac, visceral, and somatic pain. However, the following factors should be considered in any discussion of a possible role for cardiovascular-pain regulatory interactions in SIAs.

The basic tenet of the model is that under conditions of baroreceptor activation there is a suppression of nociceptive reflexes and a production of circulatory adjustments. However, the reflex circulatory changes brought about by experimental activation of the baroreceptor reflex arcs are not necessarily postulated to serve any type of mediational role in the primary production of analgesia, although they may exert secondary effects that oppose the conditions for the production of analgesia since they are typically compensatory in nature. For example, an elevation of arterial blood pressure will result in the activation of baroreceptor afferents to produce analgesia and a reflex slowing of the heart or bradycardia. In turn, bradycardia would result in a reduction of cardiac output, and thereby counteract the initial elevation in arterial blood pressure as well as the stimulus for the production of analgesia, i.e., baroreceptor activation. We have acknowledged that certain limitations of interpretation are necessary in view of these factors associated with experimental activation of a closed-loop system.[4] In addition, it remains an open issue where cardiovascular stimulus input actually transfers information to systems that inhibit pain, but the resultant hypoalgesia is assumed to be a reflex end-point in the same manner as the circulatory adjustments. Finally, the model makes no predictions about the nociceptive changes that follow unloading of the baroreceptors from levels of activity that maintain normal hemodynamic function, although some preliminary thoughts will be discussed later.

OPIOID-LIKE SUBSTANCES

Opioid-like substances are co-stored and co-secreted with the adrenal medullary catecholamines and are present in some peripheral nerve terminals.[7-10] There is some evidence that adrenal medullary opioid-like substances are released following exposure to stressors and may mediate the production of SIA resulting from prolonged exposure to a stressor.[11] The problem, however, has been to identify a mechanism by which circulating enkephalins and/or endorphins could produce analgesia, since they do not readily cross the blood-brain barrier[12,13] (excluding the possibility that the permeability of the barrier may be affected by any number of stimuli associated with stress). In addition, met-enkephalin and many met-enkephalin analogs are extensively metabolized on the first pass through the lungs.[14] As the following studies will show, however, these substances do not have to gain access to the CNS, since peripheral vagal afferents input to endogenous CNS substrates that inhibit pain and have associated peripheral receptors that most likely bind opioid-like substances. This mechanism was suggested by demonstrations that the cardiorespiratory effects of peripherally administered enkephalin analogs and morphine are mediated by cardiopulmonary baroreceptors with associated vagal afferents.[15,16] We have inferred that the cardiopulmonary region is also a likely site for opioid receptors[17] mediating antinociception because a major endogenous source of opioid-like substances is the adrenal medullae and degradation of opioid-like substances is substantial prior to entry into the arterial circulation.[14] However, this would not preclude other sites of opioid receptors in the periphery with associated visceral or vagal afferents, e.g., the mesentery.

Three groups of Sprague-Dawley rats ($N = 5$ in each group) were implanted with both a right common carotid artery catheter for obtaining measurements of arterial blood pressure and heart rate and an external jugular vein catheter for intravenous (i.v.) bolus infusions of vehicle or drug. Rats in one group received sham operations, rats in a second group received bilateral sinoaortic deafferentations (SAD), and rats in a third group received unilateral resections of the right cervical vagal nerve trunk. The latter two treatments were included to assess the role of sinoaortic and vagal afferents, respectively, in the hypoalgesia and cardiovascular responses produced by the drug. Unilateral vagal resection was used because a rat cannot live for any substantial length of time in the conscious state following bilateral cervical vagal resection. The day following implantation of the catheters, each rat received successive i.v. bolus infusions of isotonic saline with 5, 50, and 500 µg/kg of [D-ala²]methionine enkephalinamide (DALA, Sigma Co.), an analog of methionine enkephalin that does not readily pass the blood-brain barrier.[12] Saline vehicle and drug solutions were infused in a volume of 1 ml/kg at a rate of approximately 200 µl/sec. Each saline or drug administration was followed by a 400 µl saline flush. Tail-flick test trials were administered 0.25, 1, 2, and 3 min after each infusion. Each tail-flick latency was converted to a tail-flick index (TFI) by the equation [(test trial latency − baseline latency)/(10 seconds − baseline latency) × 100], where 10 seconds was the upper cut-off point. Cardiovascular measures of heart rate and blood pressure were taken at the corresponding times and in addition, a peak response measure was calculated that represented the largest response observed between the saline flush and the 0.25 minute trial. Cardiovascular measures are all reported as percentage change from baseline values. Figure 1 shows the outcomes of these manipulations. Figure 1 reveals a significant dose-dependent inhibition of the tail-flick reflex in sham-operated rats during early test trials followed by a recovery towards baseline values during late test trials. However, neither bilateral SAD nor right cervical vagotomy significantly altered the hypoalgesic action of DALA as compared to sham-operated rats. The SAD data clearly indicate that carotid sinus and aortic depressor nerves are not mediating the hypoalgesic actions of DALA, but the unilateral right vagotomy data do not rule out possible mediation by vagal afferents, which is demonstrated later. Extremely rapid and short-lived bradycardic and hypotensive responses were also manifested by rats in all three groups following DALA administration.

The failure to obtain an attenuation of DALA-induced hypoalgesia in the

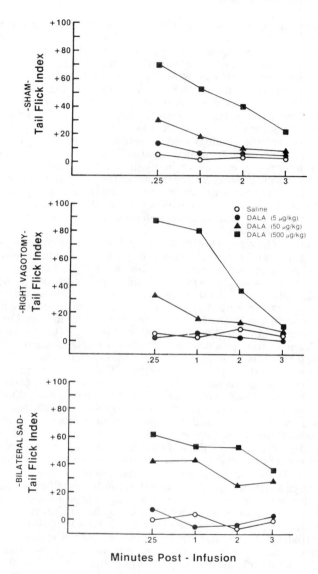

FIGURE 1. Mean tail-flick indices for sham, right vagotomy, and bilateral SAD groups following saline or DALA administration.

conscious right-vagotomized rat required us to examine the bilaterally vago-tomized rat using the lightly anesthetized preparation.[17-19] A rat with a bilateral cervical vagotomy can survive in the lightly anesthetized state. In this experiment, two groups of rats ($N = 5$ in each group) received an intraperitoneal (i.p.) injection of pentobarbital sodium (50 mg/kg), and implantation of arterial and venous catheters as described previously. Forty min after the induction of anesthesia the rats received either a sham vagotomy or a bilateral cervical vagotomy. Within three min of either the sham vagotomy or the resection, each rat received a bolus i.v. infusion of 500 µg/kg of DALA and tail-flick test trials as described previously. The outcomes of these manipulations are shown in FIGURE 2. This figure shows that lightly anesthetized sham-operated rats manifested strong inhibition of the tail-flick reflex and TFI values did not significantly differ from those shown in FIGURE 1 for conscious sham-operated rats receiving the same dose of DALA. However, lightly anesthetized bilaterally vagotomized rats showed no hypoalgesia following administration of DALA and their TFI values differed significantly from those of sham-operated rats. The middle and bottom panels of FIGURE 2 also reveal that bilateral vagotomy totally abolished the reflex bradycardic and hypotensive effects of DALA, which is consistent with the established role of the vagi in mediating the cardiorespiratory effects of other enkephalin analogs.[15,16] Thus, the hypoalgesic and cardiovascular actions of DALA clearly depend upon the integrity of only a single vagal nerve trunk, although these studies do not necessarily localize the receptor to the cardio-pulmonary region.

The specificity of DALA in producing these changes via an interaction with an opioid receptor is suggested by the outcomes of the following experiment. Two groups of rats ($N = 5$ in each group) served as subjects and were implanted with catheters as described previously. One group of rats received successive admin-istration of isotonic saline and a 500 µg/kg dose of DALA followed by repeated tail-flick test trials as described previously. Their data are presented in the upper panel of FIGURE 3. The second group of rats received successive administration of isotonic saline, 500 µg/kg of i.v. naloxone (followed by another 500 µg/kg of naloxone 5 minutes after this testing), and 500 µg/kg of DALA. Their data are presented in the bottom panel of FIGURE 3. The upper panel of this figure reveals the usual robust hypoalgesic action of DALA and the absence of any effect with the saline vehicle. The bottom panel of this figure reveals that a total of 1 mg/kg of naloxone completely eliminates this hypoalgesic action of DALA. Although not presented, this dose of naloxone also totally eliminated the reflex bradycardia and hypotension produced by 500 µg/kg of DALA. Thus, the hypoalgesia and cardiovascular responses produced by i.v. DALA administration involve media-tion by opioid receptors, although the present opioid receptor antagonist manipulation does not distinguish between the possible physiological action of DALA on a peripheral opioid receptor versus the possible pharmacological action of DALA in engaging a CNS system that utilizes opioids in the production of hypoalgesia.

Finally, the inhibition of the tail-flick reflex induced by administration of DALA involves some pathway coursing in the dorsolateral funiculus (DLF) of the spinal cord. Two groups of rats ($N = 6$ in each group) received either bilateral lesions of the DLF or sham operations approximately seven days prior to catheter implantation and testing of the tail-flick reflex in the conscious state. Each rat then received i.v. administration of saline followed by 500 µg/kg of DALA as generally described previously. FIGURE 4 presents the outcomes of these manipu-lations. In general, the top panel of this figure reveals that rats receiving DLF lesions did not show hypoalgesia in response to 500 µg/kg of DALA, while sham-

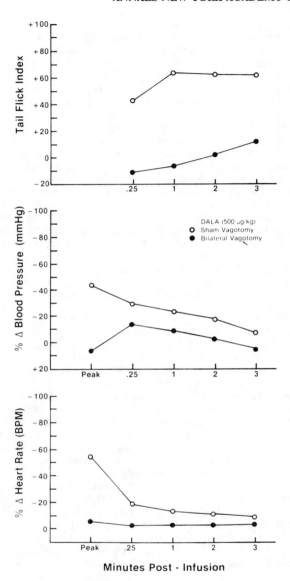

FIGURE 2. Mean tail-flick index, mean percent change in arterial blood pressure, and mean percent change in heart rate resulting from DALA administration (500 µg/kg) in bilateral vagotomized rats and sham controls.

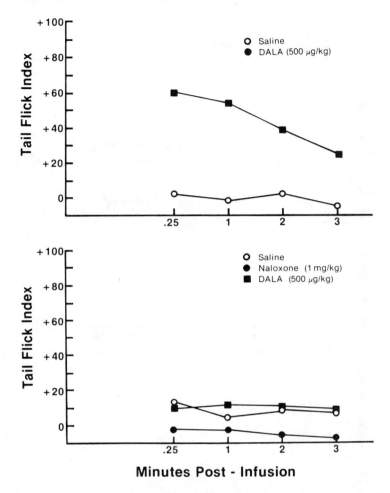

FIGURE 3. Mean tail-flick indices following either saline or DALA administration (500 μg/kg) in the absence (top panel) or the presence (bottom panel) of naloxone.

lesioned rats did show hypoalgesia. The middle and bottom panels of this figure show arterial blood pressure and heart rate changes induced by DALA in these animals. It is of interest that the hypotensive response to DALA remains intact after the bilateral DLF lesion, although the present study did not assess whether the hypotension was a consequence of bradycardia-induced reductions in cardiac output or a withdrawal of sympathetic tone. However, it is presently thought that the final common pathways for depressor responses originate in cell bodies located in the nucleus raphe magnus (NRM), the ventromedial reticular formation, and the ventral part of the lateral reticular nucleus (LRN), and

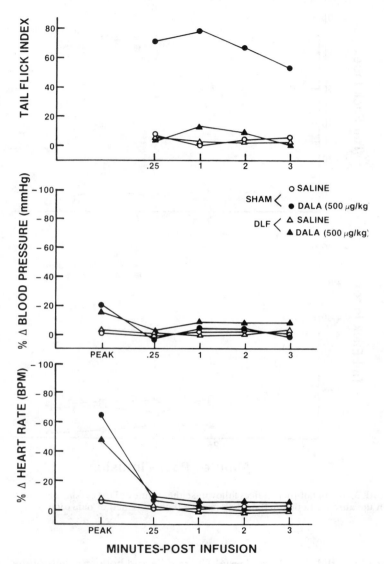

FIGURE 4. Mean tail-flick index, mean percent change in arterial blood pressure, and mean percent change in heart rate resulting from saline or DALA (500 μg/kg) administration in bilateral DLF lesioned rats and sham controls.

descend in both the ventral DLF and ventral funiculus.[1] This would account for the failure to affect reflex hypotension by bilateral DLF lesions if only sympathetic withdrawal was involved.

In summary, the experimental data suggest that circulating opioid-like substances could induce hypoalgesia by activating peripheral opioid receptors whose afferents travel in the vagi to then engage endogenous centrifugal pain inhibition systems sending fibers in the DLF to the spinal cord. Although the limitations of this interpretation have been noted and large amounts of DALA were required to produce hypoalgesia, we believe this vagal mechanism remains viable as a physiological substrate of pain inhibition since (1) opioids and opioid-like substances may be secreted in multiple and protected forms from adrenal medullae, cardiac tissue, and other yet-to-be identified tissues leaving the actual circulating amounts an unknown quantity at this point in time, (2) these substances may exert their effect directly upon receptors trafficked by the coronary circulation, and only a fraction of the amounts of DALA would reach the coronary circulation given the present route of administration through the external jugular vein, and (3) few studies have delineated the boundary conditions for the amounts of opioid-like substances that are released under severe stress.

ARTERIAL BLOOD PRESSURE

Stress reactions also involve an elevation of arterial blood pressure, primarily effected through increased sympathetic tone to the vasculature and secondarily through the release of adrenal medullary catecholamines. An experimental elevation in arterial blood pressure is capable of producing hypoalgesia[4,20] and sympathomimetics have been used as analgesics in humans.[21] It is also of interest to note that humans with essential hypertension and animals with either genetic or experimentally induced hypertension manifest analgesia to at least some forms of tissue-damaging stimuli.[22-24]

In one of our early studies,[4] a group of rats ($N = 5$) received implantation of catheters as previously described and successive bolus infusions of saline or 31.25, 62.50, and 125.00 µg/kg of phenylephrine, a peripherally acting vasoconstrictor. Tail-flick test trials were administered as previously described. FIGURE 5 presents the TFI values and cardiovascular responses resulting from these manipulations. The 62.50 and 125.00 µg/kg doses of phenylephrine did result in significant inhibition of the tail-flick reflex when compared to saline control values, although the most efficacious conditions only resulted in 60% inhibition of the tail-flick reflex. However, our previous work[20] using continuous infusion of small amounts of phenylephrine resulted in the production of profound hypoalgesia that lasted at least 30 min following termination of the infusion, and these effects could not be obtained in rats with bilateral SADs. The middle panel presents the percent increases in blood pressure produced by phenylephrine, and there is noticeable overlap of the functions. However, this may be a consequence of the action of the vasoconstrictor masking the action of the reflex inhibition of sympathetic tone. More orderly functions are shown with respect to heart rate in the bottom panel of FIGURE 5.

In another study, separate groups of rats ($N = 7$ in each group) received implantation of only an external jugular vein catheter. Each rat then received a bolus i.v. infusion of either saline or 31.25, 62.50, or 125.00 µg/kg of phenylephrine

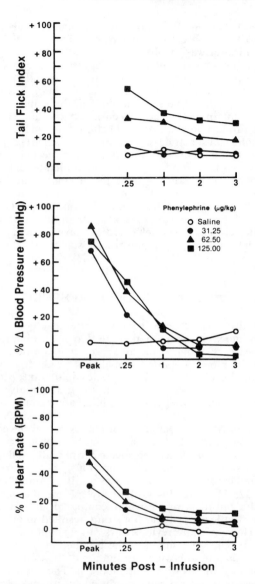

FIGURE 5. Mean tail-flick index, mean percent change in arterial blood pressure, and mean percent change in heart rate as a function of saline or phenylephrine administration.

followed by hot-plate testing 0.25 min after the infusion (plate temperature was 52°C). Figure 6 indicates that there is an orderly increase in latencies to lick the hind paw or jump from the plate, although statistical analyses indicated that only the latencies of rats in the 125.00 µg/kg condition differed significantly from saline control values. This hypoalgesic effect was unaffected by the prior administration of naloxone. Thus, at least under some conditions the hypoalgesic action of phenylephrine can be demonstrated with a supraspinal nociceptive reflex.

In summary, if we combine the outcomes obtained with continuous infusion and bolus infusion procedures then the following conclusions can be drawn. The hypoalgesic action of phenylephrine is (1) mediated by activation of arterial baroreceptors because bilateral SAD blocks the effect,[20] (2) specific to activation of either peripheral or central alpha-adrenergic receptors since phentolamine administration blocks the effect,[4] (3) enhanced by administration of either methyl atropine or atropine sulfate, but this outcome is presumably due to the larger increases in arterial blood pressures that are generated in the absence of reflex heart rate decreases,[4] and (5) unaffected by naloxone administration when a paw-lick response is used to assay pain sensitivity and possibly enhanced by naloxone administration when a tail-flick response is used, although the latter outcome was obtained using a within-subject manipulation that failed to include a control for repeated testing of the animals.[4] It is interesting to note that electrical stimulation of the carotid sinus nerve in humans has been cited as eliminating cardiac pain.[25]

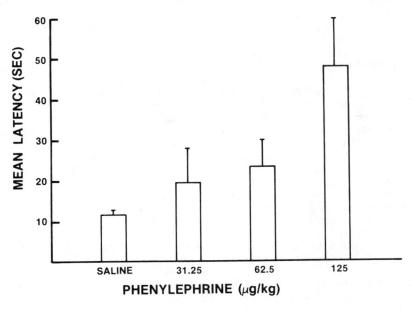

FIGURE 6. Mean latencies to paw-lick as a function of saline or phenylephrine administration.

However, some problems with this work on arterial blood pressure are that (1) the very high pressures in the bolus infusion studies may have produced an afterload on the heart resulting in both activation of and contribution by cardiopulmonary receptors with vagal afferents, (2) there is some evidence in rabbits that phenylephrine has a CNS effect that can alter arterial baroreflex control of sympathetic renal nerves following sustained but not transient pressure elevations, and this effect depends upon simultaneous peripheral activation of the baroreflexes thereby posing some possible interpretive difficulties even for the SAD data,[26] and (3) restrained animals receiving application of noxious radiant heat already have extremely high basal levels of sympathetic activity.

VOLUME EXPANSION

During conditions of both exercise and stress, blood volume is shifted centrally to the heart.[1] This can result in the activation of cardiac mechanoreceptors and the cardiopulmonary baroreceptor reflex arc.[2] We have demonstrated that experimental activation of the cardiopulmonary reflex arc by volume expansion results in reflex hypotension, bradycardia, and hypoalgesia.[27]

In these experiments, two groups of rats with sham operations and one group of rats with right cervical vagotomies received implantation of catheters as previously described. One sham-operated group was pre-treated with naltrexone (20 mg/kg i.p.) ten minutes prior to testing. All groups then received a volume expansion treatment in which a 5% Ficoll-saline solution was infused through the jugular catheter at a rate of 1.97 ml/min for 2 min epochs. Tail-flick test trials were administered every 2 min and when a 10 sec latency was manifested (upper cutoff) the infusion procedure was stopped and tail-flick trials were administered every 3 min for the ensuing 30 min. FIGURE 7 shows the outcomes obtained after termination of the infusion procedure.

All groups showed hypoalgesia that persisted for the 30 min observation period, but the right vagotomized animals showed significantly faster recovery than either sham-operated rats or sham-operated rats pre-treated with naltrexone, where the latter did not differ. This difference was not attributable to any between-group differences in the amount of volume received prior to termination of the infusion procedure. However, this vagal reflex mechanism of pain inhibition must in some fashion differ from the vagal reflex mechanism that is activated by DALA (opioid-like outcomes also occur with veratrine)[28] indicating that mechanoreceptors activated by volume expansion represent either a different population of receptors from those activated by DALA or a subpopulation of those receptors activated by DALA.

Nonetheless, a vagal reflex mechanism of pain inhibition can be demonstrated to play a role in SIA.[27] Four groups of rats received exposure to 30 minutes of inescapable footshocks (2 mA, 1 sec in duration, 1 shock delivered every 5 seconds) followed by tail-flick test trials every 5 minutes for a 30 minute observation period. Group vagotomy–shock ($N = 15$) had prior resection of the right cervical vagal nerve trunk; Group naltrexone–shock ($N = 16$) had received pre-treatment with 10 mg/kg of naltrexone 10 minutes prior to the shock treatment; Group nal-vag–shock ($N = 8$) received both prior resection of the right cervical vagal nerve trunk and pre-treatment with 10 mg/kg of naltrexone; and Group sham–shock ($N = 23$) received an injection of saline vehicle 10 minutes prior to the shock treatment. Two groups of rats received no exposure to shock,

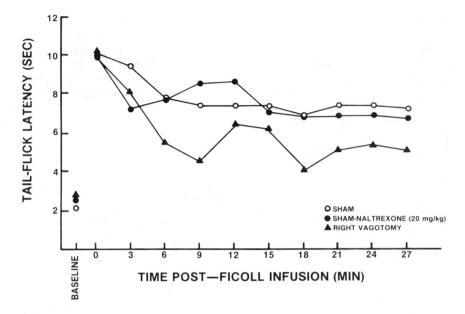

FIGURE 7. Mean latencies to tail-flick during the post-infusion observation period following volume-expansion. Baseline response latencies are denoted in the figure.

but did receive the tail-flick testing procedure. Group sham–no shock ($N = 8$) received a sham operation and Group vagotomy–no shock ($N = 8$) received prior resection of the right vagal nerve trunk. FIGURE 8 shows the outcomes of these manipulations during the 30 minute observation period. Group sham–shock showed a typical SIA when compared to the control groups sham–no shock and vagotomy–no shock. The latter two groups also did not significantly differ indicating that thresholds were not altered by the right vagotomy. Group naltrexone–shock showed significant attenuation of the SIA. Group vagotomy–shock also showed significant attenuation of the SIA and did not differ from Group naltrexone. Finally, the combination of both naltrexone and vagotomy in Group nal-vag–shock did not enhance the attenuation of SIA observed with either treatment alone. It might also be noted that bilateral SAD was not effective in altering this form of SIA.

We orginally interpreted these outcomes in the following manner. Changes in blood volume (as modeled by volume expansion) and/or peripherally released opioid-like substances (as modeled by the DALA treatment) may occur during times of stress (as modeled by the SIA procedure) and be independently capable of activating peripheral receptors whose afferents travel in the vagi. This activity engages CNS systems that inhibit pain. The only interpretive problem for this view with the present data sets is that if opioid-like substances were released during our SIA procedure and contributed to the hypoalgesia, then a right cervical vagotomy should not have been effective in attenuating this effect given

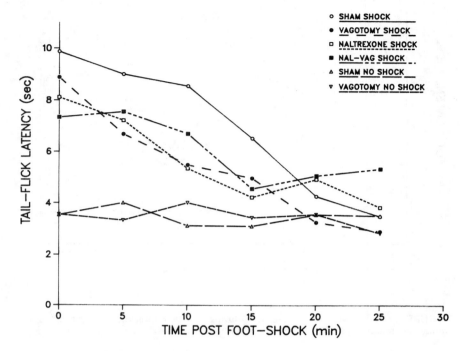

FIGURE 8. Mean latencies to tail-flick for the various treatment groups during the observation period following 30 minutes of exposure to inescapable electric footshock.

our negative outcomes of this manipulation with DALA-induced hypoalgesia. This could be accounted for by attributing the entire SIA attenuation effect to a redistribution of blood volume, but then naltrexone should have been either ineffective based upon our volume load data or additive if another system were involved.

SUMMARY

The intent of this chapter was to present the outcomes of studies using three types of experimental treatments (DALA, phenylephrine, and volume expansion) that can be thought of as modeling three types of physiologic reactions to stressors (release of opioid-like substances, elevations of arterial blood pressure, and mobilization of blood towards the heart). These experimental treatments activated cardiopulmonary and sinoaortic baroreceptors to induce bradycardia, hypotension, and suppression of nociceptive reflexes. We have previously outlined a number of potential CNS loci that may integrate and modulate cardiovascular and somatosensory events.[4] Many cells in these CNS sites receive input from the baroreceptor afferents relaying in the nucleus tractus solitarius (NTS) and then send projections to spinal loci that integrate somatosensory input and preganglionic autonomic nervous system output. However, the overall neural organization of central nuclei that integrate both cardiovascular and somato-sensory information is probably very complex and focal stimulation of any one of these sites may not result in a strong correlation between depression of cardiac function and antinociception. For instance, focal stimulation of loci that receive peripheral baroreceptor input and constitute part of the baroreceptor reflex pathway may suppress cardiac dynamics and impair nociceptive reflexes. In contrast, stimulation of central sites that augment sympathoadrenal function to increase cardiac dynamics may also impair nociceptive reflexes, but due to sympathoadrenal-induced elevations of arterial blood pressure, venous blood pressure, and/or the release of opioid-like substances into the circulation; all of which stimulate baroreceptor afferents. In our view, the best predictor of impaired reactions to noxious stimulation is not arterial or venous blood pressure per se, but rather the functional status of the baroreceptors. Under conditions of baroreceptor activation, our model predicts that responses to noxious stimuli are depressed.

In the presence of either emotional stress or certain pathological states (e.g., hypertension), the relationship between autonomic and nociceptive responses may also be difficult to interpret. For example, hypertensive rats and humans show blunted cardiac responses to baroreceptor activation, yet still display hypoalgesia to most forms of noxious stimuli. Similarly, the reflex bradycardia that might be expected in response to baroreceptor activation during psychogenic stress is also altered. In this regard, psychogenic stressors produce a unique set of cardiovascular responses that have been referred to as the defense reaction or the visceral alerting response. This response is characterized by cardiac stimulation, which increases heart rate and cardiac output; neurogenic constriction of the resistance and capacitance vessels, which increases arterial and venous pressure; and selective neurogenic or humoral dilatation of skeletal, myocardial, and cerebral vessels, which increases blood flow to these regions.[29] As noted previously, increases in arterial pressure and central venous pressure are stimuli that activate sinoaortic and cardiopulmonary baroreceptors to produce reflex bradycardia, yet the tachycardia observed during the defense reaction indicates that the baroreceptor reflex is "clamped" at the brainstem level, presumably by information arising from limbic-hypothalamic structures. In contrast to the cardiac responses, the reflex vascular responses are not altered. Thus, it is difficult to ascribe a given cardiovascular profile with the presence of impaired noci-ceptive reflexes.

The precise relationship between the defense reaction and impairment of nociceptive reflexes remains to be determined. However, focal electrical stimula-tion of some sites in the dorsal periaqueductal grey that support stimulation-produced analgesia also support the defense reaction[30] and many stressors that elicit the defense reaction have also been independently demonstrated to produce SIA and conditioned analgesia, e.g. electric shock. It seems plausible that central elicitation of the defense reaction by stress-induced activation of limbic-hypothalamic structures may produce hypoalgesia by engaging central pathways that control baroreceptor reflexes. In addition, the elevation in arterial and venous pressures produced by the defense reaction may stimulate peripheral baroreceptors, which would also impair the behavioral responses to noxious stimuli. In this regard, the activity of unmyelinated cardiac afferents that travel in the vagi is increased during the defense reaction,[31] although more definitive studies will be required to assess their relationship to SIA.

At the present time, we have little evidence about the effect of unloading sinoaortic and cardiopulmonary baroreceptors with respect to nociceptive reflexes, but vagotomy and SAD manipulations typically failed to affect baseline levels of nociceptive responses. Administration of sodium nitroprusside (a potent vasodilator) does produce a powerful hypoalgesia, but this result appears to be either a direct central or neuromuscular action of the drug rather than an effect of hypotension-induced unloading of the baroreceptors (Randich, unpublished observations).

The previous discussion alludes to the complexities of interactions between the cardiovascular and somatosensory systems during stress. The interactions undoubtedly provide the organism with a host of adaptive responses to stressors, but clearly we have little understanding of these responses at the present stage of analysis. From a teleological point of view, however, a number of advantages to such interactions can be envisioned. Baroreceptor activation may decrease the sensory and/or affective aspects of a noxious or stressful stimulus, thereby allowing the organism to both attend to and perform more relevant goal-directed behaviors, i.e., fight or flight—protective somatic responses. Baroreceptor-mediated suppression of pain may diminish sympathetic responses evoked by tissue-damaging stimuli, thereby permitting the precise orchestration of cardiovascular adjustments that are required to initiate and sustain these appropriate goal-directed behaviors, i.e., the circulatory system defends itself against deleterious cardiovascular input. But most important, we think it likely that cardiovascular-pain regulatory interactions and the ensuing reflex adjustments of both circulation and nociception under conditions of stress represent only a small part of a much larger integrated response of the organism to potentially life-threatening situations.

REFERENCES

1. ABBOUD, F. M. & M. D. THAMES. 1984. Interactions of cardiovascular reflexes in circulatory control. *In* Handbook of Physiology-The Cardiovascular System III. J. T. Shepherd & F. M. Abboud, Eds.: 675–753. American Physiological Society. Bethesda, MD.
2. BISHOP, V. S., A. MALLIANI & P. THOREN. 1984. Cardiac mechanoreceptors. *In* Handbook of Physiology-The Cardiovascular System III. J. T. Shepherd & F. M. Abboud, Eds.: 497–555. American Physiological Society. Bethesda, MD.
3. BONICA, J. J. 1979. The need of a taxonomy. Pain **6**:247–252.
4. RANDICH, A. & W. MAIXNER. 1984. Interactions between cardiovascular and pain regulatory systems. Neurosci. Biobehav. Rev. **8**:343–367.
5. BARTORELLI, C., E. BIZZI, A. LIBRETTI & A. ZANCHETTI. 1968. Inhibitory control of sinocarotid pressoceptive afferents on hypothalamic autonomic activity and sham rage behavior. Arch. Ital. Biol. **98**:308–326.
6. KOCH, E. 1932. Die irradiation der pressoreceptorischen kreislaufreflexe. Klin. Wochenschr. **2**:225–227.
7. VIVEROS, O. H. & S. P. WILSON. 1983. The adrenal chromaffin cell as a model to study the co-secretion of enkephalins and catecholamines. J. Autonom. Nerv. Syst. **7**:41–58.
8. VIVEROS, O. H., E. J. DILIBERTO, E. HAZUM & K-J. CHANG. 1979. Opiate-like materials in the adrenal medulla: Evidence for storage and secretion with catecholamines. Mol. Pharmacol. **16**:1101–1108.
9. LIVETT, B. G., D. M. DEAN, L. G. WHELAN, S. UDENFRIEND & J. ROSSIER. 1981. Co-release of enkephalin and catecholamines from culture adrenal chromaffin cells. Nature **289**:317–319.

10. GOVONI, S., I. HANBAUER, T. D. HEXUM, H.-Y. T. YANG, G. D. KELLY & E. COSTA. 1981. In vivo characterization of the mechanisms that secrete enkephalin-like peptides stored in the dog adrenal medulla. Neuropharmacology **20**:639–645.

11. LEWIS, J. W., M. G. TORDOFF, J. E. SHERMAN & J. C. LIEBESKIND. 1982. Adrenal medullary enkephalin-like peptides may mediate opioid stress-induced analgesia. Science **217**:557–559.

12. PARDRIDGE, W. M. & L. J. MIETUS. 1981. Enkephalin and blood-brain barrier: Studies of binding and degradation in isolated brain microvessels. Endocrinology **109**:1138–1143.

13. RAPOPORT, S. I., W. A. KLEE, K. D. PETTIGREW & K. OHNO. 1980. Entry of opioid peptides into the central nervous system. Science **207**:84–86.

14. MANWARING, D. & K. MULLANE. 1984. Disappearance of enkephalins in the isolated perfused rat lung. Life Sci. **35**:1787–1794.

15. WILLETTE, R. N. & H. N. SAPRU. 1982. Pulmonary opiate receptor activation evokes a cardiorespiratory reflex. Eur. J. Pharmacol. **78**:61–70.

16. WILLETTE, R. N. & H. N. SAPRU. 1982. Peripheral versus central cardiorespiratory effects of morphine. Neuropharmacology **21**:1019–1026.

17. RANDICH, A. & W. MAIXNER. 1984. [D-Ala^2]-methionine enkephalinamide reflexively induces antinociception by activating vagal afferents. Pharmacol. Biochem. Behav. **21**:441–448.

18. SANDKUHLER, J. & G. F. GEBHART. 1984. Characterization of inhibition of spinal nociceptive reflex by stimulation medially and laterally in the midbrain and medulla in the pentobarbital-anesthetized rat. Brain Res. **305**:67–76.

19. SANDKUHLER, J. & G. F. GEBHART. 1984. Relative contributions of the nucleus raphe magnus and adjacent medullary reticular formation to the inhibition by stimulation in the periaqueductal gray of a spinal nociceptive reflex in the pentobarbital-anesthetized rat. Brain Res. **305**:77–87.

20. RANDICH, A. & C. HARTUNIAN. 1983. Activation of the sinoaortic baroreceptor reflex arc induces analgesia: Interactions between cardiovascular and endogenous pain inhibition systems. Physiol. Psychol. **11**:214–220.

21. FELLOWS, E. J. & G. E. ULLYOT. 1951. Analgesics: Aralkylamines. *In* Medicinal Chemistry. C. M. Suter, Ed.: 390–396. Wiley & Sons. New York.

22. ZAMIR, N. & E. SHUBER. 1980. Altered pain perception in hypertensive humans. Brain Res. **201**:471–474.

23. ZAMIR, N. & M. SEGAL. 1979. Hypertension-induced analgesia: Changes in pain sensitivity in experimental hypertensive rats. Brain Res. **160**:170–173.

24. RANDICH, A. & W. MAIXNER. 1981. Acquisition of conditioned suppression and responsivity to thermal stimulation in spontaneously hypertensive, renal hypertensive, and normotensive rats. Physiol. Behav. **27**:585–590.

25. BERNE, R. M. & M. N. LEVY, Eds. 1981. Cardiovascular Physiology. 4th edit. C. V. Mosby Company. St. Louis, MO.

26. IMAIZUMI, T., S. D. BRUNK, B. N. GUPTA & M. D. THAMES. 1984. Central effect of intravenous phenylephrine on baroreflex control of renal nerves. Hypertension **6**:906–914.

27. MAIXNER, W. & A. RANDICH. 1984. Role of the right vagal nerve trunk in antinociception. Brain Res. **298**:374–377.

28. RANDICH, A., T. A. SIMPSON, P. A. HANGER & R. L. FISHER. 1984. Activation of vagal afferents by veratrine induces antinociception. Physiol. Psychol. **12**:293–301.

29. FOLKOW, B. 1982. Physiological aspects of primary hypertension. Physiol. Rev. **62**:347–504.

30. LOVIK, T. A. 1985. Venterolateral medullary lesions block the antinociceptive and cardiovascular responses elicited by stimulating the dorsal periaqueductal grey matter in rats. Pain **21**:241–252.

31. THOREN, P. 1979. Role of cardiac vagal C-fibers in cardiovascular control. Rev. Physiol. Biochem. Pharmacol. **86**:1–94.

The Morality and Humaneness of Animal Research on Stress and Pain

NEAL E. MILLER

The Rockefeller University
New York, New York 10021

No scientist that I know of is in favor of subjecting experimental animals to unnecessary suffering. Elsewhere I have emphasized that we should educate our students to keep experimental animals as healthy and emotionally undisturbed as possible.[4]

Most experimental research on animals involves little or no pain.[7] But one cannot conduct controlled experiments on stress and pain without deliberately inducing stress and pain. These experiments pose a moral issue that it is important to understand clearly. Stated in one way the issue is: Is it morally justifiable to cause experimental animals to suffer in order to reduce human (and animal) suffering? The same issue conversely becomes: Is it morally justifiable to prolong human (and animal) suffering in order to reduce suffering by experimental animals?

The foregoing moral issue is made still sharper by the fact that one cannot extrapolate confidently from the effects of mild levels of stress or pain to those of intense levels. With stress, including that produced by pain, the body has a remarkable homeostatic capacity to compensate for and adapt to the effects of moderately strong levels. It is when the levels are increased further and must be endured longer, so that these mechanisms break down, that one first observes certain highly significant effects such as cardiovascular damage, stomach lesions, behavioral depression from depletion of brain norepinephrine,[2,9] and what Selye[8] has described as the transition from adaptation to exhaustion.

Similarly, on the therapeutic side, aspirin is adequate to deal with certain mild pains, but larger doses of it are ineffective against more intense pains. These pains require different, more potent pain-killers and, unfortunately, there are levels of of incapacitating the patients by anesthetizing them. Limiting research to mild pain will interfere with discovery of the more potent pain killers that we need.

Pain is a major medical problem estimated to produce a burden of $50 billion a year in the U.S.A.[6] Severe stress creates or aggravates a wide range of mental and physical problems.[2] To limit research to lower levels of pain and stress will prevent progress on understanding and treating the very conditions that produce the most intense human suffering.

To return to the moral choice between human and animal suffering, the three major religions of the West, whether one considers their source divine inspiration or distilled social wisdom, have a clear-cut answer. Christians, Jews, and Muslims share a story that crystallizes the answer. As a test of his faith, Abraham was about to sacrifice his son when God told him to spare the child and, instead, sacrifice a lamb; the answer was to spare the human and sacrifice the animal.

A variety of biological considerations all lead to the same conclusion shared by Western religions. When those who claim that it is immoral to exploit animals by experimenting on them have it called to their attention that pet cats and dogs exploit mice, birds, woodchucks, and deer by killing them, their reply is that these pet animals are merely responding to their genetically inherited instincts. But humans, even more than their cousins the primates, have inherited a strong innate curiosity that has led them along the path to knowledge and civilization. Furthermore, all mammals have strong innate motivation to protect their young from harm. It is unwise to appear to be threatening the cub of a nearby mother bear. The answer of biology to our moral issue is like that of the Bible, Torah, and Koran: "Save your child."

There is time to clarify only the key aspects of the moral question before us. The informed biologist has an enormous respect for the awesome complexity of even the simplest single-celled forms of life. Many of these simple creatures move toward conditions that are beneficial to them and away from those that are harmful. Purifying our water to prevent deadly plagues, washing our hands, or other forms of sanitation cause astronomical numbers of infectious agents to die. To move up the scale of life, people could not live, even in the simplest gathering society, without eating products that interfere with the lives of plants, insects, and the vast array of other animals that compete with people for these vegetarian foods. Many biomedical scientists are leaders in conservational measures to preserve the balance of nature. But in this world that balance inevitably involves either obvious or concealed lethal competition. One cannot live without interfering with other forms of life.

Where does one draw any line? I suggest that a biologically rational and legally practical place is at the clear-cut boundary of the human species. To give only one more of the reasons for this conclusion, people are different from animals in their greater capacity for reasoning and for passing on knowledge, especially by written language. Rabies (hydrophobia) used to produce horrible suffering in both animals and people before it inevitably killed its victim. Pasteur's experiments, which necessarily caused a relatively small number of dogs extreme suffering, have spared millions of both dogs and people from this dreadful disease. Over the years, the net reduction in overall suffering has been immense. One cannot imagine a dog or even a higher ape experimenting on people to produce similar benefits and writing up the results so that the knowledge would benefit future generations.

The radical animal activists claim to be morally superior to the many more moderate but equally humane people who are members of groups trying to spare animals from unnecessary suffering. But even after the value of treatments for hydrophobia had been demonstrated clearly, Mr. Coleridge, the leading antivivisectionist of his day wrote: "The Pasteur Institutes in Paris and elsewhere have entirely failed to prevent people dying of hydrophobia." As Keen[3] points out with this and many other examples: "The third way in which the influence of antivivisection injures character is by diminishing the reverence for truthfulness." And the same thing is true today. Radical animal activists publish misleading pictures, e.g., cats with their heads fastened in stereotaxic instruments, quietly staring at you with wide open eyes, but fail to tell you that these cats are under surgical anesthesia. Elsewhere, the utter falsity of their statements about mindless atrocities[1] and about the worthlessness of behavioral research on animals[5] has been thoroughly documented. Is this the behavior of people with a superior sense of ethics?

Those who assert that it is immoral to cause any animal to suffer for any human benefit also assert that preventing research on animals will cause people to be more humane to each other because research on animals promotes general inhumanity. They present no proof for such an assertion; actually, there is considerable evidence to the contrary. Hindus in India treat animals with devout kindness, but this has not prevented, and in some cases has contributed to, bloody massacres. Hindu widows have been required to burn themselves to death by leaping into the flames of the funeral pyres of their husbands. While monkeys and parrots are allowed to eat large amounts of vital grain, Hindu beggars deliberately maim their children horribly to make them piteous cripples who will bring in the alms desperately needed to buy food. Certainly in India, kindness to animals has not inevitably generalized to people.

Furthermore, the behavior of many of the radical animal activists gives little evidence for their kindness to people. Seventy years ago, Keen[3] gave examples causing him to conclude about the influence of antivivisection that "the most violent and vindictive passions have been aroused and fostered." Recently, at the 1983 meeting of the American Psychological Association I heard radical animal activists who were burning the biological scientist Edward Taub in effigy chant "Burn Taub, burn! Burn slow, burn slow, Taub!" The sadistic tone of the chant did not reflect any generalization of kindness from animals to people.

In conclusion, let us return to the research on stress-induced analgesia. The evidence that there are non-opiate as well as opiate pain-inhibiting pathways in the brain leads to the hope that research of this kind may contribute to the discovery of superior non-addicting pain-killing drugs. Any such drugs, whether derived from research on stress-induced analgesia or other research involving pain, will have to be tested on animals. Have you ever known a man or woman whose life was completely devastated by unbearable, incessant, untreatable pain? Have you ever heard the heart-rending, pitiful, piercing cries of a badly burned child having its bandages changed? If you have, I believe that you will conclude that it is highly moral and humane to conduct, and highly immoral and inhumane to obstruct or delay, the research that is the hope for relief from such excruciating human suffering.

REFERENCES

1. COILE, D. C. & N. E. MILLER. 1984. How radical animal activists try to mislead humane people. Am. Psychol. **39**:700–701.
2. Institute of Medicine. 1982. Health and Behavior: A Research Agenda. National Academy Press, Washington, D.C.
3. KEEN, W. W. 1914. Animal Experimentation and Medical Progress. Houghton Mifflin. Boston.
4. MILLER, N. E. 1983. Understanding the use of animals in behavioral research: Some critical issues. Ann. N. Y. Acad. Sci. **406**:113–118.
5. MILLER, N. E. 1985. The value of behavioral research on animals. Am. Psychol. **40**:423–440.
6. National Institutes of Health. 1982. Chronic Pain: Hope through Research. NIMH Publication No. 82-2406. U. S. Government Printing Office, Washington, D. C.
7. OVERCAST, T. D. & B. SALES. 1985. Regulation of animal experimentation. J. Am. Med. Assoc.
8. SELYE, H. 1956. Stress and Disease. McGraw-Hill. New York.
9. WEISS, J. M., W. H. BAILEY, P. A. GOODMAN, L. J. HOFFMAN, M. J. AMBROSE, S. SALMAN & J. M. CHARRY. 1982. A model for neurochemical study of depression. *In* Behavioral Models and the Analysis of Drug Action. M. Y. Spiegelstein & A. Levy, Eds.: 195–223. Elsevier Scientific. Amsterdam.

Philosophical and Practical Issues in Animal Research Involving Pain and Stress

FREDERICK A. KING

Yerkes Regional Primate Research Center
Emory University
Atlanta, Georgia

The experience of pain and physical suffering consist of two major components: one is a sensory and discriminative aspect whose mechanisms lie in the peripheral receptors, spinal cord pathways, and centers of the brain that permit the detection of pain and its differentiation from other sensory experiences. The second component is a motivational and emotional one that elaborates and transforms the sensory perception of painful stimuli into an unpleasant experience that may include suffering and anguish. The neural mechanisms for this affective component are not yet fully understood, but we know that they involve complex neural circuitry in the brain and, on the behavioral side, attitudinal variables. These affectional systems, then, interact with the more purely sensory pathways to produce the total pain experience.

In humans, the quality and quantity of the pain experience varies dramatically among individuals, and from time to time in the same individual, as a function of one's emotional state, attitude toward pain, anticipation of the stimulus and experience, perception of the situational context in which the pain is produced, and the degree of voluntary control one is capable of, or willing to exert.

These complexities make it difficult to define satisfactorily the experience of pain in humans, and even more so in non-human animals where verbal expression of sensory and affective experience is not possible. There is still considerable discussion and disagreement as to whether pain is perceived in the same manner in animals as in humans.

It has been pointed out by S. G. Dennis that distinct behavioral responses to stimuli capable of damaging tissue can be demonstrated in almost all species down to the level of protozoa.[3] This suggests that certain primitive behaviors related to what we refer to as "pain responses" in higher species, had their adaptive origins very early in animal evolution. This does not, however, imply either awareness of noxious stimuli or consciousness of suffering in these lower organisms.

Central nervous system structures responsible for higher order cognitive and affective aspects of behavior are obviously more fully developed and complex in phylogenetically advanced species. Hence, it is not unreasonable to expect a more marked capacity for suffering in those vertebrates with much more complex nervous systems. Indeed, when we consider higher species, especially certain mammals, we find that they show important behavioral similarities to human pain responses, in spite of a lack of verbal confirmation. These similar behavioral responses roughly parallel the similarities in brain development between non-human mammals and humans.

C. J. Vierck has pointed out that comparative human and animal data have established that non-human species begin to escape stimulation at approximately the same intensity levels that humans begin to report pain verbally.[3] Vierck has also quantitifed the level of pain by analyzing animal behaviors such as frequency of vocalizations, force of escape movements, and rate of operant avoidance responses. These correlate also with the intensity of the stimulation.[3]

Admittedly, our knowledge of animal pain experience is inferential and not direct. However, the elicitation in animals of skeletal motor, vocal, and autonomic responses that are similar to those displayed by humans when they are similarly stimulated, leads us to seriously consider that some higher animal species experience pain and affective experiences similar to those that are verbally reported by humans, and there may be a hierarchical arrangement for these species. For the reason that some animals are likely sentient in the sense that humans are, it is morally and scientifically fitting that scientists accept responsibility for reducing pain to the minimum consistent with the goals of the research.

I have taken here a hierarchical view of pain, which, if accepted, implies that we should exert a higher degree of concern and caution in experiments with those forms of animals possessing complex neural organizations that may permit the sensation of pain to be accompanied by the experience we know as suffering.

Supposition or acceptance of such a hierarchy that bespeaks a continuum from protozoa to humans does not, however, mean that we are morally compelled to grant rights to animals or refrain from using them in research. As ethicist Arthur Caplan has stated, there are morally relevant differences between animals and humans. Rights, in any realistic sense, are privileges granted by one group to another based upon perceived identical or highly similar properties. Throughout the history of humankind, rights have been given to individuals, to special groups, or to whole societies by some human authority. In the context of the modern philosophic foundation of science, logical positivism, there is nothing supernatural about rights. They do not materialize magically out of a void. Except in moments of revolution, rights are determined by those who wield the authorized and legal power in a particular society at any given time. In a democratic society it is the legislative branch of government, as delegated by the people that assigns rights through laws; and it is the judicial branch that interprets the intent and limits of those laws. Nothing here transcends natural processes.

Human society does not have either an absolute or an abstract obligation to grant rights to other species. Rights in any society imply responsibility; that is, understanding and compliance with the laws and expectations of that society. Animals are unable to comprehend or to comply with these demands. They clearly do not share with us the characteristics that would permit them to understand and follow the requirements of human society. To share in rights one must, as philosopher Carl Cohen has pointed out, be a moral agent in order to make moral claims; that is, one must be aware of the needs of other moral agents in the community.[4] In this sense, man is justified and moral in his denial of rights to animals and his use of them in his own self-interest. The position of the speciesist is consistent with both the logic of empirical positivism and the exploitation that presents itself throughout all societies of the animal kingdom, of which man is a part.

This does not mean, however, that we do not have a moral obligation to animals. Human awareness of the sentience of other species and our ability to empathize with suffering leads us to a responsibility, recognized by our society, to treat animals with compassion and concern for their sentience. As Cohen has stated so well, " . . . not everything to which we may have obligations, has a claim of right against us."[4] Obligations and rights, then, are not necessarily reciprocal. Cohen explains that in the context of the demands and responsibilities that human society places upon us, "if a medical researcher does not fulfill his obligations to humans by sacrificing animals when necessary, then he may fail to do his duty, to do what he has committed himself to do for the human community."[4]

Perhaps John Dewey said it best of all in a statement of clarity and humanity back in 1926[1] when discussing this same question of animal rights and experimentation,

> . . . it is the question of a certain amount of physical suffering to animals—reduced in extent to a minimum by the precautions of anesthesia, asepsis, and skill—against the bonds the relations which hold people together in society, against the conditions of social vigor and vitality, against the deepest of shocks and interferences to human love and service.

> No one who has faced this issue can be in doubt as to where the moral right and wrong lie. To prefer the claims of the physical sensations of animals to the prevention of death and the cure of disease—probably the greatest sources of poverty, distress, and inefficiency, and certainly the greatest sources of moral suffering—does not rise even to the level of sentimentalism.

> It is accordingly the duty of scientific men to use animal experimentation as an instrument in the promotion of social wellbeing; and it is the duty of the general public to protect these men from attacks that hamper their works. It is the duty of the general public to sustain them in their endeavors. For physicians and scientific men, though having their individual failings and fallibilities like the rest of us, are in this matter acting as ministers and ambassadors of the public good.

I argue here for the hierarchical and speciesist position in accepting the inequality of species. As Cohen states, "we are right to do to mosquitoes what we would not do to dogs, and to dogs what we would not do to humans."[4]

Over the past few years there has developed a powerful and rapidly increasing anti-research campaign that has its recent historical roots in the anti-intellectual and anti-scientific social movements of the 1960s and 1970s. The effectiveness of the combined forces of literally hundreds of groups opposed to animal research cannot be ignored or underestimated. If they have their way they will turn the world to their irrational and inhumane beliefs. Some states have already made it virtually impossible to obtain pound animals for research. Similar legislative movements are underway in several other states, in spite of an acute need for these animals in medical research and the fact that at least 13 million unwanted dogs are killed each year by pounds in the United States.

With regard to public understanding, the fact is that a significant segment of the population of our nation does not really recognize or understand the essentialness of animals for medical progress. Nor are they well-informed on how animals are treated and used by scientists and research laboratories. Hence, a very large number of people are vulnerable to the outright lies, distortions, and inflammatory appeals often made by anti-vivisectionist and animal rights organizations who tell them that scientists are cruel to animals and that the research they do is virtually worthless.

The time has come for scientists to be much more assertive. If we, as scientists had spoken out over the past decades, the public today would have a better understanding of what we do in our laboratories, and why and how we do it. Perhaps we would not now be facing an increasing, and often misinformed, virulent and destructive opposition. A new and major step in the right direction has been the recent formation of a coalition of several concerned scientific organizations. The coalition is developing networks of information sharing, strategic planning, legislative monitoring, and public information. There is an urgent and serious need for more active sharing in this enterprise, and orchestrated action on the part of individuals as well as scientific organizations and institutions.

It is axiomatic in the field of public communications that people do not respond positively to that which they do not understand. People rarely realize that preceding virtually every modern human medical and applied behavioral advance there have been many years of basic animal research on normal and pathological processes that was essential to that human application.

Universities and research institutions could help greatly by taking the time to explain the importance of animal research when they proudly announce to the media and the public each new advance in human medicine or surgery. That step alone could be important in raising the consciousness of the news media and the public to the critical importance of experimentation and testing with animals. Let us do everything possible to permit the public to share in our vision of the advances that lie over the horizon, and to understand how continued progress depends upon the ability and freedom of scientists to conduct animal research.

The media is science's major route to public education and opinion. I am convinced that the best assurance of fair and objective treatment by the news media is early and open contacts with reporters, writers, producers, and editors. All of us, including the media, tend to view with suspicion that which we do not understand. Understanding and confidence between scientists and the media can provide a sound framework within which the media may consider and evaluate charges of insensitivity, cruelty, and meaningless research that they will sooner or later hear from the highly vocal and emotional anti-research groups. Experience has taught us that if your organization's first contact with the media is when a crisis occurs, you are probably in trouble.

The difficulties that have been generated over the past few years will not soon go away. Therefore, we need articulate people to speak out for research with animals. We need individuals who can cope with difficult and confrontational issues in response to television, radio, and other public forum challenges. To retreat into our laboratories with the unreal hope that it will all go away, does a serious disservice to science and medicine.

Finally, there is the matter of education in our schools. I am speaking about what young people learn today about the nature and process of science. Many graduates of our high schools, colleges, and universities have little understanding of the values, goals, and methods of scientists using animals. I am not saying that graduates don't leave school without some substantive scientific knowledge, but I am saying they have little understanding of the reasons and need for animal research, the way animals are treated and research conducted, and the benefits that have accrued from it.

A concerted effort should be made by the scientific community, perhaps through its professional organizations, to provide our schools and colleges with the necessary resources on the methods and benefits of animal research. We should make every effort to see that accurate information on the use of animals in research is a part, not only of the courses of those who intend to enter the field of science, but particularly in the studies of those preparing to teach science in our public schools.

The public needs to understand that scientists and research institutions are humanely concerned with and sensitive to the needs and the sentience of animals. But it will not be known widely unless we explain it over and over again to the media, the public, government administrators, and legislators. We need to back our statements of concern with facts and examples, and most of all by responsible and positive action in our treatment of animals.

REFERENCES

1. BOYDSTON, J. A. & B. A. WALSH, Eds. 1984. John Dewey. The Later Works, 1925–1953; Vol. 2, 1925–27. Southern Illinois University Press. pp. 99–103.
2. DUBNER, R. 1983. Pain research in animals. Ann. N.Y. Acad. Sci. **406**:128–132.
3. ERICKSON, H. H. & R. L. KITCHELL. 1984. Pain Perception and Alleviation in Animals. Fed. Proc. **43**(5):1307–1312.
4. GOODWIN, L. G. 1984. The Welfare State. Nature **309**:729.
5. KATTERMAN, L. 1984. Animals in Research: Five Views The Research News **35**(10–12):8–9.
6. KITCHELL, R. L., H. H. ERICKSON, E. CARSTENS & L. E. DAVIS. 1983. Animal Pain: Perception and Alleviation. American Physiological Society. Bethesda, MD.
7. ZIMMERMAN, M. 1983. Ethical Guidelines for Investigations of Experimental Pain in Conscious Animals. Pain **16**:109–110.

Age-Related Alterations in Front-Paw Shock–Induced Analgesia

ROBERT J. HAMM AND JANET S. KNISELY

Department of Psychology
Virginia Commonwealth University
Richmond, Virginia 23284

Research on the age-related changes that occur in the central nervous system (CNS) opioid receptor system suggests that the opioid receptors appear early in embryonic development, continue to develop for a substantial period after birth, and decline during aging.[1,2] Other research[3] has demonstrated that exposure to front-paw shock produces a potent analgesic response that is opioid mediated.

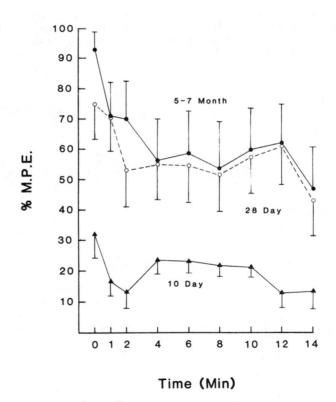

FIGURE 1. The mean %MPE (±SEM) following 90 sec of front-paw shock for rats 10 days, 28 days, and 5–7 mo old.

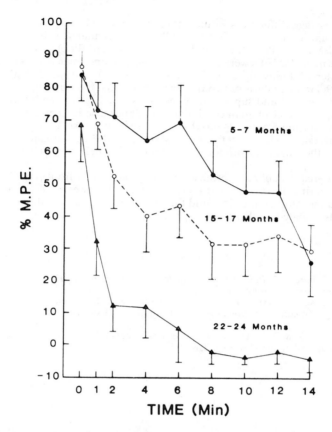

FIGURE 2. The mean %MPE (±SEM) following 90 sec of front-paw shock for rats 5–7 mo, 15–17 mo, and 22–24 mo old.

The purpose of the present study was to examine the relationship between the age-related alterations in the neurochemical indexes of the opioid system and the function of the endogenous opioid pain-inhibition system activated by front-paw shock.

Subjects were Sprague-Dawley rats 10 days old, 28 days old, 5–7 mo old, 15–17 mo old, and 22–24 mo old. Half of the rats in each age group received two intraperitoneal injections of naloxone (10 mg/kg). The remaining rats received two injections of equivolume saline. Eleven minutes following the first injection of saline or naloxone, baseline tail-flick measures were determined (three tail-flick trials separated by 2 min intervals, the maximum tail-flick latency was set at 7 sec to avoid damage to the rat's tail). After baseline measures and a second injection of saline or naloxone, all rats were exposed to 90 sec of scrambled electrical shock (60 Hz, 1.6 mA, constant current) to their front paws. Tail-flick latencies were then measured at 0, 1, 2, 4, 6, 8, 10, 12, and 14 min post-shock.

To assess age differences in the analgesia produced by front-paw shock, the percent maximum possible effect (%MPE) was calculated using the following formula: %MPE = (Post-shock tail flick − Baseline tail flick)/(7.0 − Baseline tail flick). The mean %MPEs were calculated for each saline-treated age group at each testing interval following shock (FIGURES 1 and 2) and were analyzed by a 3(Age) × 9(Time) analysis of variance (a separate analysis for each figure). As can be seen in FIGURE 1 and supported by the analysis, as age increased from 10 days to 28 days, the degree of analgesia induced by shock also increased ($p < 0.001$). As age increased from 5 mo to 24 mo (FIGURE 2), there was also a progressive decline in the analgesia produced by front-paw shock ($p < 0.001$). Naloxone significantly attenuated the analgesia produced by front-paw shock ($p < 0.001$) in both age groups.

The age-related changes in the analgesia produced by front-paw shock in the present experiment confirm that there is a parallel between the development of the opioid receptors in the CNS and the function of these receptors in producing an opioid-mediated analgesia in response to aversive stimulation.

REFERENCES

1. COYLE, J. T. & C. B. PERT. 1976. Ontogenetic development of [³H]naloxone binding in the rat brain. Neuropharmac. **15**:555–560.
2. DUPONT, A., P. SAVARD, Y. MERAND, F. LABRIE & J. R. BOISSIER. 1981. Age-related changes in central nervous system enkephalins and substance P. Life Sci. **29**:2317–2322.
3. WATKINS, L. R. & D. J. MAYER. 1982. Organization of endogenous opiate and nonopiate pain control systems. Science **216**:1185–1192.

Cold-Water-Induced Analgesia: Enhanced Function During Aging

JANET S. KNISELY AND ROBERT J. HAMM

Department of Psychology
Virginia Commonwealth University
Richmond, Virginia 23284

Recent research has revealed that various environmental stimuli are capable of activating endogenous neural and hormonal systems that are capable of blocking or attenuating pain transmission.[1] For example, cold-water immersion has been found to stimulate a hormonal/nonopioid analgesic system.[2] The purpose of the present study was to examine the function over age of the analgesia produced by cold-water swim.

Three-month-old and 23-mo-old male Sprague-Dawley rats were administered 7 mg/kg naltrexone or equivolume saline following basal nociception

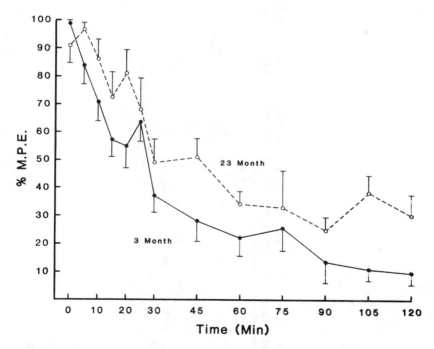

FIGURE 1. The percent maximum possible effect (%MPE ± SEM) following cold-water exposure for 3-mo- and 23-mo-old rats pretreated with saline.

413

TABLE 1. Mean Tail-Flick Latencies before Treatments and after the Injection of Saline, Naltrexone, or Adrenalectomy and Mean %MPE following Cold-Water Exposure for the Two Age Groups

	Age							
	3 mo				23 mo			
	Saline	Naltrexone	Adrenalectomy		Saline	Naltrexone	Adrenalectomy	
Basal latency	3.2	3.3	3.1		3.1	3.1	3.2	
Post-injection or post-surgery latency	3.1	3.3	3.3		3.3	3.2	3.2	
Mean %MPE of 13 testing times following cold-water exposure	44.6	45.6	71.6		58.1	57.8	69.2	

determination (three tail-flick trials, 1 min between trials). Twenty min post-injection, three tail-flick measures were repeated and rats were then placed in a 6°C water tank for 5 min. Tail-flick trials were conducted at 0, 5, 10, 15, 20, 25, 30, 45, 60, 75, 90, 105, and 120 min following cold-water immersion. Also, bilateral adrenalectomies were performed on rats from both age groups following baseline tail-flick measures. Four days following surgery, baseline latencies were repeated and rats were then exposed to cold water. Tail-flick measures following cold-water immersion were recorded as described above.

Mean basal tail-flick latencies before and after treatments were calculated and are presented in TABLE 1. As can be seen, age and treatment groups were not significantly different and the treatments did not change nociception. Tail-flick latencies following cold-water exposure were converted to percent maximum possible effect (%MPE) and mean %MPEs were calculated for each age group (FIGURE 1). These data were analyzed by a 2(Age) × 13(Time) analysis of variance. As FIGURE 1 indicates, 23-mo old animals exhibited a higher level of analgesia than 3-mo-old rats ($p < 0.02$) and the amount of analgesia decreased throughout the 120 min of testing for both age groups ($p < 0.002$). Percent MPEs following the treatments (saline, naltrexone, or adrenalectomy) were averaged over the 13 time intervals for each age group (TABLE 1) and were analyzed by separate ANOVAs (naltrexone and adrenalectomy compared with saline controls). These analyses revealed that naltrexone failed to significantly attenuate cold-water induced analgesia and adrenalectomy potentiated the analgesia observed following cold-water immersion ($p < 0.001$).

The enhanced analgesic response to cold-water immersion exhibited by aged animals is in agreement with earlier findings of other neuroendocrine indexes of increased hormonal response to stress in aged animals[3,4] and is in support of the characterization of aging as a loss of ability to adapt to stress or a reduced ability to return to homeostasis after some environmental demand.[5]

REFERENCES

1. WATKINS, L. R. & D. J. MAYER. 1982. Organization of endogenous opiate and non-opiate pain control systems. Science **216**:1185–1192.
2. BODNAR, R. J. 1984. Types of stress-inducing analgesia. *In* Stress-induced Analgesia. M. D. Trickleband & G. Curzon, Eds.:19–32. John Wiley and Sons. New York.
3. SAPOLSKY, R. M., L. C. KREY & B. S. McEWEN. 1983. The adrenocortical stress-response in the aged male rat: Impairment of recovery from stress. Exp. Gerontol. **18**:55–64.
4. McCARTY, R. 1985. Sympathetic-adrenal medullary and cardiovascular responses to acute cold stress in adult and aged rats. J. Auto. Nerv. Syst. **12**:15–22.
5. SEYLE, H. & Y. B. TUCHWEBER. 1976. Stress in relation to aging and disease. *In* Hypothalamus, Pituitary, and Aging. A. Everitt & J. Burgess, Eds.:553–569. Thomas. Springfield, IL.

Genetic Differences in Avoidance Learning Covary with Non-opioid Stress-Induced Analgesia

CAROLYN S. NAGASE AND F. ROBERT BRUSH

Department of Psychological Sciences
Purdue University
West Lafayette, Indiana 47907

Two lines of Long-Evans rats that have been selectively bred for either good or poor avoidance performance in a two-way shuttlebox also differ in conventional behavioral measures of emotionality (such as open-field defecation and Pavlovian fear conditioning)[1] and in adrenal gland weight and morphology. Low Avoidance (SLA) animals have heavier adrenal glands and are more reactive to a variety of stimuli than High Avoidance (SHA) animals. Because stress-induced analgesia (SIA) may be influenced by the animal's affective response to the

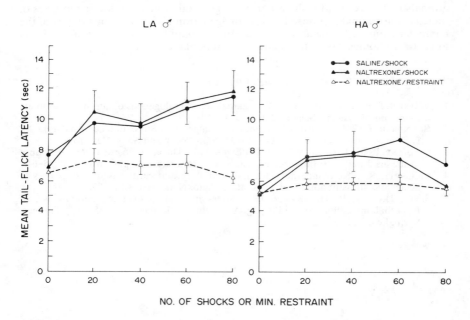

FIGURE 1. Mean (± S.E.) tail-flick response latencies as a function of number of shocks or duration of restraint in male rats of the SLA and SHA lines that received either saline or 14 mg/kg of naltrexone, s.c., 20 min before testing.

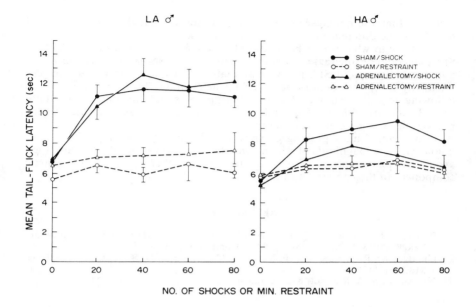

FIGURE 2. Mean (± S.E.) tail-flick response latencies as a function of number of shocks or duration of restraint in male rats of the SLA and SHA lines that were either adrenalectomized or sham adrenalectomized.

stressor or by adrenal gland activity, it seemed likely that SLA animals may be more reactive to exposure to inescapable electric shock and show greater SIA than SHA animals.

In two separate experiments, males of the SHA and SLA lines were injected s.c. with either saline vehicle or naltrexone (7 or 14 mg/kg). Twenty min later, the animals were restrained in tubes and given three tail-flick tests to establish baseline responding prior to receiving 80 inescapable shocks (1 mA, 5 sec duration, mean intershock interval of 60 sec) applied to the base of the tail or a comparable period of restraint only. Three tail-flick tests were taken after every 20 shocks or 20 min of restraint.

None of the groups differed in basal tail-flick latencies, but a reliable difference was found between the lines in the shocked groups: SLA animals exhibited a profound and long-lasting hypoalgesia whereas SHA animals displayed a moderate and short-lived SIA. Although others report sequential activation of first a non-opioid and then an opioid form of SIA using similar tail-shock procedures,[2] neither dose of naltrexone attenuated the SIA of either line, which suggests that only a non-opioid SIA was elicited in our lines[3] (FIGURE 1).

We then asked whether the adrenal gland contributed significantly to the observed line difference in SIA. Three days after adrenalectomy or sham-surgery, males of each line were exposed to the standard tail-shock procedure. Adrenal-ectomy had no effect on basal or post-shock response latencies of animals of either line, which lends further support to the idea that the SIAs are non-opioid in form and that non-opioid secretory products of the adrenal gland are not critical for SIA or the difference between the lines (FIGURE 2).

Contrary to what would be predicted, prolonged shock did not produce an SIA that could be attenuated by either opiate antagonists or adrenalectomy. The absence of an opioid SIA in these animals is not due to decreased receptor sensitivity to opiates because tail-flick latencies at 15, 30, 45, 60, and 75 min following an s.c. injection of 2 mg/kg of morphine sulfate were elevated in both lines. Injections of 7 mg/kg of naltrexone 20 min before basal tail-flick testing blocked the analgesic effects of morphine.

In our inbred lines, prolonged exposure to inescapable shock produces non-opioid SIA, the magnitude of which consistently covaries with the low and high avoidance phenotypes. These data suggest that there is a strong genetic component in the expression of SIA.

REFERENCES

1. BRUSH, F. R., S. BARON, J. C. FROEHLICH, J. R. ISON, L. J. PELLEGRINO, D. S. PHILLIPS, P. SAKELLARIS & V. N. WILLIAMS. 1985. J. Comp. Psych. **99**:66–73.
2. GRAU, J. W., R. L. HYSON, S. F. MAIER, J. MADDEN & J. D. BARCHAS. 1981. Science **213**:1409–1411.
3. NAGASE, C. S., A. RANDICH & F. R. BRUSH. 1985. Peptides **6**(Suppl. 1):29–35.

Prolongation of Vaginal Stimulation–Produced Analgesia by Leupeptin, A Protease Inhibitor

STEPHEN B. HELLER, BARRY R. KOMISARUK,
ALAN R. GINTZLER, AND ALFRED STRACHER

Institute of Animal Behavior
Rutgers University
Newark, New Jersey, 07102

Department of Biochemistry
Downstate Medical Center, SUNY
Brooklyn, New York, 11203

Vagino-cervical mechanical stimulation of the rat (VS) decreases behavioral responsivity to noxious stimuli, including leg flexion in response to foot pinch, vibrissa retraction to ear pinch, eyeblink to stimulation of the cornea, vocalization to noxious tail shock, and tail withdrawal to noxious heat.[1-3] VS is more powerful in decreasing responsivity to noxious stimuli than a standard dose of morphine sulfate (2 mg/kg).[4]

A spinal mechanism is implicated in the suppression by VS of behavioral responses to noxious stimuli. In spinal rats, VS is effective in attenuating leg withdrawal to foot pinch.[1] VS increases levels of norepinephrine (NE) and serotonin (5-HT) in spinal perfusates,[3] and transection of the dorsolateral funiculus attenuates the effect of VS.[5] Intrathecal administration of NE and 5-HT receptor antagonists attenuates the effect of VS.[5] Protease inhibitors (e.g. Thiorphan) administered to the spinal cord have been shown to potentiate the analgesic effect of endogenously released and exogenously administered opioid peptides.[6-8]

The present study was designed to determine whether leupeptin, a naturally occurring, calcium-activated serine protease inhibitor,[9] injected intrathecally, would augment the effect of VS in the tail-flick test. Following ovariectomy and implantation of an intrathecal catheter into the lumbo-sacral region, female rats were placed into one of four groups ($N = 10$ per group); leupeptin plus VS (L + VS), saline plus VS (S + VS), leupeptin without VS (L+ no VS), or saline without VS (S+ no VS). Prior to post-injection testing, all subjects were given three pre-injection baseline (B) trials. Injections (L groups, 200 µg leupeptin in 7 µl saline followed by a 7 µl saline flush; saline groups, 7 µl saline followed by a 7 µl saline flush) and testing were performed using a double-blind procedure. For Groups L + VS and S + VS, following injection, animals were given three post-injection B trials, followed by three trials with the plunger of a 1 cc glass syringe pressed against the vaginal cervix at a calibrated force of 75 grams (VS). Thirty sec following the termination of the third VS trial, subjects were given three post-VS trials (PVS). This B, VS, PVS sequence was repeated 3, 5, 10, 20, 40, and 60 min following injection of leupeptin or saline. For Groups L+ no VS and S+ no VS, following injection, animals were given three groups of three post-injection B trials at the same time intervals as Groups L + VS and S + VS, however, no VS or PVS trials were given to these groups. In all animals, the tail region exposed to the radiant heat source was systematically varied over the 60 min of testing in order to minimize tail damage.

Results show that tail-flick latencies during pre-injection B trials did not differ significantly among the four groups. Tail-flick latencies in the first post-injection B trials (preceding the first VS trials) also did not differ significantly among the four groups (FIGURE 1). Tail-flick latencies during VS trials did not differ significantly at any time between Groups L + VS and S + VS, nor did values differ significantly between Groups L+ no VS and S+ no VS during the corresponding test periods (FIGURE 1). However, latencies for Groups L + VS and S + VS during VS trials were, at each time period, significantly greater than for Groups L+ no VS and S+ no VS, respectively, in the corresponding test periods. In the PVS trials at 5, 10, and 20 min post-injection, tail-flick latencies for Group S + VS were significantly greater than those for Group S+ no VS by 50%, 90%, and 62%, respectively (FIGURE 2). In the PVS trials 3, 5, and 40 min post-injection,

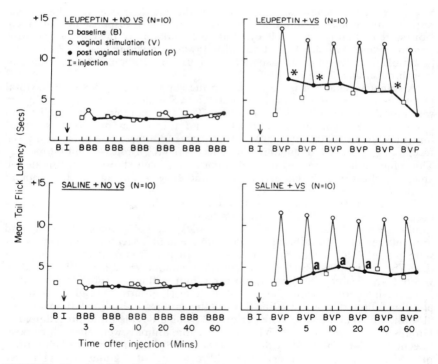

FIGURE 1. Results of baseline (B), vaginal stimulation (VS), and post-vaginal stimulation (PVS) trials for the four groups tested.
(a) S + VS > S+ no VS; $p < .05$; Duncan Test.
(*) L + VS > S + VS; $p < .05$; Duncan Test.

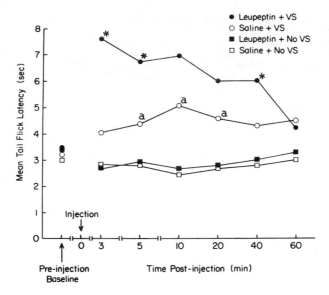

FIGURE 2. Results of post-vaginal stimulation (PVS) trials of Groups L + VS and S + VS and the corresponding baseline (B) trials of Groups L+ no VS and S+ no VS.
(a) S + VS > S+ no VS; p < .05; Duncan Test.
(*) L + VS > S + VS; p < .05; Duncan Test.

tail-flick latencies were significantly greater for Group L + VS versus Group S + VS by 82%, 53%, and 39%, respectively (FIGURE 2). In the intermediate trials at 10 and 20 min, the differences between these two groups approached significance. By 60 min post-injection, the trend towards a decreasing difference was evident in a non-significant negative difference of 6%. Ten min post injection, the baseline tail-flick latencies for Group L + VS were significantly greater (52%) than those of Group S + VS (Duncan Test, p < .05) suggesting that leupeptin produced a prolongation of analgesia in response to the VS applied 5 or more min earlier.

We conclude that administration of the protease inhibitor leupeptin intrathecally, significantly prolonged the analgesia produced by VS. This suggests that VS releases analgesic-triggering neuropeptides in the spinal cord. Apparently, tonic release of the neuropeptide(s) does not occur, since administration of leupeptin alone (i.e. in the absence of VS) did not produce analgesia.

REFERENCES

1. KOMISARUK, B. R. & K. LARSSON. 1971. Brain Res. **35**:231.
2. KOMISARUK, B. R. & J. WALLMAN. 1977. Brain Res. **137**:85.
3. STEINMAN, J. L. *et al.* 1983. Pain **16**:155.

4. KOMISARUK, B. R. *et al*. 1976. Adv. Pain Res. Ther. **1**:439.
5. WATKINS, L. *et al*. 1984. Brain Res. **294**:59.
6. CHIPKIN, R. E. *et al*. 1982. Eur. J. Pharmacol. **83**:283.
7. CHIPKIN, R. E. *et al*. 1982. Life Sci. **31**:1189.
8. YAKSH, T. L. & G. J. HARTY. 1982. Eur. J. Pharmacol. **79**:293.
9. MALIK, M. N. *et al*. 1983. J. Biol. Chem. **258**:8955.

Prenatal Exposure to Alcohol Modifies Central Opioid Analgesia Systems in the Rat[a]

L. R. NELSON,[b] J. W. LEWIS,[b] J. C. LIEBESKIND,[b,c,d]
B. J. BRANCH,[e] AND A. N. TAYLOR[c,e,f]

Departments of [b]Psychology and [f]Anatomy, and the
[c]Brain Research Institute
University of California, Los Angeles

and

[e]West Los Angeles Veterans Administration Medical Center
Brentwood Division
Los Angeles, California 90024

Prenatal exposure to alcohol in humans or animals can produce a variety of effects, including growth deficits, facial dysmorphologies, aberrant neuro-anatomical organization, and cognitive impairment.[1,2] Our laboratory has been studying long-term behavioral and neuroendocrine alterations in adult rats, prenatally exposed to ethanol (for methodological details see Taylor *et al.*[3]) Two of the most pronounced effects of this prenatal experience are altered responsiveness to stress and pharmacological agents. The present studies demonstrate that rats exposed to ethanol *in utero* demonstrate potentiated opioid-mediated stress-induced analgesia and augmented responsiveness to morphine when tested as adults.

We have assessed the analgesic response to two paradigms of footshock stress in prenatally ethanol-exposed (E) offspring. A naloxone-sensitive (opioid) form of stress-induced analgesia (SIA) followed presentation of 10 min of intermittent footshock (1 sec on every 5 sec, 2.5 mA, 60 Hz sine wave scrambled current), whereas a naloxone-insensitive (nonopioid) form of SIA resulted from 2 min of the same footshock presented continuously. Pain responsiveness was assessed with the tail-flick test. E rats had significantly potentiated opioid SIA but were not different from controls in expressing nonopioid SIA.[4] Thus, prenatal exposure to alcohol modifies opioid stress-induced analgesia, not pain inhibitory systems in general.

This finding is congruent with our previous report that E rats demonstrate enhanced activation of the hypothalamo-pituitary-adrenal (HPA) axis in response to some, but not all, stressors.[3] In fact, we have shown that the intermittent,

[a]Supported by Veterans Administration Medical Research Service (ANT) and by National Institutes of Health grant NS-07628.

[d]Address correspondence to: J. C. L., Department of Psychology, 1283 Franz Hall, UCLA, Los Angeles, CA 90024.

423

but not the continuous, footshock stress causes augmented HPA axis activation in E rats.[5]

Several responses to morphine are also potentiated in prenatal ethanol-exposed rats.[6] Analgesia (as indexed by the tail-flick test) was assessed at 30 min intervals for 2 hr following 2.5 or 5.0 mg/kg morphine. E rats had potentiated analgesia compared to controls after both doses. At a higher dose of morphine (20 mg/kg), E rats also manifested a significantly greater potentiation of HPA axis activation, as indexed by plasma corticosterone levels 60 min postdrug. Thermoregulatory responses were also altered when core temperature was measured at 30 min intervals for 4 hr postmorphine. E rats showed augmented hypothermia to morphine at 10 and 30 mg/kg, but no difference was seen in the hyperthermia caused by 1.25, 2.5, or 5.0 mg/kg.

To explore the mechanisms for the augmentation in opioid responses seen in E rats in adulthood, we examined brain levels of β-endorphin and enkephalins in early postnatal life. We and others have found elevated levels of β-endorphin in the midbrain and hindbrain of E rats, which persist to at least day 21.[7,8] Also, we examined opiate receptors of the mu and delta type in regional dissections of adult brains, but no differences were seen in E rats.[9]

Thus, we have found potentiation of several responses to stress and morphine in adult rats prenatally exposed to ethanol. It is important to note that E rats do not differ from controls on basal measures of these responses, e.g., pain sensitivity, plasma corticosterone, and body temperature. The alterations in these functions are unmasked, however, when these rats are challenged by stress or drug administration. These results indicate that prenatal ethanol exposure leads to widespread and enduring alterations in the endogenous opioid systems.

REFERENCES

1. ABEL, E. L. 1984. Fetal Alcohol Syndrome and Fetal Alcohol Effects. Plenum Press. New York.
2. STREISSGUTH, A. P., S. LANDESMAN-DWYER, J. C. MARTIN & D. SMITH. 1980. Science 209:353-361.
3. TAYLOR, A. N., B. J. BRANCH, S. H. LIU & N. KOKKA. 1982. Pharmacol. Biochem. Behav. 16:585-589.
4. NELSON, L. R., A. N. TAYLOR, J. W. LEWIS, B. J. BRANCH & J. C. LIEBESKIND. 1985. Psychopharmacology 85:92-96.
5. NELSON, L. R., A. N. TAYLOR, E. REDEI, B. J. BRANCH & J. W. LEWIS. 1984. Alcoholism 8:109.
6. NELSON, L. R., J. W. LEWIS, J. C. LIEBESKIND, N. KOKKA, D. RANDOLPH, B. J. BRANCH & A. N. TAYLOR. 1983. Soc. Neurosci. Abstr. 9:1242.
7. SHOEMAKER, W. J., G. BAETAGE, R. AZAD, V. SAPIN & F. E. BLOOM. 1983. Monogr. Neural Sci. 9:130-139.
8. WEINBERG, J., L. R. NELSON & A. N. TAYLOR. 1985. In Alcohol and Brain Development. J. West, Ed. Oxford University Press. New York.
9. NELSON, L. R., A. N. TAYLOR, B. J. BRANCH, J. C. LIEBESKIND & J. W. LEWIS. 1984. Soc. Neurosci. Abstr. 10:964.

Rotation Speed Can Determine Whether the Resulting Stress-Induced Analgesia Is Blocked by Naloxone

J. TIMOTHY CANNON, YEHUDA SHAVIT,[a] AND
JOHN C. LIEBESKIND[a]

Department of Psychology
University of Scranton
Scranton, Pennsylvania 18510

[a]Department of Psychology
University of California, Los Angeles
Los Angeles, California 90024

When considering even a single stressor, footshock, a number of parameters have been proposed as being important for selective activation of opioid or non-opioid analgesic states. These parameters of shock include: duration, pattern, number, intensity, escapability, and location (i.e., the body region to which it is applied).[1]

Recently, we showed that briefly exposing rats to footshock can cause either opioid or non-opioid forms of analgesia depending on variations in footshock intensity or duration.[1] For example, opioid analgesia can be evoked at moderate shock intensities, whereas non-opioid analgesia results from higher, presumably more noxious, shock levels. Based upon such observations, Terman et al.[1] proposed that for brief footshock durations moderate stress triggers an opioid analgesic state; whereas, more severe stress produces non-opioid analgesia.

In this study we sought to determine if a similar relationship exists between the intensity of stress and the pharmacological basis of stress analgesia when a stressor other than footshock is employed. We have reexamined rotation, one of the original stressors used to produce analgesia,[2] to determine if variations in rotation speed alter the ability of naloxone to block the resulting analgesic state.

METHODS

Sixty Fisher 344 female rats (approximately 250 g) had food and water freely available and were group housed on a 12/12 hr light/dark cycle. All testing occurred during the dark phase of this cycle. The animals were randomly assigned to five groups of 12 animals each. Naloxone (5 mg/kg ml) or saline was injected 20 min prior to testing.

Animals injected with naloxone or saline were exposed to 1 min rotation at either 110 or 150 rpm. An additional group of saline-injected animals was placed in a sack for 1 min (sham rotation). A cloth sack that provided a rotation radius of 51 cm was used for both rotation and sham conditions.

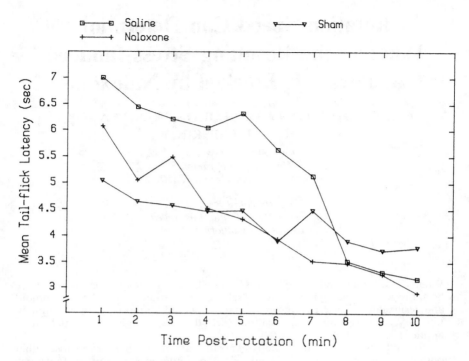

FIGURE 1. Mean tail-flick latencies after 1 min of sham (saline) and 110 rpm rotation (saline and naloxone). In comparison to the sham condition, rotation significantly elevated tail-flick latencies in saline-injected animals. Naloxone significantly reduced this elevation of tail-flick latencies to a level not significantly greater than that of the sham condition.

After rotation or sham conditions, the animals were placed in Plexiglas tubes and their tail-flick latencies were determined at 1 min intervals for 10 min. The heat source was terminated at 7 sec to minimize tissue damage.

RESULTS AND CONCLUSION

For saline-injected animals, rotation at 110 and 150 rpm significantly elevated tail-flick latencies in comparison to sham animals. Naloxone significantly reduced this elevation of latencies in the 110 rpm condition to a level not significantly different from animals that were not rotated (FIGURE 1). At 150 rpm naloxone did not reduce post-rotation analgesia. At this speed, post-rotation tail-flick latencies were not significantly different for saline- versus naloxone-injected animals (FIGURE 2).

These data appear to extend the generality of the relationship that we have suggested exists between the severity of stress and the opioid or non-opioid nature

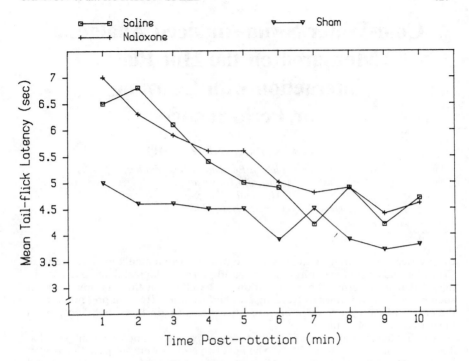

FIGURE 2. Mean tail-flick latencies after 1 min of sham (saline) and 150 rpm rotation (saline and naloxone). In comparison to the sham condition, rotation significantly elevated tail-flick latencies in animals injected with either saline or naloxone. There was no significant difference between the latter two groups after rotation.

of the subsequent analgesic state.[1] As with footshock, increasing the intensity of rotation (from 110 to 150 rpm) can change stress analgesia from naloxone blockable to naloxone insensitive.

REFERENCES

1. TERMAN, G. W., Y. SHAVIT, J. W. LEWIS, J. T. CANNON & J. C. LIEBESKIND. 1984. Intrinsic mechanisms of pain inhibition: activation by stress. Science **226**:1270–1277.
2. HAYES, R. L., G. J. BENNETT, P. G. NEWLON & D. J. MAYER. 1978. Behavioral and physiological studies of non-narcotic analgesia in rat elicited by certain environmental stimuli. Brain Res. **155**:69–90.

Cold-Water Swim–Induced Analgesia Measured on the Hot Plate: Interaction with Learning or Performance

Z. H. GALINA AND Z. AMIT

Center for Studies in Behavioral Neurobiology
Concordia University
Montreal, Quebec
Canada H3G 1M8

Cold-water swim–induced analgesia is both well documented and characterized. Considerable anatomical, physiological, and pharmacological data have accumulated that now permit the examination of the effects of this manipulation on such behavioral variables as learning and performance. Here we present data on the effects of cold-water swim on three measures of pain threshold detection as measured on the hot plate.

We divided 30 male Wistar rats into six groups. Two groups were subjected to 3.5 min of cold-water swim (CWS) The next two groups were subjected to a swim in water at room temperature (RTS) and the last two groups did not swim and were maintained in their home cages. Immediately following the swim each two groups received an i.p. injection of either naltrexone (10 mg/kg) or saline vehicle. All animals were returned to their home cages for 30 min and then brought back to the testing room for pain threshold tests. A hot-plate heated to 57°C was used and three measures were recorded: latency to paw lick, latency to jump, and latency to escape. Testing was terminated when animals escaped or after 90 sec on

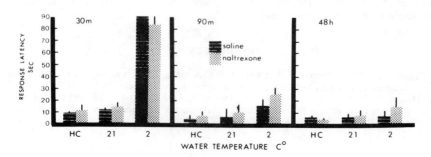

FIGURE 1. Latency to the first of any one of three responses recorded at three time periods (30 min, 90 min, and 48 hr) after 3.5 min swim in various water temperatures. The three responses were: paw lick, jump, or escape.

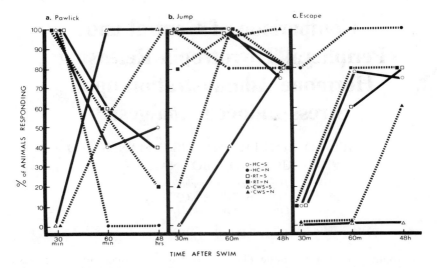

FIGURE 2. Percent of animals that respond with a given behavioral response. HC = home cage (no swim stress). RT = room temperature swim (18°C). CWS = cold water swim (2°C). N = naltrexone, S = saline.

the hot-plate without escaping. Following the testing session animals were returned to their home cages. The second testing session occurred one hour after the first session. A third and final testing session was conducted 48 hours after the first session.

The CWS animals were clearly analgesic (FIGURE 1) and displayed deficits on all three measures in a time-dependent fashion (FIGURE 2). Typically they did not paw-lick, jump, or escape during the first testing session. In the second session they recovered the paw-licking response but did not jump or escape. In the third session 48 hr after the CWS experience they partially recovered the jumping response but still did not escape. Some CWS animals were allowed to stay on the hot-plate for up to 4 min. During the entire period they exhibited only exploration and none of the responses that we measured. There was no significant difference between the RTS and home cage controls. In the first session they paw-licked and then jumped and escaped. In the second and third sessions the animals from both these groups hardly exhibited analgesia, they jumped or escaped almost immediately after being placed on the hot-plate. The failure to paw-lick observed in the CWS animals during the first session was not naltrexone reversible. On the other hand, naltrexone partially reversed the deficit in jumping and escaping observed in the CWS animals during the second and third sessions.

The data indicated an interaction between the CWS experience, of which analgesia was clearly a component, and learning or performance deficits. Opiate receptor involvement in this interaction is suggested by the data.

Comparison of Central and Peripheral Thyrotropin Releasing Hormone Administration upon Stress-Induced Analgesia[a]

PAMELA D. BUTLER, PHYLLIS E. MANN, AND
RICHARD J. BODNAR

Department of Psychology
Queens College, CUNY
Flushing, New York 11367

Thyrotropin releasing hormone (TRH) has variable effects upon analgesic responses: it reduces neurotensin analgesia, yet fails to affect either morphine analgesia or basal pain thresholds. However, TRH potentiates nonopiate analgesia elicited by 20 or 80 footshocks.[1] The present experiments compared central and peripheral TRH administration upon analgesia following forepaw shock (FPS), hindpaw shock (HPS), and cold-water swims (CWS).[2,3]

METHODS

Three groups of rats ($N = 8$) received TRH (0, 10, or 50 µg, i.c.v.) 20 min prior to both FPS and HPS (1.6 mA for 90 sec) with tail-flick latencies assessed before

TABLE 1. Alterations in Forepaw Shock Analgesia on the Tail-Flick Test following either Intracerebroventricular or Intravenous Administration of TRH

TRH	Baseline	Post-Shock (min)				
		0	4	8	12	18
i.c.v. (µg)						
0	2.7	7.5	4.7	3.7	3.5	3.0
10	2.7	8.6	5.0	4.0	3.9	2.8
50	2.8	9.3[a]	6.9[a]	6.2[a]	5.6[a]	5.2[a]
i.v. (mg/kg)						
0	2.6	9.6	7.2	6.1	6.9	5.2
2	2.7	9.9	5.4	4.9	5.9	4.9
8	2.9	9.4	6.2	5.0	4.7	3.5

[a]Significant difference ($p < .05$) from saline.

[a]Supported by PSC/City University of New York grant 6-64187.

TABLE 2. Alterations in Cold-Water Swim (21°C) Analgesia on the Tail-Flick Test following Intracerebroventricular or Intravenous Administration of TRH.

TRH	Baseline	21°C	30 Min Post-Swim		
			15°C	8°C	2°C
i.c.v. (µg)					
0	2.7	4.5	4.0	4.8	4.6
10	2.9	4.6	5.0[a]	5.0	6.9[a]
50	2.7	6.1[a]	5.8[a]	7.3[a]	7.1[a]
i.v. (mg/kg)					
0	2.6	4.7			
2	2.8	4.9			
8	2.9	5.6[a]			

[a]Significantly different ($p < .05$) from saline.

injection and for up to 20 min after shock. Separate groups ($N = 8$) received TRH (0, 2, or 8 mg/kg, i.v.) 20 min prior to FPS to assess peripheral effects. In a second paradigm, separate groups ($N = 8$) received TRH (0, 10, or 50 µg, i.c.v.) 20 min prior to a 3.5 min swim with tail-flick latencies and jump thresholds determined before injection and 30, 60, and 120 min after swims. Four swim temperatures (21, 15, 8, 2°C) were tested at weekly intervals. Finally, other groups ($N = 8$) received TRH (0, 2, or 8 mg/kg, i.v.) 20 min prior to a 21°C swim to assess peripheral effects.

RESULTS

TABLE 1 shows that while the 50 µg dose of central TRH significantly potentiated FPS analgesia over the time course, intravenous TRH failed to alter this effect. In contrast, HPS analgesia was unaffected by central TRH. TABLE 2 shows that the high central TRH dose potentiated CWS analgesia on the tail-flick test 30 min following all swim conditions. Central TRH transiently increased CWS analgesia on the tail-flick test at the low dose and on the jump test at both doses. In contrast, only the 8 mg/kg intravenous dose of TRH potentiated CWS analgesia on the tail-flick, but not the jump test at 30 and 60 min after the swim. TRH-induced changes in hypothermia did not accompany analgesic potentiations.

CONCLUSIONS

Central administration of TRH potentiates FPS analgesia and CWS analgesia in a dose-dependent manner, but fails to affect HPS analgesia. These effects appear to be centrally mediated given the relative ineffectiveness of intravenous TRH. These data indicate the modulatory actions of nonanalgesic levels of TRH to facilitate various forms of environmental analgesia.

REFERENCES

1. BUTLER, P. D. & R. J. BODNAR. 1984. Potentiation of foot shock analgesia by thyrotropin releasing hormone. Peptides 5:635–639.
2. BODNAR, R. J. 1984. Types of stress which induce analgesia. *In* Stress-induced Analgesia. M. Tricklebank & G. Curzon, Eds. John Wiley & Sons. New York.
3. WATKINS, L. R. & D. J. MAYER. 1982. The neural organization of endogenous opiate and nonopiate pain control systems. Science 216:1185–1192.

Age-Related Decrements in Stress-Induced Analgesia[a]

E. KRAMER AND R. J. BODNAR

Department of Psychology
Queens College, CUNY
Flushing, New York 11367

The aging process in rodents has been characterized by impaired coping responses, including glucose tolerance and thermoregulation.[1,2] Since acute exposure to both 2-deoxy-D-glucose (2DG) glucoprivation and cold-water swims (CWS) produce analgesia in young adult rats,[3] the present study examined whether systematic variations in these responses occurred as a function of age.

METHOD

Five age cohorts of female albino Sprague-Dawley rats (4, 9, 14, 19, 24 months) were assessed for baseline tail-flick latencies and jump thresholds over seven days. A first group of cohorts was exposed to a no swim condition and a 3.5 min CWS at a water temperature of 2°C with tail flick latencies and jump thresholds assessed 30, 60, and 90 minutes thereafter. Core body temperatures were also measured immediately prior to and 0, 30, 60, and 90 minutes following each condition. The second group of cohorts received, at 4-day intervals, ascending doses of 2DG (0, 50, 250, 450, and 650 mg/kg, i.p.) with tail flick and jump thresholds assessed 30, 60, and 120 minutes thereafter. Subsequently, food intake (0.1 g) was determined 5 hr following 2DG (0, 650, 1200 mg/kg).

RESULTS

FIGURE 1 shows that whereas the four younger cohorts displayed significant CWS analgesia on the tail-flick test, CWS analgesia was eliminated in the 24-month cohort. Further, while significant CWS analgesia was observed on the jump test in the three younger cohorts, it was significantly attenuated in the 19-month cohort and eliminated in the 24-month cohort. The reductions in CWS analgesia could not be attributed to hypothermic changes since CWS hypothermia was more pronounced in the three older cohorts. FIGURE 2 shows that the magnitude of 2DG analgesia significantly declined as a function of age on the tail flick test, with maximal effects observed at the highest dose. 2DG analgesia also showed a progressive reduction as a function of age on the jump test; this effect was less

[a]Supported by National Institute of Aging Grant 04425.

433

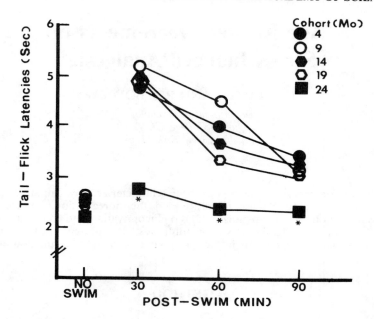

FIGURE 1. Age-related decline in the analgesic response on the tail-flick test following cold-water swims (2°C for 3.5 min). (*$p < .05$, Dunnett comparison).

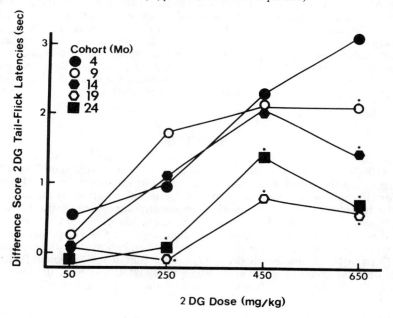

FIGURE 2. Age-related decline in the analgesic response on the tail-flick test 60 min following 2-deoxy-D-glucose administration (*$p < .05$, Dunnett comparison).

robust. In addition, 2DG hyperphagia was systematically altered; significant hyperphagia was noted in the 4 and 9 month cohorts, no change in intake was noted in the 14-month cohort, and significant hypophagia was noted in the 19 and 24 month cohorts.

DISCUSSION

These results indicate that impairments in the analgesic responses following 2DG and CWS stress accompany impairments in other physiological responses such as glucose tolerance[1] and thermoregulation.[2] However, the decline in the analgesic responses following these stressors is not merely an epiphenomenon of changes in glucoprivation or hypothermia per se, but rather appears to represent an age-dependent effect upon endogenous pain-inhibition.

REFERENCES

1. SARTIN, J., M. CHAUDHURI, M. OBENRADER & R. C. ADELMAN. 1980. The role of hormones in changing adaptive mechanisms during aging. Fed Proc. **39**:3163–3167.
2. MCDOUGAL, J. N., P. R. MARQUES & T. F. BURKS. 1981. Reduced tolerance to morphine thermoregulatory effects in senescent rats. Life Sci. **28**:137–145.
3. BODNAR, R. J., D. D. KELLY, M. BRUTUS & M. GLUSMAN. 1980. Stress-induced analgesia: Neural and hormonal determinants. Neurosci. Biobehav. Rev. **4**:87–100.

Differential Actions of Scopolamine upon the Analgesic Responses to Stress and Pilocarpine[a]

ELLEN S. SPERBER, TERRI G. SPERBER, AND
RICHARD J. BODNAR

Department of Psychology
Queens College, CUNY
Flushing, New York 11367

The muscarinic receptor blocker, scopolamine, reduces some forms of inescapable foot shock analgesia.[1-3] The present study evaluated whether scopolamine or its quarternary form, methylscopolamine, altered cold-water swim (CWS) and 2-deoxy-D-glucose (2DG) analgesia in a similar manner to its effects upon pilocarpine analgesia. As controls, the effects of scopolamine upon basal pain thresholds, CWS hypothermia, and 2DG hyperphagia were also examined.

METHODS

Separate groups of rats received scopolamine (0.01–10 mg/kg, i.p.), methylscopolamine (1–10 mg/kg, i.p.), or vehicle 5 min before CWS (2°C for 3.5 min)

TABLE 1. Reduction in Cold-Water Swim Analgesia on the Jump Test (mA) Following Scopolamine or Methylscopolamine Pretreatment

Dose (mg/kg)	Condition	Baseline	Post-Swim (min) 30	60	120
0	No Swim	.306	.281	.305	.312
0	CWS	.291	.463^a	.399^a	.390^a
Scopolamine					
0.01	CWS	.304	.353^{a,b}	.365^a	.313^b
0.1	CWS	.297	.274^b	.301^b	.308^b
1.0	CWS	.309	.382^{a,b}	.325^b	.308^b
10.0	CWS	.306	.384^{a,b}	.306^b	.335
Methylscopolamine					
1.0	CWS	.304	.328^b	.333^b	.346
10.0	CWS	.307	.423^a	.345	.331

Significantly higher (Dunnett comparison, $p < .05$) than 0/No Swim condition^a or lower than 0/CWS condition^b.

[a]Supported by PSC/City University of New York Grant 6-64187.

TABLE 2. Reduction in Pilocarpine (10 mg/kg) Analgesia on the Jump Test by Scopolamine but not Methylscopolamine

Dose (mg/kg)	Condition	Baseline	Post-Injection (min) 30	60	120
Vehicle					
0	vehicle	.338	.346	.325	.344
0	pilocarpine	.338	.468	.432	.373
Scopolamine					
0.01	pilocarpine	.281	.491	.333	.311
0.1	pilocarpine	.271	.446	.407	.357
1.0	pilocarpine	.285	.337	.319	.327
10.0	pilocarpine	.311	.250	.310	.353
Methylscopolamine					
1.0	pilocarpine	.307	.471	.474	.469
10.0	pilocarpine	.313	.426	.422	.399

with tail-flick latencies, jump thresholds, and core body temperatures assessed 30, 60, and 120 min later. 2DG analgesia (600 mg/kg, i.p.) was evaluated in the same paradigm, as were scopolamine and methylscopolamine effects upon food intake 6 hr following the same 2DG dose. Separate experiments determined whether scopolamine and methylscopolamine altered baseline tail-flick latencies and jump thresholds as well as pilocarpine (10 mg/kg, i.p) analgesia.

RESULTS

TABLE 1 indicates that scopolamine and methylscopolamine significantly reduced (30 min) and eliminated (60 and 120 min) CWS analgesia on the jump test without affecting baseline pain thresholds, CWS analgesia on the tail-flick test, or CWS hypothermia. Scopolamine and methylscopolamine failed to alter 2DG analgesia, but dose-dependently suppressed 2DG hyperphagia, an effect attributed to basal scopolamine and methylscopolamine hypophagia. TABLE 2 shows that scopolamine, but not methylscopolamine, significantly reduced pilocarpine analgesia on both the tail-flick test and the jump test.

CONCLUSIONS

In addition to the selective reduction by scopolamine of certain forms of footshock analgesia,[1-3] both scopolamine and methylscopolamine selectively reduce CWS, but not 2DG analgesia on the jump test. The reductions in CWS analgesia were test-specific and not due to either shifts in baseline pain thresholds or hypothermic changes. While scopolamine and methylscopolamine reduced CWS analgesia on the jump test alone, pilocarpine analgesia was reduced on both tests by scopolamine, suggesting that similar, but not identical endogenous processes modulate both forms of analgesia.

REFERENCES

1. LEWIS, J. W., J. T. CANNON & J. C. LIEBESKIND. 1983. Involvement of central muscarinic cholinergic mechanisms in opioid stress analgesia. Brain Res. **270**:289–293.
2. MACLENNAN, A. J., R. C. DRUGAN & S. F. MAIER. 1983. Long-term stress-induced analgesia blocked by scopolamine. Psychopharm. **80**:267–268.
3. WATKINS, L. R., Y. KATAYAMA, I. B. KINSCHENK, D. J. MAYER & R. L. HAYES. 1984. Muscarinic cholinergic mediation of opiate and non-opiate environmentally induced analgesias. Brain Res. **300**:231–242.

Stress-Induced Analgesia and Feeding in the Slug, *Limax maximus*

MARTIN KAVALIERS

Department of Psychology
University of Alberta
Edmonton, Alberta
Canada T6G 2E9

and

MAURICE HIRST

Department of Pharmacology and Toxicology
University of Western Ontario
London, Ontario
Canada

Initially it was proposed that endogenous opioid peptides and their receptors existed only within mammalian systems, but subsequent investigations have demonstrated that they have a much broader phylogenetic distribution.[1-3] Several behavioral, electrophysiological, and pharmacological investigations in molluscs have shown that opiate agonists and antagonists have actions resembling those induced in mammals.[1,2] Slugs and snails injected with low doses of the exogenous opiate agonist, morphine, display analgesic and ingestive responses that are analogous to the effects observed in mammals.[3,4] In addition, the opioid peptides, methionine- and leucine-enkephalin were isolated from neural tissue of a marine mollusc,[1] while immunohistochemical studies have revealed the presence of opioid peptides in a number of species of molluscs, including the terrestrial slug, *Limax maximus*.[2] Thus it appears reasonable to propose that opioid systems participate in the regulation of a variety of basic functions in invertebrates, in a manner similar to that evident in mammals.

Substantial evidence exists to indicate that exposure to either physical or psychological stress can increase endogenous opioid activity in mammals and induce a variety of behavioral and physiological responses, including analgesia and increased feeding.[4-6] These stress-induced responses can be suppressed by the exogenous opiate antagonist, naloxone, and are similar to the effects observed after administration of endogenous and exogenous opiates.[6] Accordingly, the activation of endogenous opioid systems by stressful procedures arising during natural and laboratory situations may form part of an intrinsic mechanism of basic survival value.[4-6]

The generality of this hypothesis was examined with *Limax*. Slugs were stressed by gently pinching the posterior or tail portion of their body. This tail-pinch stress increased their thermal nociceptive thresholds as well as increasing food intakes over three hours. These stress-induced changes in nociceptive responses and food intakes are similar to the analgesic and feeding responses obtained in mammals after imposition of a variety of stressors, including tail pinch. Pre-treatment with naloxone (1.0 mg/kg) blocked stress-induced feeding and analgesia in *Limax* in a manner similar to that observed in mammals, supporting the hypothesis that endogenous opioids are activated in slugs by stress and become involved in the mediation of stress-induced analgesia and feeding. Additionally, these observations suggest that there may have been an early evolutionary development and phylogenetic continuity of opioid involvement in the mediation of basic stress-induced behavioral and physiological responses.

REFERENCES

1. LEUNG, M. K. & G. B. STEFANO. 1984. Isolation and identification of enkephalins in pedal ganglia of *Mytilus edulis* (Mollusca). Proc. Natl. Acad. Sci. USA **81**:955–958.
2. MARCHAND, C. R., P. G. SOKOLOVE & M. P. DUBOIS. 1984. Immunocytochemical localization of a somatostatin-like substance in the brain of the giant slug, *Limax maximus*. L. Cell Tiss. Res. **238**:349–353.
3. KAVALIERS, M., M. HIRST & G. C. TESKEY. 1985. Opioid systems and feeding in the slug. *Limax maximus*: similarities to and implication for mammalian feeding. Brain Res. Bull. **14**:681–685.
4. KAVALIERS, M., M. HIRST & G. C. TESKEY. 1983. A functional role for an opiate system in snail thermal behavior. Science **220**:99–101.
5. BODNAR, R. J., D. D. KELLY, N. BRUTUS & M. GLUSMAN. 1980. Stress-induced analgesia: a review of neural and hormonal mechanisms. Neurosci. Biobehav. Rev. **4**:87–100.
6. TESKEY, G. C., M. KAVALIERS & M. HIRST. 1984. Social conflict activates opiate analgesic and ingestive behaviors in male mice. Life Sci. **35**:305–315.

Inheritance of Stress-Induced Analgesia in Mice

I. PANOCKA AND P. MAREK

Institute of Genetics and Animal Breeding
Department of Behavioral Physiology
Polish Academy of Sciences
Jastrzebiec, 05-551 Mroków, Poland

According to several reports, various mouse strains display different degrees of analgesia upon opioid treatment and of that produced by noxious stimulation. These data and also the genotype-dependent reversibility of the analgesias by

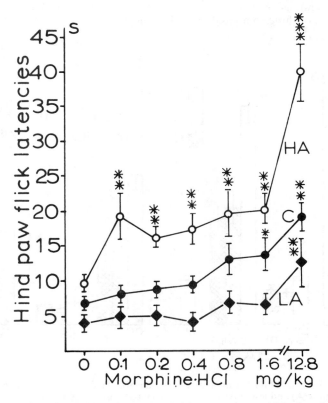

FIGURE 1. Effect of increasing doses of morphine on pain sensitivity in mice selectively bred for high (HA) and low (LA) analgesia and in controls (C). HA and C mice pretreated *($p < 0.05$), **($p < 0.001$), ***($p < 0.0001$) significantly different from saline (0 mg/kg morphine), three-way analysis of variance.

naloxone suggest genetically conditioned differentiation of the mouse endorphin system(s).[1] It was hypothesized that selective breeding of mice for high and low opioid-mediated analgesia could produce lines with high and low activity of the endorphin systems. Randomly mated six-week-old Swiss mice served as the basic stock for selection. They were exposed to 3 min swimming at 20°C and thereafter allowed to dry off for 2 min. Pain threshold accepted as hind paw flick latency was determined on a hot plate at 56°C. Mice with the shortest ($\leqslant$ 10 sec) and the longest ($\geqslant$ 50 sec) post-swim latencies were assigned as progenitors of the low (LA) and high (HA) analgesia line, respectively. For further reproduction, the LA mice with the shortest latencies, and the HA with the longest latencies only were selected. Controls were bred randomly as in the stock generation. The result of selection was a significant increase in the percentage of low and long latencies in the LA and HA lines, respectively, compared to control offspring generations. This result suggested a difference in the activity of the endorphin systems between the two lines. The next experiments were planned to verify this assumption. One group of offspring belonging to the fifth generation of the LA and HA lines were given 0–12.8 mg/kg of morphine hydrochloride in saline. Hot plate latencies were measured 30 min after the injection. As shown in FIGURE 1, the HA line was more sensitive to morphine compared to the LA line and controls. Another group was

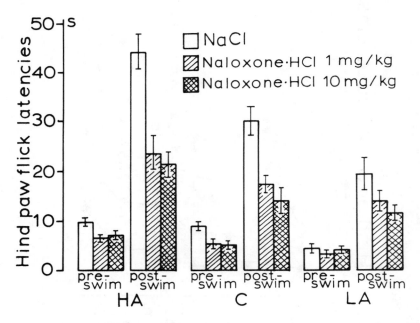

FIGURE 2. Reversal of post-swim analgesia by naloxone hydrochloride in mice selectively bred for high (HA) and low (LA) analgesia and in controls (C). HA and C mice pretreated with the two doses of naloxone displayed shorter post-swim latencies compared to those treated with saline ($p < 0.001$), whereas in the LA group a significant decrease was seen only after 10 mg of naloxone ($p < 0.05$). Post-swim latencies in all naloxone-treated mice were still significantly longer compared to the pre-swim ones ($p < 0.001$).

injected with 1 and 10 mg/kg of naloxone hydrochloride and allowed to swim for 3 min at 20°C 30 min after injection. Pain threshold was determined on a hot plate at 56°C. FIGURE 2 shows that naloxone partially reversed post-swim analgesia, more in the HA than in the LA mice. So far it is not possible to conclude whether the above between-line differences depend on different rates of opiate release upon stressful stimuli or on different development of opiate receptors.[2] The partial reversal of post-swim analgesia by naloxone indicates possible participation of two mechanisms, an opiate and a non-opiate one (similar phenomenon as revealed in rats[3]).

ACKNOWLEDGMENT

The authors thank Endo Laboratories for a gift of naloxone hydrochloride.

REFERENCES

1. RAMABADRAN, K., G. MICHAUD & J. J. JACOB. 1982. Indian J. Exp. Biol. **20**:74–76.
2. REGGIANI, A., F. BATTANI, H. KOBAYASHI, P. SPANO & M. TRABUCCHI. 1980. Brain Res. **189**:289–294.
3. WATKINS, L. R. & D. J. MAYER. 1982. Science **216**:1185–1192.

Relation of Stress-Induced Analgesia to Acupuncture Analgesia

BRUCE POMERANZ

Departments of Zoology and Physiology
University of Toronto
Toronto, Ontario, Canada M5S 1A1

INTRODUCTION

I will present the thesis that acupuncture analgesia (AA) and stress-induced analgesia (SIA) are different phenomena. It is important to emphasize this point for several reasons. First, we should not be looking for common mechanisms, although there may be many similarities. Secondly, when doing experiments on acupuncture, we should be careful to avoid stressing the animal or human subject to avoid confounding the two phenomena. Thirdly, when treating patients with acupuncture we should avoid stressing them unnecessarily, as acupuncture can achieve its effects without superimposed stress. Fourthly, researchers studying SIA may be looking at two phenomena, SIA plus AA.

I will present six reasons to support my contention that AA and SIA are different phenomena. (1) Sham acupuncture (needles placed in non-acupuncture points) fails to produce analgesia whereas true acupuncture (needles placed in true points as designated by Chinese atlases) produces analgesia in awake animals[1] and human subjects.[2] Both sham and true acupuncture produce the same amount of stress. (2) Electroacupuncture given at three different frequencies in awake rodents produces different effects, yet all three should be equally stressful. At 0.2 Hz no analgesia is observed.[3] At 4 Hz there is an analgesia mediated by endorphins.[1,3] At 200 Hz there is an analgesia mediated by serotonin.[4] Similar results have been observed in humans.[5] (3) Acupuncture in awake horses releases cortisol. However, sham acupuncture has no cortisol effect even though it should be equally stressful.[6] (4) AA has been observed in anesthetized animals.[7,8] As the animals are not conscious, there is very little stress involved. (5) AA occurs when stimulating A beta afferent fibers[9,10] and hence is non-painful and non-stressful. (6) Anecdotally, the AA is targeted to specific painful sites. For example, stimulation of LI 4, which is in the first dorsal interosseus muscle in the web between the thumb and the index finger, produces analgesia of the face and neck, but not of the lower extremities.[11] SIA should produce analgesia over the entire body equally in a fight-or-flight response.

In the remaining paper, each of these points will be elaborated on under separate headings.

Sham Acupuncture Does Not Produce Analgesia whereas True Acupuncture Causes AA

Sham acupuncture can be done because there are specific points in the body that are purported to be effective in producing AA. Acupuncture sites have been empirically and anecdotally mapped by the Chinese for thousands of years in humans (and in animals for veterinarian use). Sham acupuncture is done by stimulating non-acupuncture points, using similar intensities of stimulation as that used at true acupuncture sites. The stress produced by both sites should be constant. If SIA were involved, then both sites should produce the same effect. In fact sham acupuncture gives no analgesia, while true acupuncture in a matched group of animals[1] (or patients[2]) gives AA. In the animal study,[1] true acupuncture was administered to LI 4 for 20 min at 4 Hz, using intensities sufficient to activate A beta fibers but below pain levels. This produced AA. Sham acupuncture was given on the back of the animal far away from known acupuncture points, using the same intensity of stimulation. No AA resulted. A similar study was done in awake human volunteers.[2] Stimulating LI 4 (in the first dorsal interosseus muscle of the hand) raised pain threshold of dental pain; sham acupuncture in the fifth dorsal interosseus muscle produced no AA in these human volunteers.

Electroacupuncture Given at Three Different Frequencies Produces Different Effects, Yet All Three Should Be Equally Stressful

In these experiments awake rats were used. As rats are easily stressed by needle insertion, "electroacupuncture" was given by transcutaneous electrical nerve stimulation (TENS) without the use of needles., This is often referred to as acupuncture-like TENS. The TENS electrode was placed over UB 60, which is near the achilles tendon of the hindpaw, and low intensities were used to activate only A beta afferent fibers. At 0.2 Hz no AA results, at 4 Hz AA is observed and can be prevented by naloxone., At 200 Hz AA is observed and can not be affected by naloxone.[3] Using awake mice we have observed similar results with needles inserted into LI 4,[1,4] whereby 4 Hz produced endorphinergic AA,[1] and 200 Hz produced AA mediated largely by serotonin.[4] Similar results have been reported in humans, whereby 2 Hz acupuncture-like TENS produced AA that was reversed by naloxone, while 100 Hz produced analgesia that was not affected by naloxone.[5] As all frequencies are equally stressful they should all produce the same kind of SIA.

Acupuncture in Horses Releases Cortisol, whereas Sham Acupuncture Has No Effect

Our results with AA in mice have implicated pituitary endorphins.[12] Since ACTH and endorphins are co-released, we decided to measure blood cortisol levels in awake horses before and after 30 minutes of acupuncture treatment: True acupuncture raised cortisol levels, whereas sham needling did not. The horses were not visibly stressed by the procedures and in any case, the sham treatment should have been equally stressful. Clearly this release of cortisol is not related to the fight-or-flight response of an integrated stress reaction.

AA Has Been Observed in Anesthetized Animals

One must be careful when using the term analgesia in anesthetized animals, as it is a behavioral/psychological term. Antinociception is preferable here, so AA in this section will be used to mean acupuncture antinociception. Several years ago we showed that electroacupuncture in chloralose-anesthetized cats suppressed the firing of lamina 5 interneurons in the dorsal horn of the spinal cord. Moreover acupuncture specifically blocked nociceptive responses, while leaving brush and touch responses unaffected in neurons receiving a convergence of the various inputs.[7] These antinociceptive effects were prevented by naloxone. Recently we have produced AA in rats anesthetized with Nembutal.[8] These rat experiments are particularly interesting since we monitored blood pressure throughout and observed no changes to indicate stress responses of the autonomic system by the acupuncture procedure.

AA Occurs When Stimulating A Beta Afferent Fibers

As mentioned above, we produced AA in awake mice by stimulating LI 4 (the first dorsal interosseus muscle). To do so we used stimulus intensities above the level to produce muscle twitches in the hand, but below pain levels. These mice were "squeekers," producing vocalizations readily, hence we were able to easily determine the pain threshold and to stay well below that level. In order to determine the afferent fibers that mediated AA, we anesthetized a group of mice and recorded the compound action potential from nerves serving LI 4 using stimulus intensities comparable to those used for AA in awake mice.[9] From conduction velocity measurements and threshold measurements we determined that A beta (or type I and II muscle) afferents were involved. Of course, stronger stimulation that recruits A delta and C fibers could contribute additionally to the analgesia. But we deliberately avoided using stronger stimulation to avoid stressing the animals, as we felt this would confound the two phenomena, SIA and AA. Similarly, Toda has shown that AA will suppress the jaw-opening reflex in rats at A beta levels.[10] Anecdotally in the clinic, patients usually do not experience pain or stress during acupuncture needling. Hence AA can be produced without stressing the animal (or patient) by using mild stimulation to activate the low threshold non-pain afferents.

Anecdotally AA Is Targeted to Specific Painful Sites

A prominent feature of acupuncture is the purported specificity of the acupuncture points. For example, stimulation of LI 4, which is located in the first dorsal interosseus muscle in the web between the thumb and the index finger produces targeted analgesia of the face and neck but not the lower extremities.[11] SIA should produce analgesia over the entire body equally and should be nontargeted. This (targeted) aspect of AA is not well studied.

DISCUSSION

I would like to emphasize that AA and SIA are separate distinguishable phenomena only if precautions are taken to avoid stressing the animal/or patient. In all of our studies we have been very careful to avoid painful stimulation, and to calm the animals (under anesthesia there is no problem). But the following caveat is necessary. Many papers on AA do not mention these precautions. Indeed many of my colleagues use strong (painful) stimuli to obtain stronger effects, which are more robust and easier to study. While I fully sympathize with the need to study robust effects (e.g., a 90% rise in pain threshold is easier to study than a 30% rise), I am sorry to see these researchers confounding the two phenomena (SIA and AA) that I am convinced are separate and distinct. Moreover there is no need to hurt the patient in chronic pain who already is suffering considerable anguish.

A great source of confusion in this field arises from what is meant by the word stress, in the term SIA. I assume SIA is produced by a strong aversive (painful) stimulus, which produces a fight-or-flight response in conscious animals, with associated activation of the sympathetic nervous system and the pituitary adrenal axis. How can we talk about stress in a deeply anesthetized rat in which there is no change in blood pressure associated with the stressful stimulus? In a recent paper, Liebeskind *et al.*[13] show SIA in rats deeply anesthetized with Nembutal. They freely admit in that paper that there is a problem referring to this phenomenon as SIA, but they call it a semantic problem. I think of it as a more serious conceptual problem, perhaps a paradigmic problem. This should be thoroughly discussed at meetings such as this one.

I am also concerned about an SIA result from the group of Mayer *et al.*,[14] in which footshock of the forepaw produced an opioid analgesia, while shock of the hindpaw caused a non-opioid analgesia. How can a generalized stress response (of the fight-or-flight type) be so specific as to distinguish between forepaw and hindpaw stressors? This result sounds more like AA than SIA. However, milder non-stressful stimuli (to activate only A beta afferents) are needed to unravel this overlap between AA and SIA. I have published 20 papers over the past eight years using these subtle stimuli in both awake and anesthetized animals. From my results I feel that SIA researchers may be confounding the two phenomena: SIA and AA.

REFERENCES

1. POMERANZ, B. H. & D. CHIU. 1976. Life Sci. **19**:1757–1762.
2. CHAPMAN, C. R., M. E. WILSON & J. D. GEHRIG. 1976. Pain **2**:265–283.
3. PEETS J. & B. POMERANZ. 1985. *In* Advances in Pain Research and Therapy. **9**:519–525. Raven Press. New York.
4. CHENG, R. & B. POMERANZ. 1981. Brain Res. **215**:77–92.
5. ERIKSSON, M. B. E., B. H. SJOLUND & S. NIELZEN. 1979. Pain **6**:335–341.
6. CHENG, R., L. MCKIBBIN, B. ROY & B. POMERANZ. 1980 Int.J. Neurosci. **10**:95–97.
7. POMERANZ, B. & R. CHENG. 1979. Exp. Neurol. **64**:327–341.
8. WARMA, N. & B. POMERANZ. 1986. (Manuscript in preparation.)
9. POMERANZ, B. & D. PALEY. 1979. Exp. Neurol. **66**:398–402.
10. TODA, K., M. ICHIOKA, H. SUDA & A. IRIKI. 1979. Exp. Neurol. **64**:898–904.
11. Beijing Institute of Traditional Chinese Medicine, Shanghai. Science and Technology Press. 1978.
12. CHENG, R., B. POMERANZ & G. YU. 1979. Life Sci. **24**:1481–1486.
13. TERMAN, G. W., Y. SHAVIT, J. W. LEWIS, J. T. CANNON & J. C. LIEBESKIND. 1984. Science **226**:1270–1277.
14. WATKINS, L. R., & D. J. MAYER. 1982. Science **216**:1185–1192.

Index of Contributors